CRANIOPHARYNGIOMAS

CRANIOPHARYNGIOMAS: COMPREHENSIVE DIAGNOSIS, TREATMENT AND OUTCOME

Edited by

James J. Evans
Thomas Jefferson University Hospital, Philadelphia, PA, USA

Tyler J. Kenning
Albany Medical Center, Albany, NY, USA

ELSEVIER

AMSTERDAM • BOSTON • HEIDELBERG • LONDON
NEW YORK • OXFORD • PARIS • SAN DIEGO
SAN FRANCISCO • SINGAPORE • SYDNEY • TOKYO
Academic Press is an imprint of Elsevier

Academic Press is an imprint of Elsevier
The Boulevard, Langford Lane, Kidlington, Oxford, OX5 1GB
525 B Street, Suite 1800, San Diego, CA 92101-4495, USA
225 Wyman Street, Waltham, MA 02451, USA
The Boulevard, Langford Lane, Kidlington, Oxford OX5 1GB, UK

ISBN: 978-0-12-416706-3

British Library Cataloguing in Publication Data
A catalogue record for this book is available from the British Library

Library of Congress Cataloging-in-Publication Data
A catalog record for this book is available from the Library of Congress

For information on all Academic Press publications
visit our website at http://store.elsevier.com/

Typeset by TNQ Books and Journals
www.tnq.co.in

Dedications

To my wife Deborah, my daughters Sophia and Vivienne, and my parents Claire and Leonard:

Thank you for your patience, understanding, and endless support. You have all helped to make my endeavors, as well as life in general, more enjoyable and meaningful. Thanks for always being there.

Jim

To my mentors, including Jim Evans and my father, Jim Kenning, who have provided me with the foundation to do meaningful work. To my parents, Phyllis and Jim, who have always supported me. To my children, Jackson and Lauren, who are an endless source of joy. Ultimately, to my wife, Sarah, for her love and patience, allowing me to do what I do.

TJK

Contents

VIII
CONTROVERSIES

List of Contributors

Paulo Abdo do Seixo Kadri Department de Neurocirurgia, Universidade Federal de Mato Grosso do Sul, Campo Grande-Mato Grosso do Sul, Brasil

Matthew A. Adamo Department of Neurosurgery, Albany Medical Center, Albany, NY, USA

Jennifer Adamski Division of Haematology/Oncology, The Hospital for Sick Children, Toronto, Ontario, Canada

Osama Al-Mefty Department of Neurosurgery, Brigham and Women's Hospital, Boston, MA, USA

Arif N. Ali Department of Radiation Oncology and Winship Cancer Institute, Emory University, Atlanta, GA, USA

Kristian Aquilina Department of Neurosurgery, Great Ormond Street Hospital for Children NHS Foundation Trust, London, UK

James A. Balogun Division of Neurosurgery, the Hospital for Sick Children, The University of Toronto, Toronto, Canada

Garni Barkhoudarian Brain Tumor Center, John Wayne Cancer Institute at Saint John's Health Center, Santa Monica, CA, USA

Ute Bartels Division of Haematology/Oncology, The Hospital for Sick Children, Toronto, Ontario, Canada

Wenya Linda Bi Department of Neurosurgery, Brigham and Women's Hospital and Harvard Medical School, Boston, MA, USA

Eric Bouffet Division of Haematology/Oncology, The Hospital for Sick Children, Toronto, Ontario, Canada

Julie A. Bradley University of Florida Proton Therapy Institute, Jacksonville, FL, USA

Henry Brem Johns Hopkins School of Medicine, Baltimore, MD, USA

Paolo Cappabianca Department of Neurosciences and Reproductive and Odontostomatological Sciences, Division of Neurosurgery, Università degli Studi di Napoli Federico II, Naples, Italy

Ricardo L. Carrau Department of Otolaryngology – Head and Neck Surgery, The Ohio State University Wexner Medical Center, Columbus, OH, USA

William T. Couldwell Department of Neurosurgery, Clinical Neurosciences Center, University of Utah, Salt Lake City, UT, USA

Walter J. Curran Department of Radiation Oncology and Winship Cancer Institute, Emory University, Atlanta, GA, USA

Maria Laura Del Basso De Caro Department of Advanced Biomedical Sciences, Division of Pathology, Università degli Studi di Napoli Federico II, Naples, Italy

Dale Ding Lars Leksell Gamma Knife Center, Department of Neurological Surgery, University of Virginia Health System, Charlottesville, VA, USA

Alberto Di Somma Department of Neurosciences and Reproductive and Odontostomatological Sciences, Division of Neurosurgery, Università degli Studi di Napoli Federico II, Naples, Italy

Leo F.S. Ditzel Filho Department of Neurological Surgery, The Ohio State University Wexner Medical Center, Columbus, OH, USA

Brian J. Dlouhy Department of Neurosurgery, University of Iowa Hospitals and Clinics, Iowa City, IA, USA; Centre for Minimally

Invasive Neurosurgery, Prince of Wales Hospital, Sydney, New South Wales, Australia

Ian F. Dunn Department of Neurosurgery, Brigham and Women's Hospital and Harvard Medical School, Boston, MA, USA

James J. Evans Department of Neurological Surgery, Thomas Jefferson University Hospital, Philadelphia, PA, USA

Manuel Ferreira, Jr. Department of Neurological Surgery, University of Washington, Harborview Medical Center, Seattle, WA, USA

David P. Friedman Jefferson Medical College and Thomas Jefferson University Hospital, Philadelphia, PA, USA

Takeshi Funaki Department of Neurosurgery, University of Florida, Gainesville, FL, USA

Ashish R. Gandhe Jefferson Medical College and Thomas Jefferson University Hospital, Philadelphia, PA, USA

Ravi H. Gandhi Goodman Campbell Brain and Spine, Indiana University School of Medicine, IN, USA

M. Reid Gooch Department of Neurosurgery, Albany Medical Center, Albany, NY, USA

Daniel J. Indelicato University of Florida Proton Therapy Institute, Jacksonville, FL, USA

George Jallo Johns Hopkins School of Medicine, Baltimore, MD, USA

Ali O. Jamshidi Department of Neurological Surgery, The Ohio State University Wexner Medical Center, Columbus, OH, USA

John Jane, Jr. Department of Neurosurgery, University of Virginia Health Sciences Center, University of Virginia, Charlottesville, VA, USA

Rachel Jimenez Radiation Oncology, Massachusetts General Hospital/Harvard Medical School, Boston, MA, USA

David Jones Department of Pathology and Laboratory Medicine/Affiliated Pathology Services, Albany Medical College/Center Hospital, Albany, NY, USA

Daniel F. Kelly Brain Tumor Center, John Wayne Cancer Institute at Saint John's Health Center, Santa Monica, CA, USA

Tyler J. Kenning Department of Neurosurgery, Albany Medical Center, Albany, NY, USA

Edward E. Kerr Department of Neurological Surgery, The Ohio State University Wexner Medical Center, Columbus, OH, USA

Irene Kim Department of Neurosurgery, NYU Langone Medical Center, New York, NY, USA; Division of Pediatric Neurosurgery, NYU Langone Medical Center, New York, NY, USA

Anne Klibanski Neuroendocrine Unit, Massachusetts General Hospital, Boston, MA, USA; Harvard Medical School, Boston, MA, USA

Douglas Kondziolka Department of Neurosurgery, NYU Langone Medical Center, New York, NY, USA

Khaled M. Krisht Department of Neurosurgery, Clinical Neurosciences Center, University of Utah, Salt Lake City, UT, USA

Edward R. Laws, Jr. Department of Neurosurgery, Brigham and Women's Hospital and Harvard Medical School, Boston, MA, USA

Cheng-Chia Lee Lars Leksell Gamma Knife Center, Department of Neurological Surgery, University of Virginia Health System, Charlottesville, VA, USA

Robert G. Louis Brain Tumor Center, John Wayne Cancer Institute at Saint John's Health Center, Santa Monica, CA, USA; Department of Anatomical Sciences, St George's University School of Medicine, Grenada

L. Dade Lunsford Center for Image Guided Neurosurgery, Department of Neurological Surgery, University of Pittsburgh Medical Center, Pittsburgh, PA, USA

Shannon M. MacDonald Department of Radiation Oncology, Massachusetts General

Hospital, Harvard Medical School, Boston, MA, USA; Radiation Oncology, Massachusetts General Hospital/Harvard Medical School, Boston, MA, USA

Alessandra Mantovani Department of Neurological Surgery, University of Washington, Harborview Medical Center, Seattle, WA, USA

Konstantinos Margetis Department of Neurological Surgery, Weill Cornell Medical College, New York, NY, USA; Department of Neurological Surgery, Memorial Sloan-Kettering Cancer Center, New York, NY, USA

Luigi Maria Cavallo Department of Neurosciences and Reproductive and Odontostomatological Sciences, Division of Neurosurgery, Università degli Studi di Napoli Federico II, Naples, Italy

Carolina Martins Department of Neurosurgery, University of Florida, Gainesville, FL, USA

Heather J. McCrea Departments of Neurosurgery, Weill Cornell Medical College, New York Presbyterian Hospital, New York, NY, USA

Gautam U. Mehta Surgical Neurology Branch, National Institutes of Neurological Disorders and Stroke, National Institutes of Health, Bethesda, MD, USA; Department of Neurosurgery, University of Virginia Health Sciences Center, University of Virginia, Charlottesville, VA, USA

Edward A. Monaco, III Center for Image Guided Neurosurgery, Department of Neurological Surgery, University of Pittsburgh Medical Center, Pittsburgh, PA, USA

Hermann L. Müller Department of Pediatrics, Klinikum Oldenburg, Oldenburg, Germany

Ajay Niranjan Center for Image Guided Neurosurgery, Department of Neurological Surgery, University of Pittsburgh Medical Center, Pittsburgh, PA, USA

Guilian Niu Department of Pathology and Laboratory Medicine/Affiliated Pathology Services, Albany Medical College/Center Hospital, Albany, NY, USA

Edward H. Oldfield Surgical Neurology Branch, National Institutes of Neurological Disorders and Stroke, National Institutes of Health, Bethesda, MD, USA; Department of Neurosurgery, University of Virginia Health Sciences Center, University of Virginia, Charlottesville, VA, USA

Bradley A. Otto Department of Otolaryngology – Head and Neck Surgery, The Ohio State University Wexner Medical Center, Columbus, OH, USA

Troy D. Payner Goodman Campbell Brain and Spine, Indiana University School of Medicine, IN, USA

Maria Peris-Celda Department of Neurosurgery, University of Florida, Gainesville, FL, USA

Carlos D. Pinheiro-Neto Division of Otolaryngology, Albany Medical Center, Albany, NY, USA

Daniel M. Prevedello Department of Neurological Surgery, The Ohio State University Wexner Medical Center, Columbus, OH, USA

Jiang Qian Department of Pathology and Laboratory Medicine/Affiliated Pathology Services, Albany Medical College/Center Hospital, Albany, NY, USA

Albert L. Rhoton Department of Neurosurgery, University of Florida, Gainesville, FL, USA

Benjamin A. Rubin Division of Pediatric Neurosurgery, NYU Langone Medical Center, New York, NY, USA

James T. Rutka Division of Neurosurgery, the Hospital for Sick Children, The University of Toronto, Toronto, Canada

Theodore H. Schwartz Departments of Neurosurgery, Otolaryngology, Head and Neck Surgery, Weill Cornell Medical College, New York Presbyterian Hospital, New York, NY, USA

Laligam N. Sekhar Department of Neurological Surgery, University of Washington, Harborview Medical Center, Seattle, WA, USA

Robert C. Sergott Wills Eye Hospital and Thomas Jefferson University, Philadelphia, PA, USA

Roshan V. Sethi Department of Radiation Oncology, Massachusetts General Hospital, Harvard Medical School, Boston, MA, USA

Jason P. Sheehan Lars Leksell Gamma Knife Center, Department of Neurological Surgery, University of Virginia Health System, Charlottesville, VA, USA

Eugenia Shekhtman Department of Neurosurgery, NYU Langone Medical Center, New York, NY, USA

Walavan Sivakumar Department of Neurosurgery, Clinical Neurosciences Center, University of Utah, Salt Lake City, UT, USA

Domenico Solari Department of Neurosciences and Reproductive and Odontostomatological Sciences, Division of Neurosurgery, Università degli Studi di Napoli Federico II, Naples, Italy

Mark Souweidane Department of Neurological Surgery, Weill Cornell Medical College, New York, NY, USA; Department of Neurological Surgery, Memorial Sloan-Kettering Cancer Center, New York, NY, USA

Zachary Tempel Center for Image Guided Neurosurgery, Department of Neurological Surgery, University of Pittsburgh Medical Center, Pittsburgh, PA, USA

Charles Teo Centre for Minimally Invasive Neurosurgery, Prince of Wales Hospital, Sydney, New South Wales, Australia

Philip V. Theodosopoulos Department of Neurological Surgery, University of California San Francisco, San Francisco, CA, USA

Dominic Thompson Department of Neurosurgery, Great Ormond Street Hospital for Children NHS Foundation Trust, London, UK

Nicholas A. Tritos Neuroendocrine Unit, Massachusetts General Hospital, Boston, MA, USA; Harvard Medical School, Boston, MA, USA

Rafael Uribe Pontificia Universidad Javeriana, Bogotá, Colombia

Rowan Valentine Department of Neurosurgery, University of Florida, Gainesville, FL, USA

Hung Tzu Wen Department of Neurosurgery, University of Florida, Gainesville, FL, USA

Jeffrey H. Wisoff Department of Neurosurgery, NYU Langone Medical Center, New York, NY, USA; Division of Pediatric Neurosurgery, NYU Langone Medical Center, New York, NY, USA

Anthony T. Yachnis Neuropathology Section, Department of Pathology, Immunology, and Laboratory Medicine, University of Florida College of Medicine, Gainesville, FL, USA

Tong Yang Departments of Neurosurgery, Weill Cornell Medical College, New York Presbyterian Hospital, New York, NY, USA

Foreword

Craniopharyngiomas is the first complete resource for physicians involved in the care of patients with one of the most challenging brain tumors. The list of authors is world-class and the contents are outstanding. It is one of the most exciting and comprehensive volumes focused on one of the most complicated problems that I have encountered during my career. This book provides access to the world's masters in dealing with craniopharyngiomas. It truly stands as a model for other academicians and clinicians wanting to bring focus to a complicated clinical problem.

Management of craniopharyngiomas requires the focus of many medical specialists, with the neurosurgeon taking a leading role. Drs. Evans and Kenning have brought together the world experts in every aspect of the evaluation and treatment of these difficult tumors. The book is divided into 36 chapters within eight sections, and the authors of each chapter are academic and clinical leaders in their specialty. In addition to having excellent chapters on surgical techniques, radiation, and intracavitary therapy, it also addresses the management of recurrent craniopharyngiomas, pediatric considerations, and surgical approach controversies.

Congratulations to Drs. James Evans and Tyler Kenning on this outstanding contribution to one of the most complex problems with which we deal. This book is a "must have volume" for every clinician involved in the care of patients with craniopharyngiomas. It highlights Drs. Evans' and Kenning's passion for perfection and their desire to make the treatment of craniopharyngiomas more accurate, precise, gentle, and safe.

Albert L. Rhoton, Jr., M.D.
R.D. Keene Family Professor and
Chairman Emeritus
University of Florida

Preface

Craniopharyngiomas are widely considered to be among the most formidable and challenging intracranial tumors, despite being considered benign histologically. Their anatomical location, propensity for adherence to critical neurovascular structures, and the devastating spectrum of clinical symptoms that may occur not only with their growth but also with their treatment make these tumors extremely problematic to manage.

Once considered a purely surgical disease, largely due to the inefficacy of adjuvant treatment, the management of craniopharyngiomas has continually emphasized the need for equanimity and humility in the cranial base surgeon. Ever since their initial recognition as a distinct pathological entity, these tumors have confounded surgeons for over a century. Harvey Cushing, Walter Dandy, and countless others have repeatedly expressed their frustration, and often hopelessness, in managing these lesions.

Currently, the treatment of craniopharyngiomas has evolved to include teams of specialists from multiple medical disciplines with the neurosurgeon still taking the lead role. Although these complicated tumors and their treatment have been widely addressed in the literature, a text dedicated to their multidisciplinary management had yet to be compiled. We have brought together global leaders from the fields of neurosurgery, radiation oncology, pathology, ophthalmology, neuro-oncology, endocrinology, neuroanatomy, and neuroradiology in order to create a comprehensive resource for physicians involved in the treatment of these difficult tumors. We are extremely grateful to each of our contributing authors, all renowned experts in their respective fields, for enthusiastically accepting our invitation and contributing to this effort. Finally, we are indebted to Elsevier Academic Press and their superb editorial staff for their guidance and assistance in producing this text. We hope that this will be a valuable resource to those involved in treating patients with craniopharyngiomas.

James J. Evans, MD
Tyler J. Kenning, MD

SECTION I

INTRODUCTION

CHAPTER

1

Introduction

M. Reid Gooch*, James J. Evans†, Tyler J. Kenning*

*Department of Neurosurgery, Albany Medical Center, Albany, NY, USA; †Department of Neurological Surgery, Thomas Jefferson University Hospital, Philadelphia, PA, USA

One would expect these congenital epithelial tumors to be capable of enucleation like dermoid cysts elsewhere in the body, but they so definitely adhere to the adjacent structures neighboring on their place of origin, it is rarely possible to shell them out of their bed without the production of serious secondary symptoms. To be sure, one may occasionally succeed in stripping out a thin-walled cyst, and examples of this have been reported, but when the tumor is partly solidified and calcareous, sad experience warns the surgeon to leave it pretty much alone. ***Harvey Cushing, 1932.***

"Though this tumor is still an ominous disease, it seems fair to say, that the outlook has improved considerably." ***J. Lindholm and EH Nielsen, 2009***

INTRODUCTION

Craniopharyngiomas are rare brain tumors defined by the World Health Organization as "benign, partly cystic epithelial tumor[s] of the sellar region presumably derived from Rathke pouch epithelium" (Louis Dn, 2007). While technically benign growths, craniopharyngiomas and their subsequent treatment can cause damage or destruction to critical sellar and parasellar structures, leading some clinicians to call this entity a "benign tumor in a malignant location." Indeed for a WHO grade 1 lesion the management can be quite complicated and controversial.

EPIDEMIOLOGY

A 2011 study reviewed 15 population-based studies of craniopharyngiomas including over 1000 cases, and estimated a world incidence of 1.34 patients per one million people (Nielsen et al., 2011). In the United States, there were approximately 2680 cases of craniopharyngiomas diagnosed between 2005–2009, representing 0.9% of new central nervous system tumors. Among patients aged 0–14, the percentage was significantly higher, at 4.1% (Dolecek et al.,

Craniopharyngiomas
http://dx.doi.org/10.1016/B978-0-12-416706-3.00001-5

2012). This bimodal age distribution is well described with approximate peaks at ages 5–14 and then again in adulthood around age 65 (Haupt et al., 2006), but the tumor has been diagnosed from the prenatal period to the ninth decade (Lederman et al., 1987; Arai et al., 2003).

Internationally, the highest rates of craniopharyngiomas have been reported in African and Asian countries (Haupt et al., 2006). A review of childhood intracranial neoplasms seen at a university teaching hospital in Nigeria from 1960–1982 found that 8/89 (9%) tumors were craniopharyngiomas (Aghadiuno et al., 1985). A second Nigerian study found 38% of their children with intracranial neoplasms harbored craniopharyngiomas (Izuora et al., 1989). These numbers are likely biased by a less advanced medical infrastructure whereby university clinicians are more likely to witness the drastic presentations of a slowly growing benign tumor, but they are impressive nonetheless. A Japanese study reported the incidence of craniopharyngiomas as 5.8% among all new CNS brain tumors and 12.5% in children (Mori and Kurisaka, 1986). In China, a review that examined 12,785 brain tumors, including metastatic lesions, found that 6.5% were craniopharyngiomas (Cheng, 1982). This geographic tendency remains unexplained and the ethnic disparity does not appear to exist in studies conducted within the United States (Dolecek et al., 2012). Finally, the tumor does not demonstrate a predilection with respect to gender.

There are no known environmental risk factors for developing craniopharyngiomas, including prior radiation therapy. Additionally, there is no clear familial tendency, although three case reports documenting craniopharyngiomas in siblings (Vargas et al., 1981; Combelles et al., 1984; Boch et al., 1997) and one in first cousins (Thomsett et al., 1980) suggest the possibility of an autosomal recessive trait, which may sometimes be associated with tumor formation. Overall, craniopharyngioma occurrence appears to be a rare, spontaneous event.

PATHOPHYSIOLOGY

There are two histologically defined subtypes of craniopharyngioma: adamantinomatous (the majority of cases across all age groups) and papillary. Both are derived from Rathke pouch epithelium, yet the origin of these epithelial cells is thought to distinguish the subtype. Adamantinomatous craniopharyngiomas occur predominantly in the pediatric population and are frequently calcified and cystic in nature. The cysts can become quite large and contain a cholesterol-rich, "motor-oil"-like fluid that is caustic if it contacts normal brain tissue. The tumor's solid components consist of a pallisading columnar cell layer encasing loose stellate epithelial and desquamated cells called "wet keratin" (Figure 1.1). Rosenthal fibers are often found at the interface of the tumor with the brain – a manifestation of astrocytic gliosis (Prabhu and Brown, 2005). Adamantinomatous craniopharyngiomas are believed to arise due to neoplastic changes of epithelial cells originating from the developing stomodeum, which become trapped in the craniopharyngeal duct during pituitary development. This is called the "embryogenetic theory" and may account for the adamantinomatous subtype being the one most commonly found in children: the epithelial cells are present in an improper location from the patient's earliest development (Prabhu and Brown, 2005; Garre and Cama, 2007).

Papillary craniopharyngioma, on the other hand, is primarily an adult disease. Histologically, these tumors also can include wet keratin, but the squamous epithelial cells are well differentiated, the tumor is more solid and uniform in nature with a fibrovascular core,

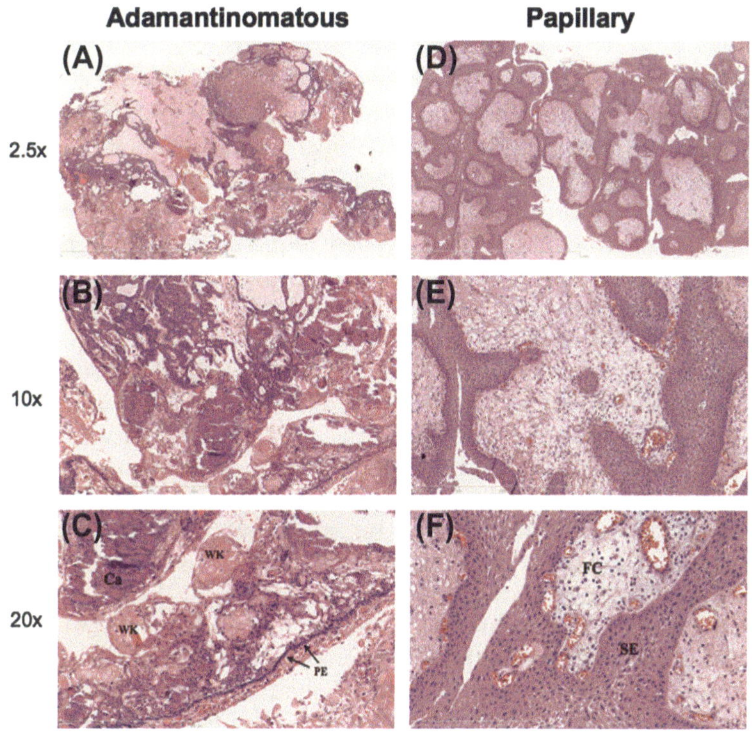

FIGURE 1.1 **Histological sections of craniopharyngioma. A–C**, Adamantinomatous type consisting of epithelial lobules with loose stroma, wet keratin (WK), calcifications (Ca) and peripheral palisading epithelium (PE). **D–F**, Papillary type consisting of sheets of well-differentiated non-keratinizing squamous epithelium (SE) in a papillary configuration, with a broad fibrovascular core (FC). Magnification is indicated on the left. *(Courtesy of Jiang Qian, MD, PhD; Albany Medical Center Department of Pathology.)*

and there is typically a lack of calcifications, cystic elements or intratumoral fluid (Figure 1.1). Papillary craniopharyngiomas may be explained by the "metaplastic theory," which suggests that the tumors arise secondary to metaplasia of adenohypophyseal cells in the pars tuberalis. Therefore, adamantinomatous craniopharyngiomas are masses that occur after neoplastic changes to epithelial cells in the craniopharyngeal duct, whereas papillary craniopharyngiomas arise after cells in the craniopharyngeal duct undergo metaplasia and transform into abnormal epithelial cells. Thus, the papillary subtype is exceedingly rare in younger patients, as the development of these tumors requires more time to have the normal cells undergo metaplastic transformation and subsequent growth (Prabhu and Brown, 2005; Karavitaki et al., 2006; Garre and Cama, 2007).

Recent data suggest that the true origin of craniopharyngiomas may comprise a combination of these theories. A large pathology-based review found that of 131 craniopharyngioma specimens, 20 (15%) contained both squamous epithelial and adamantinomatous features. As the authors note, this suggests that the subtypes may exist within a "craniopharyngioma spectrum" (Szeifert et al., 1993).

HISTORY

The modern scientific understanding of craniopharyngiomas began in the second half of the 19th century. Friedrich Albert von Zenker, a German pathologist, is credited with the first pathological description of the tumor in 1857 (Zenker, 1857; Barkhoudarian and Laws, 2013) and the first histological description is attributed to Mott and Barratt in 1899 (Mott Fa, 1899). Mott and Barratt described three patients with third ventricular tumors who died likely secondary to complications from hydrocephalus. They found epithelial cells in two of the tumor specimens and their report of one patient's histology closely resembles that of a papillary craniopharyngioma. Interestingly, the authors noted "It is unfortunate that the hypophysis…was not examined, for the anterior lobe of this organ is said to be developed from a diverticulum of the nasal mucous membrane extending through the base of the skull toward the hollow infundibulum which grows to meet it, and it is possible to conceive that this may explain these misplaced epidermal cells" (Mott Fa, 1899). The authors were likely referring to the embryological work of Rathke, whose studies on the formation of the pituitary gland were published in 1839 (Rathke, 1839; Lindholm and Nielsen, 2009). Yet, it was another German pathologist, Jakob Erdheim, who did study hypophyseal tumors, and in 1904, convincingly proposed the existence of a distinct class of sellar tumors originating from epithelial cells trapped along the embryonic craniopharyngeal duct. For many years these would be referred to as "Erdheim tumors" (Lindholm and Nielsen, 2009).

A. E. Halstead performed the first known operation for a craniopharyngioma in Chicago during the summer of 1909. A 39-year-old patient referred to as HR presented with a 2-year history of headaches and subsequently developed a progressive bitemporal hemianopsia. This history and clinical exam, coupled with complaints of intermittent polyuria led Halstead to perform a transsphenoidal operation where a "blue colored pulsating [hypophyseal] mass" was found and resected. Postoperatively the patient suffered from pyrexia and a state of "shock" attributed to gauze packing. Following surgical removal of that packing, the patient eventually did well and 5 weeks after the initial operation, HR was discharged from the hospital in good health, with improving vision and ultimately returned to work (Figure 1.2). The pathological description of the tumor led the surgical team to conclude that this was an "epithelial tumor developing in the sella turcica from fragments of undifferentiated epithelium developing from the craniopharyngeal duct" – an Erdheim tumor (Halstead, 1910).

In 1932, Harvey Cushing published his experience of 2000 brain tumors and included 92 "craniopharyngiomas." He was not the first to use this term and stated immediately that the "cumbersome" word encompassed the "kaleidoscopic tumors, solid and cystic, which take their origin from epithelial rests ascribable to an imperfect closure of the hypophyseal or craniopharyngeal duct". In Cushing's series, five patients died before an intervention, and 19 of the remaining 87 patients died after a total of 130 operations. Thus, his case-based mortality was 21.8% and the operative mortality was 14.6%. Compared to modern standards, both of these rates are relatively high but nevertheless this was an impressive feat in the early 20th century. This set the standard for craniopharyngioma surgery and the term describing the mass would endure.

Throughout the ensuing decades, craniopharyngioma surgery benefited from improvements in general surgical care, including electrocautery and antibiotics. Improvements in

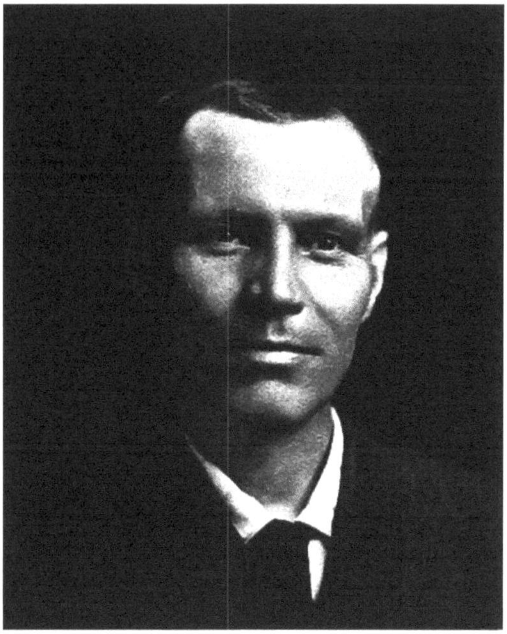

FIGURE 1.2 Photograph of HR taken two and a half months after his operation by Dr. Halstead. He is the first patient known to have undergone surgery for a craniopharyngioma. *(Reprinted from: Halstead AE. Remarks on the Operative Treatment of Tumors of the Hypophysis, Surgery, Gynecology and Obstetrics 1910; 5:501, with permission.)*

the understanding of the physiology of the sellar region and its pathology, including diabetes insipidus and corticosteroid use, contributed to better surgical outcomes as well (Ingraham et al., 1952; Tytus et al., 1955). In the 1970s, the advent of better imaging techniques, using CT and then MRI, provided invaluable information to aid in the diagnosis, planning, and post-operative care of these patients.

Advancements in radiological visualization resulted in a renewed interest in the various surgical approaches to sellar lesions. For Halstead's patient HR, he chose a transsphenoidal route presumably due to his belief that the patient had a pituitary adenoma. While Cushing utilized transsphenoidal approaches early in his career he eventually abandoned them in favor of transcranial resections of craniopharyngiomas. He ultimately concluded that the morbidity of the transnasal technique was unacceptably high (Figure 1.3). Transcranial approaches were then favored for many years and became increasingly popular as descriptions of skull base techniques were applied to craniopharyngiomas, including supraorbital-pterional (Al-Mefty, 1987), transpetrosal-transtentorial (Hakuba et al., 1985), and subfrontal (Samii and Tatagiba, 1997) approaches.

A renewed interest in transsphenoidal surgery began in the 1960s, led by Jules Hardy and Gerard Guiot with their utilization of video fluoroscopy (Hardy and Wigser, 1965; Barkhoudarian and Laws, 2013). The endonasal approach for craniopharyngiomas was further supported by a 1980 case series by Edward Laws, consisting of 26 transsphenoidal

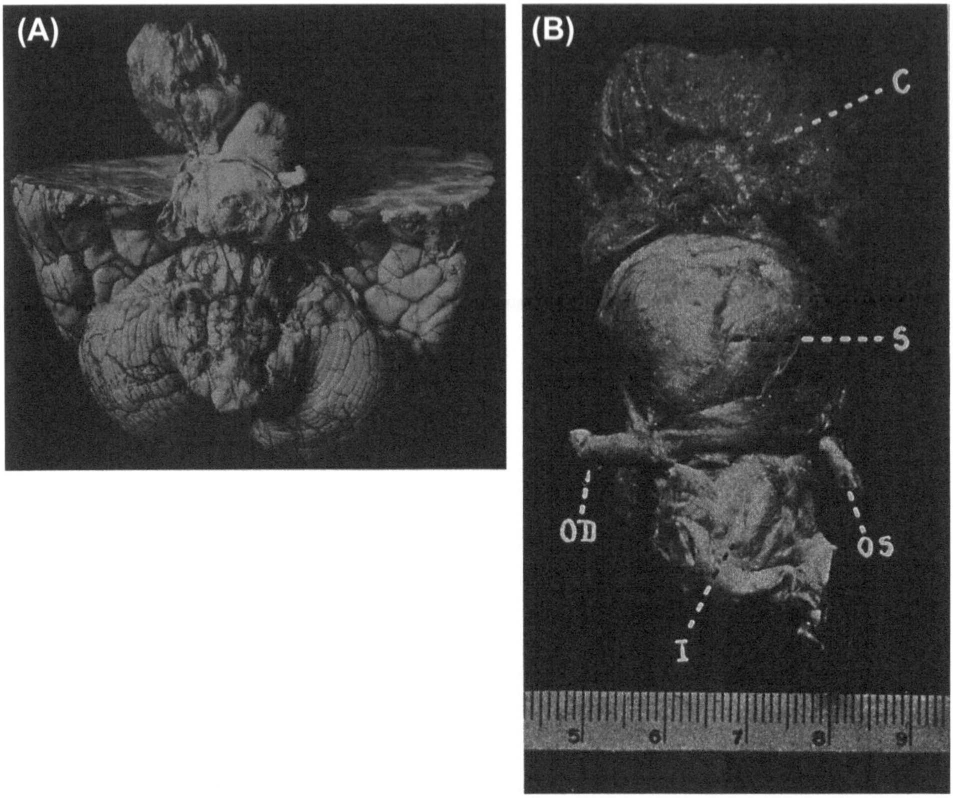

FIGURE 1.3 This gross specimen from Cushing's 1932 review demonstrates a complication of transsphenoidal resection prior to the advent of modern imaging techniques: **A**. "To show the intracranial extension of a primarily intrasellar craniopharyngioma operated upon from below owing to a mistaken diagnosis of adenoma." **B.** "The same tumor...detached to show its relation to stretched chiasm and optic nerves. O.D., right optic nerve. O.S., left optic nerve. I., intrasellar portion of tumor. S., suprasellar expansion of same. C., superimposed cyst." *(Reprinted from: Cushing H Intracranial tumors. (1932) Notes upon a series of two thousand verified cases with surgical mortality percentages pertaining thereto. Thomas, Springfield, p 95–96.)*

craniopharyngioma resections (Laws, 1980). The expanded endonasal endoscopic approach has since widened this corridor and its application (Gardner et al., 2008).

The strategy behind craniopharyngioma surgery has also evolved, driven by the early realization that aggressive resection – while potentially providing excellent oncological control and limiting recurrence – could result in significant morbidity and mortality. In a 1949 review of 51 consecutive craniopharyngioma patients, 41% did not survive beyond the early post-operative period (Figure 1.4). While the authors noted that in these cases, "[they had] undoubtedly erred on the side of being too radical as is attested by our operative mortality," they ultimately concluded that "too few attempts have been made by competent surgeons to remove these tumors totally." (Gordy et al., 1949). These contradictory statements embody the dilemma surrounding the management of craniopharyngiomas: while complete surgical excision may provide a cure, it may also be accompanied by significant morbidity. The

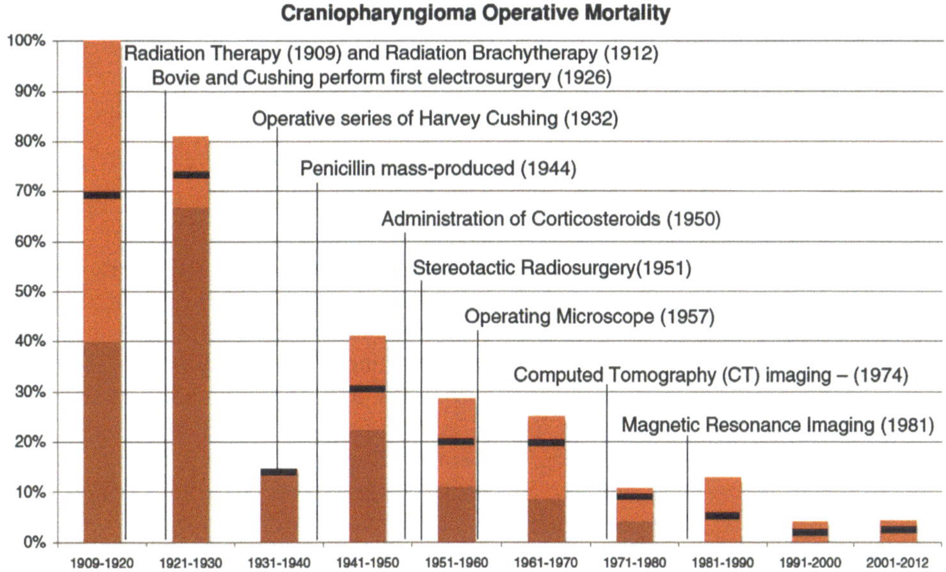

FIGURE 1.4 Rates of peri-operative mortality based on selected series of craniopharyngioma patients ($n > 10$), published within the date range provided. Black bar = average rate; shaded region = range. *(Reprinted with permission from: Barkhoudarian, G and Laws, ER. Craniopharyngioma: history. (2013). Pituitary 16, p. 4.)*

surgical paradigm has therefore shifted so that, when obtainable, gross total resection remains the goal, but adjuvant therapies have come to play a larger role in treatment.

The first report of utilizing radiation in the management of craniopharyngiomas was in the 1930s (Carpenter, 1937; Lindholm and Nielsen, 2009), but it was not until the 1960s and 1970s that the benefits of radiation in limiting tumor recurrence were consistently demonstrated (Hoff and Patterson, 1972). Today, conventional radiotherapy has been clearly shown as effective in helping to control tumor growth when given either immediately after a subtotal resection or when used as salvage therapy (Stripp et al., 2004; Minniti et al., 2009). Minniti et al. note that craniopharyngioma recurrence after subtotal resection may approach 85%, however several large series document 10-year local control of 77–89% and 20-year control of 54–79% when radiotherapy is administered after surgery (Minniti et al., 2009). Just as surgical techniques have evolved, so too have radiation techniques. Fractionated stereotactic radiotherapy and stereotactic radiosurgery have the potential benefit of less damage to surrounding tissue (an important consideration for sellar lesions) and fewer long-term side effects from irradiation. Further studies will be needed, however, to establish their benefit over conventional radiation methods (Minniti et al., 2009; Iannalfi et al., 2013). Intracavitary irradiation can also be utilized for predominantly cystic craniopharyngiomas (Hasegawa et al., 2004; Julow, 2013).

Chemotherapy, both systemic and intracavitary, has demonstrated promise as another adjunctive treatment for craniopharyngioma (Takahashi et al., 2005; Yeung et al., 2012). Overall, its application remains limited. Again, intracavitary administration is reserved for patients with large cystic components, while systemic therapy is generally used for patients with particularly aggressive tumors who have exhausted traditional treatments (Mortini et al., 2013). Finally, work investigating the molecular mechanisms behind craniopharyngioma formation will hopefully lead to future therapies (Pettorini et al., 2010), but this is largely speculative at this point.

PRESENTATION AND THE MODERN DISEASE COURSE

Craniopharyngioma patients typically present with symptoms caused by mass effect and tumor invasion. This leads to disruption of structures within the sellar and parasellar space, namely the optic apparatus, pituitary gland, hypothalamus, and ventricular system. As a result, the most common presenting symptoms are vision changes, endocrine abnormalities, and symptoms of increased intracranial pressure (Duff et al., 2000; Van Effenterre and Boch, 2002; Karavitaki et al., 2005; Mallucci et al., 2012). While adult patients typically present with visual deficits, children more frequently present with symptoms of increased intracranial pressure and hydrocephalus, including headache, nausea, and vomiting (Karavitaki et al., 2005; Nielsen et al., 2012). Visual deficits and endocrine abnormalities are often detected during the initial evaluation even if not appreciated clinically (Fahlbusch et al., 1999; Van Effenterre and Boch, 2002). Overall, those patients with primarily endocrinopathies seek medical attention after a much longer duration of symptoms. In a review of 122 such patients including both children and adults, the median time between initial symptom onset and diagnosis was 27 months with a maximum of 15 years (Van Effenterre and Boch, 2002). Other frequent symptoms at presentation include short stature, diabetes insipidus, impaired sexual function, cold intolerance, and hemiparesis.

The evaluation for a suspected craniopharyngioma is similar to the workup for any mass within the sellar or suprasellar space: an enhanced MRI with thin cuts dedicated through the region of the sella and anterior cranial base, pituitary hormone assessment, and an ophthalmologic examination with automated visual field analysis. In a minority of cases, the presentation requires urgent surgical intervention, usually due to hydrocephalus. For these patients, hydrocephalus can be managed with either a ventriculostomy or shunt while surgery addressing the tumor can be postponed until the patient stabilizes. Surgery may entail biopsy, cyst decompression and fenestration, debulking, resection or a combination of the above. An Ommaya reservoir is sometime placed in a cyst cavity for future chemotherapy administration (Dastoli et al., 2011). Observation is always an option, however there are no data in the literature to support a "wait and see" approach for a symptomatic sellar lesion suspected to be a craniopharyngioma. For asymptomatic patients harboring an incidentally found craniopharyngioma, there are insufficient data to definitively predict the true natural history. It does appear that most lesions likely become symptomatic with time. A case series from 2005 included 13 patients who were initially managed non-operatively with serial radiologic follow-up. Twelve of the 13 patients did eventually require surgery due to an increase in tumor size and the resultant development of clinical symptoms. For the final patient, one surgery was performed for diagnostic purposes (Karavitaki et al., 2006, personal communication with the author).

With a better understanding of the morbidity that may potentially attend an aggressive resection, some have advocated for more conservative surgical approaches (De Vile et al., 1996).

Outcome studies have begun to emphasize quality of life measures, rather than simply survival and radiological evidence of recurrence (Duff et al., 2000; Poretti et al., 2004; Dekkers et al., 2006; Fjalldal et al., 2013). Duff et al., examined 121 patients with a mean follow-up of 10 years to identify those patients with a "good outcome," as defined by several factors including school status, employability, and psychological and emotional health. While 83% (101/121) of the patients were alive at follow-up, only 60% (73/121) achieved a "good outcome" (Duff et al., 2000).

In the interest of achieving this "good outcome" some clinicians have developed various classification systems in attempts to stratify patients and select the appropriate level of aggressive care. Puget et al. divided patients into three categories based on the extent of hypothalamic involvement, and tailored their treatment paradigm accordingly. In their prospective cohort, no patient demonstrated new hypothalamic injury after treatment or had a decreased quality of life, even without any significant oncologic recurrences demonstrated in their follow-up period (Puget et al., 2007). Other groups have developed similar grading systems and treatment paradigms (Mallucci et al., 2012). Still, some large series continue to advocate for aggressive resection as the best, most definitive treatment for this disease process (Yasargil et al., 1990; Fahlbusch et al., 1999; Elliott et al., 2010; Lee et al., 2012). Nevertheless, with the development of advanced radiation techniques and effective adjuvant treatments for residual or recurrent disease, the emphasis on a radical surgical resection has somewhat lessened (Figure 1.5).

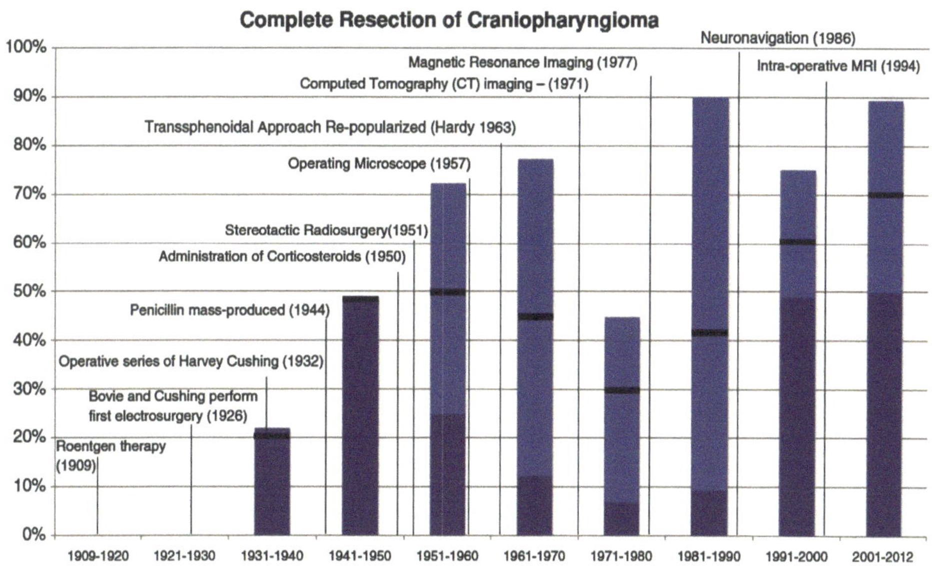

FIGURE 1.5 Rates of self-reported "gross total" or "complete" resection of craniopharyngiomas in selected series ($n > 10$), published with the date range provided. Black bar = average rate; shaded region = range. *(Reprinted with permission from: Barkhoudarian, G and Laws, ER. Craniopharyngioma: history. (2013). Pituitary 16, p. 6.)*

CONCLUSION

Craniopharyngioma care encompasses some of the most challenging aspects of neurosurgery. The tumor's unforgiving location and the need for interdisciplinary management of this complex disease demand that the clinical decision-making must strike the proper balance between aggressive resection of a benign mass with cautious restraint so as not to induce unsatisfactory morbidity. Furthermore, the benefits of adjunctive therapies, while unquestionably valuable, have not been clearly defined. The treatment paradigm has progressively shifted from one focused on complete surgical resection and the limitation of recurrence to that of oncologic control while limiting morbidity and preserving quality of life. The best way to optimize this balance is still unclear and likely an individualized approach must be tailored to both the patient's disease and the treating physician's ability.

References

Aghadiuno, P.U., Adeloye, A., Olumide, A.A., Nottidge, V.A., 1985. Intracranial neoplasms in children in Ibadan, Nigeria. Childs Nerv. Syst 1 (1), 39–44.

Al-Mefty, O., 1987. Supraorbital-pterional approach to skull base lesions. Neurosurgery 21 (4), 474–477.

Arai, T., Ohno, K., Takada, Y., Aoyagi, M., Hirakawa, K., 2003. Neonatal craniopharyngioma and inference of tumor inception time: case report and review of the literature. Surg. Neurol. 60 (3), 254–259; discussion 259.

Barkhoudarian, G., Laws, E.R., 2013. Craniopharyngioma: history. Pituitary 16 (1), 1–8.

Boch, A.L., Van Effenterre, R., Kujas, M., 1997. Craniopharyngiomas in two consanguineous siblings: case report. Neurosurgery 41 (5), 1185–1187.

Carpenter Rc, C.G., Frazier, Ch, 1937. The treatment of hypophyseal stalk tumors by evacuation and irradiation. AJR Am. J. Roentgenol. 38, 162–177.

Cheng, M.K., 1982. Brain tumors in the People's Republic of China: a statistical review. Neurosurgery 10 (1), 16–21.

Combelles, G., Ythier, H., Wemeau, J.L., Cappoen, J.P., Delandsheer, J.M., Christiaens, J.L., 1984. [Craniopharyngioma in the same family]. Neurochirurgie 30 (5), 347–349.

Dastoli, P.A., Nicacio, J.M., Silva, N.S., Capellano, A.M., Toledo, S.R., Ierardi, D., Cavalheiro, S., 2011. Cystic craniopharyngioma: intratumoral chemotherapy with alpha interferon. Arq. Neuropsiquiatr. 69 (1), 50–55.

De Vile, C.J., Grant, D.B., Kendall, B.E., Neville, B.G., Stanhope, R., Watkins, K.E., Hayward, R.D., 1996. Management of childhood craniopharyngioma: can the morbidity of radical surgery be predicted? J. Neurosurg. 85 (1), 73–81.

Dekkers, O.M., Biermasz, N.R., Smit, J.W., Groot, L.E., Roelfsema, F., Romijn, J.A., Pereira, A.M., 2006. Quality of life in treated adult craniopharyngioma patients. Eur. J. Endocrinol. 154 (3), 483–489.

Dolecek, T.A., Propp, J.M., Stroup, N.E., Kruchko, C., 2012. CBTRUS statistical report: primary brain and central nervous system tumors diagnosed in the United States in 2005–2009. Neuro. Oncol. 14 (Suppl. 5), v1–49.

Duff, J., Meyer, F.B., Ilstrup, D.M., Laws Jr., E.R., Schleck, C.D., Scheithauer, B.W., 2000. Long-term outcomes for surgically resected craniopharyngiomas. Neurosurgery 46 (2), 291–302; discussion 302–305.

Elliott, R.E., Sands, S.A., Strom, R.G., Wisoff, J.H., 2010. Craniopharyngioma Clinical Status Scale: a standardized metric of preoperative function and posttreatment outcome. Neurosurg. Focus 28 (4), E2.

Fahlbusch, R., Honegger, J., Paulus, W., Huk, W., Buchfelder, M., 1999. Surgical treatment of craniopharyngiomas: experience with 168 patients. J. Neurosurg. 90 (2), 237–250.

Fjalldal, S., Holmer, H., Rylander, L., Elfving, M., Ekman, B., Osterberg, K., Erfurth, E.M., 2013. Hypothalamic involvement predicts cognitive performance and psychosocial health in long-term survivors of childhood craniopharyngioma. J. Clin. Endocrinol. Metab. 98 (8), 3253–3262.

Gardner, P.A., Kassam, A.B., Snyderman, C.H., Carrau, R.L., Mintz, A.H., Grahovac, S., Stefko, S., 2008. Outcomes following endoscopic, expanded endonasal resection of suprasellar craniopharyngiomas: a case series. J. Neurosurg. 109 (1), 6–16.

Garre, M.L., Cama, A., 2007. Craniopharyngioma: modern concepts in pathogenesis and treatment. Curr. Opin. Pediatr. 19 (4), 471–479.

Gordy, P.D., Peet, M.M., Kahn, E.A., 1949. The surgery of the craniopharyngiomas. J. Neurosurg. 6 (6), 503–517.

Hakuba, A., Nishimura, S., Inoue, Y., 1985. Transpetrosal-transtentorial approach and its application in the therapy of retrochiasmatic craniopharyngiomas. Surg. Neurol. 24 (4), 405–415.

Halstead, A., 1910. Remarks on the operative treatment of 256 tumors of the hypophysis. Surg. Gynecol. Obstet. 10, 494–502.

Hardy, J., Wigser, S.M., 1965. Trans-sphenoidal surgery of pituitary fossa tumors with televised radiofluoroscopic control. J. Neurosurg. 23 (6), 612–619.

Hasegawa, T., Kondziolka, D., Hadjipanayis, C.G., Lunsford, L.D., 2004. Management of cystic craniopharyngiomas with phosphorus-32 intracavitary irradiation. Neurosurgery 54 (4), 813–820; discussion 820–822.

Haupt, R., Magnani, C., Pavanello, M., Caruso, S., Dama, E., Garre, M.L., 2006. Epidemiological aspects of craniopharyngioma. J. Pediatr. Endocrinol. Metab. 19 (Suppl. 1), 289–293.

Hoff, J.T., Patterson Jr, R.H., 1972. Craniopharyngiomas in children and adults. J. Neurosurg. 36 (3), 299–302.

Iannalfi, A., Fragkandrea, I., Brock, J., Saran, F., 2013. Radiotherapy in craniopharyngiomas. Clin. Oncol. (R. Coll. Radiol.).

Ingraham, F.D., Matson, D.D., Mc, L.R., 1952. Cortisone and ACTH as an adjunct to the surgery of craniopharyngiomas. N. Engl. J. Med. 246 (15), 568–571.

Izuora, G.I., Ikerionwu, S., Saddeqi, N., Iloeje, S.O., 1989. Childhood intracranial neoplasms Enugu, Nigeria. West Afr. J. Med. 8 (3), 171–174.

Julow, J.V., 2013. Intracystic irradiation for craniopharyngiomas. Pituitary 16 (1), 34–45.

Karavitaki, N., Brufani, C., Warner, J.T., Adams, C.B., Richards, P., Ansorge, O., Shine, B., Turner, H.E., Wass, J.A., 2005. Craniopharyngiomas in children and adults: systematic analysis of 121 cases with long-term follow-up. Clin. Endocrinol. (Oxf) 62 (4), 397–409.

Karavitaki, N., Cudlip, S., Adams, C.B., Wass, J.A., 2006. Craniopharyngiomas. Endocr. Rev. 27 (4), 371–397.

Laws Jr, E.R., 1980. Transsphenoidal microsurgery in the management of craniopharyngioma. J. Neurosurg. 52 (5), 661–666.

Lederman, G.S., Recht, A., Loeffler, J.S., Dubuisson, D., Kleefield, J., Schnitt, S.J., 1987. Craniopharyngioma in an elderly patient. Cancer 60 (5), 1077–1080.

Lee, M.H., Kim, S.H., Seoul, H.J., Nam, D.H., Lee, J.I., Park, K., Kim, J.H., Kong, D.S., 2012. Impact of maximal safe resection on the clinical outcome of adults with craniopharyngiomas. J. Clin. Neuro. sci. 19 (7), 1005–1008.

Lindholm, J., Nielsen, E.H., 2009. Craniopharyngioma: historical notes. Pituitary 12 (4), 352–359.

Louis Dn, O.H., Od, Wietsler, Wk, Cavenee, 2007. WHO Classification of Tumours of the Central Nervous System, Fourth. Ed. 238.

Mallucci, C., Pizer, B., Blair, J., Didi, M., Doss, A., Upadrasta, S., Newman, W., Avula, S., Pettorini, B., 2012. Management of craniopharyngioma: the Liverpool experience following the introduction of the CCLG guidelines. Introducing a new risk assessment grading system. Childs Nerv. Syst. 28 (8), 1181–1192.

Minniti, G., Esposito, V., Amichetti, M., Enrici, R.M., 2009. The role of fractionated radiotherapy and radiosurgery in the management of patients with craniopharyngioma. Neurosurg. Rev. 32 (2), 125–132; discussion 132.

Mori, K., Kurisaka, M., 1986. Brain tumors in childhood: statistical analysis of cases from the Brain Tumor Registry of Japan. Childs Nerv. Syst. 2 (5), 233–237.

Mortini, P., Gagliardi, F., Boari, N., Losa, M., 2013. Surgical strategies and modern therapeutic options in the treatment of craniopharyngiomas. Crit. Rev. Oncol. Hematol. 88 (3), 514–529.

Mott Fa, B.J., 1899. Three cases of tumour of the third ventricle. Arch. Neurol. Psychiatry 1, 417–440.

Nielsen, E.H., Feldt-Rasmussen, U., Poulsgaard, L., Kristensen, L.O., Astrup, J., Jorgensen, J.O., Bjerre, P., Andersen, M., Andersen, C., Jorgensen, J., Lindholm, J., Laurberg, P., 2011. Incidence of craniopharyngioma in Denmark (n = 189) and estimated world incidence of craniopharyngioma in children and adults. J. Neurooncol. 104 (3), 755–763.

Nielsen, E.H., Jorgensen, J.O., Bjerre, P., Andersen, M., Andersen, C., Feldt-Rasmussen, U., Poulsgaard, L., Kristensen, L.O., Astrup, J., Jorgensen, J., Laurberg, P., 2012. Acute presentation of craniopharyngioma in children and adults in a Danish national cohort. Pituitary 16 (4), 528–535.

Pettorini, B.L., Frassanito, P., Caldarelli, M., Tamburrini, G., Massimi, L., Di Rocco, C., 2010. Molecular pathogenesis of craniopharyngioma: switching from a surgical approach to a biological one. Neurosurg. Focus 28 (4), E1.

Poretti, A., Grotzer, M.A., Ribi, K., Schonle, E., Boltshauser, E., 2004. Outcome of craniopharyngioma in children: long-term complications and quality of life. Dev. Med. Child. Neurol. 46 (4), 220–229.

Prabhu, V.C., Brown, H.G., 2005. The pathogenesis of craniopharyngiomas. Childs Nerv. Syst. 21 (8–9), 622–627.

Puget, S., Garnett, M., Wray, A., Grill, J., Habrand, J.L., Bodaert, N., Zerah, M., Bezerra, M., Renier, D., Pierre-Kahn, A., Sainte-Rose, C., 2007. Pediatric craniopharyngiomas: classification and treatment according to the degree of hypothalamic involvement. J. Neurosurg. 106 (Suppl. 1), 3–12.
Rathke, M.H., 1839. Uber die Entstehung der Glandula pituitaria. Arch. Anat. Physiol. Wiss. Med. 5, 482–485.
Samii, M., Tatagiba, M., 1997. Surgical management of craniopharyngiomas: a review. Neurol. Med. Chir. (Tokyo) 37 (2), 141–149.
Stripp, D.C., Maity, A., Janss, A.J., Belasco, J.B., Tochner, Z.A., Goldwein, J.W., Moshang, T., Rorke, L.B., Phillips, P.C., Sutton, L.N., Shu, H.K., 2004. Surgery with or without radiation therapy in the management of craniopharyngiomas in children and young adults. Int. J. Radiat. Oncol. Biol. Phys. 58 (3), 714–720.
Szeifert, G.T., Sipos, L., Horvath, M., Sarker, M.H., Major, O., Salomvary, B., Czirjak, S., Balint, K., Slowik, F., Kolonics, L., et al., 1993. Pathological characteristics of surgically removed craniopharyngiomas: analysis of 131 cases. Acta Neurochir. (Wien) 124 (2–4), 139–143.
Takahashi, H., Yamaguchi, F., Teramoto, A., 2005. Long-term outcome and reconsideration of intracystic chemotherapy with bleomycin for craniopharyngioma in children. Childs Nerv. Syst. 21 (8–9), 701–704.
Thomsett, M.J., Conte, F.A., Kaplan, S.L., Grumbach, M.M., 1980. Endocrine and neurologic outcome in childhood craniopharyngioma: review of effect of treatment in 42 patients. J. Pediatr. 97 (5), 728–735.
Tytus, J.S., Seltzer, H.S., Kahn, E.A., 1955. Cortisone as an aid in the surgical treatment of craniopharyngiomas. J. Neurosurg. 12 (6), 555–564.
Van Effenterre, R., Boch, A.L., 2002. Craniopharyngioma in adults and children: a study of 122 surgical cases. J. Neurosurg. 97 (1), 3–11.
Vargas, J.R., Pino, J.A., Murad, T.M., 1981. Craniopharyngioma in two siblings. JAMA 246 (16), 1807–1808.
Yasargil, M.G., Curcic, M., Kis, M., Siegenthaler, G., Teddy, P.J., Roth, P., 1990. Total removal of craniopharyngiomas. Approaches and long-term results in 144 patients. J. Neurosurg. 73 (1), 3–11.
Yeung, J.T., Pollack, I.F., Panigrahy, A., Jakacki, R.I., 2012. Pegylated interferon-alpha-2b for children with recurrent craniopharyngioma. J. Neurosurg. Pediatr. 10 (6), 498–503.
Zenker, F., 1857. Enorme Cystenbildung im Gehirn, vom Hirnanhang ausgehend. Virchows Arch. 12, 454–466.

CHAPTER

2

Craniopharyngiomas: Anatomical Considerations

Maria Peris-Celda, Rowan Valentine*, Carlos D. Pinheiro-Neto†, Takeshi Funaki*, Carolina Martins*, Hung Tzu Wen*, Albert L. Rhoton**

***Department of Neurosurgery, University of Florida, Gainesville, FL, USA;**
†Division of Otolaryngology, Albany Medical Center, Albany, NY, USA

"The anatomical structures that come in relation to the operative field are many and of great importance." **AE Halstead, 1902**

INTRODUCTION

The anterior pituitary or adenohypophysis develops from Rathke's pouch, an evagination of epithelial ectoderm of the oropharynx. The posterior pituitary or neurohypophysis derives from a downward evagination of the neuroectoderm from the floor of the third ventricle. Craniopharyngiomas originate from residual cells of the Rathke's pouch. The original cavity of Rathke's pouch remains first as a cleft, and later as scattered vesicles that can be readily identified in sagittal sections through the mature gland. The dorsal wall of Rathke's pouch remains thin and fuses with the adjoining part of the neurohypophysis as the pars intermedia. Craniopharyngiomas tend to arise from the anterior superior margin of the pituitary gland and grow into the sellar and parasellar areas involving the pituitary gland, infundibulum, hypothalamus, optic nerves and chiasm, and third ventricle (Figure 2.1). The tumor usually receives its arterial supply from perforating branches originating from the internal carotid, posterior and anterior communicating, and anterior cerebral arteries. These tumors may extend into the third ventricle or be primarily intraventricular. Surgical classifications of craniopharyngiomas are based on their location in relation to the chiasm (Hoffman, 1990), diaphragma sellae (Wang et al., 2005), third ventricle (Steno et al., 2004), or infundibulum (Kassam et al., 2008; Park et al., 2013). An understanding of the surgical anatomy of the cranial base and adjacent structures is essential to

Craniopharyngiomas
http://dx.doi.org/10.1016/B978-0-12-416706-3.00002-7

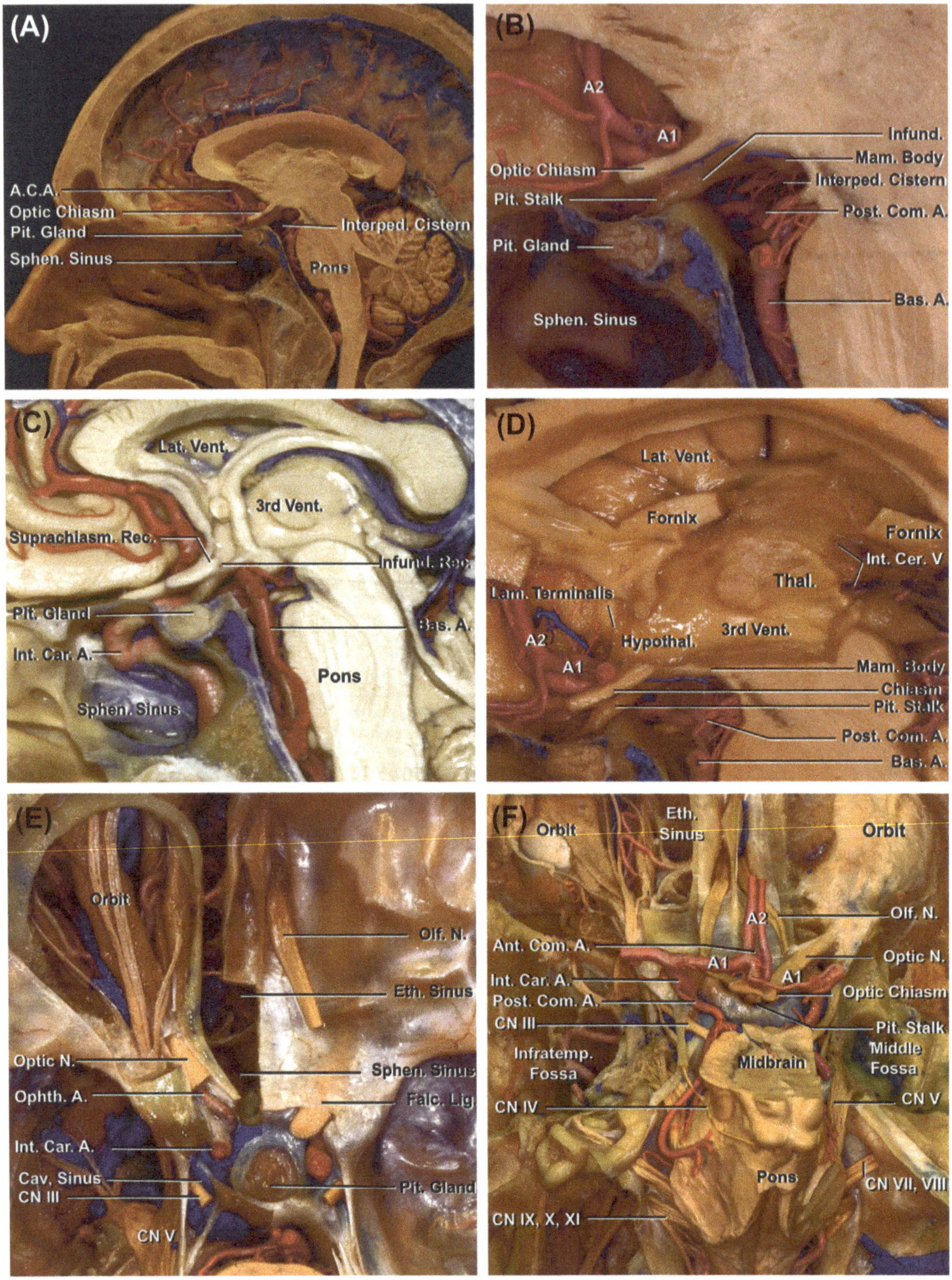
(A)
A.C.A.
Optic Chiasm
Pit. Gland
Sphen. Sinus
Interped. Cistern
Pons
(B)
A2
A1
Optic Chiasm
Pit. Stalk
Pit. Gland
Sphen. Sinus
Infund.
Mam. Body
Interped. Cistern
Post. Com. A.
Bas. A.
(C)
Lat. Vent.
3rd Vent.
Suprachiasm. Rec.
Infund. Rec.
Pit. Gland
Bas. A.
Int. Car. A.
Pons
Sphen. Sinus
(D)
Lat. Vent.
Fornix
Fornix
Int. Cer. V
Thal.
Lam. Terminalis
3rd Vent.
A2
Hypothal.
A1
Mam. Body
Chiasm
Pit. Stalk
Post. Com. A.
Bas. A.
(E)
Orbit
Olf. N.
Eth. Sinus
Optic N.
Sphen. Sinus
Ophth. A.
Falc. Lig.
Int. Car. A.
Cav. Sinus
CN III
Pit. Gland
CN V
(F)
Orbit
Eth. Sinus
Orbit
A2
Olf. N.
Ant. Com. A.
A1
Optic N.
Int. Car. A.
A1
Optic Chiasm
Post. Com. A.
CN III
Pit. Stalk
Infratemp. Fossa
Midbrain
Middle Fossa
CN IV
CN V
Pons
CN VII, VIII
CN IX, X, XI

accurately planning and completing craniotomies or expanded endoscopic endonasal approaches to craniopharyngiomas.

ANATOMY OF THE CRANIAL BASE

The cranial base has an endocranial surface, which faces the brain, and an exocranial surface, which faces the nasal cavity and sinuses, orbits, pharynx, infratemporal and pterygopalatine fossae, and the parapharyngeal and infrapetrosal spaces. The sella turcica, where the pituitary gland sits, is located in the center of the middle cranial base, and constitutes the focal point for approaches to craniopharyngiomas. Understanding the anatomy of the sphenoid sinus and its intracranial relationships is of paramount importance in completing the endoscopic endonasal approaches to craniopharyngiomas.

The Endocranial and Exocranial Surfaces

The endocranial surface of the anterior cranial base, formed by the ethmoid, sphenoid, and frontal bones, is divided into medial and lateral portions (Figures 2.2, 2.3, and 2.4). The medial part, covering the upper nasal cavity and the sphenoid sinus, is formed by the crista galli and the cribriform plate of the ethmoid bone anteriorly, and the planum of the sphenoid body posteriorly. The lateral part, which covers the orbit and the optic canal, is formed by the frontal bone and the lesser wing of the sphenoid bone, which blends medially into the anterior clinoid process. The foramen caecum in the midline serves as the site of passage of an emissary vein and the cribriform plate is pierced by the filaments of the olfactory nerve.

FIGURE 2.1 Craniopharyngiomas are tumors originating from Rathke's pouch, an evagination of ectoderm that forms the adenohypophysis. Craniopharyngiomas tend to arise in the superior aspect of the pituitary and in their growth may involve the sellar, parasellar, retrosellar, and suprasellar areas. **A,** Midsagittal view of an anatomical specimen showing the pituitary gland and its relationship to the sphenoid sinus and nasal cavity inferiorly, the optic chiasm and anterior cerebral artery superiorly, and the interpeduncular cistern posteriorly. **B,** Neurovascular relationships. The distal A1 and proximal A2 are located above the optic chiasm, the posterior communicating artery and the basilar artery are located posterior to the infundibulum in the interpeduncular cistern. **C,** Midsagittal section showing the third and lateral ventricles. Craniopharyngiomas may extend into the ventricles or be primarily intraventricular, and frequently involve the optic chiasm, and hypothalamus. **D,** Midsagittal section of the third ventricle. The septum pellucidum has been removed and the fornix has been transected posterior to the foramen of Monro to show the lateral ventricle. The hypothalamus extends from the lamina terminalis to the mamillary bodies posteriorly. The lamina terminalis is posterior to the A1 and A2 in midline and the anterior communicating artery. The mamillary bodies are superior to the posterior communicating and basilar arteries. **E,** Superior view of the anterior and middle cranial fossae, and sellar and parasellar areas. The dura mater and bone on the left side have been removed to show the relationship of the pituitary gland with the orbit and sphenoid sinus anteriorly, and cavernous sinus laterally. **F,** Posterior-superior view showing the brainstem in the posterior fossa. The pituitary stalk and infundibulum lie in the middle fossa inferior to the optic chiasm. Note the vascular relationships with the A1-A2, and anterior and posterior communicating arteries. A., artery; A.C.A., anterior cerebral artery; Bas., basilar; CN, cranial nerve; Car., carotid; Cav., cavernous; Cer., cerebral; Com., communicating; Eth., ethmoid; Falc., falciform; Hypothal., hypothalamus; Infratemp., infratemporal; Infund., infundibular; Int., internal; Interped., interpeduncular; Lat., lateral; Lig., ligament; Mam., mammillary; Olf., olfactory; Ophth., ophthalmic; Pit., pituitary; Post., posterior; Rec., recess; Sphen., sphenoid; Suprachiasm., suprachiasmatic; Thal., thalamus; V., vein; Vent., ventricle.

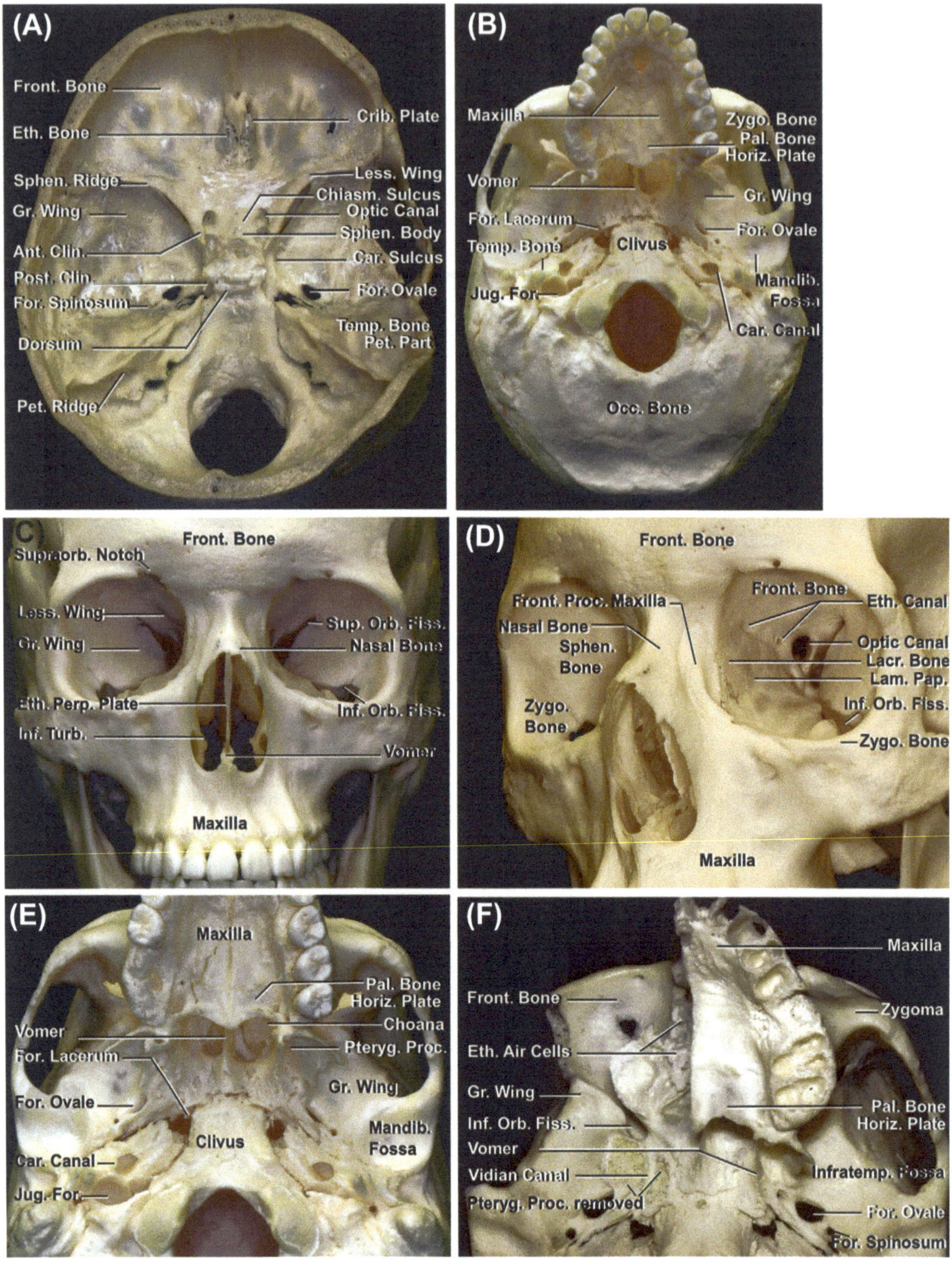
(A)
Front. Bone
Eth. Bone
Crib. Plate
Sphen. Ridge
Less. Wing
Chiasm. Sulcus
Gr. Wing
Optic Canal
Sphen. Body
Ant. Clin.
Car. Sulcus
Post. Clin.
For. Spinosum
For. Ovale
Temp. Bone Pet. Part
Dorsum
Pet. Ridge
(B)
Maxilla
Zygo. Bone
Pal. Bone Horiz. Plate
Vomer
Gr. Wing
For. Lacerum
For. Ovale
Clivus
Temp. Bone
Mandib. Fossa
Jug. For.
Car. Canal
Occ. Bone
(C)
Front. Bone
Supraorb. Notch
Less. Wing
Sup. Orb. Fiss.
Gr. Wing
Nasal Bone
Eth. Perp. Plate
Inf. Orb. Fiss.
Inf. Turb.
Vomer
Maxilla
(D)
Front. Bone
Front. Proc. Maxilla
Front. Bone
Eth. Canal
Nasal Bone
Sphen. Bone
Optic Canal
Lacr. Bone
Lam. Pap.
Zygo. Bone
Inf. Orb. Fiss.
Zygo. Bone
Maxilla
(E)
Maxilla
Pal. Bone Horiz. Plate
Choana
Vomer
For. Lacerum
Pteryg. Proc.
Gr. Wing
For. Ovale
Mandib. Fossa
Clivus
Car. Canal
Jug. For.
(F)
Maxilla
Front. Bone
Zygoma
Eth. Air Cells
Gr. Wing
Pal. Bone Horiz. Plate
Inf. Orb. Fiss.
Vomer
Vidian Canal
Infratemp. Fossa
Pteryg. Proc. removed
For. Ovale
For. Spinosum

The optic canal transmits the optic nerve and the ophthalmic artery. The anterior cranial base faces the frontal lobes with the gyri recti medially and the orbital gyri laterally, along with the branches of the anterior cerebral arteries medially and middle cerebral arteries laterally. On the exocranial side, the anterior cranial base is divided into a medial part related to the frontal, ethmoid, and the sphenoid sinuses with the nasal cavity below and a lateral part that corresponds to the orbit and maxilla (Figures 2.2–2.4) (Rhoton, 2002).

The endocranial surface of the middle cranial base, formed by the sphenoid and temporal bones, has medial and lateral parts (Figures 2.3 and 2.5). The medial part is formed by the body of the sphenoid bone, the site of the tuberculum sellae, pituitary fossa, middle and posterior clinoid processes, carotid sulcus, and the dorsum sellae (Figures 2.3 and 2.6).

FIGURE 2.2 **Osseous structure of the anterior and middle cranial base. A,** The anterior fossa is separated from the middle fossa by the sphenoid ridge and the chiasmatic sulcus. The middle cranial fossa is separated from the posterior cranial fossa by the dorsum sellae and the petrous ridges. The upper surface of the anterior cranial base is formed by the frontal bones which roof the orbits, the ethmoid bone which is interposed between the frontal bones and is the site of the cribriform plate, and the lesser wings and anterior part of the body of the sphenoid which form the posterior part of the floor of the anterior fossa. The upper surface of the middle cranial base floor is formed by the greater sphenoid wing and posterior two-thirds of the sphenoid body anteriorly and the upper surface of the temporal bone posteriorly. The posterior part of the cranial base is formed by the posterior aspect of the sphenoid body and the temporal and occipital bones. The cribriform plate, sella, and clivus are located in the medial part of the cranial base. The lateral part of the cranial base is located above the orbits, pterygopalatine and infratemporal fossae, and the subtemporal and lateral part of the suboccipital areas. **B,** Exocranial surface of the cranial base. This surface is more complicated than the endocranial surface. It is not demarcated into three well-defined fossae as is the endocranial surface. The exocranial surface is formed by the maxilla, zygomatic, palatine, sphenoid, temporal, and occipital bones, and the vomer. The maxilla, orbits, and nasal cavity are located below the anterior fossa. The anterior part of the hard palate is formed by the maxilla and the posterior part is formed by the palatine bone. The anterior part of the zygomatic arch is formed by the zygomatic bone and the posterior part by the squamosal part of the temporal bone. The mandibular fossa on the lower surface of the temporal squama is located below the posterior part of the middle fossa. The vomer attaches to the lower part of the body of the sphenoid and the perpendicular plate of the ethmoid to form the posterior part of the nasal septum. **C** and **D,** Anterior and anterolateral views of the skull. The orbital rim is formed by the frontal bone, zygoma, and maxilla. The roof of the orbit is formed by the frontal and sphenoid bones, the lateral wall by the greater sphenoid wing and the zygomatic bone, the floor by the maxilla, except for a small part of the posterior floor formed by the palatine bone, and the medial wall of the orbit by the maxilla, and lacrimal and ethmoid bones. The nasal bone is interposed above the anterior nasal aperture between the maxillae. The nasal cavity is located between the ethmoid bones above and the maxillae and palatine bones, and the sphenoid pterygoid process below. It is roofed by the frontal and ethmoid bones, and the floor is formed by the maxillae and palatal bones. The osseous nasal septum is formed by the perpendicular ethmoid plate and the vomer. The inferior turbinate is a separate bone, and the middle and superior turbinates are appendages of the ethmoid bone. The orbit opens through the superior orbital fissure into the middle fossa and through the inferior orbital fissure into the pterygopalatine and infratemporal fossae. **E,** Inferior view of the maxillae and palatine bones forming the floor of the nasal cavity. The nasal cavity opens onto the nasopharynx through two apertures called choanae, formed laterally by the pterygoid processes. **F,** The right half of the maxilla and zygomatic arch have been removed. The inferior orbital fissure is located between the greater sphenoid wing and the maxilla. The right orbital roof and ethmoid air cells have been preserved. The right pterygoid process has been removed at its junction with the sphenoid body. The roof of the vidian canal, which extends through the base of the pterygoid process, has been preserved. Ant., anterior; Car., carotid; Chiasm., chiasmatic; Clin., clinoid; Crib., cribriform; Eth., ethmoid; Fiss., fissure; For., foramen; Front., frontal; Gr., greater; Horiz., horizontal; Inf., inferior; Infratemp., infratemporal; Jug., jugular; Less., lesser; Mandib., mandibular; Occip., occipital; Orb., orbital; Pal., palatine; Perp., perpendicular; Pet., petrous; Post., posterior; Proc., process; Pteryg., pterygoid; Sphen., sphenoid; Sup., superior; Supraorb., supraorbital; Temp., temporal; Turb., turbinate.; Zygo., zygomatic.

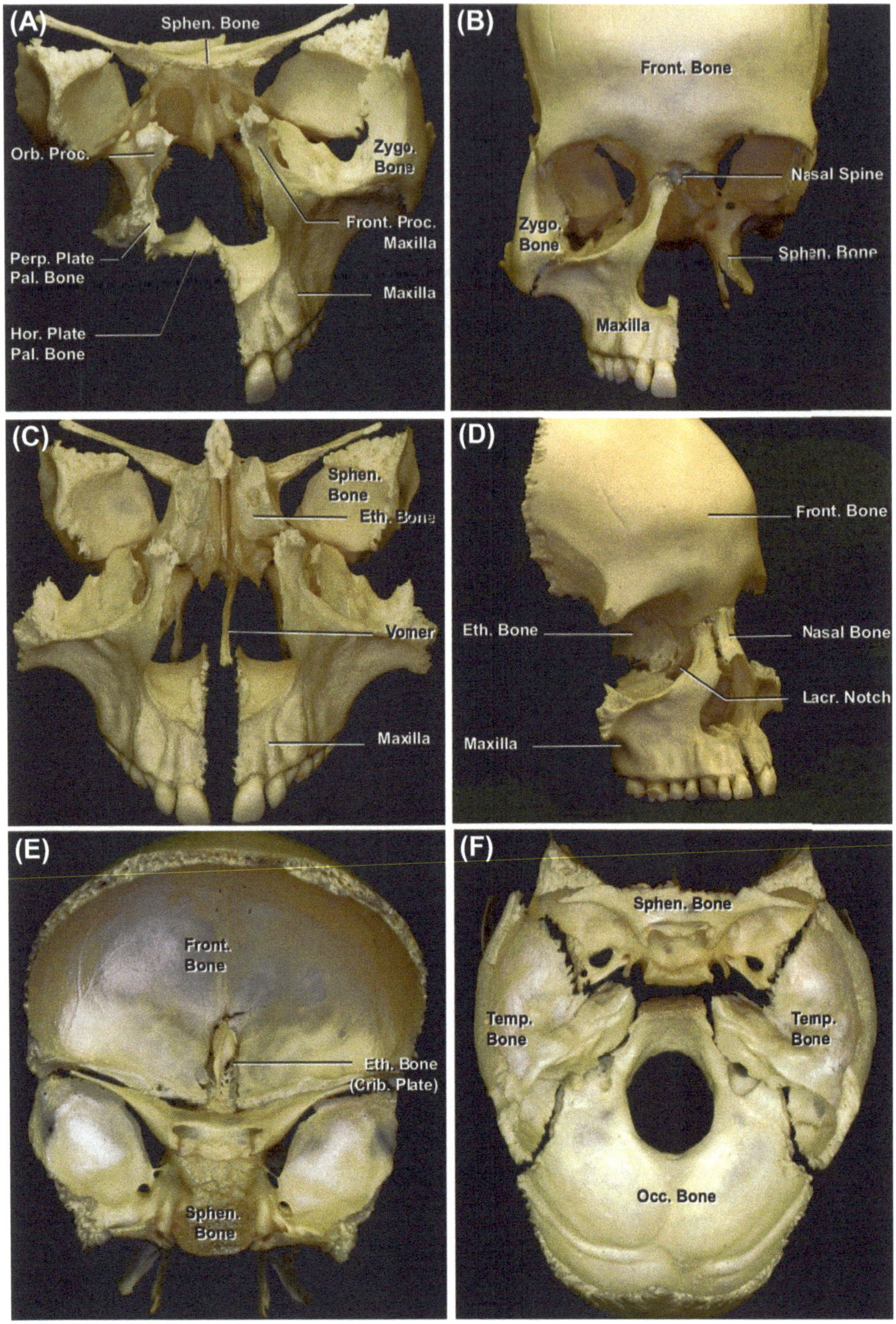
(A)
Sphen. Bone
Orb. Proc.
Zygo. Bone
Front. Proc. Maxilla
Perp. Plate Pal. Bone
Maxilla
Hor. Plate Pal. Bone
(B)
Front. Bone
Nasal Spine
Zygo. Bone
Sphen. Bone
Maxilla
(C)
Sphen. Bone
Eth. Bone
Vomer
Maxilla
(D)
Front. Bone
Eth. Bone
Nasal Bone
Lacr. Notch
Maxilla
(E)
Front. Bone
Eth. Bone (Crib. Plate)
Sphen. Bone
(F)
Sphen. Bone
Temp. Bone
Temp. Bone
Occ. Bone

The lateral part is formed by the lesser and greater sphenoid wings, with the superior orbital fissure between them. The lesser wing is connected to the body of the sphenoid bone by an anterior root, which forms the roof of the optic canal, and a posterior root, also called the optic strut, which forms the floor of the optic canal and separates the optic canal from the superior orbital fissure (Figure 2.6). The greater wing forms the largest part of the endocranial surface of the middle fossa, with the squamosal and the petrosal parts of the temporal bone completing this surface. The superior orbital fissure transmits the oculomotor, trochlear, ophthalmic, and abducens nerves, a recurrent meningeal artery, and the superior and inferior ophthalmic veins. The maxillary and mandibular nerves pass through the foramen rotundum and ovale, respectively, both located in the greater wing of the sphenoid. The not infrequently occurring sphenoidal emissary foramen, located anteromedial to the foramen spinosum, gives passage to a vein connecting the cavernous sinus and the pterygoid venous plexus. The upper surface of the petrous bone is grooved along the course of the greater and lesser petrosal nerves (Figure 2.5) (Rhoton, 2000). The carotid canal extends upward and medially and provides passage to the internal carotid artery and carotid sympathetic nerves in their course to the cavernous sinus. The posterior trigeminal root reaches an impression on the upper surface of the petrous bone, where Meckel's cave and the semilunar ganglion sit. The carotid canal opens below the trigeminal ganglion near the distal end of the carotid canal, where the carotid artery becomes intracavernous (Figure 2.5). The arcuate eminence approximates the position of the superior semicircular canal.

The lateral portion of the middle cranial base is formed by the endocranial surface of the greater wing of the sphenoidal bone and upper surface of the temporal bone. The basal surface of the temporal lobe rests against the endocranial surface of the middle cranial fossa. The medial portion contains the sellar and the parasellar regions, where the pituitary gland and cavernous sinus are located (Figure 2.1E) (Rhoton, 2002). The basal temporal lobe, formed by the parahippocampal, occipitotemporal, and inferior temporal gyri, and uncus, is supplied by branches of the internal carotid, anterior choroidal, and posterior and middle cerebral arteries. The cavernous sinus is situated between an outer or meningeal layer of dura facing the brain, and an inner or periosteal layer attached to the bone of the middle fossa (Rhoton, 2002). The inner layer splits into two parts when it reaches the cavernous sinus. One layer invests the nerves and forms the inner layer of the lateral wall, and the medial layer faces the body of the sphenoid bone and forms the medial wall of the sinus.

FIGURE 2.3 **Osseous structure of the nasal cavity and skull base. A,** Anterior view of the left maxilla, right palatine, and sphenoid bones. The hard palate, the floor of the nasal cavity, is formed by the palatine process of the maxilla anteriorly and horizontal plate of the palatine bone posteriorly. **B,** The frontal bone articulates anteriorly with the frontal process of the maxilla and its nasal spine forms part of the roof of the nasal cavity. **C,** The ethmoid bone articulates posteriorly with the body of the sphenoid to form part of the medial orbital wall, septum, and roof of the nose. **D,** The roof of the nasal cavity is formed by the nasal bones, nasal spine of the frontal bone, cribriform plate of the ethmoid, and sphenoid (not shown in this picture). **E,** Posterior view of the frontal, ethmoid, and sphenoid bones forming the intracranial surface of the anterior cranial base. The frontal bone forms the roof of the ethmoid cells. **F,** The middle fossa is formed by the sphenoid and temporal bones. The posterior fossa is formed by the temporal and occipital bones. Crib., cribriform; Eth., ethmoid; Front., frontal; Horiz., horizontal; Lacr., lacrimal; Orb., orbital; Pal., palatine; Perp., perpendicular; Proc., process; Sphen., sphenoid; Sup., superior; Zygo., zygomatic.

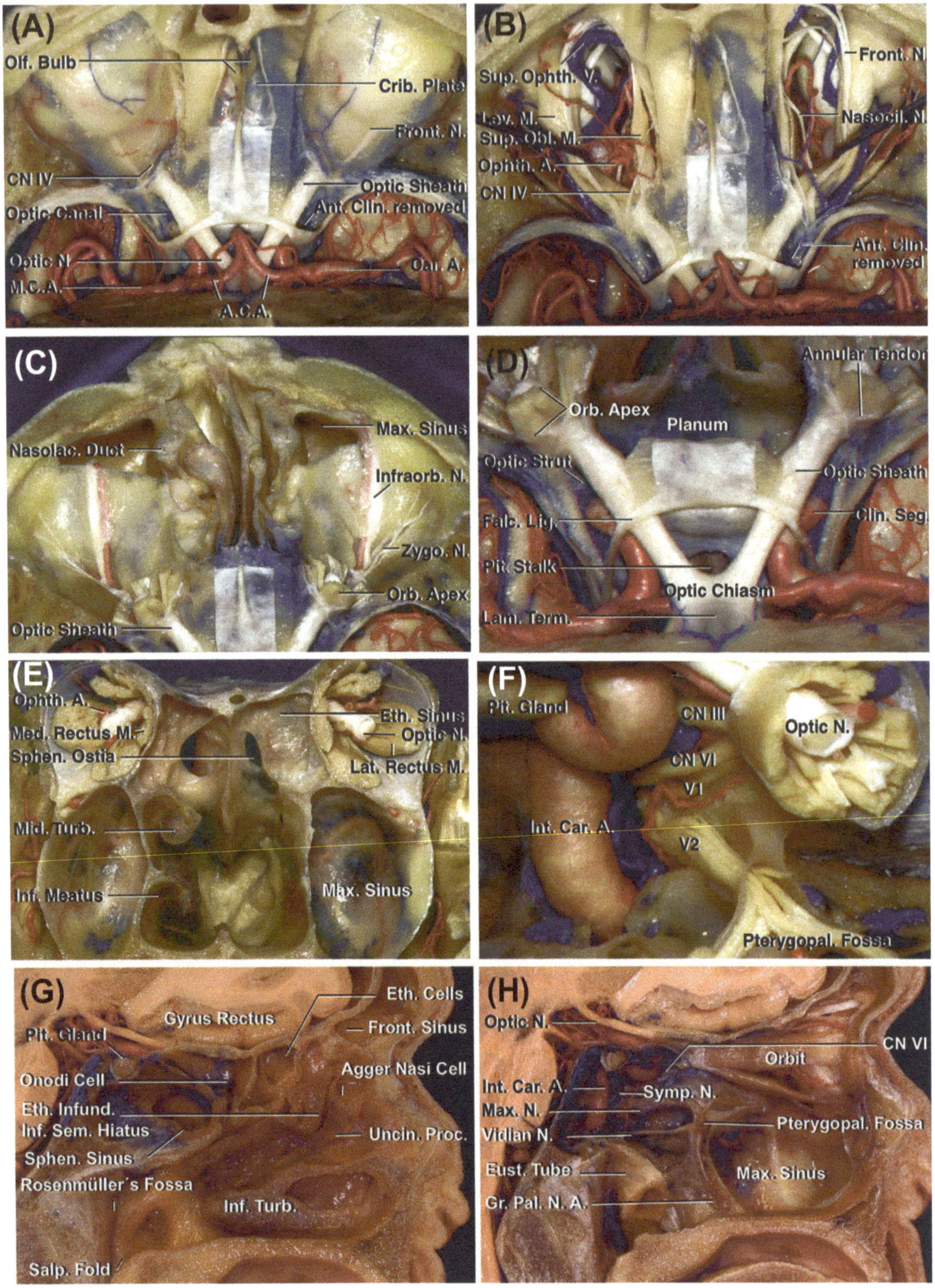

(A)
Olf. Bulb
Crib. Plate
Front. N.
CN IV
Optic Sheath
Optic Canal
Ant. Clin. removed
Optic N.
Car. A.
M.C.A.
A.C.A.
(B)
Front. N.
Sup. Ophth. V.
Lev. M.
Nasocil. N.
Sup. Obl. M.
Ophth. A.
CN IV
Ant. Clin. removed
(C)
Max. Sinus
Nasolac. Duct
Infraorb. N.
Zygo. N.
Orb. Apex
Optic Sheath
(D)
Annular Tendon
Orb. Apex
Planum
Optic Strut
Optic Sheath
Falc. Lig.
Clin. Seg.
Pit. Stalk
Optic Chiasm
Lam. Term.
(E)
Ophth. A.
Eth. Sinus
Med. Rectus M.
Optic N.
Sphen. Ostia
Lat. Rectus M.
Mid. Turb.
Inf. Meatus
Max. Sinus
(F)
Pit. Gland
CN III
Optic N.
CN VI
V1
Int. Car. A.
V2
Pterygopal. Fossa
(G)
Eth. Cells
Gyrus Rectus
Front. Sinus
Pit. Gland
Agger Nasi Cell
Onodi Cell
Eth. Infund.
Inf. Sem. Hiatus
Uncin. Proc.
Sphen. Sinus
Rosenmüller's Fossa
Inf. Turb.
Salp. Fold
(H)
Optic N.
CN VI
Orbit
Int. Car. A.
Symp. N.
Max. N.
Pterygopal. Fossa
Vidian N.
Eust. Tube
Max. Sinus
Gr. Pal. N. A.

The same inner layer invests the oculomotor, trochlear, and ophthalmic nerves, and the distal part of the abducens nerve in their course through the lateral wall of the cavernous sinus. The internal carotid artery with its posterior bend, horizontal segment, anterior bend, and clinoidal segments courses inside the cavernous sinus. The clinoidal segment of the internal carotid artery, located between the distal and proximal dural rings, is covered by a layer of dura, which forms a collar (the carotid collar) around the artery. In a previous study we found that the venous plexus, forming the cavernous sinus, extends through the lower ring inside the carotid collar and around the clinoid segment to the level of the upper ring. The meningohypophyseal trunk, with its tentorial, inferior hypophyseal, and dorsal meningeal branches, and the inferolateral trunk, also called the artery of the inferior cavernous sinus, arise from the intracavernous carotid artery. The proximal abducens nerve passes through Dorello's canal, located below the petrosphenoid ligament, and receives sympathetic branches from the internal carotid nerve that pass to the ophthalmic nerve to enter the orbit (Rhoton, 1996). The sella houses the pituitary gland and is partially closed above by the diaphragma sellae. Anterolateral to the diaphragm, the carotid cave, a

FIGURE 2.4 **Relationships of the anterior cranial base. A,** Both orbits have been unroofed to expose the periorbita. The optic canals have been unroofed and the anterior clinoids removed to expose the optic nerves, which are enclosed in the optic sheath within the optic canal. The frontal and trochlear nerves can be seen through the periorbita. The roof of the ethmoid sinuses and the olfactory bulbs sitting on the cribriform plate have been preserved. The anterior cerebral arteries course above the optic chiasm. **B,** The intraorbital fat has been removed and the levator and superior rectus muscles have been retracted laterally to expose both globes, ophthalmic arteries, superior ophthalmic veins, and nasociliary nerves. **C,** The orbital contents have been removed to expose the lateral wall and floor of the orbit. The maxillary sinuses are exposed below the orbital floors. The maxillary nerves give rise to both the infraorbital nerve, which courses along the floor of the orbit to reach the cheek, and the zygomatic nerve, which courses along the lateral wall of the orbit to reach the malar eminence and temple. **D,** Enlarged view. The optic nerves are enclosed within the optic sheath as they course through the optic canal. The annular tendon, from which the rectus muscles arise, surrounds the optic nerve and medial portion of the superior orbital fissure. Removal of the anterior clinoid exposes the clinoid segment of the carotid artery. The optic strut, which separates the optic canal and superior orbital fissure, has also been removed. The segment of anterior cerebral arteries passing above the chiasm has been removed to expose the lamina terminalis. The falciform dural fold extends across the optic nerve at the entrance into the optic canal. **E,** Anterior view of a coronal section anterior to the sphenoid sinus, through the nasal cavity, orbits, and maxillary sinuses. The upper part of the nasal cavity is separated from the orbits by the ethmoidal sinuses. The lower part of the nasal cavity is bounded laterally by the maxillary sinuses. The middle turbinate projects medially from the lateral nasal wall at the junction of the roof of the maxillary and ethmoidal sinuses. The posterior ethmoid air cells are located in front of the lateral part of the sphenoid sinus. **F,** The lateral wall of the sphenoid and ethmoid sinuses, and the posterior wall of the maxillary sinus have been removed to expose the orbital apex, pterygopalatine fossa, and the internal carotid artery and nerves coursing through the cavernous sinus. Note the relationship of CNs III, VI, V1, and V2 lateral to the internal carotid artery in the cavernous sinus. The maxillary nerve exits the foramen rotundum to enter the pterygopalatine fossa where it gives rise to the infraorbital and greater palatine nerves and communicating rami to the pterygopalatine ganglion. **G** and **H,** Specimen divided in the midsagittal plane to show the paranasal sinuses. Note the relationships of the frontal, ethmoid and sphenoid sinuses with the gyrus rectus and the posterior extension of the posterior-superior ethmoid (Onodi) cell into the upper part of the sphenoid sinuses. **H,** Further lateral dissection exposes the carotid artery in the cavernous sinus, and the orbit and maxillary sinus. A., artery; A.C.A., anterior cerebral artery; Ant., anterior; CN, cranial nerve; Car., carotid; Clin., clinoid; Crib., cribriform; Eth., ethmoid; Front., frontal; Inf., inferior; Infraorb., infraorbital; Infundib., infundibulum; Int., internal; Lev., levator; M., muscle; M.C.A., middle cerebral artery; Max., maxillary; Med., medial; N., nerve; Nasocil., nasociliary; Nasolac., nasolacrimal; Obl., oblique; Olf., olfactory; Ophth., ophthalmic; Orb., orbital; Pit., pituitary; Pterygopal., pterygopalatine; Proc., process; Salp., salpingopharyngeal; Sem., semilunar; Sup., superior; Symp., sympathetic; Uncin., uncinate; V., vein; Zygo., zygomatic.

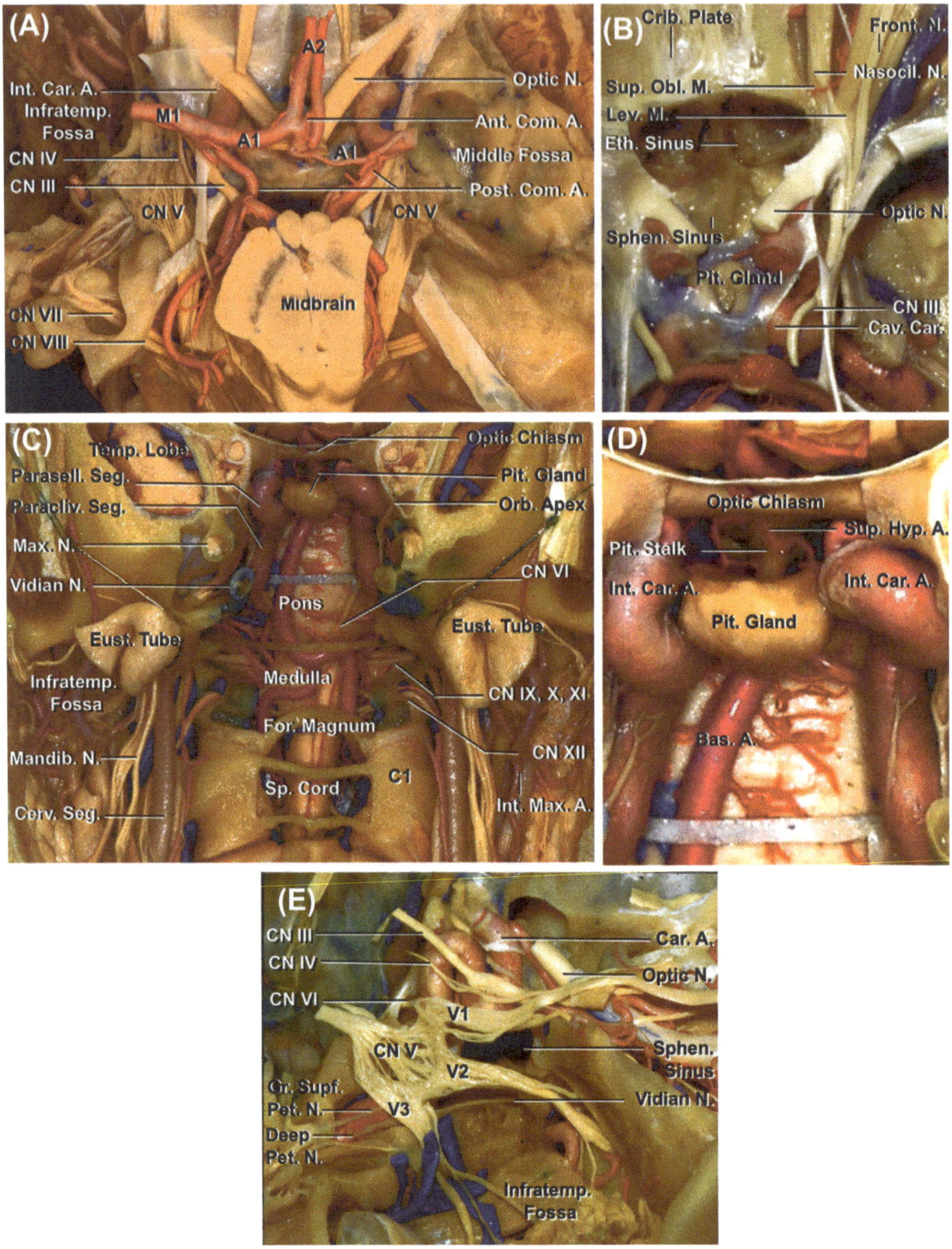

FIGURE 2.5 Relationships of the middle cranial base. Craniopharyngiomas are typically located in the medial part of the middle cranial base. **A,** Endocranial view of the middle cranial base showing the neurovascular elements of the medial and lateral parts. The left middle fossa has been drilled to expose the infratemporal fossa. The anterior cerebral arteries course above the optic nerves and chiasm. **B,** Endocranial view of the sellar and parasellar areas. The cavernous sinus has been dissected on the right side to expose the cavernous carotid lateral to the pituitary gland. The optic canal and sphenoid sinus have been unroofed, and the anterior clinoid removed. **C,** Coronal section to show

the pituitary gland, and parasellar and paraclival segments of the carotid artery. The clivus has been completely removed to expose the brainstem. The temporal lobe is located in the middle fossa, lateral to the pituitary gland and superior to the infratemporal fossa. **D,** Enlarged view of the pituitary gland, with the optic chiasm superiorly, and carotid arteries laterally. The superior hypophyseal arteries supply the pituitary stalk and optic chiasm. **E,** Lateral view of the right cavernous sinus and the infratemporal fossa. CNs III, IV, and V1 are located in the lateral wall of the cavernous sinus, whereas CN VI runs inside the sinus. **F,** Superior endocranial view of middle cranial base. The floor of the middle fossa has been preserved. The anterior part of the floor of the middle fossa is formed by the greater sphenoid wing, which roofs the infratemporal fossa, and the posterior part of the floor is formed by the upper surface of the temporal bone. The internal acoustic meatus, mastoid antrum, and tympanic cavities have been unroofed. The dural roof and lateral wall of the cavernous sinus have been removed. The petrous segment of the internal carotid artery is exposed lateral to the trigeminal nerve. The temporalis muscle is exposed in the temporal fossa lateral to the greater sphenoid wing. **G,** The floor of the middle fossa has been removed to show the relationships below the floor. The temporalis muscle descends medial to the zygomatic arch in the temporal fossa to insert on the coronoid process of the mandible. The infratemporal fossa is located medial to the temporal fossa, below the greater sphenoid wing, and contains the pterygoid muscles and venous plexus and branches of the mandibular nerve and maxillary artery. The mandibular condyle is located below the posterior part of the middle fossa floor, which is formed by the temporal bone. **H,** Enlarged view of the posterior part of the area below the middle fossa floor. The roof of the temporal bone, which forms the posterior part of the floor of the middle fossa, has been opened to expose the mastoid antrum, eustachian tube, semicircular canals, cochlea, nerves in the internal acoustic meatus, and the mandibular condyle. **I,** The trigeminal nerve has been reflected forward. The abducens nerve passes below the petrosphenoid ligament and through Dorello's canal. The petrous segment of the carotid passes below the petrolingual ligament to enter the cavernous sinus. The greater petrosal nerve is joined by the deep petrosal branch of the carotid sympathetic plexus to form the vidian nerve, which passes forward in the vidian canal that has been unroofed. The lesser petrosal nerve arises from the tympanic branch of the glossopharyngeal nerve, which ascends on the promontory in the tympanic nerve plexus and regroups to cross the floor of the middle fossa, exiting the cranium to provide parasympathetic innervation through the otic ganglion to the parotid gland. The tensor tympani muscle and eustachian tube are layered, with the former above the latter, along and separated from the anterior surface of the petrous carotid by a thin layer of bone. **J,** Inferior view of axial section of a cranium at the level of the maxillary sinus. The pterygopalatine fossa is located between the posterior wall of the maxillary sinus and the pterygoid process. The roof of the maxillary sinus forms the floor of the orbit. The infratemporal fossa is located below the greater wing of the sphenoid and opens medially into the pterygopalatine fossa. The medial wall of the pterygopalatine fossa is formed by the perpendicular plate of the palatine bone, which has an opening, the sphenopalatine foramen, through which branches of the maxillary artery and nerve reach the nasal cavity. The ethmoid air cells are located medial to the orbit. **K,** Inferior views of an axial section of the cranial base. The infratemporal fossa is surrounded by the maxillary sinus anteriorly, the mandible laterally, the pterygoid process anteromedially, and the parapharyngeal space posteromedially. It contains the mandibular nerve and maxillary artery and their branches, the medial and lateral pterygoid muscles, and the pterygoid venous plexus. The posterior nasopharyngeal wall is separated from the lower clivus by the longus capitis, and the nasopharyngeal roof rests against the upper clivus and floor of the sphenoid sinus. **L,** Enlarged view with highlighting of the pre- (red) and poststyloid (yellow) compartments of the parapharyngeal space. The styloid diaphragm, formed by the anterior part of the carotid sheath, separates the parapharyngeal space into pre- and poststyloid parts. The prestyloid compartment, a narrow fat-containing space between the medial pterygoid and tensor veli palatini muscle, separates the infratemporal fossa from the medially located lateral nasopharyngeal region containing the tensor and levator veli palatini and the eustachian tube. The poststyloid compartment contains the internal carotid artery, internal jugular vein, and CNs IX through XII. **M,** The right carotid canal has been drilled to show the petrous segment of the internal carotid artery, and the right half of the clivus has been drilled to show the sphenoid sinus and sella. A., artery; Ac., acoustic; CN, cranial nerve; Cap., capitis; Car., carotid; Cav., cavernous; Cond., condyle; Crib., cribriform; Eth., ethmoid; Eust., eustachian; Ext., external; Fiss., fissure; For., foramen; Gang., ganglion; Gl., gland; Gr., greater; Inf., inferior; Infraorb., infraorbital; Infratemp., infratemporal; Int., internal; Jug., jugular; Lat., lateral, lateralis; Less., lesser; Lev., levator; Lig., ligament; Long., longus; M., muscle; Max., maxillary; Mid., middle; N., nerve; Nasolac., nasolacrimal; Orb., orbital; Pal., palatini; Palat., palatine; Perp., perpendicular; Pet., petrosal, petrous; Petroling., petrolingual; Petrosphen., petrosphenoid; Plex., plexus; Post., posterior; Proc., process; Pteryg., pterygoid; Pterygopal., pterygopalatine; Rec., rectus; Seg., segment; Semicirc., semicircular; Sig., sigmoid; Sphen., sphenoid; Sulc., sulcus; Temp., temporalis; Tens., tensor; Tymp., tympani; V., vein; Vel., veli; Zygo., zygomatic.

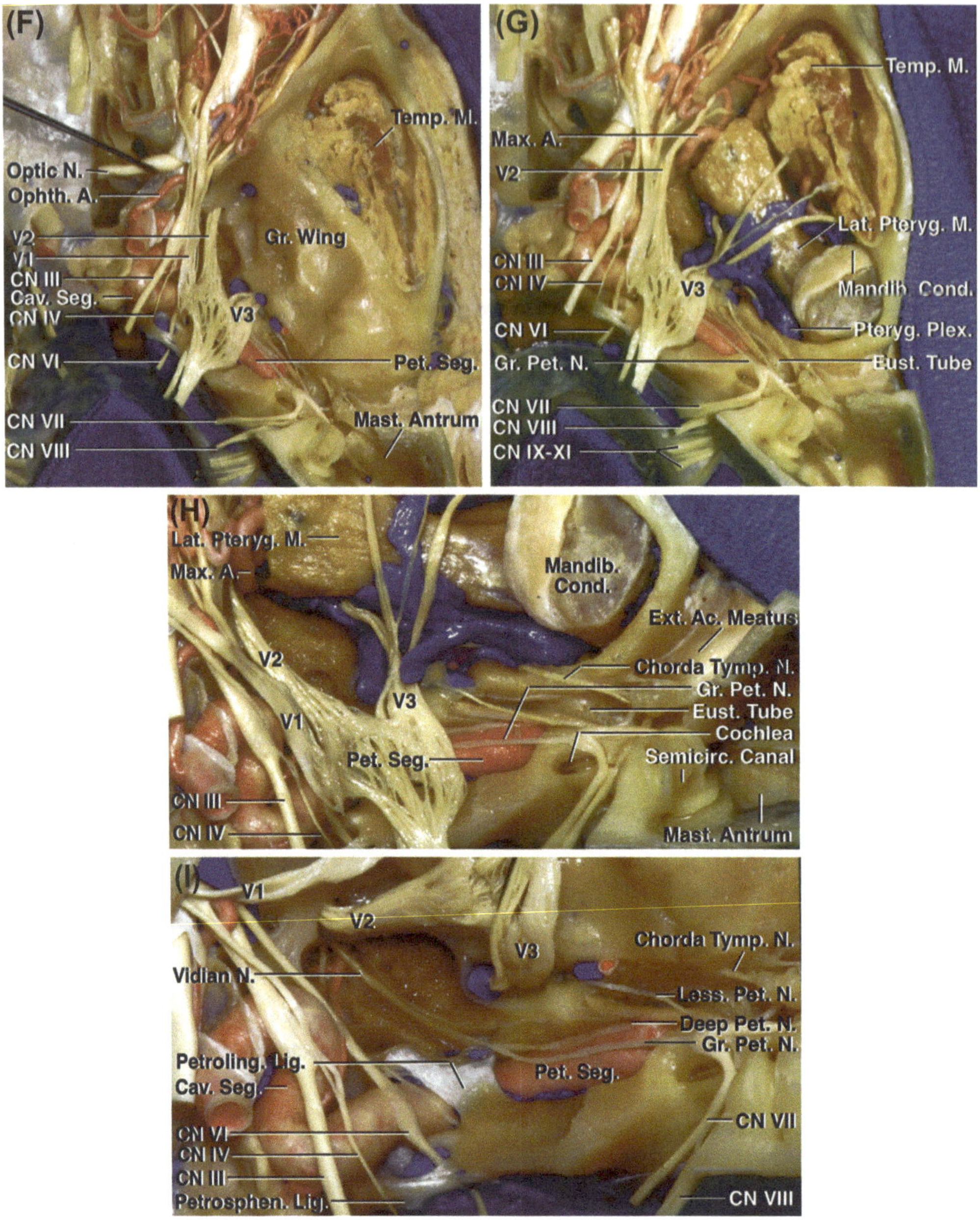

FIGURE 2.5 cont'd

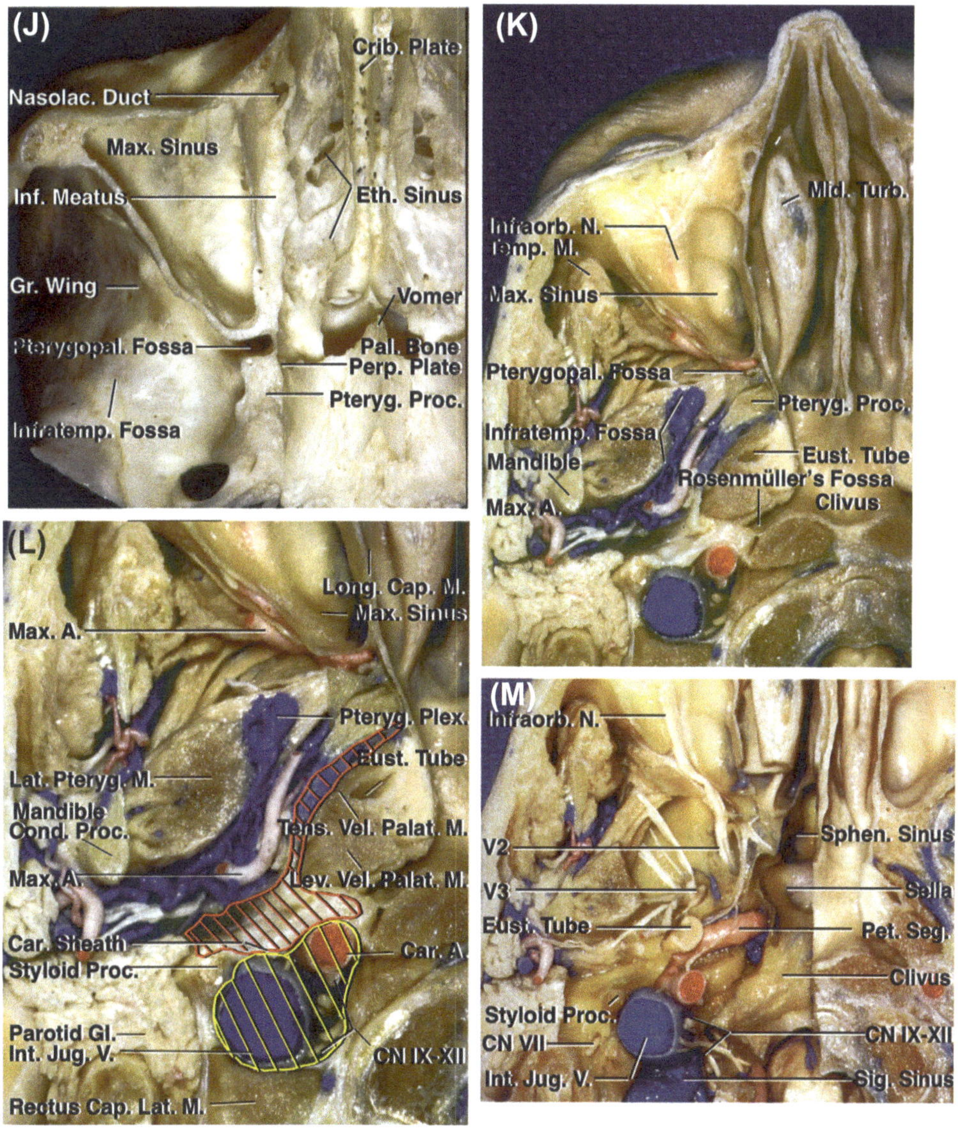

FIGURE 2.5 cont'd

dural depression at the level of the distal dural ring, extends downward medial to the initial intradural segment of the internal carotid artery.

The main venous afferents to the cavernous sinus are the superior and inferior ophthalmic veins and the sphenoparietal sinus. Several venous compartments, named according to their relationship to the cavernous carotid artery, empty mainly in the basilar, and superior and inferior petrosal sinuses, or, by way of the foramina in the middle fossa floor, into the pterygoid venous plexus.

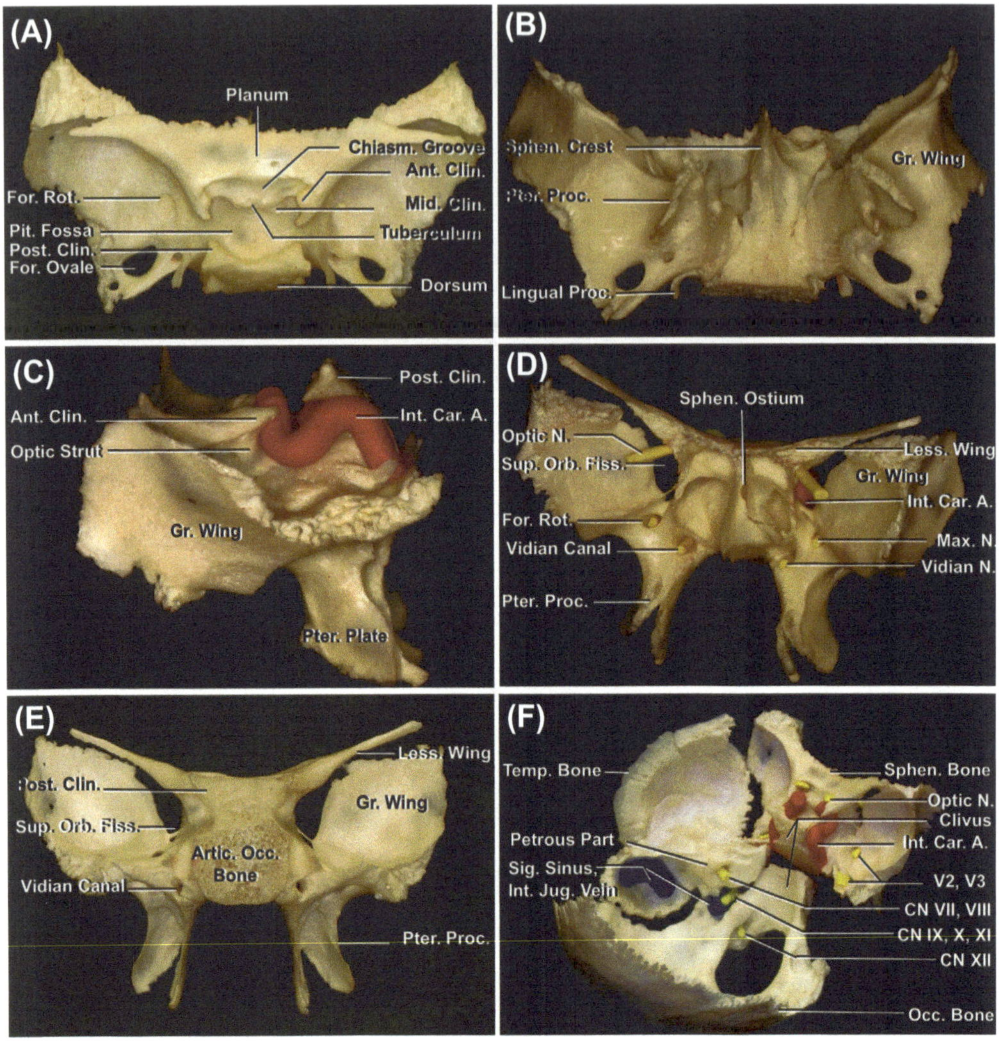

FIGURE 2.6 **Sphenoid bone and its relationships. A,** Superior view. The pituitary fossa is located in the upper aspect of the sphenoid body. The anterior boundary of the pituitary fossa is the tuberculum and the posterior boundary is the dorsum and posterior clinoids. The chiasmatic groove is located between the planum and the pituitary fossa. **B,** Inferior view. The greater wing forms part of the middle fossa floor. **C,** Lateral view. The internal carotid artery courses along the carotid sulcus. **D,** Anterior view of the sphenoid bone. The optic nerve passes through the optic canal, the maxillary nerve through the foramen rotundum, and the vidian nerve through the vidian canal. **E,** Posterior view of the sphenoid and the articulation with the occipital bone. **F,** The sphenoid bone articulates posteriorly with the occipital and temporal bones. The clivus is formed by the sphenoid body superiorly and the clival part of the occipital bone inferiorly. A., artery; Ant., anterior; Artic., articulation; CN, cranial nerve; Car., carotid; Chiasm., chiasmatic; Clin., clinoid; Fiss., fissure; For., foramen; Int., internal; Jug., jugular; Mand., mandibular; Max., maxillary; Mid., middle; N., nerve; Post., posterior; Proc., process; Pter., pterygoid; Rot., rotundum; Sig., sigmoid; Sphen., sphenoid.

The exocranial surface of the middle cranial base is also divided into medial and lateral parts (Figures 2.2, 2.5, and 2.6F) (Rhoton, 2002). The medial part encompasses the sphenoid body and sinus and the upper part of the basal (clival) part of the occipital bone, positioned above the nasopharynx. The lateral part is formed by the greater sphenoid wing, the petrous, tympanic, styloid, and squamous parts of the temporal bone, and the zygomatic, palatine, and maxillary bones. The medial and lateral parts are separated at a parasagittal plane passing through the medial pterygoid plate (Rhoton, 2002).

The posterior cranial base corresponds to the floor of the posterior fossa and the area around the foramen magnum (Rhoton, 2000). It is formed by the sphenoid, temporal, and occipital bones (Figures 2.2, 2.3, and 2.6F). Medially, it is formed by the dorsum sellae, basilar (clival) portion of the occipital bone, and the foramen magnum. Laterally, the endocranial surface is formed by the temporal and the occipital bones, with the petro-occipital fissure and the jugular foramen lying between the occipital and temporal bones.

The Recesses in the Sphenoid Sinus and Their Intracranial Relationships

The neurovascular relationships of the sphenoid bone are among the most complex of any bone, and the intracranial relationships of the recesses of the sphenoid sinus are key to planning and completing endoscopic endonasal approaches (Figures 2.6 and 2.7). The sphenoid sinus is located at the center of the endonasal approaches to the sellar and parasellar areas.

The sphenoid sinus separates the paired cavernous sinuses, cavernous segments of the internal carotid arteries, and the optic, extraocular, and trigeminal nerves. The anterior wall of the sinus faces the nasal cavity. The posterior wall is formed by the part of the clivus between the dorsum sellae and the basilar part of the occipital bone. The lateral wall of the sphenoid sinus borders the medial wall of the cavernous sinus and can extend laterally beyond the line connecting the vidian canal and foramen rotundum. The superior wall of the sphenoid sinus is formed by the planum and the sellar floor, whereas the inferior wall of the sphenoid sinus faces the nasopharynx.

The sphenoid sinus opens through the sphenoid ostia into the nasal cavity. The anterior wall of the sphenoid sinus is convex anteriorly with the paired ostia medial and superior. The posterior part of the ethmoid bone, containing the posterior ethmoid cells, articulates with the anterior sphenoid face lateral to the ostia. The recess formed at this articulation between the body of the sphenoid and the posterior aspect of the ethmoid bone is called the sphenoethmoidal recess. Occasionally, and of importance in surgery, the most posterior ethmoid cell may extend into the sphenoid sinus and is called an Onodi cell (Figure 2.4G). It is important to identify an Onodi cell because the optic canal may cross it, and if unrecognized during surgery may result in optic nerve injury (Snyderman et al., 2009). The relationships of the superior wall of the sphenoid sinus are very complex. The superior wall of the sphenoid sinus is formed by the planum and the sellar wall. The sellar wall covers the sellar and parasellar areas, including the surface between the superior limit of the optic prominences and the sellar floor (Figures 2.5 and 2.7). There are different patterns of pneumatization of the sphenoid sinus of importance in surgery that can be divided into three major types in the adult: conchal (the inferior part of the sella is solid bone, 1–5%), presellar

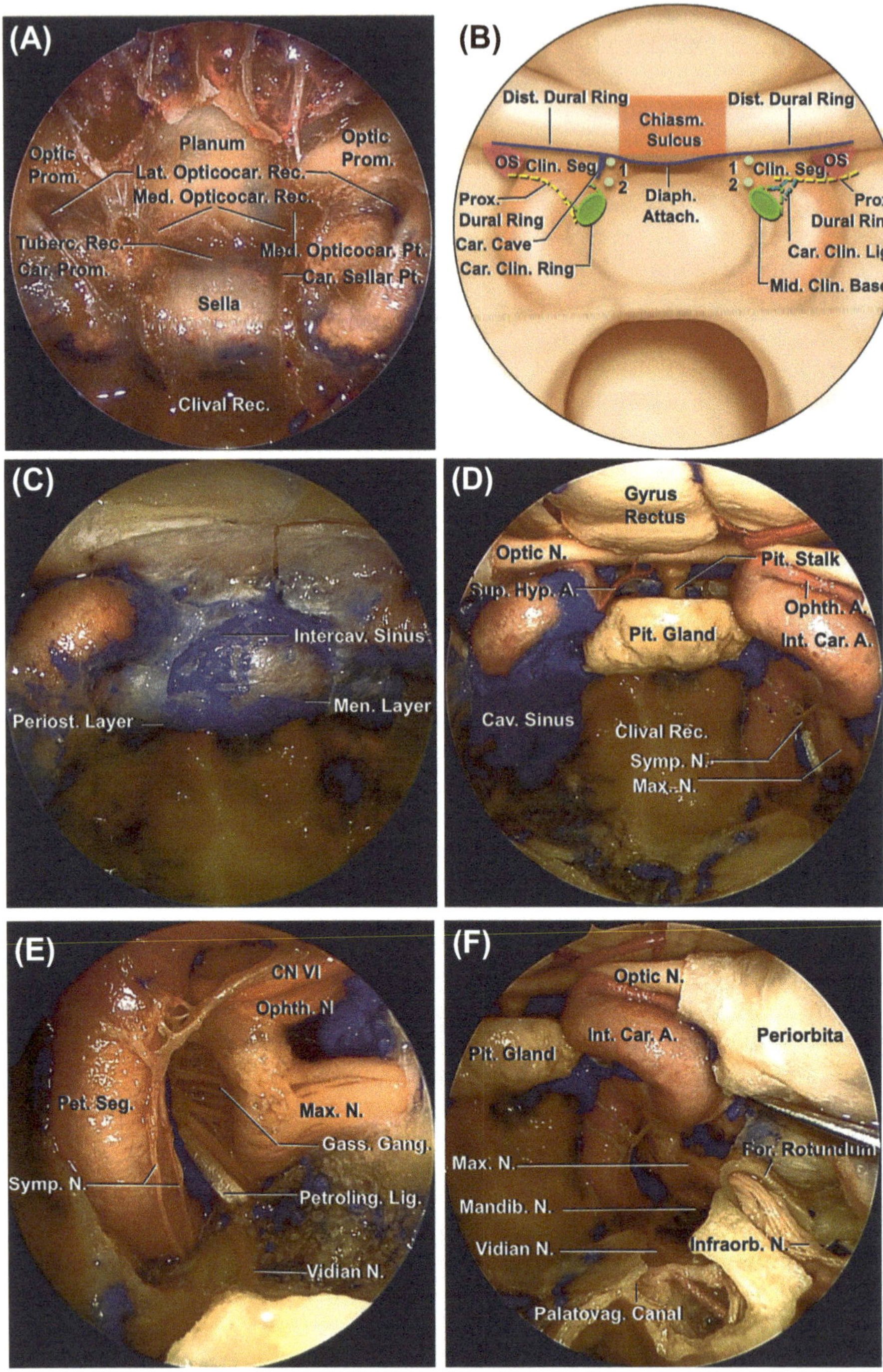
(A)
Planum
Optic Prom.
Optic Prom.
Lat. Opticocar. Rec.
Med. Opticocar. Rec.
Tuberc. Rec.
Car. Prom.
Med. Opticocar. Pt.
Car. Sellar Pt.
Sella
Clival Rec.
(B)
Dist. Dural Ring
Dist. Dural Ring
Chiasm. Sulcus
OS
Clin. Seg.
1
2
Clin. Seg.
OS
Prox. Dural Ring
Diaph. Attach.
Prox. Dural Ring
Car. Cave
Car. Clin. Ring
Car. Clin. Lig.
Mid. Clin. Base
(C)
Intercav. Sinus
Men. Layer
Periost. Layer
(D)
Gyrus Rectus
Optic N.
Pit. Stalk
Sup. Hyp. A.
Ophth. A.
Pit. Gland
Int. Car. A.
Cav. Sinus
Clival Rec.
Symp. N.
Max. N.
(E)
CN VI
Ophth. N
Pet. Seg.
Max. N.
Gass. Gang.
Symp. N.
Petroling. Lig.
Vidian N.
(F)
Optic N.
Int. Car. A.
Periorbita
Pit. Gland
For. Rotundum
Max. N.
Mandib. N.
Vidian N.
Infraorb. N.
Palatovag. Canal

(the air cavity does not penetrate beyond a vertical plane parallel to the anterior sellar wall, 23–24%) and the most common, the sellar type in which the pneumatization extends posteriorly below the sellar floor up to the clivus (67–76%). Endonasally in the sellar type of sphenoid sinus, the pituitary fossa forms a bulging oval prominence in the midline of the sinus roof, surrounded laterally by the prominence overlying the anterior loop of the intracavernous carotid artery (presellar carotid) and superiorly by the clinoid segment of the carotid artery. The carotid artery can form prominences in the anterior part of the sella (presellar segment) in 98%, below the sellar floor (infrasellar segment) in 80%, and in the posterolateral part of the sinus (retrosellar segment or vertical segment) in 78% of cases. Any part of the carotid prominences can be present and the others absent. Only the presellar segment is present in the presellar type of sphenoid sinus. The bone over the cavernous carotid just below the tuberculum can be dehiscent in 10% of cases and less than 0.5 mm

FIGURE 2.7 Endoscopic transphenoidal view of the superior wall of the sphenoid sinus, formed by the planum and the sellar wall. **A,** Superior wall of the sphenoid sinus. The important anatomic features of the sphenoid sinus include the sellar prominence in the center, carotid prominences laterally, and optic canals superiorly. The medial and lateral opticocarotid recesses are located along the medial and lateral sides of the prominences overlying the optic nerve and carotid artery, respectively. The recess just superior to the sellar prominence, called the tuberculum recess, is located between both medial opticocarotid recesses. The medial opticocarotid point and the caroticosellar point are seen in the edges of the medial opticocarotid recess. The base of the middle clinoid process, when present, is positioned inferolateral to the caroticosellar point. **B,** Diagram showing the intracranial relationships of the recesses and prominences of the sphenoid sinus. The lateral opticocarotid recess extends into the optic strut in most specimens. The lateral aspect of the distal dural ring is located approximately 1 mm above the tuberculum recess and is medially continuous with the diaphragm attachment that is located at the level or slightly inferior to this recess (blue line). The proximal dural ring is located along the inferior border of the lateral opticocarotid recess and its projection extends medially toward the tuberculum recess (yellow dotted line). The base of the middle clinoid (green shadowed area), when present, protrudes inside the cavernous sinus toward the anterior clinoid and inferior and lateral to the medial opticocarotid point (point 1) and caroticosellar point (point 2). The caroticoclinoid ligament (dark green interrupted line), when present, extends from the inferior aspect of the anterior clinoid to the middle clinoid. If a caroticoclinoid ring is present, the proximal dural ring extends posterior to the carotid artery below the osseous ring and blends into the medial wall of the cavernous sinus (right side of the sellar wall). The middle clinoid base is located at the midsuperior level of the sellar prominence directed posterior and superior to the anterior clinoid at approximately the center of the carotid prominence. When present, the carotid cave is located between points 1 and 2. The chiasmatic sulcus is positioned above the tuberculum recess and between the optic prominences. **C,** Dissection of the sellar area. The periosteal layer of the dura mater has been partially removed over the anterior surface of the pituitary gland. The intercavernous sinus that connects paired cavernous sinuses, runs between the meningeal and periosteal layers of the dura. **D,** The dura covering the pituitary gland and sellar diaphragm has been removed to show the sellar and suprasellar regions, and cavernous sinus. **E,** Anteromedial view of the left cavernous sinus. The sympathetic nerves ascend on the internal carotid artery and send a branch to the orbit. The gasserian ganglion and the V1 and V2 are exposed lateral to the internal carotid artery. CN VI is located medial to V1. The vidian nerve arises along the inferolateral aspect of the lacerum segment of the internal carotid artery. **F,** Anteromedial view of the left cavernous sinus. The infraorbital nerve can be followed posteriorly through the foramen rotundum to the maxillary nerve and gasserian ganglion. The vidian nerve passes forward to enter the pterygopalatine fossa. During transsphenoidal surgery, the maxillary nerve can be followed to the gasserian ganglion and the vidian nerve can be followed to the internal carotid artery. The palatovaginal canal extends posteriorly on the medial side of the vidian canal to the nasopharynx. A., artery; CP, carotid prominence; Car., carotid; Cav. cavernous; Clin., clinoid; Infraorb., infraorbital; Intercav., intercavernous; Hyp., hypophyseal; Med., medial; Men., meningeal; Opticocar., opticocarotid; Lat., lateral; Lig., ligament; Mand., mandibular; Max., maxillary; OS, optic strut; Periost., periosteal; Seg., segment; Sph., sphenoid; Sup., superior; Symp., sympathetic; Turb., turbinate; Rec., recess.

thick in 90%. The shortest distance between carotids in the sinus wall is located just below the tuberculum in 72% of cases, at the level of the floor of the sella in 20%, and at the clivus in 8% (Rhoton, 2002). The segment of the carotid artery adjacent to the pituitary gland is also referred to as parasellar, and the segment adjacent to the clivus as paraclival. The optic nerves in the optic canals protrude into the superolateral part of the sinus and are directed from posteromedial to anterolateral. The bone forming the optic canals is dehiscent in up to 8% of cases (Stamm, 2000).

The lateral opticocarotid recess is located lateral to the carotid prominence, between the optic canal and carotid prominences. The recess has a triangular shape and corresponds to the cross-sectional shape of the optic strut base. This recess may pneumatize through the strut into the anterior clinoid process. This pneumatization is responsible for cerebrospinal fluid leaks into the sphenoid sinus and nose following anterior clinoidectomy. The tuberculum recess is located between the sellar prominences and the planum, and in most cases corresponds to the tuberculum endocranially. The diaphragma sellae attachment is located at the level of the tuberculum recess or slightly inferior (Figure 2.7B). The lateral extensions of the tuberculum recess have been described as the medial opticocarotid recesses, where the optic prominence meets the carotid prominence medial to the carotid artery. Two junction points can be recognized in the medial opticocarotid recess: the medial opticocarotid point, where the optic nerve prominence meets the carotid prominence medially, and the caroticosellar point, where the carotid prominence meets the sellar prominence superiorly. A clinically relevant middle clinoid process (greater than 1.5 mm) is present in 21.1% of cases and can form a caroticoclinoid ring, a bony ring joining the anterior and middle clinoid processes, in 2.94% of cases. The base of the middle clinoid process is most frequently located approximately 1 mm inferior and lateral to the caroticosellar junction point and its highest point is further inferior and lateral. On average, the middle clinoid is 4.75 mm inferior to the medial opticocarotid point (Peris-Celda et al., 2013). The average distance between the medial edges of the optic nerves at their first entry into the part of the optic canal in the sinus wall is 15.75 mm and this does not seem to be affected by the pneumatization of the recesses. There is no recess or prominence that represents the chiasmatic groove inside the sphenoid sinus, although its site can be estimated to be between both optic prominences (Wang et al., 2010).

VASCULAR RELATIONSHIPS

The arterial relationships in the suprasellar area are among the most complex intracranially, because this area contains all the components of the circle of Willis. The anterior part of the circle of Willis, formed by the anterior cerebral and anterior communicating arteries, is intimately related to the anterior wall of the third ventricle; the posterior part of the circle of Willis and the apex of the basilar artery are located in the anterior incisural space below the floor of the third ventricle. Both the anterior and posterior cerebral arteries send branches into the roof of the third ventricle. The internal carotid, anterior choroidal, anterior and posterior cerebral, and anterior and posterior communicating arteries give rise to perforating branches that reach the walls of the third ventricle and anterior incisural space. All the arterial components of the circle of Willis and the adjacent segments of the carotid and basilar arteries and their perforating branches may be stretched around suprasellar extensions of pituitary tumors and craniopharyngiomas (Rhoton, 2002). Gentle and accurate dissection is needed to preserve them during craniopharyngioma surgery (Figures 2.8–2.10). Deep venous structures that might be involved are mainly the basal veins of Rosenthal, which surround the midbrain and drain into the vein of Galen.

The supraclinoid portion of the internal carotid artery or C4 segment enters the cranial cavity by passing along the medial side of the anterior clinoid process and below the optic nerve (Figures 2.8 and 2.9). It courses posterior, superior, and slightly lateral to reach the lateral side of the optic chiasm and bifurcates below the anterior perforated substance at the medial end of the sylvian fissure to give rise to the anterior and middle cerebral arteries. The C4 is divided into three segments based on the site of origin of the ophthalmic, posterior communicating, and anterior choroidal arteries. The ophthalmic segment extends from the roof of the cavernous sinus and the origin of the ophthalmic artery to the origin of the posterior communicating artery; the communicating segment extends from the origin of the posterior communicating artery to the origin of the anterior choroidal artery; and the choroidal segment extends from the origin of the anterior choroidal artery to the terminal bifurcation of the internal carotid artery. The ophthalmic segment is the longest, and the communicating segment the shortest (Gibo et al., 1981). An average of eight (range 3–12) perforating arteries (excluding the ophthalmic, posterior communicating, and anterior choroidal arteries) arise from the C4 segment.

The ophthalmic artery usually arises from the medial one-third of the superior surface of the C4 immediately distal to the cavernous sinus in the area below the optic nerve. It arose above the medial one-third of the superior surface of the C4 in 78% of hemispheres and above the middle one-third of the superior surface in 22% of cases in our prior study (Gibo et al., 1981). An average of four (range 1–7) perforating arteries arise from the ophthalmic segment. There is a group of one to five (average, 2) small branches that terminate on the pituitary stalk and gland, but also branches go to the optic nerves and chiasm and the floor of the third ventricle. The largest of the branches is often referred to as the superior hypophyseal artery. Most of these branches arise from the posteromedial, medial, or posterior aspects of the ICA.

The posterior communicating artery, which forms the lateral boundary of the circle of Willis, arises from the posteromedial surface of the C4 about midway between the origin of the ophthalmic artery and the terminal bifurcation. It sweeps backward and medially below the tuber cinereum, above the sella turcica, and slightly above and medial to the oculomotor nerve to join the posterior cerebral artery. In the embryo, the posterior communicating artery continues as the posterior cerebral artery, but in the adult, the latter artery is annexed by the basilar system. If the posterior communicating artery remains the major origin of the posterior cerebral artery, the configuration is termed "fetal." An average of eight (range, 4–14) perforating branches arise from the posterior communicating artery, mostly from the superior and lateral surfaces, and course superiorly to penetrate in decreasing order of frequency, the tuber cinereum, premamillary part of the floor of the third ventricle, posterior perforated substance, interpeduncular fossa, optic tract, pituitary stalk, and optic chiasm. These branches also supply the thalamus, hypothalamus, subthalamus, and internal capsule (Saeki & Rhoton, 1977). Branch origins are distributed relatively evenly along the course of the artery. The infundibular arteries are a group of arteries that originate from the posterior communicating artery and are distributed to the infundibulum. There are fewer infundibular arteries than superior hypophyseal

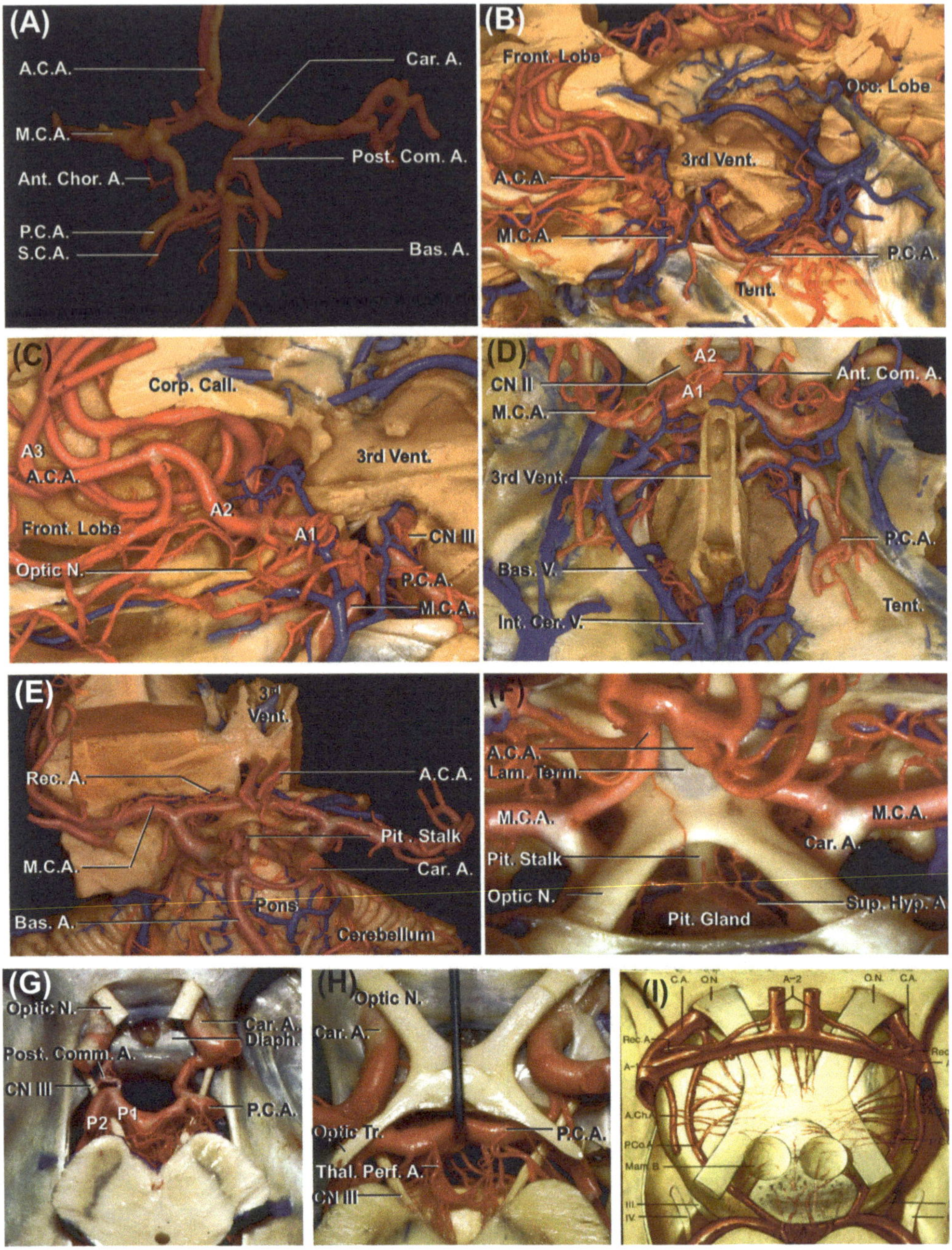

FIGURE 2.8 **Vascular relationships important in craniopharyngioma surgery. A,** Isolated circle of Willis. Craniopharyngiomas may displace or encase any or all of the components of the circle of Willis. **B,** Left lateral view of the third ventricle. The anterior, middle, and posterior cerebral arteries have been preserved. These arteries often supply or are closely related to craniopharyngiomas. **C,** Enlarged view of B. Note the course of the A1, A2, and A3 in relation

arteries. One-quarter of hemispheres have one or two infundibular arteries and the remainder have none. The superior hypophyseal and infundibular arteries pass medially below the chiasm to reach the tuber cinereum. They intermingle and form a fine anastomotic plexus around the pituitary stalk called the "circuminfundibular anastomosis." These arteries and the circuminfundibular plexus are distributed to the pituitary stalk and anterior lobe (Figure 2.9B). The inferior hypophyseal branch of the meningohypophyseal trunk of the intracavernous carotid perfuses the posterior lobe. The capsular arteries also arise from the intracavernous carotid and supply the capsule of the pituitary gland (Harris & Rhoton, 1975). This circuminfundibular plexus gives rise to ascending and descending arteries. The descending arteries include short-stalk and superficial arteries. The short-stalk arteries penetrate the infundibulum and form capillaries that lead into sinusoids running down the stalk. The superficial arteries course inferiorly on the outside of the stalk in the subarachnoid space and penetrate the anterior lobe. The ascending arteries supply the tuber cinereum, median eminence, and the inferior surface of the optic chiasm. The superior hypophyseal arteries also send branches to the chiasm and proximal portions of the optic nerves. The premamillary artery is the largest branch that arises from the posterior communicating artery. It enters the floor of the third ventricle in front of or beside the mamillary body between the mamillary body and optic tract. The premamillary artery has also been referred to as the anterior thalamoperforating artery. The premamillary artery most commonly originates on the middle one-third of the communicating artery but can also arise on the anterior or posterior one-third. It supplies the posterior hypothalamus, anterior thalamus, posterior limb of the internal capsule, and subthalamus. The anterior group of posterior communicating artery perforating branches supplies the hypothalamus, ventral thalamus, anterior one-third of the optic tract, and posterior limb of the internal capsule; the posterior group reaches the posterior perforated substance and subthalamic nucleus. Occlusion of the branches to the subthalamic nucleus leads to contralateral hemiballism. No perforating branches arise from the communicating segment of the C4 in more than half of hemispheres, and if present, only one to three are found.

The anterior choroidal artery usually arises from the C4 as a single artery with the majority arising nearer the origin of the posterior communicating artery than to the carotid bifurcation. The origin of the artery is lateral to the optic tract, but the initial segment crosses from the lateral to the medial side of the optic tract in many hemispheres, only infrequently remaining lateral to the optic tract throughout its course. It passes below or along the medial side of the

to the optic nerves and chiasm, and corpus callosum. **D,** Superior view of the third ventricle, circle of Willis, and the basal vein surrounding the midbrain. **E,** Anterior view of the cerebellum, brainstem, and right basal ganglia. Note the relationships of the internal carotid, and middle and anterior cerebral arteries to the pituitary stalk. **F,** Anterior view of the suprasellar area. The anterior communicating artery courses superior to the optic chiasm and anterior to the lamina terminalis. **G,** Superior view of the posterior part of the circle of Willis formed by the posterior communicating arteries and posterior cerebral arteries. **H,** Numerous perforating arteries arise from the P1 segment of the posterior cerebral artery and basilar apex and cross the interpeduncular cistern. **I,** Superior view. Circle of Willis and its perforating branches stretched around a suprasellar tumor. A., artery; A.C.A., anterior cerebral artery; Bas., basilar; CN, cranial nerve; Car., carotid; Chor., choroidal; Com., communicating; Diaph., diaphragm; Front., frontal; Int., internal; Lam., lamina; M.C.A., middle cerebral artery; P.C.A., posterior cerebral artery; Perf., perforating; Pit., pituitary; Post., posterior; Rec., recurrent; S.C.A., superior cerebellar artery; Tent., tentorium; Term., terminalis; Thal., thalamo; Tr., tract; Vent., ventricle. Abbreviations in **I.** A. Ch. A., anterior choroidal artery; CA, carotid artery; Mam. B., mamillary bodies; ON, optic nerve; P. Co. A., posterior communicating artery; Rec. A., recurrent artery.

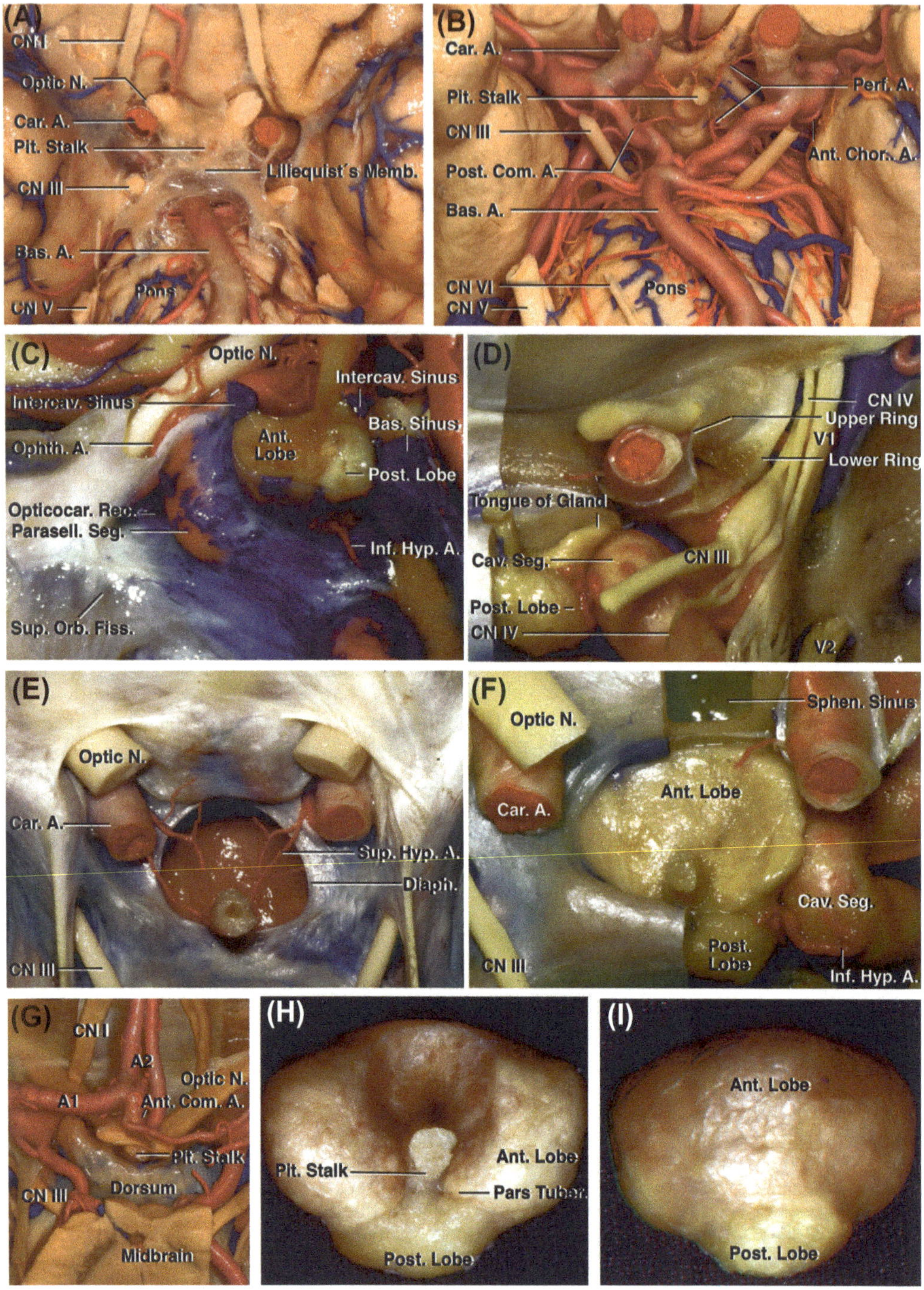
(A)
CN I
Optic N.
Car. A.
Pit. Stalk
Liliequist's Memb.
CN III
Bas. A.
Pons
CN V
(B)
Car. A.
Perf. A.
Pit. Stalk
CN III
Ant. Chor. A.
Post. Com. A.
Bas. A.
CN VI
CN V
Pons
(C)
Optic N.
Intercav. Sinus
Intercav. Sinus
Bas. Sinus
Ant. Lobe
Ophth. A.
Post. Lobe
Opticocar. Rec.
Parasell. Seg.
Inf. Hyp. A.
Sup. Orb. Fiss.
(D)
CN IV
Upper Ring
V1
Lower Ring
Tongue of Gland
CN III
Cav. Seg.
Post. Lobe
CN IV
V2
(E)
Optic N.
Car. A.
Sup. Hyp. A.
Diaph.
CN III
(F)
Optic N.
Sphen. Sinus
Ant. Lobe
Car. A.
Cav. Seg.
CN III
Post. Lobe
Inf. Hyp. A.
(G)
CN I
A2
Optic N.
A1
Ant. Com. A.
Pit. Stalk
CN III
Dorsum
Midbrain
(H)
Pit. Stalk
Ant. Lobe
Pars Tuber.
Post. Lobe
(I)
Ant. Lobe
Post. Lobe

optic tract to reach the lateral margin of the cerebral peduncle. The average length that the artery follows the optic tract is 12 mm (range, 5–25 mm) (Rhoton et al., 1979). At the anterior margin of the lateral geniculate body, the anterior choroidal artery again crosses the optic tract from medial to lateral and passes posterolateral through the crural cistern, located between the cerebral peduncle and uncus, to arrive superomedial to the uncus where it passes through the choroidal fissure to enter the choroid plexus within the temporal horn. It courses along the medial border of the choroid plexus in close relation to the lateral posterior choroidal branches of the posterior cerebral artery. It can pass dorsally along the medial border of the plexus, reaching the foramen of Monro in some cases. The branches from the cisternal segment penetrate, in decreasing order of frequency, the optic tract, uncus, cerebral peduncle, temporal horn, lateral geniculate body, hippocampus, dentate gyrus and fornix, and anterior perforated substance. These branches more commonly supply the optic tract, the lateral part of the geniculate body, the posterior two-thirds of the posterior limb of the internal capsule, most of the globus pallidus, the origin of the optic radiations, and the middle one-third of the cerebral peduncle. Less commonly supplied are part of the head of the caudate nucleus, pyriform cortex, uncus, posterior medial part of the amygdaloid nucleus, substantia nigra, red nucleus, subthalamic nucleus, and superficial aspect of the ventrolateral nucleus of the thalamus. However, none of these structures are always supplied by the artery but, in approximately two-thirds of the hemispheres, it supplies the medial part of the globus pallidus, the posterior limb and retrolenticular part of the internal capsule, the optic tract, and the lateral geniculate body. An average of four (range, 1–9) perforating branches arise from the choroidal segment. Most arise from the posterior half of the arterial wall and terminate, in descending order of frequency, in the anterior perforated substance, optic tract, and uncus.

The internal carotid artery bifurcates in the middle and anterior cerebral arteries. The anterior cerebral artery forms part of the anterior circle of Willis. The anterior cerebral artery, the smaller

FIGURE 2.9 **Relationships of the pituitary gland. A,** Inferior view of the suprasellar area with intact arachnoid membranes. The interpeduncular cistern is located posterior to the pituitary stalk, between the diencephalic and mesencephalic divisions of Liliequist's membrane. Both divisions of the membranes attach to the dorsum sella and divide posteriorly into two membranes. The diencephalic membrane attaches to the mamillary bodies and separates the chiasmatic and interpeduncular cisterns. The mesencephalic membrane separates the interpeduncular and the prepontine cisterns. **B,** Similar view to A after resection of the arachnoid membranes. Numerous perforating branches arising from the circle of Willis supply the pituitary stalk, infundibulum, optic chiasm and tract, and hypothalamus. **C,** Pituitary gland and sphenoid sinus divided in the midsagittal plane. The parasellar segment of the cavernous carotid artery courses anterior and lateral to the pituitary gland. **D,** Posterior-superior view of the right cavernous sinus. The anterior clinoid process has been removed. The cavernous carotid is located lateral to the pituitary gland. CNs III, IV, and VI are exposed in the lateral wall of the cavernous sinus. **E,** Superior view. The superior hypophyseal arteries arise from the internal carotid artery and pass to the pituitary stalk. **F,** Superior view with the left dorsum and dural wall of the left cavernous sinus removed. The anterior and posterior lobes of the pituitary gland are exposed. The inferior hypophyseal artery is a branch of the cavernous segment of the carotid artery. **G,** Superior view of the dorsum sella. The anterior communicating artery passes above the optic chiasm. **H,** Superior view of the pituitary gland. The anterior lobe or adenohypophysis is larger and originates from the ectoderm. The posterior lobe or neurohypophysis originates from the neuroectoderm and is continuous with the pituitary stalk and hypothalamus. **I,** Inferior view of the anterior and posterior lobe of the pituitary gland. Ant., anterior; Bas., basilar; Car., carotid; CN, cranial nerve; Cav., cavernous; Com., communicating; Diaph., diaphragm; Fiss., fissure; Hyp., hypophyseal; Intercav., intercavernous; N., nerve; Ophth., ophthalmic; Opticocar., opticocarotid; Orb., orbital; Parasell., parasellar; Perf., perforating; Pit., pituitary; Post., posterior; Sphen., sphenoid; Sup., superior.

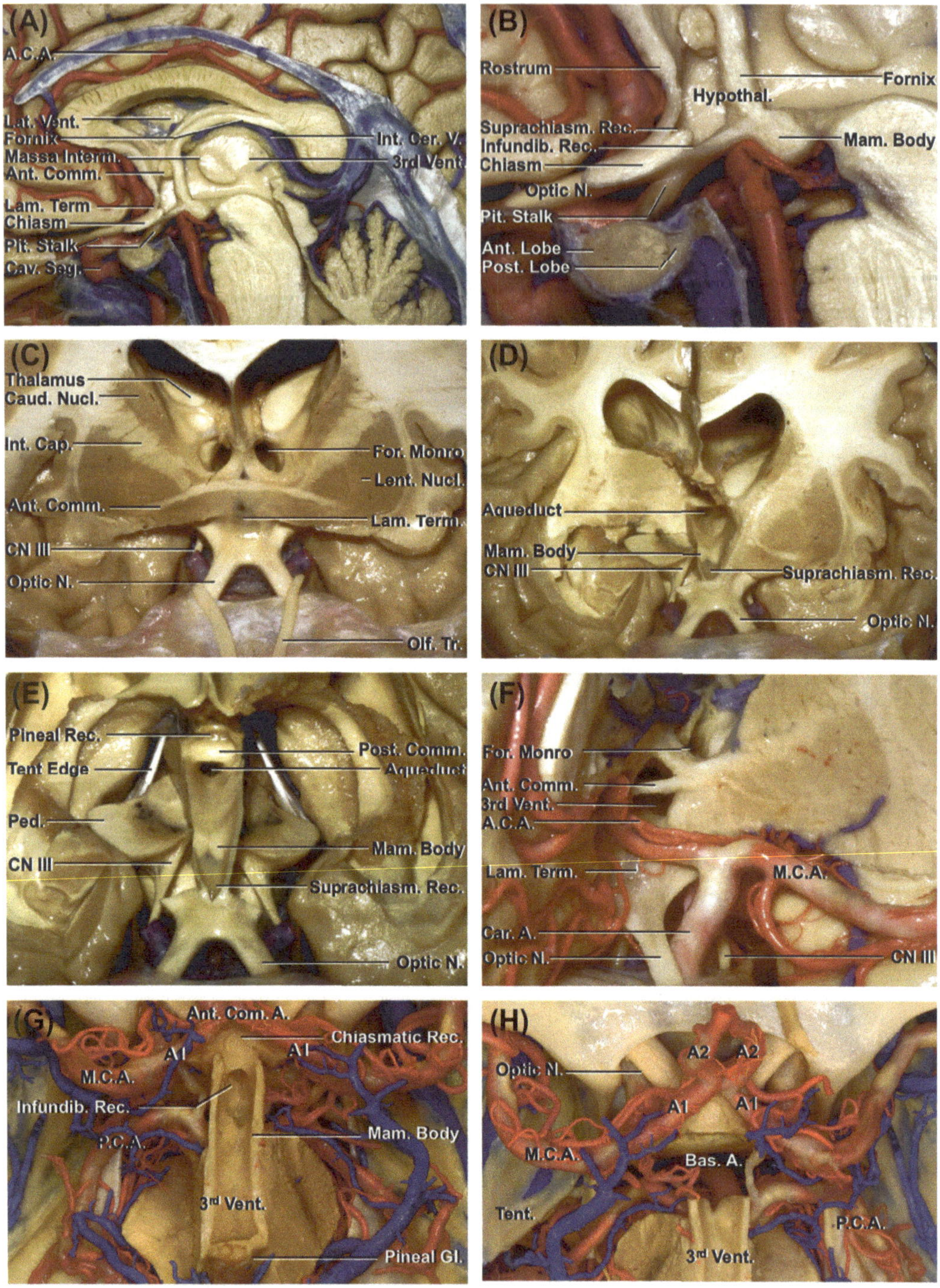

(A)
A.C.A.
Lat. Vent.
Fornix
Massa Interm.
Ant. Comm.
Lam. Term
Chiasm
Pit. Stalk
Cav. Seg.
Int. Cer. V.
3rd Vent.
(B)
Rostrum
Fornix
Hypothal.
Suprachiasm. Rec.
Infundib. Rec.
Chiasm
Optic N.
Mam. Body
Pit. Stalk
Ant. Lobe
Post. Lobe
(C)
Thalamus
Caud. Nucl.
Int. Cap.
For. Monro
Lent. Nucl.
Ant. Comm.
Lam. Term.
CN III
Optic N.
Olf. Tr.
(D)
Aqueduct
Mam. Body
CN III
Suprachiasm. Rec.
Optic N.
(E)
Pineal Rec.
Post. Comm.
Tent Edge
Aqueduct
Ped.
Mam. Body
CN III
Suprachiasm. Rec.
Optic N.
(F)
For. Monro
Ant. Comm.
3rd Vent.
A.C.A.
Lam. Term.
M.C.A.
Car. A.
Optic N.
CN III
(G)
Ant. Com. A.
Chiasmatic Rec.
A1
A1
M.C.A.
Infundib. Rec.
Mam. Body
P.C.A.
3rd Vent.
Pineal Gl.
(H)
A2
A2
Optic N.
A1
A1
M.C.A.
Bas. A.
Tent.
P.C.A.
3rd Vent.

of the two terminal branches of the internal carotid artery, arises at the medial end of the sylvian fissure, lateral to the optic chiasm and below the anterior perforated substance. It courses anteromedially above the optic nerve or chiasm and below the medial olfactory striae to enter the interhemispheric fissure. Near its entrance into the fissure, it is joined to the opposite anterior cerebral artery by the anterior communicating artery, and ascends in front of the lamina terminalis to pass into the longitudinal fissure between the cerebral hemispheres. The anterior cerebral artery is divided at the anterior communicating artery into two parts, proximal (precommunicating) and distal (post-communicating). The proximal part, extending from the origin to the anterior communicating artery, constitutes the A1 segment. The distal part is formed by the A2 (infracallosal), A3 (precallosal), A4 (supracallosal), and A5 (posterocallosal) segments. The A1 courses above the optic chiasm or nerves to join the anterior communicating artery. The recurrent branch of Heubner, the largest artery arising from the A1 or the proximal 0.5 mm of the A2, doubles back on its parent anterior cerebral artery and passes above the carotid bifurcation and middle cerebral artery (MCA) into the medial part of the sylvian fissure before entering the anterior perforated substance (Perlmutter & Rhoton, 1976). The recurrent artery diameter is usually less than half that of the A1, but it may infrequently be as large as or exceed the A1 diameter if the A1 is hypoplastic. The A1 and A2 and the anterior communicating artery give rise to numerous basal perforating arteries. An average of eight basal perforators (range, 2–15), exclusive of Heubner's artery, arise from each A1 (Perlmutter & Rhoton, 1976; Rhoton & Perlmutter, 1980). The lateral half of A1 is a richer source of branches than the medial half. The A1 branches terminate, in descending order of frequency, in the anterior perforated substance, dorsal surface of the optic chiasm or suprachiasmatic portion of the hypothalamus, optic tract, dorsal surface of the optic nerve, and sylvian fissure between the cerebral hemispheres and the lower surface of the frontal lobe. The A1, excluding the recurrent artery and the A2, most consistently supplies the chiasm and anterior third ventricle and hypothalamic area, but only inconsistently supplies the caudate

FIGURE 2.10 **Third ventricle and surrounding structures. A,** Midsagittal section. The roof of the third ventricle is formed by the body of the fornix, two layers of the tela choroidea, and a layer of vessels in between the layers of tela. **B,** Enlarged view of the anteroinferior aspect of the third ventricle. The hypothalamus is located between the lamina terminalis anteriorly and the posterior aspect of the mammillary bodies posteriorly. The hypothalamus and thalamus form the lateral wall of the third ventricle. The suprachiasmatic recess is located between the lamina terminalis and the optic chiasm. The infundibular recess extends downward behind the chiasm. **C,** Anterior view of a coronal section of the brain through the anterior commissure. The columns of the fornix pass around the superior and anterior margins of the foramen of Monro and behind the anterior commissure. **D,** The dissection has been advanced on the right side to the level of the thalamus. The third ventricle and aqueduct are exposed. **E,** Both thalami have been removed. The third ventricular floor extends from the optic chiasm to the aqueduct. **F,** Anterior view. The coronal section extends through the third ventricle. The anterior wall of the third ventricle below the anterior commissure has been removed. The A1 and anterior communicating artery course adjacent the anterior wall of the third ventricle. **G,** Superior view of the floor of the third ventricle. Diencephalic structures form the premamillary part of the third ventricle whereas mesencephalic structures form the postmamillary part of the third ventricle. **H,** The premamillary part of the floor of the third ventricle has been partially removed to expose the basilar artery. A., artery; A.C.A., anterior cerebral artery; Ant., anterior; Bas., basilar; CN, cranial nerve; Car., carotid; Caud., caudate; Cav., cavernous; Cist., cistern; Com., communicating; Comm., commissure; For., foramen; Gl., gland; Hypothal., hypothalamus; Infundib., infundibular; Int., interna; Interm., intermedia; Lam., lamina; Lat., lateral; M.C.A., middle cerebral artery; N., nerve; P.C.A., posterior cerebral artery; Ped., peduncle; Pit., pituitary; Post., posterior; Rec., recess; S.C.A., superior cerebellar artery; Seg., segment; Suprachiasm., suprachiasmatic; Tent., tentorium; Term., terminalis; V., vein; Vent., ventricle.

and globus pallidus. Heubner's artery, by contrast, provides a rich supply to the caudate and adjacent internal capsule, but much less to the hypothalamus. Compromise of the hypothalamic branches that arise mainly from the A1, excluding the recurrent artery, may result in emotional changes, personality disorders, and intellectual deficits, including anxiety and fear, weak spells, and symptoms referable to disordered mentation, such as dizziness, agitation, and hypokinesis without paralysis, or alterations of the conscious or waking state. The frequent inclusion of recurrent artery ischemia when the A1 branches are involved adds a hemiparesis with brachial predominance to the deficit. This contrasts with the crural weakness of distal anterior cerebral artery occlusion. The anterior communicating artery also frequently gives rise to perforating arteries that terminate in the superior surface of the optic chiasm and above the chiasm in the anterior hypothalamus. The anterior communicating artery is frequently the site of origin of one or two, but as many as four branches that terminate, in descending order of frequency, in the suprachiasmatic area, dorsal surface of the optic chiasm, anterior perforated substance, and frontal lobe, and perfuse the fornix, corpus callosum, septal region, and anterior cingulum (Dunker & Harris, 1976). Most arise from the superior or posterior surfaces of the anterior communicating artery. The A2 is also the site of origin of perforating branches terminating in the inferior frontal area, anterior perforated substance, dorsal optic chiasm, and the suprachiasmatic area. The A2 (infracallosal) segment begins at the anterior communicating artery, passes anterior to the lamina terminalis, and terminates at the junction of the rostrum and genu of the corpus callosum.

The posterior part of the circle of Willis is formed by the proximal posterior cerebral artery and posterior communicating artery and, together, in varying degrees, they provide the flow to the distal posterior cerebral artery. A hypoplastic arterial segment is defined as one having a diameter of 1 mm or less. In our study, posterior communicating artery hypoplasia was found unilaterally in 26% and bilaterally in 6%, and a fetal configuration, in which the posterior cerebral artery arises predominantly from the carotid artery, was found unilaterally in 20% and bilaterally in 2% of cases (Saeki & Rhoton, 1977). The posterior portion of the circle of Willis sends a series of perforating arteries into the diencephalon and midbrain that may become stretched around suprasellar tumors or posterior circle aneurysms. Some of the perforating branches arising from the upper part of the basilar artery overlap with some of those arising from the posterior circle. The posterior cerebral artery arises at the basilar bifurcation, is joined by the posterior communicating artery at the lateral margin of the interpeduncular cistern, encircles the brainstem passing through the crural and ambient cisterns to reach the quadrigeminal cistern, and is distributed to the posterior part of the hemisphere. The P1 segment, also called the precommunicating segment, extends from the basilar bifurcation to the junction with the posterior communicating artery. The relatively constant branches arising from the P1 are: 1) the thalamoperforating artery, which by definition enters the brain through the posterior perforated substance; 2) the medial posterior choroidal artery directed to the choroid plexus in the third and lateral ventricles; 3) the branch to the quadrigeminal plate; and 4) rami to the cerebral peduncle and mesencephalic tegmentum. The superior cerebellar artery arises from the basilar artery at a level between the P1 origin and 7 mm below (average, 2.5 mm). The superior cerebellar artery may infrequently have a common origin with the P1 or arise from P1. The initial segment gives rise to perforating vessels whose termination may overlap with those arising from the basilar apex and P1. An average of four, but as many as a dozen, perforating branches, the largest of which may have a diameter of 1.5 mm, arise mainly from the superior and posterior surfaces of the P1, course superiorly and posteriorly, and divide into numerous branches that terminate in the interpeduncular fossa, posterior perforated substance, cerebral peduncle, mamillary bodies, and posterior midbrain. Perforating branches rarely arise from the anterior side of the basilar apex, but they arise from the anterior surface in a third of P1s, and terminate in the posterior perforated substance and mamillary bodies. The largest P1 branch is a thalamoperforating artery in 42% of hemispheres, a posterior choroidal artery in 40%, or a large trunk from which both arteries arise in 18% (Saeki & Rhoton, 1977). The posterior and lateral surfaces of the upper centimeter of the basilar artery are also a rich source of perforating arteries that overlap with those arising from the P1. An average of 8 (range, 3–18) branches arise from the upper centimeter of the basilar artery.

CISTERNAL, NEURAL, AND VENTRICULAR ANATOMY

Knowledge of the cisternal and vascular anatomy allows preservation of the structures potentially encased or displaced during craniopharyngioma surgery.

Cisternal Anatomy

Depending on their size and location, craniopharyngiomas can grow in the suprasellar space towards or into the chiasmatic, lamina terminalis, carotid, pericallosal, and interpeduncular cisterns (Figures 2.9 and 2.10). The arachnoid membranes separating the cisterns form an arachnoidal plane between the tumor and important vessels or neural structures. Tumors arising in the sella often extend upward into the suprasellar cisterns to compress the floor of the third ventricle and involve the circle of Willis and deep cerebral venous system (Rhoton et al., 1981; Yamamoto et al., 1981; Rhoton, 2002).

The area involved by those tumors usually corresponds to the anterior incisural space located between the free edges of the tentorium and the front of the midbrain (Rhoton, 2000; Ono et al., 1984). The anterior incisural space corresponds roughly to the suprasellar area. From the front of the midbrain it extends obliquely forward and upward around the optic chiasm to the subcallosal area. It opens laterally into the sylvian fissure and between the uncus and the brainstem. The part of the anterior incisural space located below the optic chiasm has posterior and posterolateral walls. The posterior wall is formed by the cerebral peduncles. The posterolateral wall is formed by the anterior third of the uncus, which hangs over the free edge of the tentorium above the oculomotor nerve. The infundibulum of the pituitary gland crosses the anterior incisural space to pass through the opening in the diaphragm sellae. The part of the anterior incisural space situated above the optic chiasm is limited superiorly by the rostrum of the corpus callosum, posteriorly by the lamina terminalis, and laterally by the part of the medial surfaces of the frontal lobes located below the rostrum. The anterior incisural space opens laterally into the part of the sylvian fissure situated below the anterior perforated substance. The anterior limb of the internal capsule, the head of the caudate nucleus, and the anterior part of the lentiform nucleus are located above the anterior perforated substance. The interpeduncular cistern sits in the posterior part of the anterior incisural space between the cerebral peduncles and the dorsum sellae. This cistern is located between both leaves of Liliequist's membrane at the confluence of the supra- and infratentorial parts of the subarachnoid space and communicates anteriorly with the chiasmatic cistern located below the optic chiasm. The interpeduncular and chiasmatic cisterns are separated by the diencephalic leaf of Liliquist's membrane, an arachnoidal sheet extending from the dorsum sellae to the anterior edge of the mamillary bodies. The chiasmatic cistern communicates around the optic chiasm with the cisterna lamina terminalis, which lies anterior to the lamina terminalis. The chiasmatic cistern surrounds the optic nerves and chiasm and contains the pituitary stalk and carotid perforating branches. The interpeduncular cistern contains the basilar bifurcation, proximal part of the posterior cerebral arteries, thalamoperforating arteries, and the initial segment of the circumflex perforating and medial posterior choroidal arteries. The optic and oculomotor nerves and the posterior part of the olfactory tracts pass through the suprasellar region and anterior incisural space. Each olfactory tract runs posteriorly and splits just above the anterior clinoid process to form the medial and lateral olfactory striae, which course along the anterior margin of the anterior perforated substance.

The carotid cistern is situated between the lateral edge of the optic chiasm medially, the temporal lobes laterally, and the anterior perforated substance above, and contains the internal carotid and posterior communicating arteries, and the origin of the anterior and middle cerebral, ophthalmic, and anterior choroidal arteries. The lamina terminalis cistern is positioned above the optic chiasm and anterior to the lamina terminalis between the frontal lobes and contains the A1 and proximal A2 segments of the anterior cerebral artery, the anterior communicating and orbitofrontal arteries, some of the basal perforating arteries, and the initial segment of the recurrent artery. If the tumor has an upward extension it may involve the pericallosal cistern, situated in the interhemispheric fissure on the outer surface of the corpus callosum and contains the anterior cerebral arteries.

Pituitary Gland

The pituitary gland is a reddish-gray, ovoid body, about 12 mm in transverse and 8 mm in anteroposterior diameter, and with an average adult weight of 500 mg (Figure 2.9). It is continuous with the pituitary stalk and infundibulum, a hollow, conical process extending downward from the tuber cinereum of the hypothalamus. It lies within the pituitary fossa of the sphenoid bone, where it is covered superiorly by a circular diaphragma sellae of dura mater. The diaphragma is pierced centrally by an aperture for the infundibulum, and separates the anterior superior aspect of the pituitary from the optic chiasm. Inferiorly, the pituitary is separated from the floor of the fossa by a venous sinus that communicates with the circular sinus. The infundibulum contains neural hypophyseal connections and is continuous with the median eminence of the tuber cinereum. When exposed from above by opening the diaphragm, the posterior lobe of the pituitary gland is lighter in color than the anterior lobe. The anterior lobe wraps around the lower part of the pituitary stalk to form the pars tuberalis. The posterior lobe is softer, almost gelatinous, and is more densely adherent to the sellar wall. The anterior lobe is firmer and is more easily separated from the sellar walls. The gland's width is the same or more than either its depth or its length in most patients. Its inferior surface usually conforms to the shape of the sellar floor, but its lateral and superior margins vary in shape because these walls are composed of soft tissue rather than bone. If there is a large opening in the diaphragma, the gland tends to be concave superiorly in the area around the stalk. The superior surface may become triangular as a result of being compressed laterally and posteriorly by the carotid arteries. As the anterior lobe is separated from the posterior lobe, there is a tendency for the pars tuberalis to be retained with the posterior lobe. Small intermediate lobe cysts are frequently encountered during separation of the anterior and posterior lobes (Rhoton et al., 1979; Rhoton, 2002).

Optic Nerves and Chiasm

The optic nerves and chiasm are often displaced or compressed by the tumor, which may result in progressive vision loss. Their location in relation to the tumor may play a major role in selecting the operative approach to a craniopharyngioma. The optic nerves and chiasm and the anterior part of the optic tracts cross the anterior incisural space (Figures 2.4, 2.5, 2.8, and 2.9). The optic nerves emerge from the optic canals medial to the attachment of the free edges of the tentorium to the anterior clinoid processes and are directed posteriorly, superiorly, and medially toward the optic chiasm. From the chiasm, the optic tracts continue in a posterolateral direction around the cerebral peduncles to enter the middle incisural spaces. The upper surface of the optic nerve proximal to its entrance into the optic canal is covered by a leaf of dura mater, the falciform ligament (Figure 2.1E), which extends medially from the anterior clinoid process. The length of nerve covered only by the dura of the falciform process at the intracranial end of the optic canal may vary from less than 1 mm to as much as 1 cm (Renn & Rhoton, 1975). Coagulation of the dura above the optic nerve just proximal to the optic canal on the assumption that bone separates the dura mater from the nerve could lead to nerve injury. Compression of the optic nerve against the sharp edge of the falciform process may result in a visual field deficit, even if the compressing lesion does not damage the nerve enough to cause visual loss. Normally, the optic nerve is separated medially from the sphenoid sinus by a thin layer of bone, but if the sinus is well pneumatized, this bone is absent, and the optic nerves may protrude directly into the sphenoid sinus, separated from the sinus by only mucosa and the dural sheath of the nerve (Gibo et al., 1981). The optic chiasm is situated at the junction of the anterior wall and floor of the third ventricle. The anterior cerebral and anterior communicating arteries, the lamina terminalis, and the third ventricle are located above the chiasm. The tuber cinereum and the infundibulum are posterior, the internal carotid arteries are lateral, and the diaphragm sellae and pituitary gland are inferior to the optic chiasm. The suprachiasmatic recess of the third ventricle is located between the chiasm and lamina terminalis. The infundibular recess extends into the base of the pituitary stalk behind the optic chiasm (Figure 2.10B). The relationship of the chiasm to the sella is an important determinant of the ease with which the pituitary fossa can be exposed by the transfrontal surgical route, and also for the endoscopic endonasal approaches. The normal chiasm overlies the diaphragma sellae and the pituitary gland, the prefixed chiasm overlies the tuberculum, and the postfixed chiasm overlies the dorsum. In approximately 70% of our cases, the chiasm is in the normal position; of the remaining 30%, approximately half are "prefixed" and half "postfixed." A prominent tuberculum sellae may restrict access to the sella, even in the presence of a normal chiasm. The tuberculum may vary from being almost flat to protruding upward as much as 3 mm, and it may project posteriorly to the margin of a normal chiasm. A prefixed chiasm, a normal chiasm with a small area between the tuberculum and the chiasm, and a superior protruding tuberculum sellae do not limit exposure by the transsphenoidal approach, but they limit access to the suprasellar area provided by the transcranial approach. There are several methods of gaining access to the suprasellar area when these variants are present. One is to expose the sphenoid sinus from above by opening through the tuberculum and planum sphenoidale, thus converting the approach to a transfrontal-transsphenoidal exposure. If the chiasm is prefixed and the tumor is seen through a thin, stretched anterior wall of the third ventricle, the lamina terminalis may be opened to expose the tumor, an approach used for craniopharyngiomas involving the third ventricle. If the space between the carotid artery and the optic nerve has been enlarged by a lateral or parasellar extension of tumor, the tumor may be removed through this space. An understanding of the relationship of the carotid artery, optic nerve, and anterior clinoid process is fundamental to all surgical approaches to the sellar and parasellar areas. The carotid artery and the optic nerve are medial to the anterior clinoid process. The artery exits the cavernous sinus beneath and slightly lateral to the optic nerve. The optic nerve pursues a posteromedial course toward the chiasm, and the carotid artery pursues a posterolateral course toward its bifurcation below the anterior perforated substance (Rhoton, 2002).

Hypothalamus

Often involved in craniopharyngiomas, the hypothalamus extends from the lamina terminalis to posterior to the mamillary bodies, and from the hypothalamic sulcus to the floor of the third ventricle. It lies beneath the thalamus and anterior to the tegmental part of the subthalamus and the mesencephalic tegmentum. Laterally, it is bordered by the anterior part of the subthalamus, internal capsule, and optic tract (Figures 2.1 and 2.10).

Third Ventricle

The third ventricle is located in the center of the head, below the corpus callosum and the body of the lateral ventricle, above the sella turcica, pituitary gland, hypothalamus, and midbrain, and between the cerebral hemispheres, and the paired thalami (Figures 2.1, 2.8, and 2.10). It is intimately related to the circle of Willis and its branches and the great vein of Galen and its tributaries. Craniopharyngiomas may have an intraventricular extension or be primarily intraventricular, and are among the most difficult tumors to expose and remove. Manipulation of the walls of the third ventricle may cause hypothalamic dysfunction, as manifested by disturbances of consciousness, temperature control, respiration, hypophyseal secretion, visual loss due to damage of the optic chiasm and tracts, and memory loss due to injury to the columns of the fornix in the walls of the third ventricle (Rhoton et al., 1981; Yamamoto et al., 1981; Rhoton, 2002).

The third ventricle is a narrow, funnel-shaped, unilocular, midline cavity. It communicates at its anterosuperior margin with each lateral ventricle through the foramen of Monro and posteriorly with the fourth ventricle through the aqueduct of Sylvius. It has a roof, a floor, and an anterior, posterior, and two lateral walls.

The roof of the third ventricle forms a gentle upward arch, extending from the foramen of Monro anteriorly to the suprapineal recess posteriorly. The roof has four layers: one neural layer formed by the fornix, two thin membranous layers of tela choroidea, and a layer of blood vessels between the sheets of tela choroidea. The choroidal fissure extends into the lateral margins of the roof. The upper layer of the anterior part of the roof of the third ventricle is formed by the body of the fornix, and the posterior part of the roof is formed by the crura and the hippocampal commissure. The septum pellucidum is attached to the upper surface of the body of the fornix (Figures 2.1C and D). The tela choroidea forms two of the three layers in the roof below the layer formed by the fornix. The tela choroidea consists of two thin, semiopaque membranes derived from the pia mater, which are interconnected by loosely organized trabeculae. The final layer in the roof is a vascular layer located between the two layers of tela choroidea. The vascular layer consists of the medial posterior choroidal arteries and their branches and the internal cerebral veins and their tributaries. Parallel strands of choroid plexus project downward on each side of the midline from the inferior layer of tela choroidea into the superior part of the third ventricle. The velum interpositum is the space between the two layers of tela choroidea in the roof of the third ventricle. It is located on the medial side of the body portion of the choroidal fissure in the roof of the third ventricle below the body of the fornix and between the superomedial surfaces of the thalami. The upper layer of the tela choroidea is attached to the lower surface of the fornix and the hippocampal commissure. The lower wall has an anterior part that is attached to the small ridges on the free edge of the fiber tracts, called the striae medullaris thalami, which extend along the superomedial borders of the thalami from the foramen of Monro to the habenular commissure. The posterior part of the lower wall is attached to the superior surface of the pineal body. The suprapineal recess of the third ventricle is located between the lower layer of tela choroidea and the upper surface of the pineal body. The paired parallel strands of choroid plexus in the roof of the third ventricle are attached to the lower layer of tela choroidea. Many of the veins draining the frontal horn and body converge on the velum interpositum to form the internal cerebral veins. The internal cerebral veins arise in the anterior part of the velum interpositum, just behind the foramen of Monro, and they exit the velum interpositum above the pineal body to enter the quadrigeminal cistern and join the great vein. The velum interpositum is usually a closed space that tapers to a narrow apex just behind the foramen of Monro, but it may infrequently have an opening situated between the splenium and pineal body that communicates with the quadrigeminal cistern to form the cisterna velum interpositum. There also may be a space above the velum interpositum between the hippocampal commissure and splenium called the cavum vergae.

The floor extends from the optic chiasm anteriorly to the orifice of the aqueduct of Sylvius posteriorly. The anterior half of the floor is formed by diencephalic structures, and the posterior half is formed by mesencephalic structures. When viewed inferiorly, the structures forming the floor include, from anterior to posterior, the optic chiasm, infundibulum of the hypothalamus, tuber cinereum, mamillary bodies, posterior perforated substance, and the part of the tegmentum of the midbrain located above the medial aspect of the cerebral peduncles. The optic chiasm is located at the junction of the floor and the anterior wall of the third ventricle. The chiasm slopes posteriorly and superiorly from its junction with the optic nerves. The inferior surface of the chiasm forms the anterior part of the floor, and the superior surface forms the lower part of the anterior wall. The optic tracts arise from the posterolateral margin of the chiasm and course obliquely away from the floor toward the lateral margin of the upper part of the midbrain. The infundibulum, tuber cinereum, mamillary bodies, and posterior perforated substance are located in the space limited anteriorly and laterally by the optic chiasm and tracts, and posteriorly by the cerebral peduncles. The infundibulum of the hypothalamus is a hollow, funnel-shaped structure located between the optic chiasm and the tuber cinereum. The pituitary gland (hypophysis) is attached to the infundibulum, and the axons in the infundibulum extend to the posterior lobe of the hypophysis. The tuber cinereum is a prominent mass of hypothalamic gray matter located anterior to the mamillary bodies. The tuber cinereum merges anteriorly into the infundibulum. The tuber cinereum around the base of the infundibulum is raised to form a prominence called the median eminence. The mamillary bodies form paired, round prominences posterior to the tuber cinereum. The posterior perforated substance is a depressed, punctuated area of gray matter located in the interval between the mamillary bodies anteriorly and the medial surface of the cerebral peduncles posteriorly. The posterior part of the floor extends posterior and superior to the medial part of the cerebral peduncles and superior to the tegmentum of the midbrain.

When viewed from above and inside the third ventricle, the optic chiasm forms a prominence at the anterior margin of the floor (Figure 2.10G). The infundibular recess extends into the infundibulum behind the optic chiasm. The mamillary bodies form paired prominences on the inner surface of the floor posterior to the infundibular recess. The part of the floor between the mamillary bodies and the aqueduct of Sylvius has a smooth surface that is concave from side to side. This smooth surface lies above the posterior perforated substance anteriorly and the medial part of the cerebral peduncles and the tegmentum of the midbrain posteriorly.

The anterior margin of the third ventricle extends from the foramina of Monro above to the optic chiasm below. Only the lower two-thirds of the anterior surface are seen on the external surface of the brain; the upper third is hidden posterior to the rostrum of the corpus callosum. The part of the anterior wall visible on the surface is formed by the optic chiasm and the lamina terminalis. The lamina terminalis is a thin sheet of gray matter and pia mater that attaches to the upper surface of the chiasm and stretches upward to fill the interval between the optic chiasm and the rostrum of the corpus callosum.

When viewed from within, the boundaries of the anterior wall are formed, from superior to inferior, by the columns of the fornix, foramina of Monro, anterior commissure, lamina terminalis, optic recess, and optic chiasm. The foramen of Monro on each side is located at the junction of the roof and the anterior wall. The foramen is a duct-like canal that opens between the fornix and the thalami into each lateral ventricle and extends inferiorly below the fornix into the third ventricle as a single channel. The foramen of Monro is bounded anteriorly by the junction of the body and the columns of the fornix and posteriorly by the anterior pole of the thalamus. The size and shape of the foramina of Monro depend on the size of the ventricles: if they are small, each foramen is a crescent-shaped opening bounded anteriorly by the concave curve of the fornix and posteriorly by the convex anterior tubercle of the thalamus. As the ventricles enlarge, the foramen on each side becomes rounder. The structures that pass through the foramen are the choroid plexus, the distal branches of the medial posterior choroidal arteries, and the thalamostriate, superior choroidal, and septal veins. The anterior commissure is a compact bundle of fibers that crosses the midline in front of the columns of the fornix. The anterior-posterior diameter of the anterior commissure varies from 1.5 to 6.0 mm. In our specimens, the distance from the posterior end of the anterior commissure to the anterior border of the foramen of Monro ranged from 1.0 to 3.5 mm (average, 2.2 mm), and the distance from the upper edge of the optic chiasm to the anterior border of the anterior commissure ranged from 8 to 12 mm (average, 10 mm). The lamina terminalis fills the interval between the anterior commissure and the optic chiasm. The lamina attaches to the midportion of the superior surface of the chiasm, leaving a small cleft between the upper half of the chiasm and the lamina, called the optic recess.

The posterior wall of the third ventricle extends from the suprapineal recess above to the aqueduct below. When viewed from anteriorly and within the third ventricle, it consists, from above to below, of the suprapineal recess, habenular commissure, pineal body and its recess, posterior commissure, and aqueduct of Sylvius. The suprapineal recess projects posteriorly between the upper surface of the pineal gland and the lower layer of tela choroidea in the roof. The pineal gland extends posteriorly into the quadrigeminal cistern from its stalk, which has an upper and a lower lamina. The habenular commissure, which interconnects the habenulae, crosses the midline in the upper lamina, and the posterior commissure crosses in the lower lamina. The pineal recess projects posteriorly into the pineal body between the two laminae. The shape of the orifice of the aqueduct of Sylvius is triangular, with its base on the posterior commissure and the other two limbs formed by the central gray matter of the midbrain. When viewed from posteriorly, the only structure in the posterior wall is the pineal body. The pineal gland projects posteriorly into the quadrigeminal cisterns and is concealed by the splenium of the corpus callosum above, the thalamus laterally, and the quadrigeminal plate and the vermis of the cerebellum inferiorly.

The lateral walls are not visible on the external surface of the brain, but are hidden between the cerebral hemispheres. They are formed by the hypothalamus inferiorly and the thalamus superiorly. The lateral walls when viewed from laterally have an outline like the lateral silhouette of a bird's head with an open beak. The head is formed by the oval medial surface of the thalamus. The open beak, which projects anteriorly and inferiorly, is formed by the recesses in the hypothalamus. The pointed upper beak is formed by the optic recess and the lower beak is formed by the infundibular recess. The hypothalamic and thalamic surfaces are separated by the hypothalamic sulcus, a groove that is often ill-defined and extends from the foramen of Monro to the aqueduct of Sylvius. The superior limit of the thalamic surfaces of the third ventricle is marked by narrow, raised ridges, known as the striae medullaris thalami. These striae extend forward from the habenulae along the superomedial surface of the thalamus near the attachment of the lower layer of the tela choroidea. The habenulae are small eminences on the dorsomedial surfaces of the thalamus just in front of the pineal gland. The habenulae are connected across the midline in the rostral stalk of the pineal gland by the habenular commissure.

The massa intermedia projects into the upper half of the third ventricle and often connects the opposing surfaces of the thalamus. It is present in approximately 75% of brains, being located 2.5 to 6.0 mm (average, 3.9 mm) posterior to the foramen of Monro. The columns of the fornix form distinct prominences in the lateral walls of the third ventricle just below the foramina of Monro, but inferiorly they sink below the surface.

ANATOMY OF SURGICAL APPROACHES FOR CRANIOPHARYNGIOMAS

Craniopharyngiomas have usually been approached through craniotomies. Improvement in endoscopy and closure techniques with vascularized flaps has increased the use and safety of endoscopic endonasal approaches for craniopharyngiomas (Kassam et al., 2008; Koutourousiou et al., 2013). The approach to a craniopharyngioma is selected on the basis of the surgical anatomy and extension of the tumor as well as experience and training of the neurosurgeon. The endoscope can also be used to improve the surgical view in a craniotomy.

Surgical Anatomy of Craniotomy Approaches and Endoscopic Assistance

The subfrontal, supraorbital, pterional, frontotemporal, subtemporal, and orbitozygomatic approaches have been used to approach craniopharyngiomas (Figure 2.11) (Rhoton, 2002;

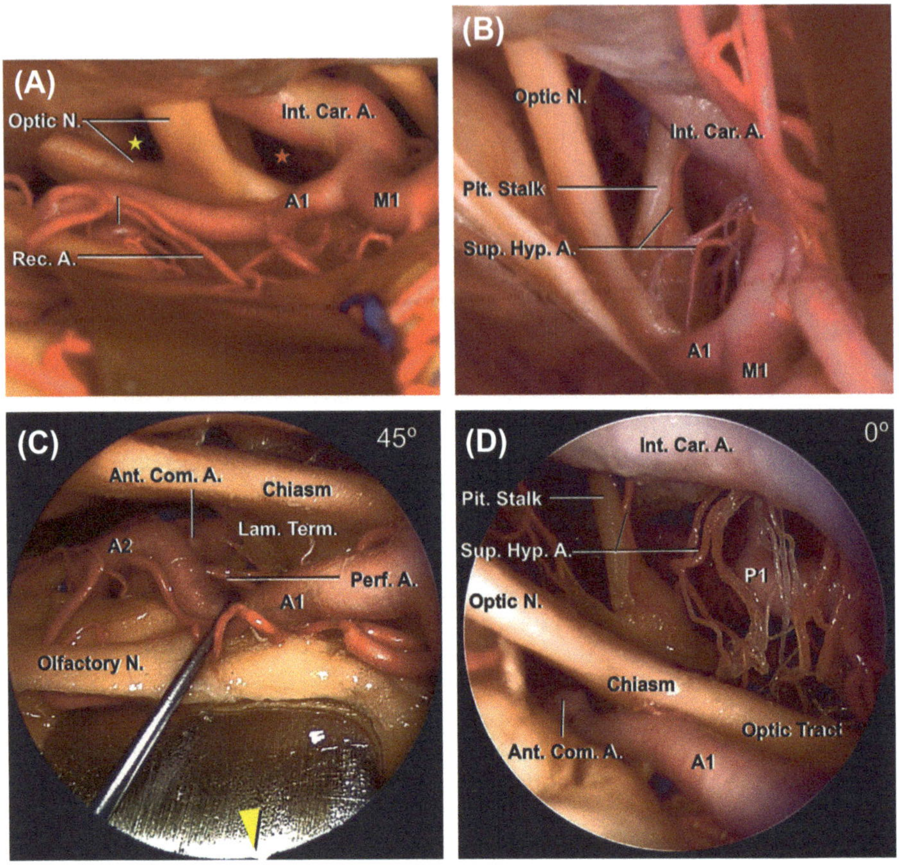

FIGURE 2.11 Surgical anatomy of craniotomy approaches for craniopharyngiomas. Microscopic and endoscopic views with pterional (**A–F**) and subfrontal interhemispheric approaches (**G–I**). **A,** Microscopic view of a pterional approach. The optic nerves and chiasm, and the carotid artery and its bifurcation are exposed. The best surgical corridor for most craniopharyngiomas is through the subchiasmatic route (yellow star) or through the opticocarotid window (red star), located between the optic nerve and carotid artery. **B,** View of the pituitary stalk and perforating arteries supplying the pituitary stalk, hypothalamus, and chiasm through the opticocarotid window. **C,** Endoscopic assisted image through a pterional approach with the 45° endoscope oriented towards the surgeon showing the chiasm, lamina terminalis, and A1 and A2. The endoscope aids in exposing the supra- and retrosellar structures and the perforating arteries. The yellow triangles indicate the orientation of the lens with the angled endoscopes. **D,** Enlarged view of the opticocarotid window with a 0° endoscope showing the superior hypophyseal arteries and P1 segment. **E,** 30° Endoscopic view showing the lamina terminalis and anterior communicating artery complex over the optic chiasm. The endoscope aids in exposing the areas above and below the optic chiasm. **F,** Endoscopic view of the medial side of the carotid artery and the area below the optic nerve with a 30° endoscope. This view, not available with the microscope, is especially useful in craniopharyngioma resection. **G,** Subfrontal interhemispheric approach exposing the optic chiasm and pituitary stalk. **H–I,** The endoscope improves the visualization of the arteries and other structures in the subchiasmatic region. A., artery; Car., carotid; Com., communicating; Hyp., hypophyseal; Int., internal; Lam., lamina; N., nerve; Pit., pituitary; Sup., superior; Term., terminalis.

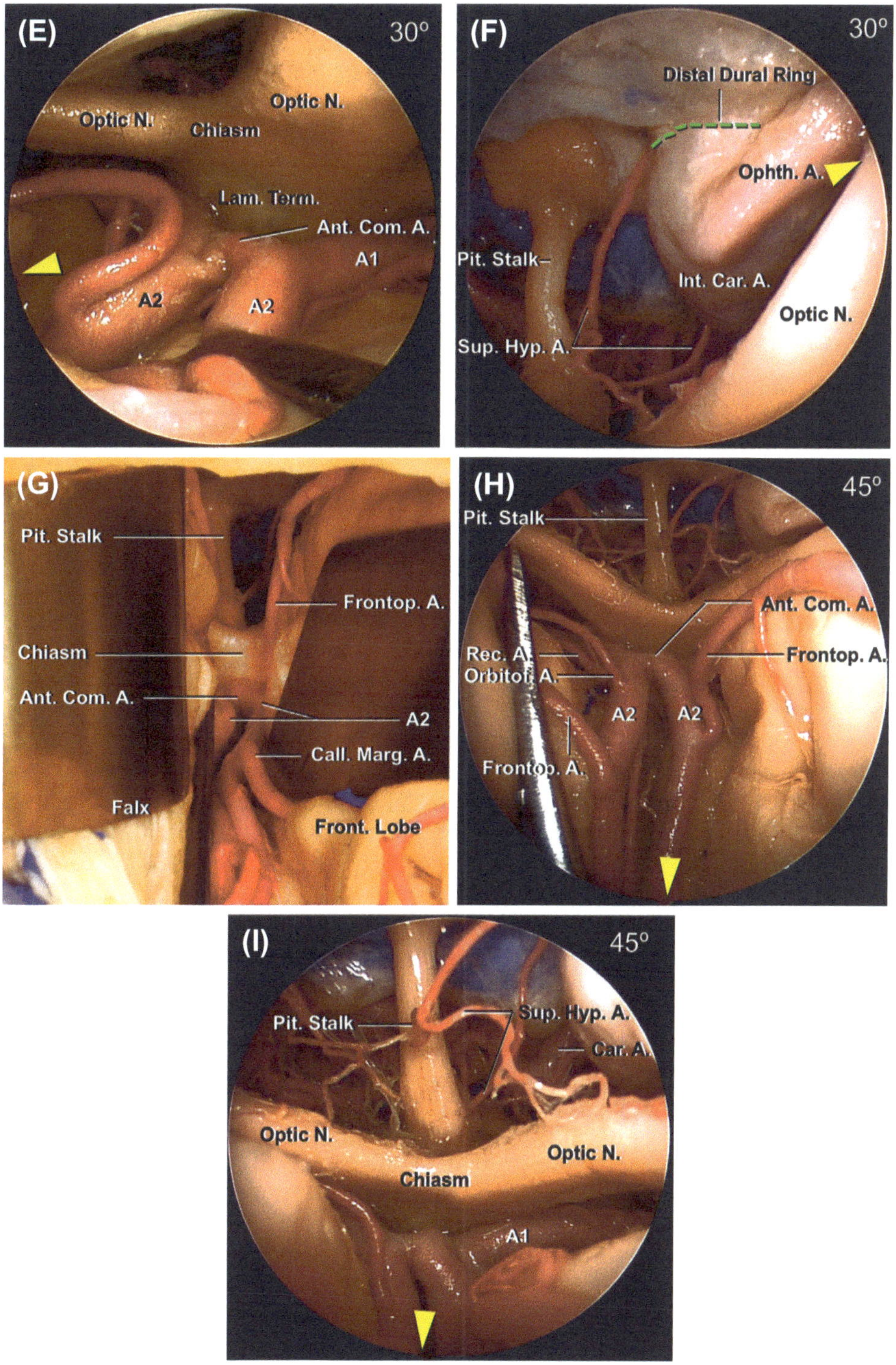

FIGURE 2.11 cont'd

Gerganov et al., 2013). A tumor situated between, above, or below the optic nerves and chiasm in the chiasmatic and lamina terminalis cisterns may be approached through a small frontal bone flap with frontal lobe elevation to expose the involved optic nerves and chiasm. The bicoronal (Souttar) scalp incision from the subfrontal approach is located behind the hairline. The scalp flap is reflected forward as a single layer and a small frontal bone flap is positioned just above the supraorbital margin and extending up to the lateral edge of the superior sagittal sinus. The lateral burr hole, above the orbital rim, is positioned at the keyhole site and the medial burr hole usually extends through the front and back wall of the frontal sinus. The craniotomy can be extended bilaterally or enlarged as needed. Elevating both frontal lobes may improve access to the interhemispheric area. The subfrontal approach is used for lesions located between the upper surface of the pituitary gland and lower surface of the optic nerves and chiasm. If there is an intraventricular extension, the tumor could be removed through the lamina terminalis. A pterional or orbitozygomatic craniotomy would be performed if there was a need to expose the area lateral to the anterior clinoid process and supraclinoid segment of the internal carotid artery. This frontotemporal route provides better access for the opticocarotid approach directed between the carotid artery and the optic nerve, while permitting access by the lamina terminalis approach directed above the chiasm and the subchiasmatic approach used if the tumor elevates the chiasm and opens the space between the optic nerves and chiasm. The opticocarotid approach would be used if the tumor opened or protruded through the space between the optic nerve and carotid artery and the tumor was difficult to reach by the subchiasmatic approach. The lamina terminalis approach would be selected if the chiasm was prefixed and the tumor presented through a thin stretched lamina terminalis. The subfrontal route provides a more direct anterior approach for the subchiasmatic and lamina terminalis exposures. However, these exposures can be accessed from a more lateral and oblique trajectory in the frontotemporal approaches. The endoscope can be used as an adjuvant in open approaches. Straight and angled endoscopes complement and improve the microscopic view in certain areas with both the subfrontal and the pterional-orbitozygomatic approaches as described for vascular surgery (Peris-Celda et al., 2013).

Surgical Anatomy of the Endoscopic Endonasal Approach

Comprehensive knowledge of the nasal anatomy is paramount for surgeons who perform endoscopic endonasal surgeries. The fundamentals of the endonasal approach and resection of craniopharyngiomas are based on the transsphenoidal approach (Figure 2.12) (Kassam et al., 2008). Small craniopharyngiomas in the sella and adjacent suprasellar space can be removed through the same type of transsphenoidal exposure directed through the anterior sellar wall that is used for small pituitary tumors. However, larger tumors with suprasellar, parasellar, or presellar extensions will require a large opening and the more complex closure described below. The identification of the natural ostium of the sphenoid sinus is the first step. With a 0° endoscope, the ostium is identified at the sphenoethmoidal recess, usually situated medial to the superior turbinate. If a supreme turbinate is present, the ostium can be located between the superior and the supreme turbinate. Rarely is it found lateral to the superior turbinate. To reach the sphenoethmoidal recess, it is important to expand the space inside the nose. Pushing or displacing the inferior and middle turbinates laterally (lateralizing) improves access, visualization, and room for the advancement of instruments inside the nasal cavity. Lateralizing

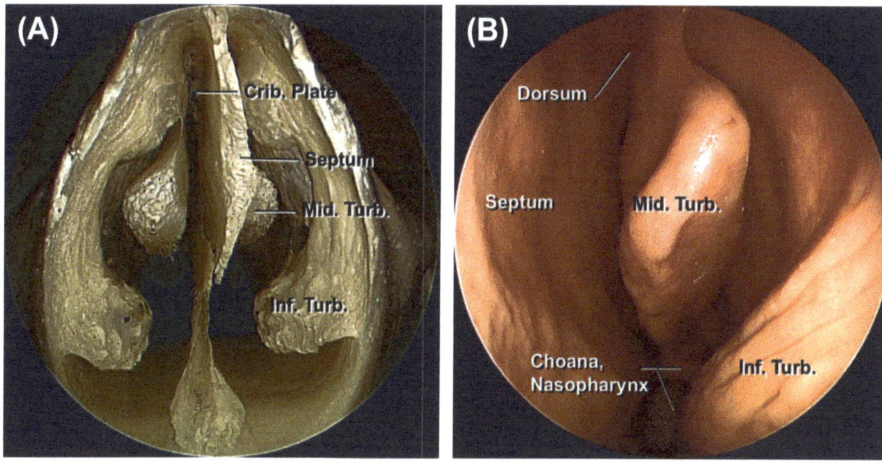

FIGURE 2.12 **Endoscopic endonasal approach for craniopharyngioma surgery. A–F,** Images of the nasal cavity obtained with a 0° endoscope in a dry skull (left) and equivalent image in an anatomical specimen (right). **A,** Anterior view through the piriform aperture. The septum separates the nasal cavity in the midline. The inferior and middle turbinates are exposed. **B,** The endoscope is introduced through the left nostril. The septum is located on the left side of the image. The middle and inferior turbinates protrude from the lateral wall of the nasal cavity. The choana or posterior nasal aperture opens into the nasopharynx. **C** and **D,** Anterior view of the middle meatus. The first prominence seen below and lateral to the middle turbinate is the uncinate process and behind it is the bulla ethmoidalis formed by the anterior ethmoid cells. The middle turbinate is usually resected or lateralized to enlarge the surgical corridor. **E** and **F,** The sphenoid ostium is exposed posteriorly between the superior turbinate and septum. **G,** The sphenoid rostrum and crest are reliable landmarks for locating the midline. The sphenoid ostia are medial to the superior turbinates. Compare how the access to the sphenoid sinus is enlarged with the left posterior ethmoidectomy. **H,** Example of bilateral Onodi cells, an anatomical variation in which the ethmoid sinus pneumatizes posteriorly above the sphenoid sinus. The optic canals protrude into the Onodi cells. Care must be taken not to damage the optic nerves in the walls of the Onodi cells. **I,** View of the anteior wall of the sphenoid sinus after bilateral posterior ethmoidectomies. **J,** View of the sphenoid septations which often cross the carotid artery prominences posteriorly. **K,** Anatomic landmarks in the sphenoid sinus. The sellar prominence is in the center, with carotid prominences laterally, and optic canals superiorly. **L,** Endonasal access to resect craniopharyngiomas often requires drilling of the bone of the sellar wall, planum, and tuberculum. In this dissection, the periosteal layer of the dura covering the gland has been resected while preserving the meningeal layer. **M,** The dura covering sellar and cavernous sinuses has been removed to expose the gland and carotid arteries. **N,** The diaphragma sellae has been removed to expose the pituitary stalk and optic chiasm. **O,** Opening the lamina terminalis allows removal of tumor in the third ventricle endoscopically. The A1 segment of the anterior cerebral artery is exposed superiorly. **P,** Enlarged view of the third ventricle. The foramina of Monro and aqueduct are exposed. **Q,** Transposition of the pituitary gland superiorly allows drilling of the dorsum and posterior clinoids. **R,** View of the interpeduncular fossa after removing the dorsum and drilling the posterior clinoids. This maneuver gives access to retroinfundibular tumors. A., artery; A.C.A., anterior cerebral artery; Ant., anterior; Bas., basilar; Car., carotid; Cav., cavernous; Clin., clinoid; CN, cranial nerve; Com., communicating; Comm., commissure; Crib., cribriform; Font., fontanelle; For., foramen; Hyp., hypophyseal; Inf., inferior; Intercav., intercavernous; Interm., intermedia; Lat., lateral; M.C.A., middle cerebral artery; Mamm., mamillary; Med., medial; Mening., meningeal; Mid., middle; N., nerve; Opticocar., opticocarotid; Ost., ostium; P.C.A., posterior cerebral artery; Periost., periosteal; Pit., pituitary; Post., posterior; Proc., process; Prom., prominence; Rec., recess; Sem., semilunar; Sphen., sphenoid; Sup., superior; Tuberc., tuberculum; Turb., turbinate; Unc., uncinate.

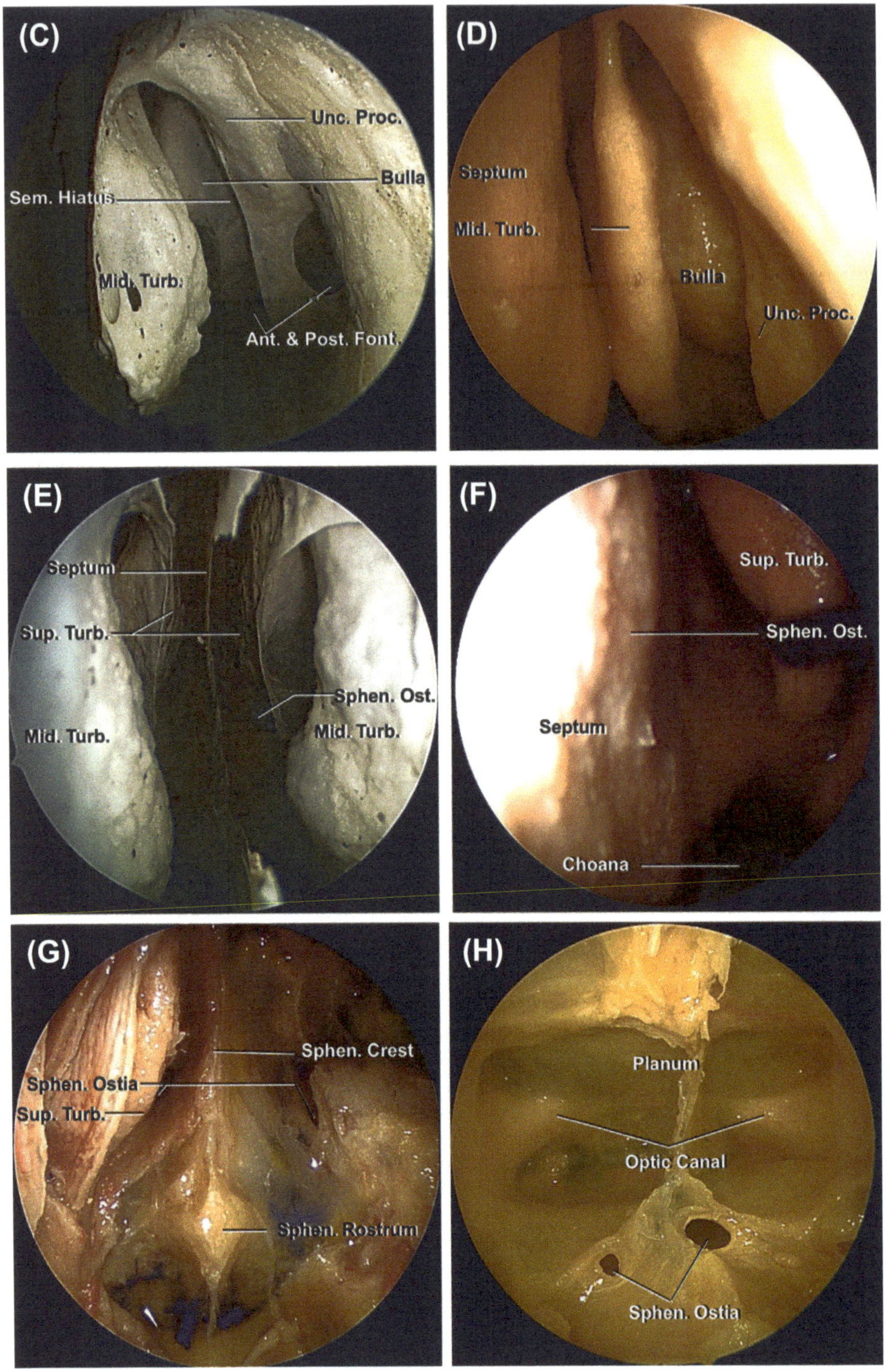

FIGURE 2.12 cont'd

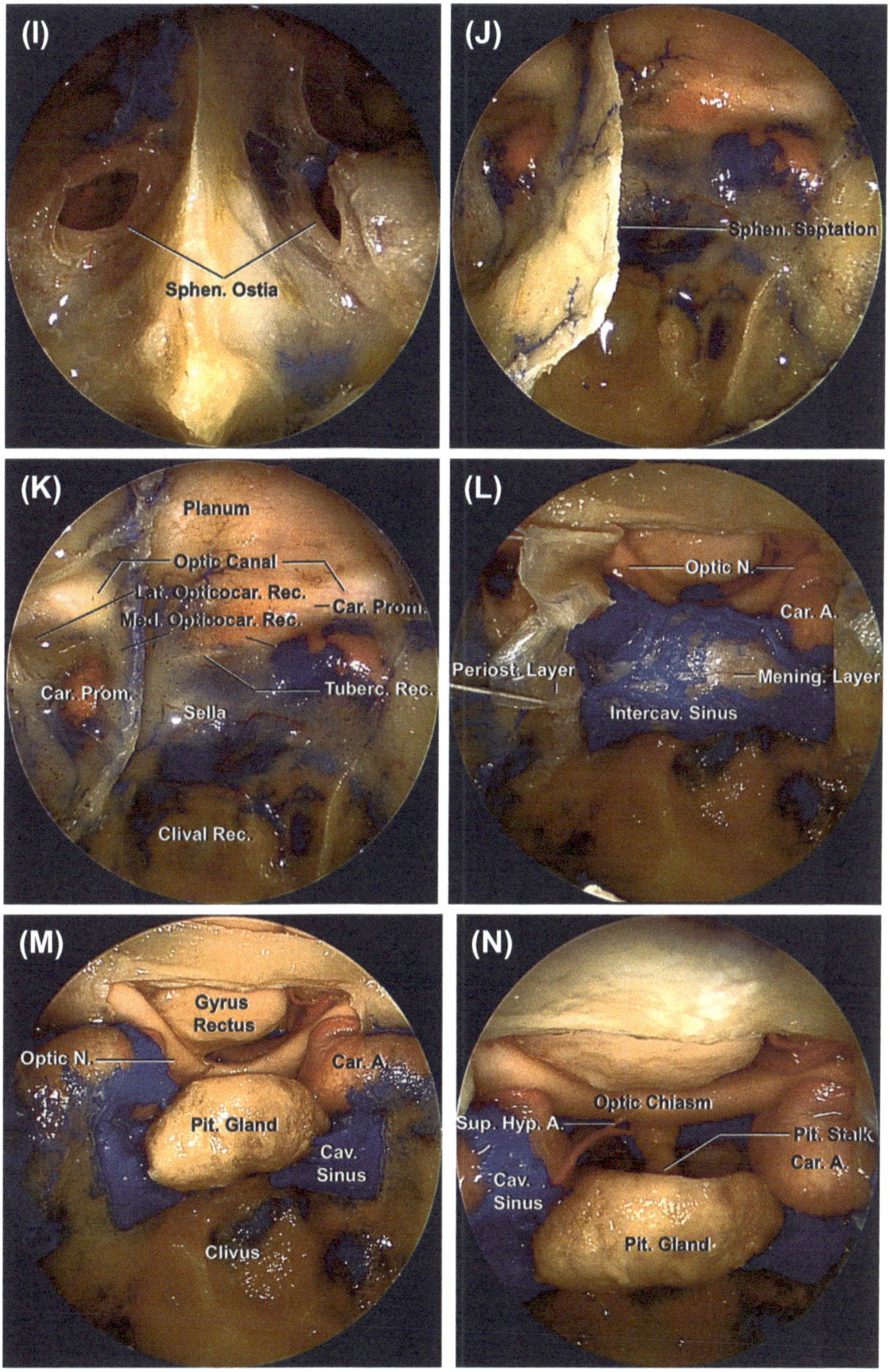

FIGURE 2.12 cont'd

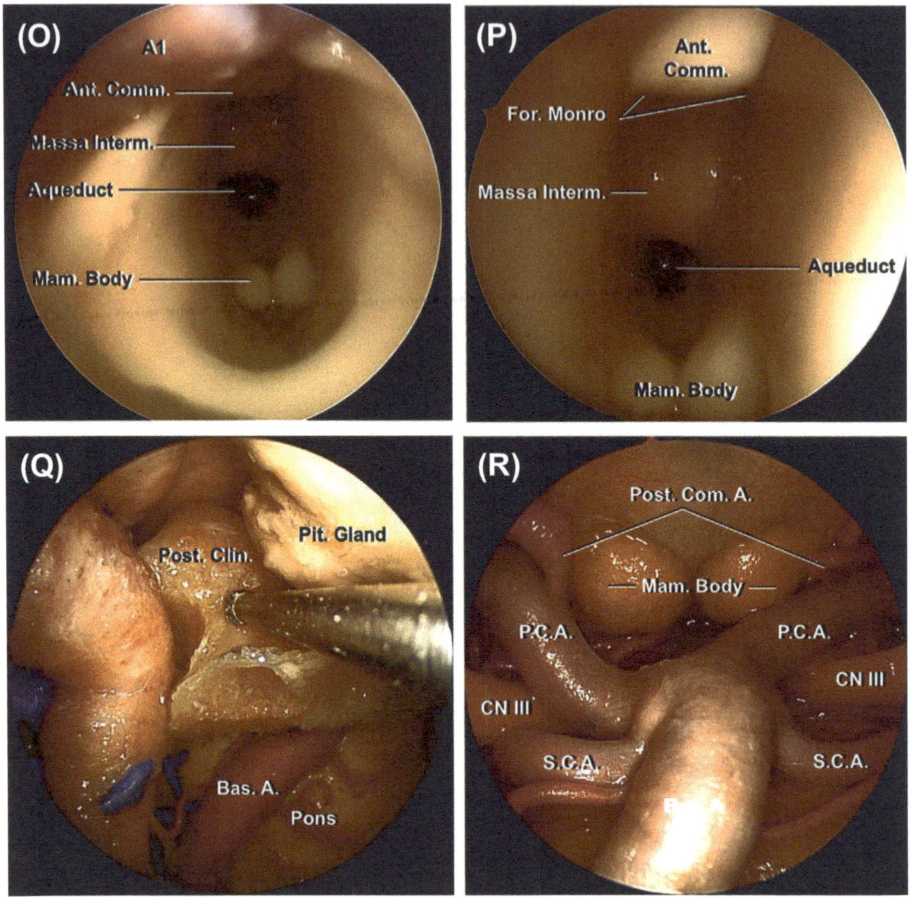

FIGURE 2.12 cont'd

the turbinates should be performed gently, since the fracture line from the inferior turbinate lateralization can extend to the nasolacrimal duct and/or orbit. The nasolacrimal duct drains to the anterior part of the inferior meatus and the bone of the inferior turbinate is usually thicker in that anterior part. The fracture line from the lateralization of the middle turbinate can extend to the skull base and cause a cerebrospinal fluid leak. The surgeon should carefully avoid the mobilization of the turbinate close to the skull base. Once more room is created, the endoscope can be advanced and placed between the nasal septum and the middle turbinate for satisfactory visualization of the sphenoethmoidal recess.

Craniopharyngiomas usually involve the suprasellar space and their resection is usually associated with high-flow intraoperative cerebrospinal fluid leak. Reconstruction with a vascularized nasoseptal flap is often needed to prevent postoperative cerebrospinal fluid leak and meningitis (Hadad et al., 2006; Pinheiro-Neto et al., 2011; Peris-Celda et al., 2013). For a suprasellar lesion like a craniopharyngioma, the decision regarding from which side of the septum to harvest the flap is made based upon the side of the wider opening and/or the absence of septal deviation. Once the flap is harvested and placed in the nasopharynx, the sphenoidotomy is performed. It may be helpful in some cases to consider resection of the superior turbinate and perform a partial retrograde posterior ethmoidectomy, if there is a need to enlarge the sphenoidotomy laterally and expose the lateral wall of the orbit (Figures 2.12G–J). The sphenoidotomy and posterior ethmoidectomy should be extended superiorly up to the skull base in order to expose the planum sphenoidale and optic canals if needed. The pedicle of the septal flap should be displaced off the sphenoid rostrum, and careful drilling of the rostrum is performed to enlarge the sphenoidotomy inferiorly. After those steps are completed, attention should be turned to the contralateral side. It is important to preserve the strip of mucosa on the sphenoid rostrum along which the posterior septal artery runs to supply the septal mucosa. The artery runs from the sphenopalatine foramen and crosses the sphenoid rostrum approximately 9 mm below the sphenoid ostium (Pinheiro-Neto et al., 2011). After the contralateral sphenoid ostium is identified, it is enlarged laterally and superiorly identically to the first side. The septal mucosa above the level of the inferior aspect of the sphenoid ostium can be partially removed to improve binostril visualization and instrumentation. A posterior septectomy should avoid extensive resection of the superior septum, which can result in hyposmia or anosmia. After a wide exposure of the sphenoid sinus is achieved, the sphenoid septations are removed with the drill. It is very important to drill all septations including the ones extending to the floor of the sphenoid sinus. This is important, not just for the approach and manipulation of instruments inside the sinus, but also to create a flat bone surface to receive the septal flap for reconstruction. Then the mucosa from the sphenoid sinus is completely removed.

The main bone that needs to be removed in order to reach the suprasellar space is the tuberculum sella. The opening of the dura of the tuberculum sella gives direct access to the suprasellar region. However it is important to extend the bone removal towards the pituitary fossa and planum sphenoidale, even if the dural opening does not include those areas in order to allow adequate movement of the instruments inside the suprasellar space during the tumor resection. The bone removal is tailored according to the size and location of the lesion and the image guidance system's determination of how much bone to remove. Drilling of the planum sphenoidale is performed in a trapezoid shape medial to the optic canals. The posterior osteotomy is positioned just anterior to the tuberculum sella, and the anterior osteotomy is placed as needed based on the image guidance. After completing all four osteotomies, the island of bone housing the planum sphenoidale is isolated and carefully dissected from the dura. Then the bone over the anterior wall of the sella turcica is removed leaving the bridge of bone on which the tuberculum sits. The tuberculum is carefully resected with a microkerrison rongeur. The lateral limit is the optic canal; however in cases of large craniopharyngiomas, part of the optic canal wall can be removed. Copious irrigation is needed to avoid spread of heat to the optic canal during drilling. Once the dura mater is well exposed, bipolar coagulation of the superior intercavernous sinus is performed and the dura is finally opened to expose the suprasellar space. Once opened, the pituitary stalk, optic chiasm, gyrus rectus, and anterior communicating complex are exposed. The lamina terminalis may be opened to expose the intraventricular portion of the tumor (Figure 2.12O– P). The pituitary gland can be transposed superiorly and medially to allow drilling of the dorsum and adjacent posterior clinoids. The retroinfundibular portion of the tumor in the interpeduncular fossa can be approached (Figure 2.12Q–R).

References

Dunker, R.O., Harris, A.B., 1976 Mar. Surgical anatomy of the proximal anterior cerebral artery. J. Neurosurg. 44 (3), 359–367.

Gerganov, V., Metwali, H., Samii, A., Fahlbusch, R., Samii, M., 2013 Nov 22. Microsurgical resection of extensive craniopharyngiomas using a frontolateral approach: operative technique and outcome. J. Neurosurg.

Gibo, H., Lenkey, C., Rhoton Jr., A.L., 1981 Oct. Microsurgical anatomy of the supraclinoid portion of the internal carotid artery. J. Neurosurg. 55 (4), 560–574.

Hadad, G., Bassagasteguy, L., Carrau, R.L., et al., 2006 Oct. A novel reconstructive technique after endoscopic expanded endonasal approaches: vascular pedicle nasoseptal flap. Laryngoscope 116 (10), 1882–1886.

Halstead, A.E., 1902. Remarks on the operative treatment of tumors of the hypophysis. Surg. Gynecol. Obstet. 494–502.

Harris, F., Rhoton Jr., A.L., 1975. Microsurgical anatomy of the cavernous sinus. Surgical forum 26, 462–463.

Hoffman, H.J., 1990 Jan. Craniopharyngiomas The role for resection. Neurosurg. Clin. N. Am. 1 (1), 173–180.

Kassam, A.B., Gardner, P.A., Snyderman, C.H., Carrau, R.L., Mintz, A.H., Prevedello, D.M., 2008 Apr. Expanded endonasal approach, a fully endoscopic transnasal approach for the resection of midline suprasellar craniopharyngiomas: a new classification based on the infundibulum. J. Neurosurg. 108 (4), 715–728.

Koutourousiou, M., Gardner, P.A., Fernandez-Miranda, J.C., Tyler-Kabara, E.C., Wang, E.W., Snyderman, C.H., 2013 Nov. Endoscopic endonasal surgery for craniopharyngiomas: surgical outcome in 64 patients. J. Neurosurg. 119 (5), 1194–1207.

Ono, M., Rhoton Jr., A.L., Barry, M., 1984 Feb. Microsurgical anatomy of the region of the tentorial incisura. J. Neurosurg. 60 (2), 365–399.

Park, S.W., Jung, H.W., Lee, Y.A., Shin, C.H., Yang, S.W., Cheon, J.E., Kim, I.O., Phi, J.H., Kim, S.K., Wang, K.C., 2013 Jul. Tumor origin and growth pattern at diagnosis and surgical hypothalamic damage predict obesity in pediatric craniopharyngioma. J. Neuro.Oncol. 113 (3), 417–424.

Peris-Celda, M., Kucukyuruk, B., Monroy-Sosa, A., Funaki, T., Valentine, R., Rhoton Jr., A.L., 2013 Feb 19. The recesses of the sellar wall of the sphenoid sinus and their intracranial relationships. Neurosurgery.

Peris-Celda, M.P.-N.C., Funaki, T., Fernandez-Miranda, J.C., Gardner, P., Snyderman, C., Rhoton, A.L., 2013. The extended nasoseptal flap for skull base reconstruction of the clival region: an anatomical and radiological study. Journal of Neurological Surgery Part B: Skull Base 74 (6), 369–386.

Peris-Celda, M., Da Roz, L., Monroy-Sosa, A., Morishita, T., Rhoton Jr., A.L., 2014. Surgical anatomy of endoscopic assisted approaches to common aneurysm sites. Neurosurgery 10 (suppl. 1), 121–144.

Perlmutter, D., Rhoton Jr., A.L., 1976 Sep. Microsurgical anatomy of the anterior cerebral-anterior communicating-recurrent artery complex. J. Neurosurg. 45 (3), 259–272.

Pinheiro-Neto, C.D., Ramos, H.F., Peris-Celda, M., et al., 2011 Dec. Study of the nasoseptal flap for endoscopic anterior cranial base reconstruction. Laryngoscope 121 (12), 2514–2520.

Renn, W.H., Rhoton Jr., A.L., 1975 Sep. Microsurgical anatomy of the sellar region. J. Neurosurg. 43 (3), 288–298.

Rhoton Jr., A.L., 2000 Sep. Jugular foramen. Neurosurgery 47 (Suppl. 3), S267–S285.

Rhoton Jr., A.L., 2000 Sep. Tentorial incisura. Neurosurgery 47 (Suppl. 3), S131–S153.

Rhoton Jr., A.L., 2000 Sep. The foramen magnum. Neurosurgery 47 (Suppl. 3), S155–S193.

Rhoton Jr., A.L., 2002 Oct. The anterior and middle cranial base. Neurosurgery 51 (Suppl. 4), S273–S302.

Rhoton Jr., A.L., 2002 Oct. The cavernous sinus, the cavernous venous plexus, and the carotid collar. Neurosurgery 51 (Suppl. 4), S375–S410.

Rhoton Jr., A.L., 2002 Oct. The lateral and third ventricles. Neurosurgery 51 (Suppl. 4), S207–S271.

Rhoton Jr., A.L., 2002 Oct. The sellar region. Neurosurgery 51 (Suppl. 4), S335–S374.

Rhoton Jr., A.L., 2002 Oct. The supratentorial arteries. Neurosurgery 51 (Suppl. 4), S53–120.

Rhoton Jr., A.L., Perlmutter, D., 1980. Microsurgical anatomy of anterior communicating artery aneurysms. Neurol. Res. 2 (3–4), 217–251.

Rhoton Jr., A.L., Fujii, K., Fradd, B., 1979 Aug. Microsurgical anatomy of the anterior choroidal artery. Surg. Neurol. 12 (2), 171–187.

Rhoton Jr., A.L., Hardy, D.G., Chambers, S.M., 1979 Jul. Microsurgical anatomy and dissection of the sphenoid bone, cavernous sinus and sellar region. Surg. Neurol. 12 (1), 63–104.

Rhoton Jr., A.L., Yamamoto, I., Peace, D.A., 1981 Mar. Microsurgery of the third ventricle: Part 2. Operative approaches. Neurosurgery 8 (3), 357–373.

Rhoton ALJN, Y., 1996. The orbit and sellar region: microsurgical anatomy and operative approaches. Thieme Medical Publishers Inc, New York, 3–25.
Rhoton, A.L.J., 2000. The temporal bone and transtemporal approaches. Neurosurgery 47 (Suppl. 3), S211–S265.
Saeki, N., Rhoton Jr., A.L., 1977 May. Microsurgical anatomy of the upper basilar artery and the posterior circle of Willis. J. Neurosurg. 46 (5), 563–578.
Snyderman, C.H., Pant, H., Carrau, R.L., Prevedello, D., Gardner, P., Kassam, A.B., 2009 Sep. What are the limits of endoscopic sinus surgery? The expanded endonasal approach to the skull base. Keio. J. Med. 58 (3), 152–160.
Stamm, A.C.D.W. (Ed.), 2000. Micro-endoscopic surgery of the paranasal sinus and the skull base. Springer, Heidelberg.
Steno, J., Malacek, M., Bizik, I., 2004 May. Tumor-third ventricular relationships in supradiaphragmatic craniopharyngiomas: correlation of morphological, magnetic resonance imaging, and operative findings. Neurosurgery 54 (5), 1051–1058 discussion 8–60.
Wang, K.C., Hong, S.H., Kim, S.K., Cho, B.K., 2005 Aug. Origin of craniopharyngiomas: implication on the growth pattern. Childs. Nerv. Syst. 21 (8–9), 628–634.
Wang, J., Bidari, S., Inoue, K., Yang, H., Rhoton Jr., A., 2010 Apr. Extensions of the sphenoid sinus: a new classification. Neurosurgery 66 (4), 797–816.
Yamamoto, I., Rhoton Jr., A.L., Peace, D.A., 1981 Mar. Microsurgery of the third ventricle: Part I. Microsurgical anatomy. Neurosurgery 8 (3), 334–356.

CHAPTER

3

Imaging of Craniopharyngiomas and Radiologic Differential Diagnosis

David P. Friedman, Ashish R. Gandhe

Jefferson Medical College and Thomas Jefferson University Hospital, Philadelphia, PA, USA

"It is hoped that improved imaging may help to determine which tumors are amenable to safe removal." ***EG Fischer et al., 1990***

INTRODUCTION

Craniopharyngiomas (Figures 3.1–3.15) are benign, epithelially derived neoplasms that arise from remnants of Rathke's pouch epithelium. This pouch appears during the fourth gestational week and arises as a dorsal diverticulum from the stomatodeum (primitive oral cavity) lined by epithelial cells of ectodermal origin. The epithelium of Rathke's pouch is the precursor of the adenohypophysis of the pituitary gland, including the anterior lobe, intermediate lobe, and pars tuberalis. Rathke's pouch extends cranially to form the craniopharyngeal duct. Obliteration of the craniopharyngeal duct is associated with involution of the pouch to a narrow Rathke's cleft, which ordinarily regresses. The embryology of Rathke's pouch mirrors the appearance and location of its most important associated lesions – craniopharyngioma and Rathke cleft cyst (Tavangar et al., 2004; Prabhu & Brown, 2005; Trifanescu et al., 2012). Indeed, it has been suggested that there is a continuum between epithelial cystic lesions of the sellar region (Harrrison et al., 1994; Wolfe & Heros, 2010).

Craniopharyngiomas have the most heterogeneous radiologic appearance of any suprasellar neoplasm. Two distinct pathologic types exist (adamantinomatous and papillary) (Prabhu & Brown, 2005). Craniopharyngiomas may be cystic, solid, or mixed cystic-solid; moreover, the cystic and to a lesser extent the solid portions can demonstrate variable density on CT imaging, and variable signal characteristics on MR imaging (Karnaze et al., 1986; Pusey et al., 1987; Eldevik et al., 1996; Wolfe & Heros, 2010). On occasion, tumor cysts may show fluid–fluid levels (Abrahams et al., 1989). Craniopharyngiomas can be calcified or noncalcified. Although a suprasellar location is most common, these neoplasms can also arise primarily in the sella; rarely, they can arise in unusual locations such as the third ventricle,

Craniopharyngiomas
http://dx.doi.org/10.1016/B978-0-12-416706-3.00003-9

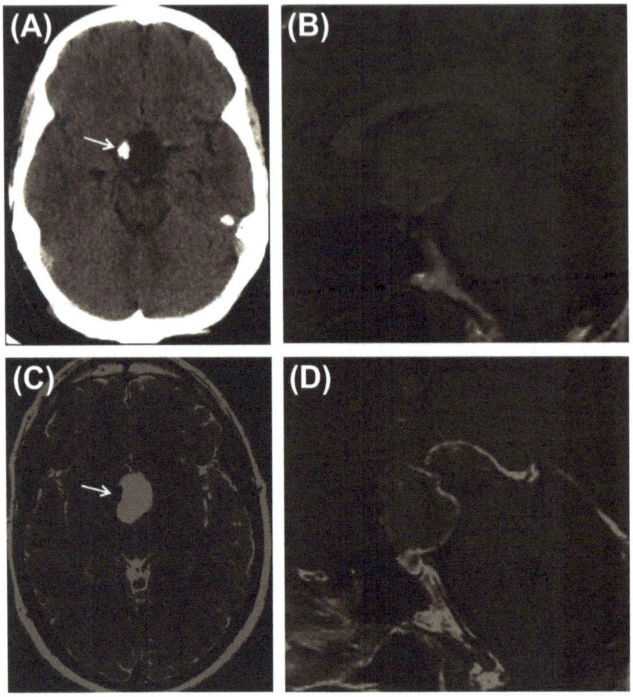

FIGURE 3.1 **A 33-year-old man with suprasellar adamantinomatous craniopharyngioma. A,** Axial, non-contrast CT image shows a hypodense, suprasellar cystic mass measuring 20 Hounsfield units in density, with a peripheral, nodular focus of calcification (arrow). The calcification is not typically seen with a Rathke cleft cyst. **B,** Sagittal, T1-weighted MR image shows a lobulated, moderately hyperintense, suprasellar mass. **C,** Axial, T2--weighted MR image shows focal hypointensity (arrow) corresponding to the calcification seen on CT imaging. **D,** Sagittal, T1-weighted enhanced MR image shows peripheral enhancement of the mass. The enhancement is not typically seen with a Rathke cleft cyst.

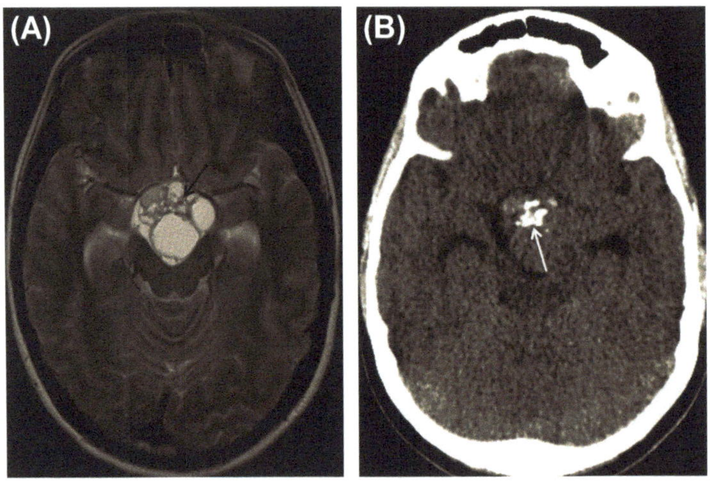

FIGURE 3.2 **A 22-year-old man with suprasellar adamantinomatous craniopharyngioma. A,** Axial, T2-weighted MR image shows a complex, multicystic, suprasellar mass. The cysts have variable signal intensity, primarily reflecting different protein concentrations. Areas of hypointensity (arrow) are related to calcification. The mass splays the cerebral peduncles. **B,** Axial, non-contrast CT image shows calcifications (arrow) corresponding to the areas of hypointensity on MR imaging.

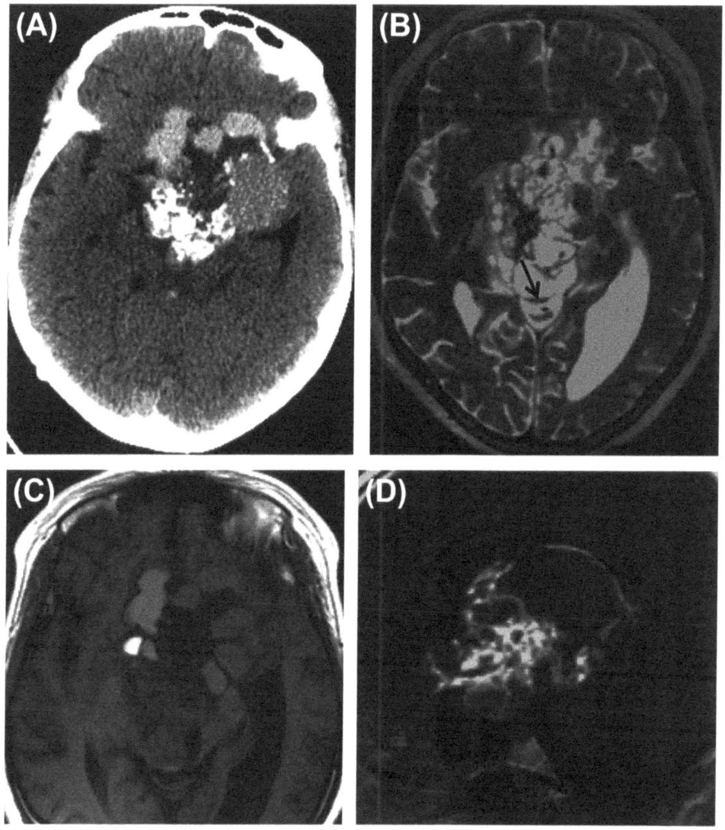

FIGURE 3.3 **An 18-year-old man with intrasellar and suprasellar adamantinomatous craniopharyngioma. A,** Axial, non-contrast CT image shows a massive, calcified, cystic, and solid suprasellar mass. The cysts have variable density, ranging from 23–60 Hounsfield units. Both the solid and cystic portions of the tumor show calcification. **B,** Axial, T2-weighted MR image shows that the hyperdense cysts are relatively hypointense, whereas the hypodense cysts are hyperintense. A posterior cyst invaginates into the midbrain, and shows a small fluid–fluid level (arrow). Edema is seen adjacent to the posterior and right lateral portion of the tumor. **C,** Axial, T1-weighted MR image also shows complex signal characteristics of the cysts. The hyperdense cysts show variable hyperintensity. **D,** Sagittal, T1-weighted, enhanced MR image shows extensive, heterogeneous enhancement of the tumor.

sphenoid sinus, or nasopharynx (Kanungo et al., 1995; Deutsch et al., 2001; Behari et al., 2003). Craniopharyngiomas can be small and clinically inconsequential, or massive and life-threatening, with large lesions simultaneously involving the anterior, middle, and posterior cranial fossae (Sener, 1993). Although histologically benign, they can locally invade the brain parenchyma and cause vasogenic edema (Saeki et al., 2003). Leakage of cyst contents into the subarachnoid space or ventricular system can result in chemical meningitis (Kulkarni et al., 2000). Rarely, remote recurrences have been reported by direct

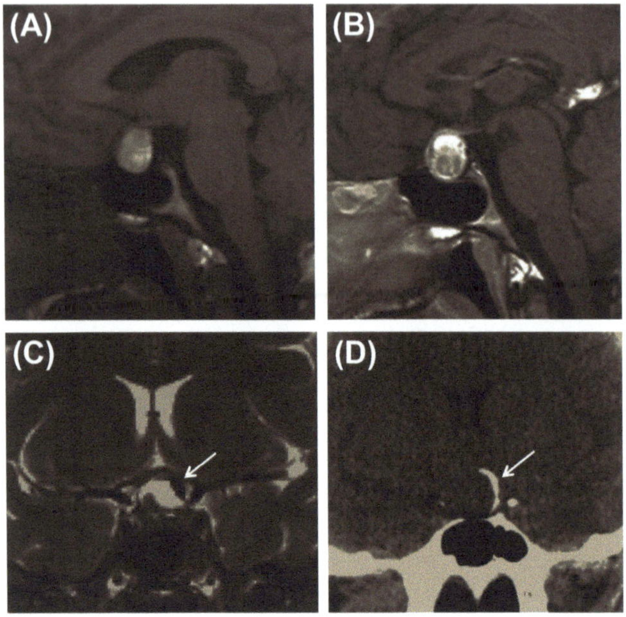

FIGURE 3.4 **A 29-year-old woman with intrasellar and suprasellar adamantinomatous craniopharyngioma.** **A,** Sagittal, T1-weighted MR image shows a hyperintense, intrasellar, and suprasellar cystic mass elevating the optic chiasm. **B,** Sagittal, T1-weighted enhanced MR image shows peripheral enhancement of the tumor; this is not typically seen with a Rathke cleft cyst. **C,** Coronal, T2-weighted MR image shows complex signal within the mass; crescentic hypointensity (arrow) along the left lateral border represents calcification, and essentially excludes the diagnosis of complex pituitary adenoma/pituitary apoplexy. **D,** Coronal, non-contrast CT image confirms the presence of crescentic, peripheral calcification (arrow). This pattern of calcification can also be seen in aneurysms, but is rare in Rathke cleft cysts.

transplantation of tumor or presumed seeding of the subarachnoid spaces (Gupta et al., 1999; Ito et al., 2001; Bianco et al., 2006). Since the suprasellar cistern is home to a large number of other neoplasms, as well as developmental, vascular, and inflammatory lesions, the multitude of potential appearances of craniopharyngioma can offer a formidable challenge in arriving at the correct diagnosis. Fortunately, knowledge of the appearances of craniopharyngiomas on imaging studies, along with the complementary roles played by CT and MR imaging in the evaluation of intrasellar and suprasellar lesions, enable the interpreting physician to arrive at an accurate and relatively short differential diagnosis in most cases.

IMAGING – GENERAL CONCEPTS

Optimal interpretation of any neuroradiologic imaging study requires knowledge of the demographics of relevant lesions. Craniopharyngiomas account for approximately 3% of all intracranial neoplasms. However, they are the most common non-glial brain tumor in children. There is no sex predominance. There is a bimodal age distribution of

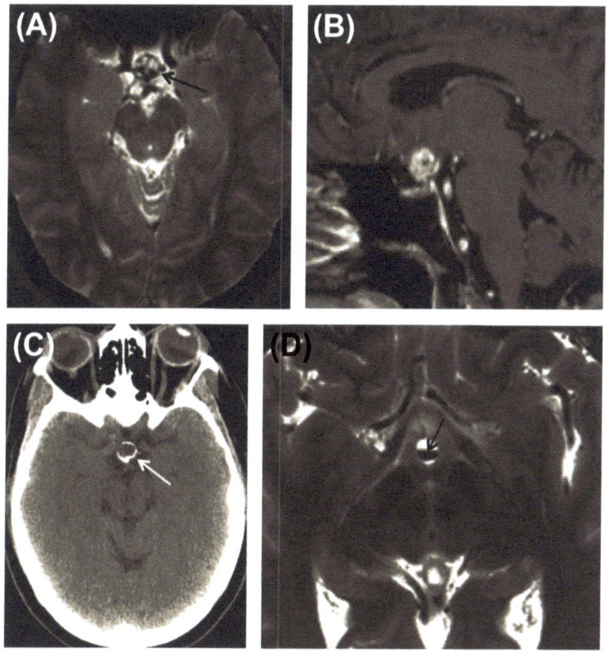

FIGURE 3.5 **A 48-year-old woman with a suprasellar adamantinomatous craniopharyngioma.** **A,** Axial gradient echo image shows a rounded, suprasellar mass with areas of punctate and crescentic hypointensity (arrow), representing calcification. **B,** Sagittal, T1-weighted, enhanced MR image shows predominantly solid enhancement of the tumor. **C,** Axial, non-contrast CT image shows peripheral calcification (arrow) of the mass; calcification is uncommon in papillary craniopharyngioma. **D,** Axial, T2-weighted MR image shows a small cyst at the posterosuperior aspect of the mass with a fluid–fluid level (arrow) and dependent hypointensity; this is not typically seen in papillary craniopharyngioma.

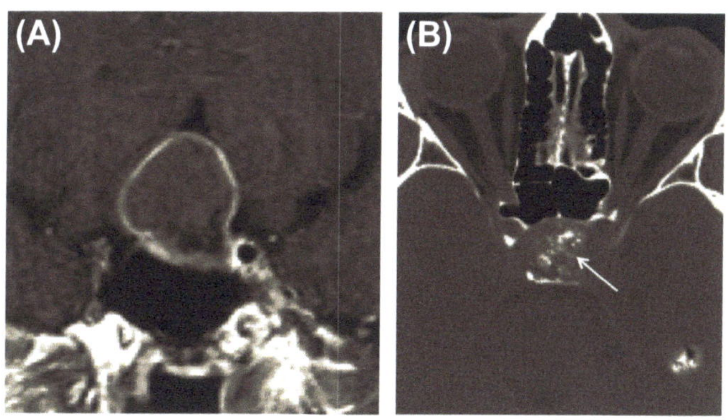

FIGURE 3.6 **A 24-year-old man with intrasellar and suprasellar adamantinomatous craniopharyngioma.** **A,** Coronal, T1-weighted, enhanced MR image shows a cystic, centrally isointense, peripherally enhancing, intrasellar, and suprasellar mass. There is constriction of the mass at the level of the diaphragma sella, and there is no evidence of cavernous sinus invasion. **B,** Axial, non-contrast CT image shows dense intrasellar calcification (arrow), essentially confirming the diagnosis of craniopharyngioma and excluding a cystic/hemorrhagic pituitary macroadenoma. There is remodeling and smooth erosion of the tuberculum and dorsum sella. CT imaging is superior to MR imaging in the detection and characterization of calcification.

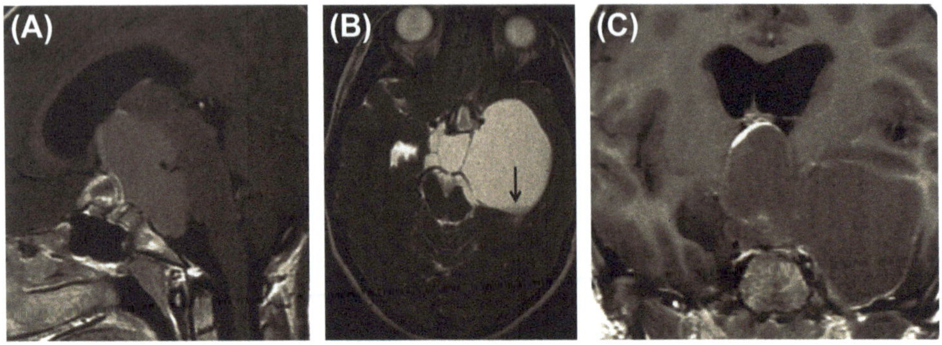

FIGURE 3.7 **A pediatric patient with adamantinomatous craniopharyngioma. A,** Sagittal, T1-weighted, enhanced MR image shows a large, cystic, and solid, intrasellar, suprasellar, and prepontine mass. The cyst is hyperintense relative to parenchyma, and the anterior, solid component shows heterogeneous enhancement. **B,** Axial, T2-weighted MR image shows a large, cystic component in the left middle cranial fossa; a small fluid–fluid level is seen (arrow). **C,** Coronal. T1-weighted, enhanced MR image shows areas of peripheral enhancement of the cystic portion of the tumor. *(Case courtesy of Joseph Piatt, MD)*

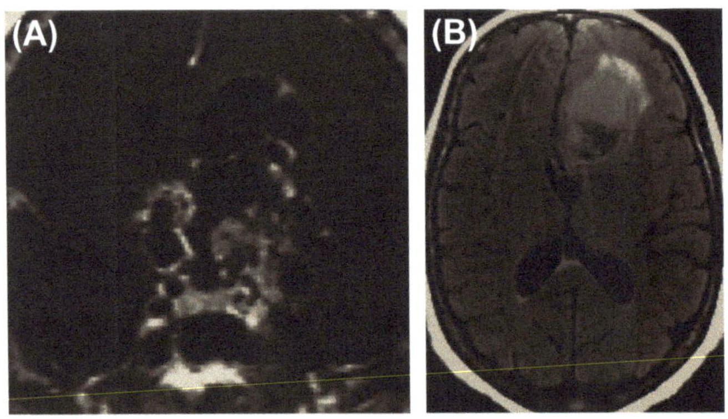

FIGURE 3.8 **A 64-year-old woman with suprasellar adamantinomatous craniopharyngioma. A,** Coronal, T1-weighted, enhanced MR image shows a massive, solid, and cystic, enhancing suprasellar mass. Enhancement is seen along all of the cyst walls, which is typical of craniopharnyngioma. **B,** Axial FLAIR image shows edema in the left frontal lobe adjacent to a large, proteinaceous cyst.

craniopharyngiomas; greater than 50% occur in childhood or adolescence, with a peak incidence at 5–10 years of age. There is a second peak in the sixth decade (Bunin et al., 1998). There are two distinct types, with different histopathologic and imaging appearances. The adamantinomatous type can occur at any age, although this type is seen in almost all pediatric patients. The papillary type occurs almost exclusively in adults. As such, the age of the patient is an important piece of information when analyzing a sellar/suprasellar lesion (Szeifert et al., 1993; Tavangar et al., 2004).

Pre- and post-contrast enhanced MR imaging with attention to the sellar region is the modality of choice when evaluating sellar/suprasellar/third ventricular lesions. The superior contrast resolution and tissue characterization, as well as the multiplanar capability of

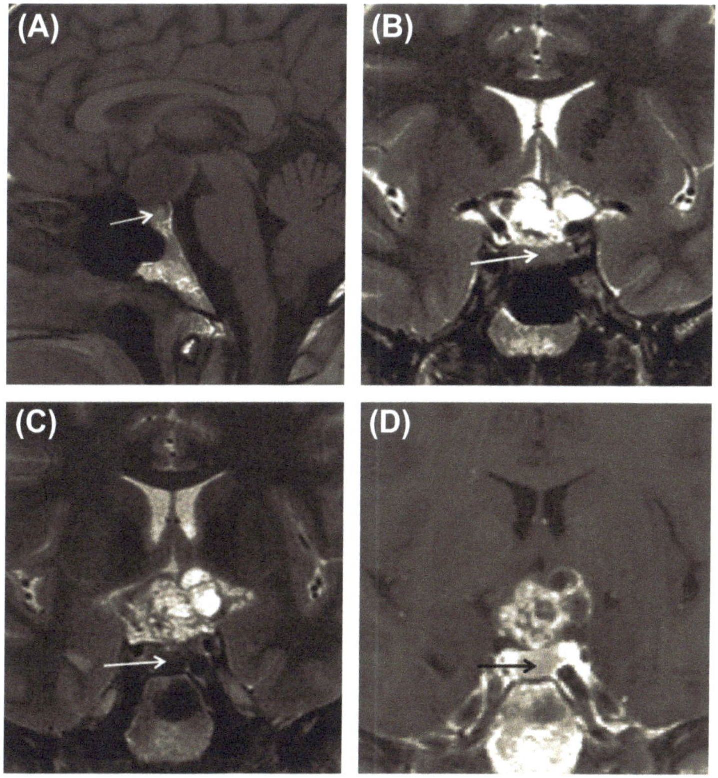

FIGURE 3.9 **A 33-year-old man with a suprasellar adamantinomatous craniopharyngioma and an incidental, presumed intrasellar Rathke cleft cyst. A,** Sagittal, T1-weighted MR image shows a lobulated, suprasellar mass that is mildly hyperintense relative to CSF. There is also a small, hyperintense focus (arrow) at the pars intermedia of the adenohypophysis that is most consistent with an incidental Rathke cleft cyst. This is the most common appearance of these cysts; although a cystic pituitary adenoma remains in the differential diagnosis, the location at the pars intermedia is typical of Rathke cleft cyst. **B,** Coronal, T2-weighted MR image shows the complex, suprasellar mass; note the normal signal (arrow) of the adenophypophysis. **C,** Coronal, T2-weighted MR image immediately posterior to **B,** shows the marked hypointensity (arrow) of the presumed Rathke cleft cyst. **D,** Coronal, T1-weighted, enhanced MR image shows enhancement of the cyst walls, as well as the solid portion of the mass; the presumed Rathke cleft cyst (arrow) does not enhance.

this technique, make it the radiologist's most indispensable tool. The study can be obtained on 1.5 Tesla or 3.0 Tesla MR scanner; lower field strength scanners (e.g., 0.3 Tesla) should be strenuously avoided if possible. An exception to this rule would be the presence of suprasellar metallic surgical material causing susceptibility artifact; the latter would be reduced on lower field strength scanners. In addition to inferior image quality and diminished detection of contrast enhancement, hemosiderin and calcification are less visible on lower field strength scanners. High-resolution, thin-section, T1-weighted imaging of the sellar region in the sagittal and coronal planes is mandatory, and should be obtained both pre- and

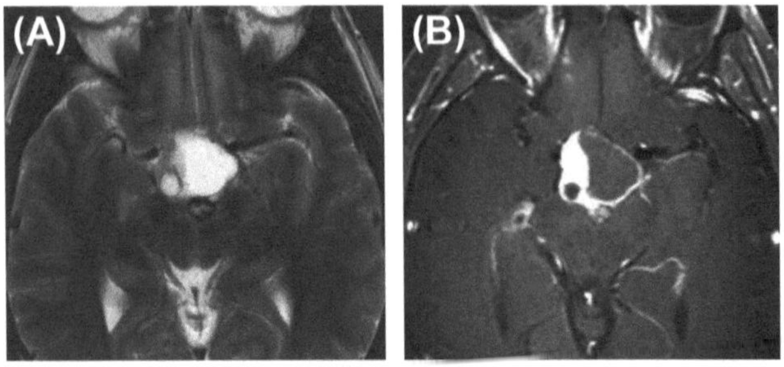

FIGURE 3.10 **A 26-year-old man with suprasellar adamantinomatous craniopharnyngioma. A,** Axial, T2-weighted MR image shows a cystic and solid suprasellar mass; the solid portion is heterogeneous in signal. **B,** Axial, T1-weighted, enhanced MR image shows peripheral enhancement of the cystic portion and relatively diffuse enhancement of the solid portion. The cystic portion is hyperintense relative to CSF.

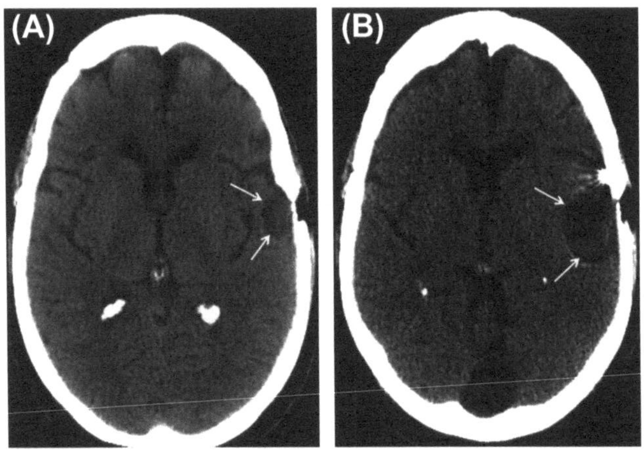

FIGURE 3.11 **A 69-year-old woman with surgically proved recurrent perisylvian craniopharyngioma 34 years after initial resection, due to presumed transplantation of tumor. A,** Axial, non-contrast CT image shows a hypodense, left perisylvian mass. **B,** Axial, enhanced CT image obtained 3 years later shows marked interval enlargement of the peripherally enhancing, left perisylvian mass (arrows).

post-contrast administration (standard dose). Dynamic enhanced imaging of the sellar region can be performed if diagnostic considerations include pituitary microadenoma or the rare parasellar cavernous hemangioma. Half dose or double dose contrast administration is almost always unnecessary in the evaluation of suspected craniopharyngioma. High-resolution, thin-section, coronal, T2-weighted images are also essential. All of the other standard pulse sequences must be carefully scrutinized, including diffusion imaging, gradient imaging (for magnetic susceptibility effects), and FLAIR (fluid-attenuated inversion recovery) imaging. Restricted diffusion is associated with epidermoid tumors, noting

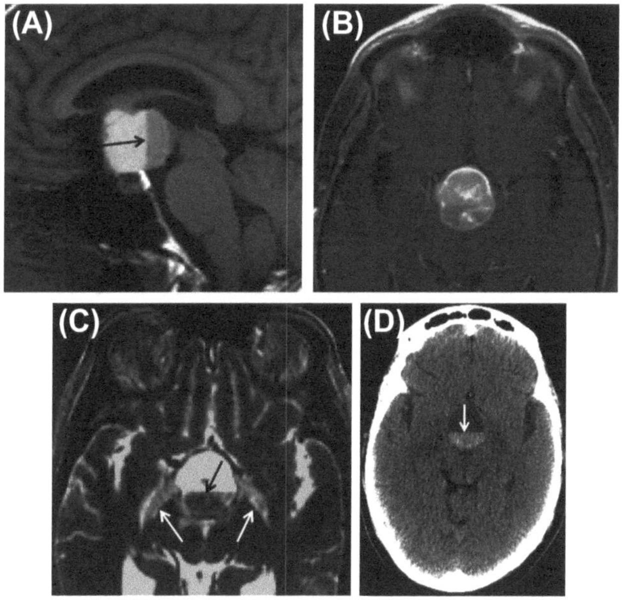

FIGURE 3.12 **A 55-year-old man with atypical suprasellar papillary craniopharyngioma. A,** Sagittal, T1-weighted MR image shows a large, cystic, hyperintense, suprasellar mass with a fluid–fluid level (arrow). **B,** Axial, T1-weighted enhanced MR image shows peripheral enhancement of the cyst, with areas of internal nodular enhancement. **C,** Axial, T2-weighted MR image shows the cystic mass with a fluid–fluid level (black arrow); the two components of fluid have markedly different signal characteristics. Edema (white arrows) is seen in the optic tracts bilaterally. **D,** Axial, non-contrast CT image shows the fluid–fluid level (arrow), but no calcification. Absence of calcification is typical of papillary craniopharyngioma, although in all other respects the CT and MR imaging characteristics are typical of adamantinomatous craniopharnyngioma. This case demonstrates that definitive histologic diagnoses of craniopharyngiomas cannot be made based upon imaging.

that diffusion-weighted imaging can be unreliable in the setting of certain stages of blood products (particularly extracellular methemoglobin) (Tsuruda et al., 1990; Smirniotopoulos & Chiechi, 1995). Gradient imaging is very sensitive in the detection of acute or chronic blood products, and to a lesser extent calcification. T1-, T2- and FLAIR sequences help characterize the cystic and solid portions of lesions; the latter can identify parenchymal edema. Because of the complexity of MR imaging, it is essential that the interpreter of the study integrate all of the findings on each sequence, and have a comprehensive understanding of artifacts and pitfalls. For example, a T1-hyperintense suprasellar cystic craniopharyngioma will appear bright on 3-D time of flight MR angiography (MRA), potentially mimicking flow signal in an anterior communicating artery aneurysm. This artifact will disappear on phase contrast MR angiography (Tsuruda et al., 1992; Ozsarlak et al., 2004).

Unlike glial tumors, advanced MR imaging techniques such as MR spectroscopy, MR perfusion imaging, and diffusion tensor imaging do not ordinarily play an important role in the assessment of sellar/suprasellar lesions (Plaza et al., 2013). If exclusion of an aneurysm or preoperative localization of arterial vasculature is warranted, 3-D time of flight or phase contrast MR angiography can be obtained.

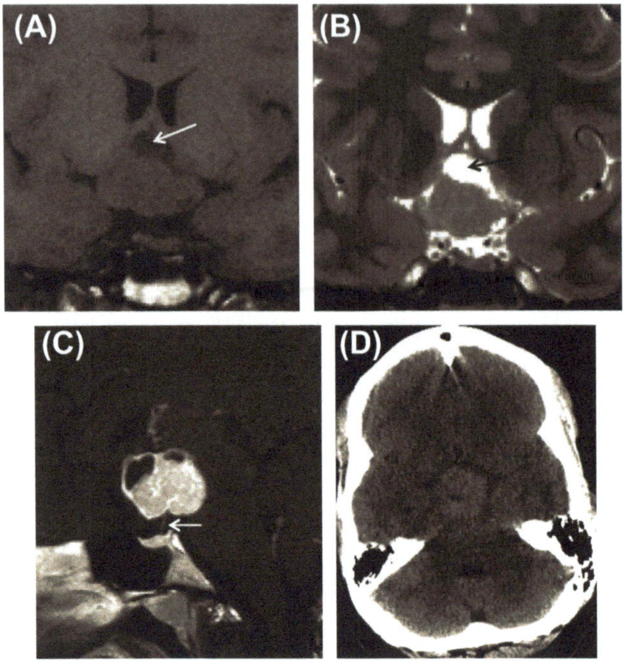

FIGURE 3.13 **A 23-year-old woman with suprasellar papillary craniopharyngioma arising in the third ventricle. A,** Coronal, T1-weighted MR image shows a lobulated, suprasellar mass that is isointense relative to parenchyma; a cystic-appearing portion (arrow) that is only mildly hyperintense relative to CSF is seen superiorly. **B,** Coronal, T2-weighted MR image also shows a lobulated, suprasellar mass that is isointense to the parenchyma; the cystic-appearing portion (arrow) is hyperintense. **C,** Sagittal, T1-weighted enhanced MR image shows mostly solid enhancement of the mass. The infundibulum (arrow) is not displaced posteriorly (compare to chordoid glioma, Figure 3.16). **D,** Axial, non-contrast CT image shows a mass that is isodense to parenchyma; no calcification is seen.

CT imaging does not merely play a passive role in surgical planning prior to transsphenoidal or transfrontal resection of a sellar or suprasellar mass. Because of its superiority (compared to MR imaging) in detecting calcification and characterizing any osseous remodeling or erosion, CT imaging can play an active role in arriving at the correct preoperative diagnosis. This is particularly true of adamantinomatous craniopharnygioma, which calcifies in up to 90% of cases. For example, identification of an expanded sella with a calcified intrasellar mass on CT imaging would warrant primary consideration of an intrasellar craniopharyngioma rather than a pituitary adenoma; the calcification would not necessarily be as apparent on MR imaging. Peripheral, rim-like calcification associated with a suprasellar mass would always warrant consideration of an aneurysm as well as craniopharyngioma; again, this calcification would not necessarily be as apparent on MR imaging. Other than a vascular lesion such as an aneurysm, craniopharyngioma is one of the few brain masses that may show this pattern of peripheral calcification. Of note, in a patient without a

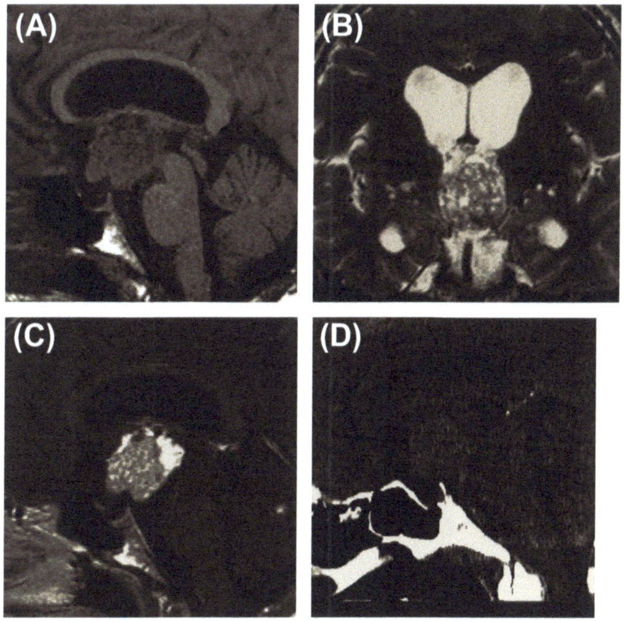

FIGURE 3.14 **A 52-year-old man with suprasellar papillary craniopharyngioma arising in the third ventricle.** **A,** Sagittal, T1-weighted MR image shows a relatively spherical, suprasellar mass that is isointense to hypointense relative to parenchyma. **B,** Coronal, T2-weighted MR image shows inhomogeneous signal in the mass. **C,** Sagittal, T1-weighted enhanced MR image shows diffuse enhancement of the mass. **D,** Sagittal, non-contrast CT image shows a mass that is isodense relative to parenchyma; no calcification is seen.

contraindication to MR imaging or administration of a gadolinium-based contrast agent, there is essentially no role for the administration of iodinated contrast for a CT brain or sinus/sellar study when evaluating a suprasellar mass. However, CT angiography can be obtained if MR angiography is insufficient to assess the regional vasculature.

CT is also extremely sensitive in the detection of fat density, which is particularly valuable in the suprasellar region. For example, suprasellar hyperintensity on T1-weighted MR imaging could potentially be related to a Rathke cleft cyst, suprasellar lipoma, fat within a dermoid or teratoma, subacute clot (methemoglobin) within a partially or completely thrombosed aneurysm, proteinaceous fluid in a cystic craniopharyngioma, metastatic melanoma, an ectopic posterior pituitary, or Pantopaque (Yousem et al., 1990; Bonneville et al., 2006; Ginat & Meyers, 2012). Although identification of chemical shift artifact in the frequency encoded direction is a signature of fat, this finding can be subtle (Hood et al., 1999). A fat-suppressed, T1-weighted sequence will cause fat to suppress, allowing accurate characterization on MR imaging. However, CT imaging allows easy identification and/or confirmation of fat density (usually measuring −30 to −100 Hounsfield units) in a lesion, which would essentially exclude the diagnosis of craniopharyngioma.

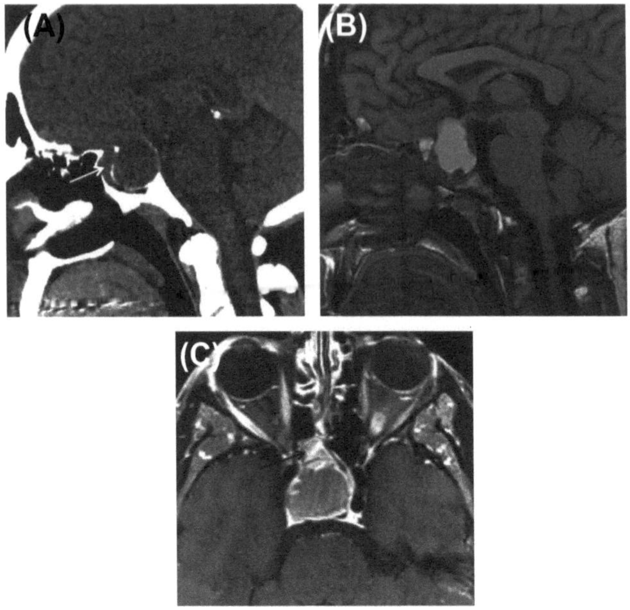

FIGURE 3.15 **A 33-year-old man with intrasellar and suprasellar adamantinomatous craniopharyngioma.** **A,** Sagittal, non-contrast CT image shows marked sellar expansion by an intrasellar and suprasellar mass. There is near complete opacification (arrow) of the remodeled sphenoid sinus anterior to the mass. Calcification in the mass is absent, a feature seen in only a minority of adamantinomatous craniopharyngiomas. **B,** Sagittal, T1-weighted MR image shows a complex appearance to the mass; the cystic portions are markedly hyperintense. **C,** Axial, T1-weighted enhanced MR image shows peripheral enhancement of the cystic component, with solidly enhancing tumor (arrow) in the right sphenoid sinus.

LOCATION, LOCATION, LOCATION

To borrow a phrase from the real estate market, a cardinal tenet in neuroradiology when evaluating a lesion is "location, location, location". The geographic center of craniopharyngiomas is the suprasellar cistern in approximately 75% of patients; approximately 20% are intrasellar and suprasellar; approximately 5% are purely intrasellar (Adamson et al., 1990; Tavangar et al., 2004). Primary third ventricular lesions are rare, and ectopic locations are extremely rare. From a surgical perspective, craniopharyngiomas involving the sella can be categorized as being purely intrasellar, intra- and suprasellar infradiaphragmatic, intra- and suprasellar transdiaphragmatic, and intra- and suprasellar supradiaphragmatic (Effenterre & Boch, 2002). Tumors may compress or expand the diaphragm, but do not usually invade it. Transdiaphragmatic tumors probably arise within the sella and extend through the diaphragma along the infundibulum. With regard to suprasellar craniopharyngioma, tumors can be categorized as being prechiasmatic, retrochiasmatic, and/or infrachiasmatic. Purely intraventricular tumors arise above the floor of the third ventricle in the region of the tuber cinereum. Partially intraventricular tumors arise below the floor of the third ventricle and penetrate the ventricle after invasion of the parenchyma. Not all of the aforementioned categorizations can be confidently discriminated on MR imaging.

As it happens, radiologists like mnemonics, and perhaps the most famous mnemonic in neuroradiology was constructed for suprasellar lesions (S-A-T-C-H-M-O). Once a mass is localized to the suprasellar region, the differential diagnosis includes: S = sellar tumor, sarcoid; A = aneurysm, arachnoid cyst; T = teratoma/dermoid, tuberculosis; C= craniopharnyngioma, cleft cyst (Rathke), choristoma, chordoid glioma; H = hypothalamic glioma, hamartoma of the tuber cinereum, histiocytosis; M = meningioma, metastasis; O = optic chiasm glioma. This mnemonic is not all-inclusive, and other lesions encountered in the suprasellar region, albeit uncommonly, include lymphocytic hypophysitis, non-Hodgkins lymphoma, germinoma, infundibuloma, and lipoma (Karnaze et al., 1986; Johnsen et al., 1991; Donovan & Nesbit, 1996).

ADAMANTINOMATOUS CRANIOPHARYNGIOMA

Adamantinomatous craniopharyngioma (Figures 3.1–3.10, 3.15) is the most common pathologic type; this tumor can occur at any age, and it accounts for almost all pediatric cases (Sorva et al., 1987; Harwood-Nash, 1994). Histologically, this type demonstrates adamantinoma-like epithelium, "wet keratin" nodules, necrotic debris, microcysts, and/or macrocysts containing cholesterol crystals and proteinaceous material, and calcifications (90%). The classic macroscopic appearance of the cyst contents has been described as "machine oil" or "crankcase oil". These tumors are associated with inflammatory changes and fibrosis; as a result, they adhere to adjacent normal structures (including the vasculature at the circle of Willis), and can even invade the parenchyma (Szeifert et al., 1993; Miller, 1994). The inflammatory and fibrotic nature of these lesions can make complete resection difficult, and recurrence common (Adamson et al., 1990; Eldevik et al., 1996; Petito, 1996). The complex radiologic appearance of adamantinomatous craniopharyngioma reflects these histologic characteristics.

The classic radiologic description of adamantinomatous craniopharyngioma on CT imaging incorporates three key characteristics: (1) cyst, (2) calcification, and (3) enhancement (Figures 3.1–3.6) (Fitz et al., 1978). The cyst(s) can be hypodense or hyperdense relative to normal parenchyma, and they can be very small or very large. The density of the cyst(s) on CT imaging is a function of the cyst contents; the higher the protein concentration, the denser the cyst. CT is superior to MR imaging in detecting calcification. Calcification tends to be more striking in pediatric as compared to adult tumors (Sorva et al., 1987; Harwood-Nash, 1994). Calcification is present in the vast majority of lesions; it may be coarse or stippled, and it can be located along the cyst walls and/or within the nodular portions. Although enhanced MR imaging has replaced enhanced CT imaging in the evaluation of the brain, the cyst walls on CT imaging typically enhance after contrast administration, as do the solid, nodular portions of the tumor. It is critically important to distinguish a hyperdense, peripherally calcified aneurysm of the circle of Willis from a hyperdense, peripherally calcified adamantinomatous craniopharyngioma (Figures 3.4, 3.5). Moreover, other suprasellar lesions (e.g., meningioma, tuberculosis, cysticercosis) can demonstrate calcification. Of note, identification of calcification in an intrasellar mass warrants strong consideration of craniopharyngioma rather than pituitary adenoma, as the latter typically do not calcify (Figure 3.6) (Johnsen et al., 1991; Choi et al., 2007).

Craniopharyngiomas are avascular on conventional angiography (Baker, 1972). If warranted, CT angiography can be obtained to most elegantly establish the relationship of the tumor to the adjacent arterial vasculature; there is little role for conventional diagnostic angiography in this setting. Larger lesions may displace the internal carotid arteries laterally, the basilar artery posteriorly, and the anterior communicating artery complex/anterior cerebral arteries superiorly. Although adamantinomatous craniopharyngioma can adhere to, or surround arterial walls, frank vascular narrowing is very rare; arterial vasospasm induced by chemical meningitis from cyst rupture has been reported (Shida et al., 1998). In the unusual circumstance where MR imaging and MR angiography are inconclusive in ruling out a suprasellar aneurysm, CT angiography can also be very helpful.

The most characteristic appearance of adamantinomatous craniopharyngioma on MR imaging is a heterogeneous, lobulated, mass with cystic and solid components, as well as calcifications (Figures 3.1–3.10) (Karnaze et al., 1986; Pusey et al., 1987; Donovan & Nesbit, 1996; Eldevik et al., 1996). The cystic components are well-defined and most commonly internally uniform. These cysts contain various amounts of cholesterol, triglycerides, methemoglobin, protein, and desquamated epithelium (Adamson et al., 1990). The signal of the cyst contents is primarily related to protein concentration and the presence of free methemoglobin, and is most commonly hyperintense on T1-weighted, T2-weighted, and FLAIR images. On T1-weighted sequences, as protein concentration increases, signal intensity changes from hypointense to hyperintense and to hypointense again. On T2-weighted sequences, as protein concentration increases, signal intensity changes from hyperintense to hypointense. The density of cysts on CT imaging correlates with the signal characteristics on MR imaging; very dense cysts will not be as hyperintense on MR imaging (particularly on T2-weighted imaging) (Figure 3.3) (Pusey et al., 1987; Ahmadi et al., 1992). Fluid–fluid levels are seen in a minority of cysts (Figures 3.3, 3.5, 3.7); when present, they are typically located in exophytic cysts, rather than within the solid portions of the tumor. Identification of a large fluid–fluid level within the substance of a sellar/suprasellar mass should prompt greater concern for a hemorrhagic pituitary adenoma/pituitary apoplexy (Abrahams et al., 1989). The solid portion of adamantinomatous craniopharyngiomas is heterogeneous in signal on different pulse sequences. Both the cyst walls and the solid nodules can calcify; calcification is best seen on T2-weighted or T2*-gradient echo imaging, and manifests as focal hypointensity (Figures 3.1, 3.2, 3.5). Calcification is seen in almost all pediatric cases, and a majority of adult cases. Uncommonly, a small tumor in adults manifests only as small, calcified, suprasellar nodule; this lesion can easily be overlooked on MR imaging unless subtle distortion of the suprasellar anatomy is identified.

Hyperintense signal on T2-weighted and FLAIR sequences in the brain parenchyma adjacent to a craniopharyngioma is uncommon (Figures 3.3, 3.8), even with very large lesions; if present, this may reflect vasogenic edema due to (1) parenchymal invasion by the tumor, (2) microscopic leakage of cyst contents, or (3) compression of the optic chiasm/tracts. Cholesterol species in cystic tumors are capable of producing an inflammatory parenchymal reaction (Ahmadi et al., 1992). Even compact fiber bundles such as the internal capsules and optic chiasm/tracts, which are relatively resistant to edema, may become edematous if they are exposed to these insults over a protracted period of time (Saeki et al., 2003). Moreover, reactive gliosis can be seen adjacent to craniopharyngiomas, which will also be hyperintense on T2-weighted and FLAIR images.

Although craniopharyngiomas can grow in all directions, frank invasion of the cavernous sinuses is very rare (unlike pituitary adenoma and meningioma). Additionally, rare manifestations of adamantinomatous craniopharyngioma include rupture of a cyst in the subarachnoid space with the resultant development of chemical meningitis (Kulkarni et al., 2000), and remote postsurgical recurrence due to presumed spread in the cerebrospinal fluid pathways or direct transplantation of tumor cells (Figure 3.11) (Gupta et al., 1999; Bianco et al., 2006).

PAPILLARY CRANIOPHARYNGIOMA

The less common papillary (squamous) craniopharyngioma (Figures 3.12–3.14) occurs almost exclusively in adults. Histologically, this type demonstrates a papillary architecture composed of mature squamous epithelium; "wet keratin" nodules, necrotic debris, cholesterol crystals, inflammatory changes, and fibrosis are not seen. Calcification is very uncommon (Szeifert et al., 1993; Miller, 1994). Although some overlap exists in the imaging characteristic of the two histologic types of craniopharyngioma (Figures 3.5, 3.12, 3.15), in most cases papillary craniopharyngioma has a distinctively different appearance than the adamantinomatous type (Figures 3.13, 3.14) (Crotty et al., 1995; Sartoretti-Schefer et al., 1997). As a point of departure, papillary craniopharyngiomas are more likely to be purely suprasellar, and they are relatively homogeneous in appearance. Typical features on MR imaging include a spherical (not lobulated), predominantly solid, heterogeneously enhancing nodule; the nodule is usually isodense (relative to parenchyma) on CT imaging, isointense in signal on T1-weighted images, and more heterogeneous in signal on T2-weighted images (Figures 3.13, 3.14). Large, T1-hyperintense proteinaceous cysts, which are a hallmark of adamantinomatous tumors, are generally not seen; the non-enhancing portions of papillary craniopharyngioma have a relatively low protein concentration and remain hypointense on T1-weighted and hyperintense on T2-weighted images (Eldevik et al., 1996). Similarly, calcification is very uncommon but can occur; as such, calcification is unfortunately not a specific feature of adamantinomatous tumors. Because of the paucity of inflammatory changes and fibrosis, papillary craniopharyngiomas are more easily separable from adjacent structures, including the vasculature, and may be less prone to recur (Miller, 1994; Petito, 1996). It is apparent from this description that papillary craniopharyngiomas will also be less likely to cause adjacent parenchymal edema or gliosis.

Alas, a minority of papillary craniopharnygiomas (Figure 3.12) can have very similar imaging characteristics compared to adamantinomatous tumors, making radiological distinction not possible. Tumors with mixed histological features also occur, although the imaging appearance of these lesions is typically that of adamantinomatous craniopharyngioma; because of this observation, some authors believe that papillary tumors that appear identical to adamantinomatous tumor on imaging are, in reality, mixed tumors that have been subjected to sampling errors on pathological examination (Sartoretti-Schefer et al., 1997). Of note, although the histologic type of craniopharyngioma may be diagnosed radiologically on preoperative imaging studies in the significant majority of cases, the single most important predictor of recurrence is the extent of tumor resection (Adamson et al., 1990; Effenterre & Boch, 2002). As such, the preoperative differentiation of these two histologic types is not absolutely critical, as the surgical goal of complete resection will not be affected.

UNUSUAL LOCATIONS OF CRANIOPHARYNGIOMA

Among the rare sites of origin of craniopharyngioma, the third ventricle (Figures 3.13, 3.14) is perhaps the most frequently encountered. Purely intraventricular craniopharyngiomas are typically seen in adults, and either histologic type may occur in this location. Symptoms of elevated intracranial pressure are more common presenting complaints than visual or endocrinologic disturbances. Because of their location, these tumors may become quite large prior to presentation. The third ventricular floor remains intact, the suprasellar cistern remains patent, the optic chiasm is displaced inferiorly, and sellar abnormalities are absent (Behari et al., 2003). The differential diagnosis of purely intraventricular third ventricular masses includes chordoid glioma, colloid cyst, choroid plexus papilloma/carcinoma, germinoma, and metastatic disease (Glastonbury et al., 2011). In particular, chordoid glioma (Figure 3.16) is a rare, slow-growing, non-invasive neoplasm (WHO Grade II) that arises from the anterior third ventricle and is frequently adherent to the hypothalamus. Radiologically, chordoid glioma appears as a well-defined, ovoid mass that is hyperdense relative to gray matter on CT imaging, isointense on T1-weighted MR imaging, slightly hyperintense on T2-weighted

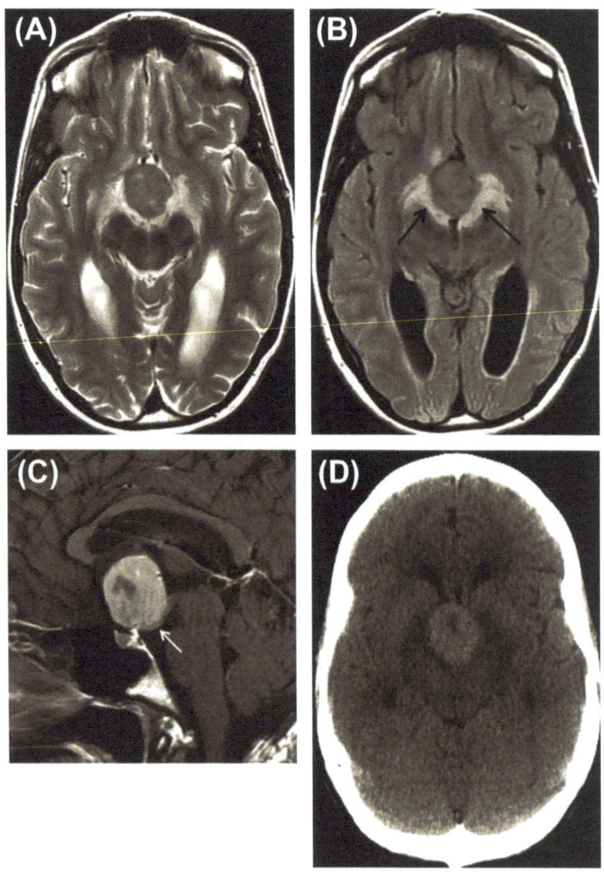

FIGURE 3.16 **A 29-year-old woman with chordoid glioma. A,** Axial, T2-weighed MR image shows a suprasellar mass which is mostly isointense relative to parenchyma. **B,** Axial FLAIR images shows mild to moderate edema (arrows) adjacent to the mass. **C,** Sagittal, T1-weighted enhanced MR images shows a mostly solidly enhancing, suprasellar (third ventricular) mass; the infundibulum (arrow) is displaced posteriorly. The degree of edema and the posterior displacement of the infundibulum are more typical of chordoid glioma than third ventricular papillary craniopharyngioma. **D,** Axial, non-contrast CT image shows a mildly hyperdense, suprasellar mass with adjacent edema.

imaging, and enhances intensely. Cystic changes and parenchymal edema can be present, but calcification is rare. The infundibulum is displaced posteriorly (Pomper et al., 2001). From this description, it is apparent that chordoid glioma can have many imaging characteristics similar to a purely intraventricular papillary craniopharyngioma.

The theory of craniopharnygioma originating from remnants of the obliterated craniopharnyngeal duct suggests that these tumors can arise anywhere along the migration of Rathke's pouch from the vomer, the roof of the nasopharynx, through the midline sphenoid bone to the sellar region. Because craniopharyngiomas can also arise in locations completely remote from this embryologic pathway, it has been postulated that certain ectopic craniopharnyngiomas might originate from multipotential or totipotential cells. Not surprisingly, craniopharyngioma has been reported in locations as diverse as the nasopharynx, sphenoid sinus, pineal gland, and fourth ventricle (Kanungo et al., 1995; Deutsch et al., 2001). In short, these tumors can potentially occur anywhere.

RATHKE CLEFT CYST

Because of embryologic and certain radiologic similarities of Rathke cleft cyst (RCC) and craniopharyngioma, a separate discussion of RCC is warranted. RCC (Figures 3.17–3.22) is a congenital, non-neoplastic cyst that develops secondary to failure of obliteration of the lumen of Rathke's pouch and subsequent enlargement of the cleft. Neoplastic degeneration does not occur. RCC is the most common, incidentally discovered sellar lesion, followed by pituitary

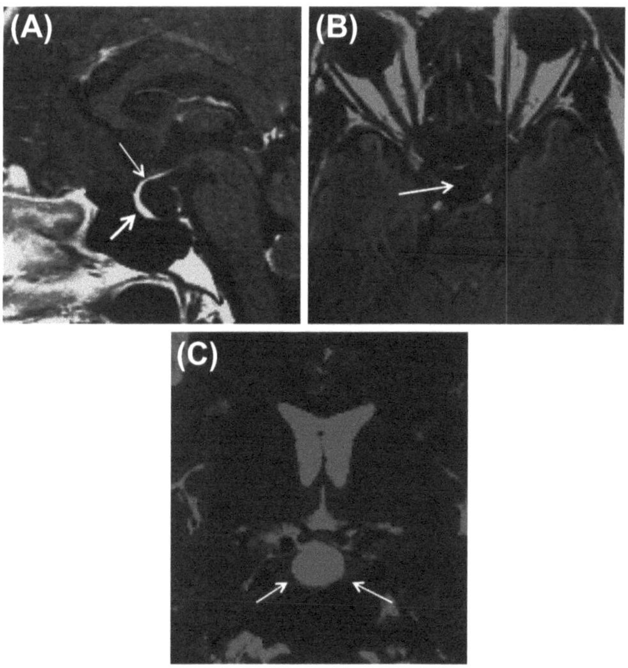

FIGURE 3.17 **A 62-year-old man with intrasellar Rathke cleft cyst. A,** Sagittal, T1-weighted, enhanced MR image shows a non-enhancing, intrasellar cystic lesion displacing enhancing pituitary tissue anteriorly ("claw" sign) (thick arrow). The cyst is isointense relative to CSF. The infundibulum (thin arrow) is displaced anteriorly in the midline. **B,** Axial FLAIR image also shows that the cyst (arrow) is isointense relative to CSF; this feature is uncommon in craniopharyngioma. **C,** Coronal, T2-weighted MR image shows the hyperintense cyst surrounded by pituitary tissue inferiorly and laterally (arrows) ("egg in cup" sign). There was no calcification on CT imaging, and the cyst was isodense relative to CSF (not shown).

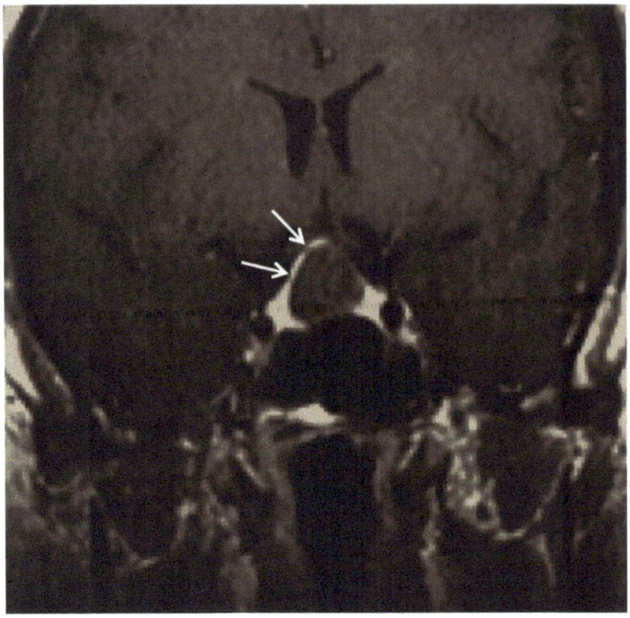

FIGURE 3.18 **A 52-year-old woman with a primarily intrasellar Rathke cleft cyst.** Coronal, T1-weighted enhanced MR image shows enhancing pituitary tissue (arrows) displaced to the right by a non-enhancing, cystic mass ("claw" sign).

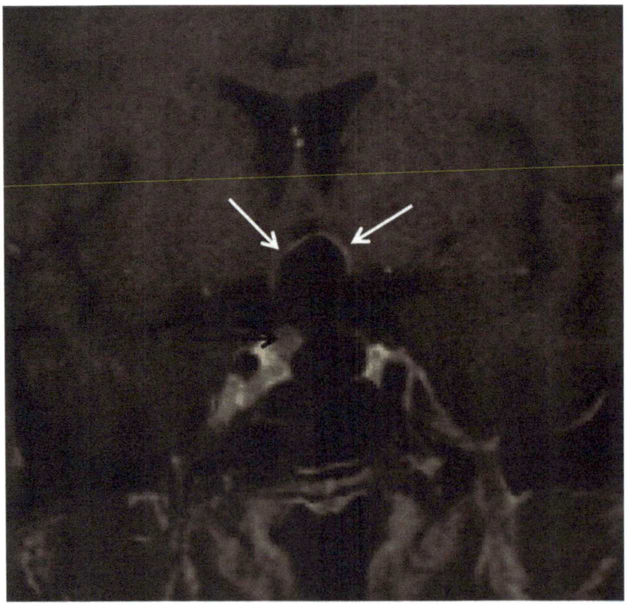

FIGURE 3.19 **A 64-year-old woman with an intrasellar and suprasellar Rathke cleft cyst.** Coronal, T1-weighted enhanced MR image shows a cystic intrasellar and suprasellar mass. There is thin, peripheral enhancement (white arrows) along the superior aspect of the lesion, which is more typical of a craniopharyngioma. Right superolateral nodular enhancement (black arrow) represents displaced pituitary tissue. CT imaging showed a non-calcified, hypodense cyst (not shown).

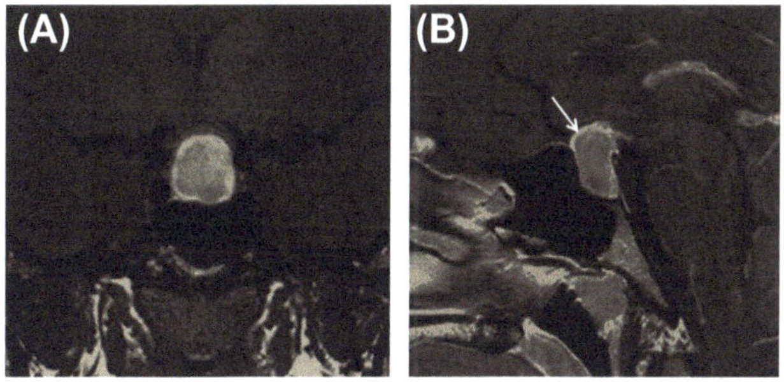

FIGURE 3.20 **A 20-year-old woman with intrasellar and suprasellar Rathke cleft cyst. A,** Coronal, T1-weighted MR image shows a hyperintense, intrasellar, and suprasellar cystic mass. **B,** Sagittal, enhanced T1-weighted MR image shows anterior midline displacement of the infundibulum (white arrow) and a posterior ledge sign (black arrow).

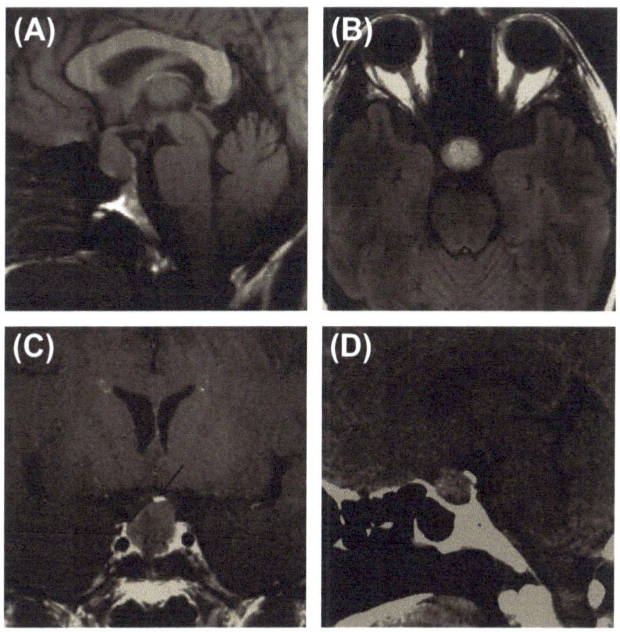

FIGURE 3.21 **A 42-year-old woman with intrasellar and suprasellar Rathke cleft cyst. A,** Sagittal, T1-weighted MR image shows a hyperintense intrasellar and suprasellar cystic lesion. **B,** Axial FLAIR image shows that the cyst is hyperintense relative to CSF. **C,** Coronal, T1-weighted enhanced MR image shows no enhancement of the lesion; the enhancing infundibulum (arrow) is seen superiorly. **D,** Sagittal, non-contrast CT image shows a non-calcified, hyperdense cyst.

adenoma; in routine autopsies, RCC is encountered in 13–33% of normal pituitary glands (Shin et al., 1999; Trifanescu et al., 2012). In neuroradiologic practice, a presumptive diagnosis of incidental intrasellar RCC is frequently made, recognizing that pathologic proof will not be forthcoming; these lesions are managed conservatively. Symptomatic RCCs may be seen in

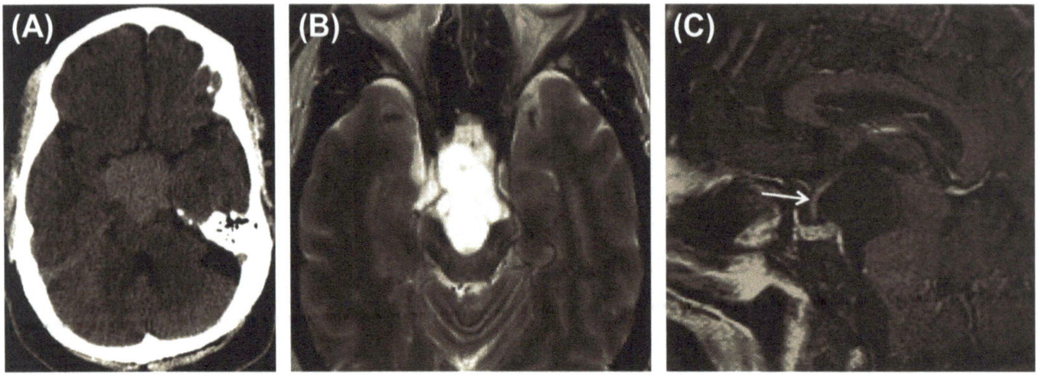

FIGURE 3.22 **A 50-year-old man with a large suprasellar Rathke cleft cyst. A,** Axial, non-contrast CT image shows a large, hyperdense, non-calcified, suprasellar mass. **B,** Axial, T2-weighted MR image shows a large, moderately hyperintense suprasellar mass splaying the cerebral peduncles. **C,** Sagittal, T1-weighted enhanced MR image shows no enhancement of the lesion. The enhancing infundibulum (arrow) is displaced anteriorly in the midline.

all age groups, with a peak frequency between the fourth and sixth decades. Pediatric cases are rare; this may be attributed to the fact that RCCs can grow slowly with time, and therefore they become clinically evident later in life. There is a slight female predominance, which may be related to earlier presentation in women due to menstrual irregularities. Most RCCs remain stable in size and imaging characteristics, and some may even become smaller. Symptomatic RCCs are uncommon; when present, symptoms are related to pituitary/hypothalamic dysfunction, visual disturbances, and/or headache (Kucharczyk et al., 1987; Shin et al., 1999). Preoperative diagnosis of RCC is important, as this lesion is typically treated with cyst drainage and removal of as much of the cyst wall as possible, while neoplasms such as craniopharyngioma require complete resection to avoid recurrence.

The vast majority of RCCs are intrasellar (Figures 3.9, 3.17, 3.18), intrasellar and suprasellar (Figures 3.19–3.21), or suprasellar (Figure 3.22) in location, and most are small (Kucharczyk et al., 1987). However, because of their embryology, and similarity to craniopharyngioma, RCCs can arise anywhere from the nasopharynx to the third ventricle; for example, an intrasphenoidal RCC has been reported (Megdiche-Bazarbachaa et al., 2006). RCC is the most common medially situated pituitary lesion; pituitary adenomas tend to be located laterally in the pituitary gland. In addition, RCCs are classically located in the posterior portion of the adenohypophysis, between the anterior and intermediate lobes (Sumida et al., 1994). The MR imaging protocol is the same as for craniopharyngioma; the principal role of CT imaging is the detection of calcification, fat, and/or osseous changes. Similar to craniopharyngioma, a T1-hyperintense suprasellar RCC can simulate an aneurysm on 3-D time of flight (but not phase contrast) MR angiography.

RCCs appear as smooth, spherical, or ovoid cysts; they are lined by a single cell layer of epithelium. The contents of the cyst vary from clear, cerebrospinal fluid (CSF)-like fluid to thick, mucoid material. Similar to craniopharyngioma, the density of a RCC on CT imaging, and the signal characteristics on MR imaging, are highly variable and relate to the protein concentration (Choi et al., 2007). However, homogeneously hypointense signal intensity on

T2-weighted images is very suggestive of RCC (Bonneville et al., 2007). Unlike adamantinomatous craniopharyngioma, calcification in RCC is rare; if present, the calcification will be curvilinear (Nakasu et al., 1999). Enhancement of the cyst wall (Figure 3.19) is also uncommon; when present, it is attributed to localized inflammatory changes related to cholesterol species and/or blood products. Importantly, an enhancing rim of normal pituitary tissue should not be confused with abnormal enhancement of the cyst wall. The normal pituitary gland may be displaced in any direction, and its position is usually around or under the cyst. Depending upon the position of the displaced pituitary tissue, this enhancing rim has been termed the "claw" or "egg in cup" sign (Figures 3.17, 3.18). When a RCC extends superiorly through the diaphragma sella, a characteristic ledge of tissue can overly the neurohypophysis; this has been termed the "posterior ledge" sign (Figure 3.20) (Kucharczyk et al., 1987; Sumida et al., 1994). Midline anterior displacement of the infundibulum (Figures 3.17, 3.20, 3.22) is also a salient feature of RCC due to the typical midline location at the pars intermedia. Some RCC have a non-enhancing, intracystic nodule; these nodules are typically hyperintense on T1-weighted images and hypointense on T2-weighted images. Grossly, these nodules are yellow, waxy, solid masses that pathologically represent a mucin clump composed of protein and cholesterol. Depending upon the signal characteristics of the RCC itself, the intracystic nodule may be difficult to discern but it is generally best seen on T2-weighted images (Byun et al., 2000). Unlike RCC, an intracystic nodule in a craniopharyngioma will show enhancement. From this discussion, it is evident that the characteristic appearance of RCC is a small, cystic, non-enhancing, non-calcified, sellar/suprasellar mass, possibly with a non-enhancing, intracystic nodule.

Symptomatic hemorrhage into a RCC is a rare event that mimics pituitary apoplexy (Chaiban et al., 2011); indeed, the distinction can be difficult or impossible to make without previous imaging demonstrating a RCC. The signal characteristics of the lesion will depend upon the stage of blood products; T1-hyperintense methemoglobin is most often encountered. The etiology for the hemorrhage is not certain.

RADIOLOGIC DIFFERENTIAL DIAGNOSIS

A complete review of the imaging appearance of all sellar/suprasellar lesions is beyond the scope of this chapter. However, in addition to Rathke cleft cyst, a number of other potentially similar-appearing lesions warrant discussion.

Pituitary adenomas (Figures 3.23–3.26) arise in the sella; suprasellar, parasellar, and/or infrasellar extension is common. These tumors are rare in prepubescent children. It also bears repeating that papillary craniopharnygiomas occur almost exclusively in adults, and tend to be purely suprasellar; as such, these tumors are less likely to be confused with pituitary adenomas (Crotty et al., 1995). Similar to adamantinomatous craniopharyngiomas, pituitary adenomas can be large, lobulated, and show complex signal and enhancement characteristics on MR imaging. Adenomas often show cystic changes (Figure 3.23) with proteinaceous/hemorrhagic contents; identification of a fluid-fluid level in a cystic portion of the tumor (Figures 3.24, 3.25) is more common with an adenoma. The cystic changes in a pituitary adenoma are located within the tumor mass; true exophytic cysts are more typical of adamantinomatous craniopharyngioma. However, pituitary adenomas are overall much more uniform in appearance

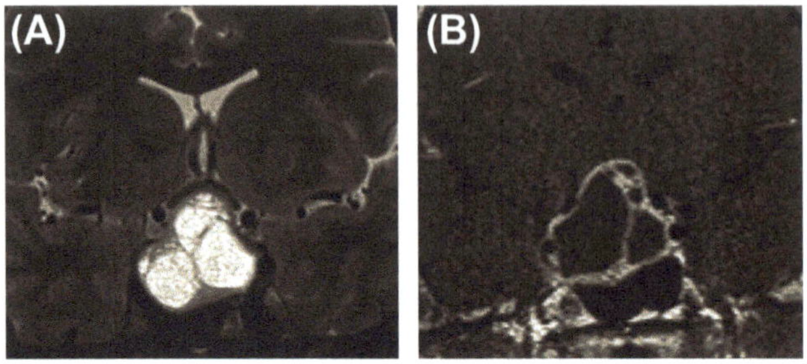

FIGURE 3.23 **A 34-year old man with cystic pituitary macroadenoma. A,** Coronal, T2-weighted MR image shows a complex, cystic intrasellar and suprasellar mass. **B,** Dynamic, T1-weighted enhanced MR image shows enhancement of the periphery of the mass, as well as internal septations. There was no calcification on CT imaging (not shown).

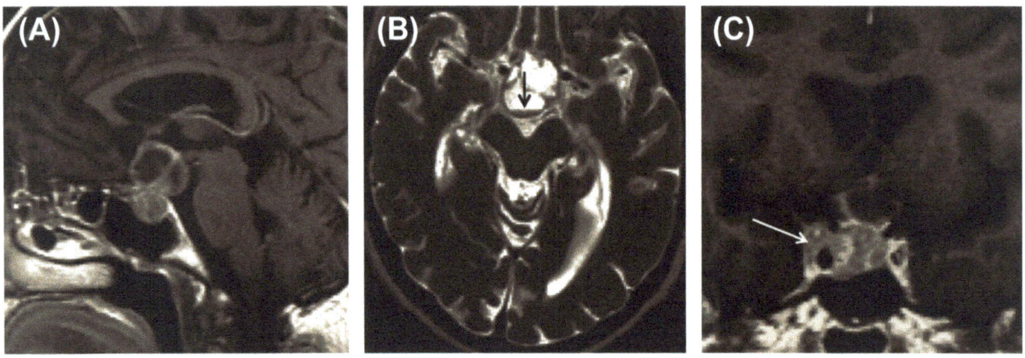

FIGURE 3.24 **A 72-year-old woman with cystic pituitary macroadenoma. A,** Sagittal, T1-weighted enhanced MR image shows a cystic and solid, heterogeneously enhancing, intrasellar, and suprasellar mass. **B,** Axial, T2--weighted MR image shows a fluid–fluid level (arrow) in a hyperintense, cystic portion of the mass. **C,** Coronal, T1-weighted enhanced MR image shows right cavernous sinus invasion (arrow), which is typical of pituitary macroadenomas and very rarely seen with craniopharyngioma. There was no calcification on CT imaging (not shown).

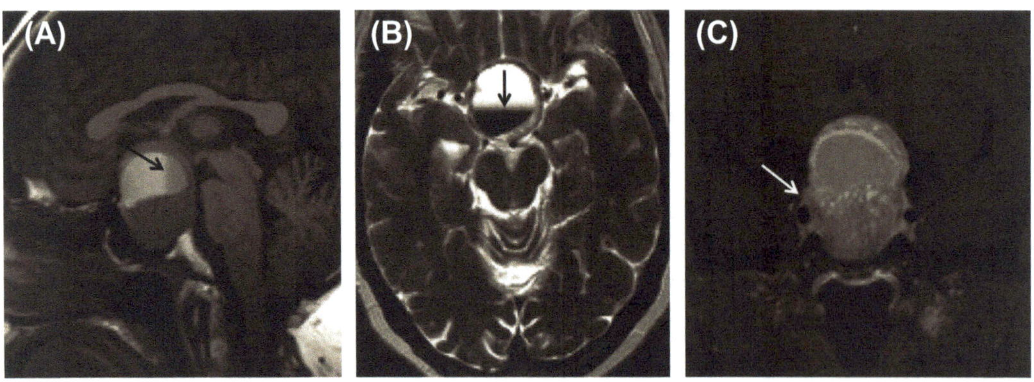

FIGURE 3.25 **A 59-year-old woman with hemorrhagic pituitary macroadenoma. A,** Sagittal, T1-weighted MR image shows a cystic and solid, intrasellar, and suprasellar mass with a fluid–fluid level (arrow). **B,** Axial, T2-weighted MR image shows the fluid–fluid level (arrow) in the mass. **C,** Coronal, T1-weighted enhanced MR image shows diffuse enhancement of the solid portions of the tumor; right cavernous sinus invasion (arrow) cannot be excluded. There was no calcification on CT imaging (not shown).

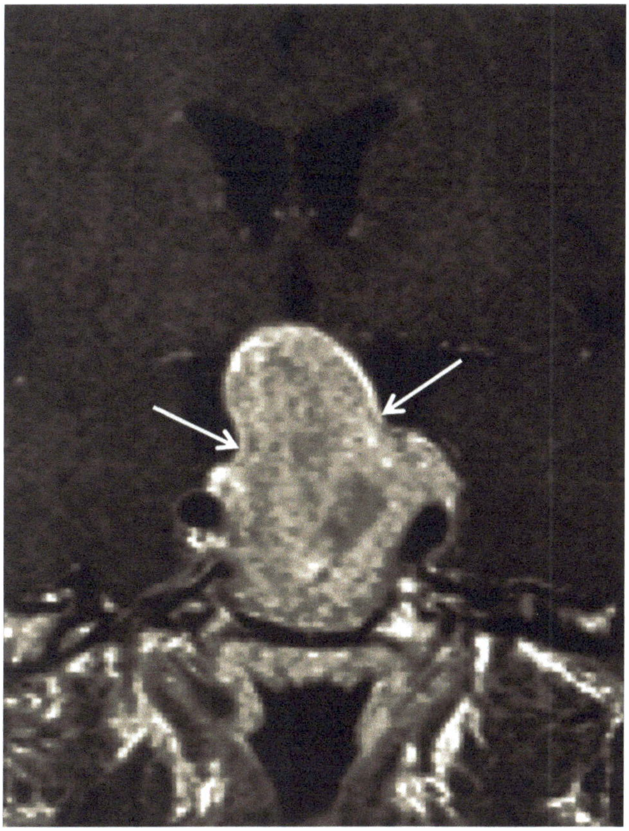

FIGURE 3.26 **A 45-year-old man with pituitary macroadenoma.** Coronal, T1-weighted enhanced MR image shows characteristic "snowman" configuration of a diffusely enhancing, intrasellar, and suprasellar mass; the constriction (arrows) occurs at the level of the diaphragma sella.

(Figure 3.26) than adamantinomatous craniopharyngioma. Unlike adamantinomatous craniopharyngioma, adenomas rarely calcify, may invade one or both cavernous sinuses, and may encase (but not narrow) the cavernous and/or supraclinoid internal carotid arteries (Lee & Deck, 1985; Karnaze et al., 1986; Johnsen et al., 1991; Donovan & Nesbit, 1996; Choi et al., 2007). Parenchymal edema is even less common in association with adenomas. Clearly, pituitary adenomas should not be confused with purely suprasellar craniopharyngiomas. From a practical perspective, it is usually not difficult to distinguish most pituitary adenomas from craniopharyngiomas on imaging studies; moreover, secretory adenomas can be diagnosed on clinical grounds. Diagnostic dilemmas perhaps most frequently occur with non-secretory, cystic tumors; it is important to remember that calcification associated with an adamantinomatous craniopharyngioma may be relatively inapparent on MR imaging.

Suprasellar arachnoid cysts (Figure 3.27) will show CT density and MR signal characteristics similar to simple cerebrospinal fluid; however, CSF pulsation artifacts in larger lesions may cause a somewhat inhomogeneous appearance on MR imaging. Nodular soft tissue, calcification, and enhancement are absent (Osborn & Preece, 2006). Racemose cysts due to neurocysticercosis (Figure 3.28) can also show CT density and MR signal characteristics similar (but not necessarily identical) to cerebrospinal fluid; the FLAIR sequence is most likely

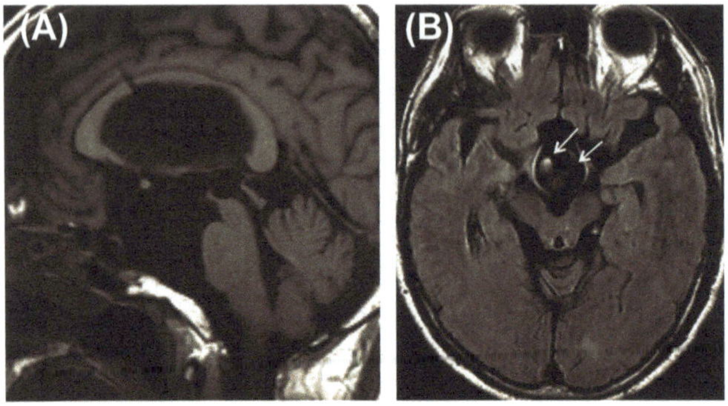

FIGURE 3.27 **A 46-year-old man with a suprasellar arachnoid cyst. A,** Sagittal, T1-weighted MR image shows a massive sellar/suprasellar/prepontine region cyst that is isointense relative to CSF. There is poor definition of normal anatomic structures, and striking osseous remodeling of the skull base due to chronic CSF pulsation. There was no abnormal enhancement, and no restricted diffusion (not shown). **B,** Axial FLAIR image shows CSF pulsation artifacts (arrows) in the cyst; otherwise, the cyst contents suppress. A Rathke cleft cyst would not show CSF pulsation artifact.

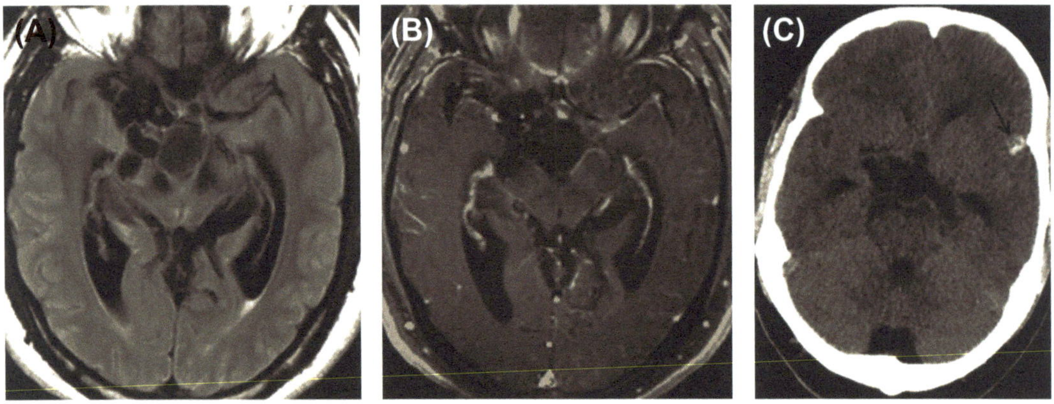

FIGURE 3.28 **A 40-year-old man with neurocysticercosis and a suprasellar racemose cyst. A,** Axial FLAIR MR image shows a multicystic suprasellar mass; the cysts are mildly hyperintense relative to CSF. **B,** Axial, T1-weighted enhanced MR image shows no abnormal enhancement of the lesion. There was no restricted diffusion (not shown). **C,** Axial, non-contrast CT image shows no calcification associated with the hypodense cystic mass; however, a calcification (arrow) is present along the anterior aspect of the left Sylvian fissure.

to highlight any difference. If present, enhancement is usually mild, and nodular soft tissue is absent. Calcification is typically present (Figure 3.29), either regional to the cyst or elsewhere within the parenchyma or subarachnoid space. Regional parenchymal gliosis can also be seen (Arriada-Mendicoa et al., 2003; Kimura-Hayama et al., 2010).

Suprasellar epidermoid tumors (Figure 3.30) typically are similar in signal to CSF on T1-weighted and T2-weighted images (but not FLAIR images), as well as showing diffusion restriction and little, if any enhancement (Tsuruda et al., 1990). Moreover, epidermoids are most commonly off midline in location. Suprasellar dermoid tumors (Figure 3.31) and

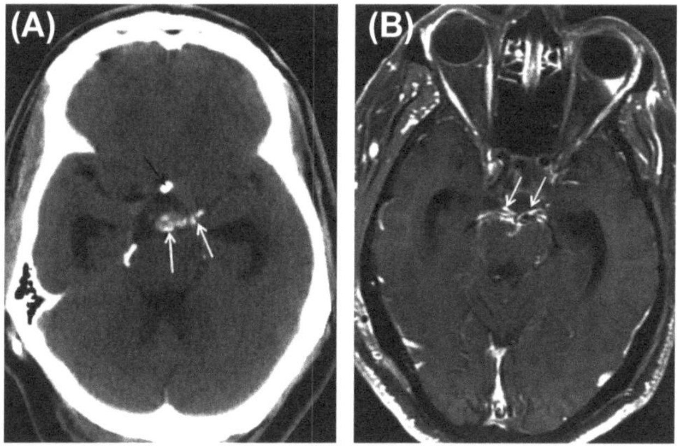

FIGURE 3.29 **A 67-year-old man with neurocysticercosis. A,** Axial, non-contrast CT image shows suprasellar and cisternal calcifications (white arrows). The tip of a shunt catheter (black arrow) is seen at the anterior aspect of the suprasellar cistern. **B,** Axial, T1-weighted enhanced MR image shows foci of crescentic enhancement (arrows) in the suprasellar and prepontine cisterns.

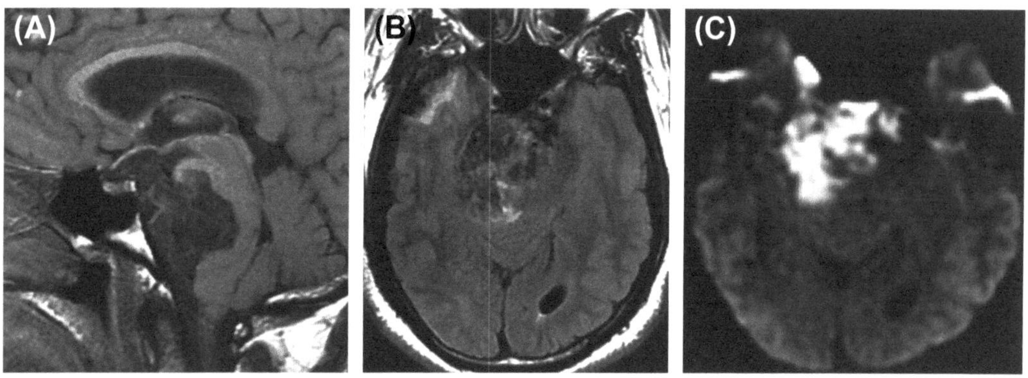

FIGURE 3.30 **A 55-year-old man with prepontine and suprasellar epidermoid. A,** Axial, T1-weighted MR image shows a large, lobulated, prepontine, and suprasellar mass. The mass is hypointense relative to parenchyma, but mildly hyperintense relative to CSF. There is no osseous remodeling of the skull base. There was no abnormal enhancement (not shown). **B,** Axial FLAIR image shows extremely heterogeneous signal within the mass. There is no CSF pulsation artifact. **C,** Axial b=1000 diffusion image shows restricted diffusion within the mass, which is characteristic of an epidermoid tumor given the other imaging characteristics.

teratomas have a more complex appearance, including calcification, but the consistent presence of fat density on CT or fat signal on MR imaging will suggest the correct diagnosis. These tumors are typically midline in location. Dermoids show little or no enhancement, and have a tendency to rupture, with resultant fat droplets dispersed throughout the ventricles or subarachnoid spaces. Teratomas are more closely associated with the pineal region (Smirniotopoulos & Chiechi, 1995). Intracranial lipomas are non-neoplastic congenital malformations that are typically midline; although hyperintense on T1-weighted images, the fat

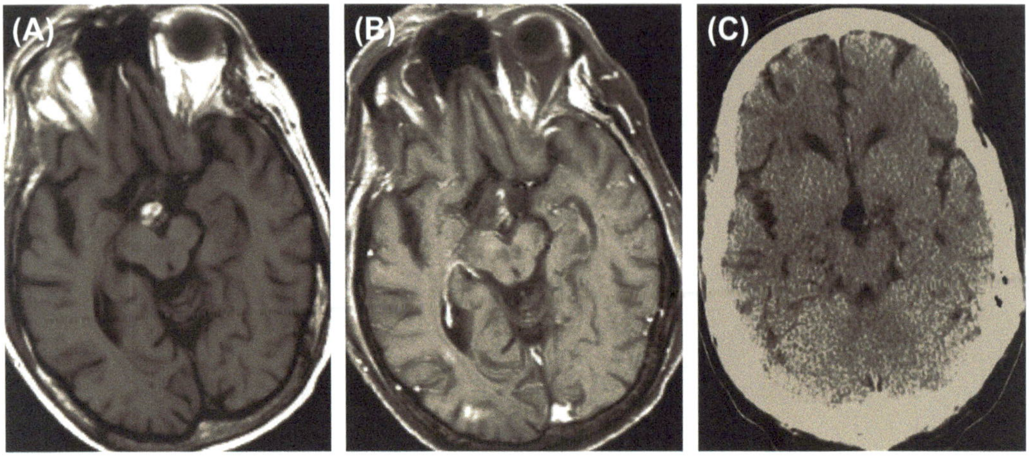

FIGURE 3.31 **A 58-year-old man with presumed dermoid cyst. A,** Axial, T1-weighted MR image shows a heterogeneous mass ventral to the interpeduncular cistern, with areas of T1 shortening. **B,** Axial, T1-weighted enhanced MR image shows suppression of the T1 hyperintense portion of the mass, in keeping with fat. **C,** Axial, non-contrast CT image confirms the presence of fat within the tumor.

signal of a suprasellar lipoma should not be confused with a craniopharyngioma. Intracranial lipomas may be associated with crescentic calcifications (Truwit & Barkovich, 1990). Of note, unlike the T1-weighted hyperintensity associated with methemoglobin, proteinaceous fluid, and melanin, the T1-weighted hyperintensity of fat in a dermoid, teratoma, or lipoma will suppress when using a variety of fat-suppression techniques. Moreover, fat will show chemical shift artifact (Figure 3.32) in the frequency-encoded direction; recognition of its presence can be used as a diagnostic signature of fat. This artifact increases with the field strength of

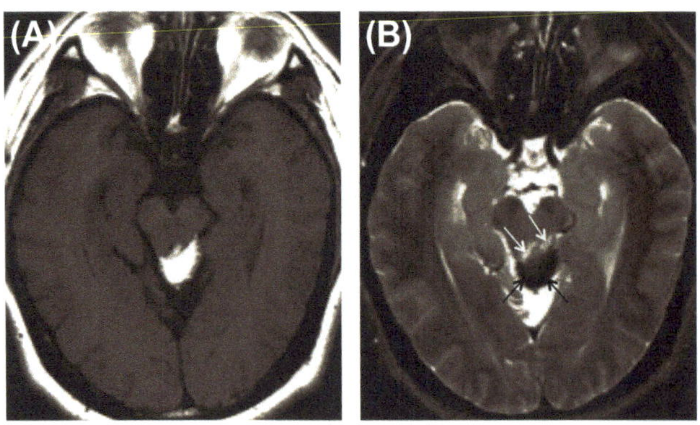

FIGURE 3.32 **A 42-year-old woman with tectal lipoma showing chemical shift artifact. A,** Axial, T1-weighted MR image shows a markedly hyperintense tectal mass; the lesion suppressed on fat-suppressed, T1-weighted enhanced imaging (not shown). **B,** Axial, T2-weighted MR image shows a band of hyperintensity (white arrows) along the anterior aspect of the mass, and a band of hypointensity (black arrows) along the posterior aspect of the mass, in keeping with chemical shift artifact in the frequency-encoded direction. This artifact identifies the tissue as fat.

the MR unit. Because of the difference in resonance frequencies between water and fat, when converting the MRI signal from the frequency to spatial domain, protons at the same location are mis-registered by the Fourier transformation. This chemical shift mis-registration causes accentuation of any fat–water interfaces along the frequency axis. Where fat and water are in the same location, this artifact can be seen as a bright or dark band at the edge of the anatomy (Hood et al., 1999).

Partially or completely thrombosed suprasellar aneurysms (Figure 3.33) can pose a significant diagnostic dilemma in anatomic imaging studies. Hence, when confronted with any suprasellar mass, particularly a mass containing T1-hyperintensity, the possibility of aneurysm should at least be considered. These round or lobulated lesions are typically variably

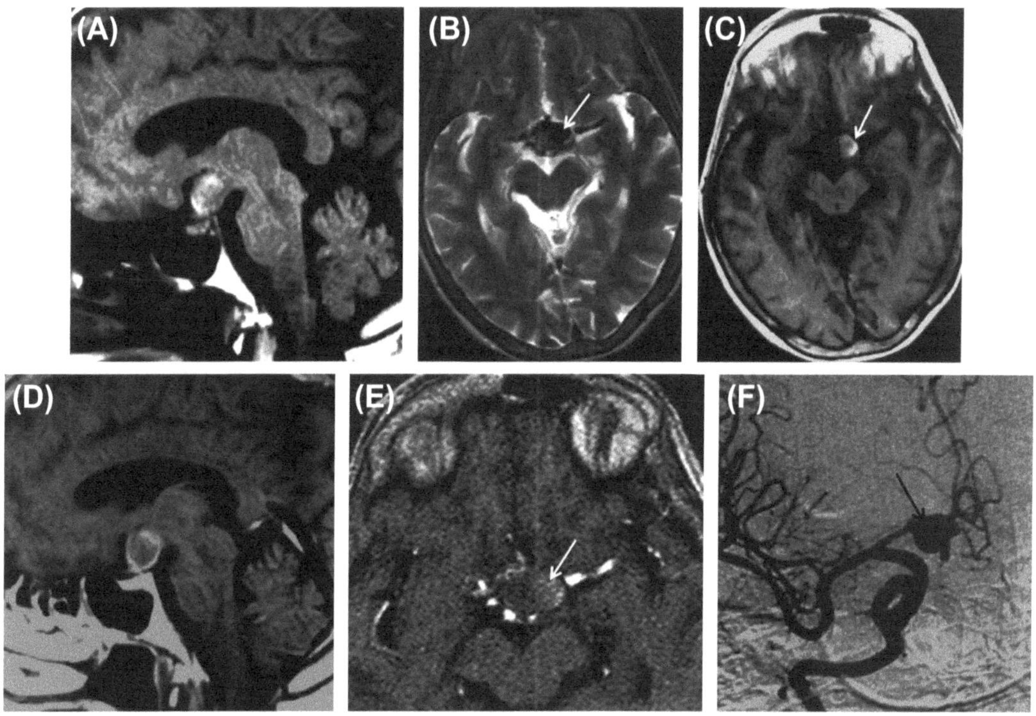

FIGURE 3.33 **A 50-year-old man with a partially thrombosed anterior communicating artery aneurysm; the MRI scan was performed on a 0.3 Tesla MR unit. A,** Sagittal, T1-weighted MR image shows an ovoid, heterogeneous signal suprasellar mass, part of which is hyperintense relative to parenchyma. **B,** Axial, T2-weighted MR image again shows heterogeneous signal within the mass, including an area of hypointensity (arrow). There is no evidence of pulsation artifact in the phase-encoded direction. **C,** Axial, T1-weighted MR image shows hyperintensity (arrow) with the T2 hypointense portion of the mass, suggesting proteinaceous contents. **D,** Sagittal, T1-weighted enhanced MR image shows peripheral enhancement of the mass. **E,** Source date from the 3-D time of flight MRA shows faint hyperintensity (arrow) within the mass, corresponding to the region of hyperintensity on the T1-weighted axial image; this precludes the diagnosis of flow-related enhancement. The overall appearance of the lesion suggests an adamantinomatous craniopharnyngioma. **F,** Conventional angiogram, frontal oblique projection, right internal carotid artery injection, shows a partially thrombosed, anterior communicating artery aneurysm (arrow). The diagnosis of aneurysm on the MRI and MRA examinations is very difficult, in part due to the low field strength of the scanner.

dense on CT imaging (reflecting clotted and/or unclotted blood), and a rim of calcification can be present in larger aneurysms. The MR imaging characteristics will depend upon the degree and age of the thrombus, but areas of T1-weighted hyperintensity, T2-weighted hypointensity, and blooming on T2*-gradient echo imaging are characteristics suggestive of a vascular abnormality. The abnormal signal may have a laminated appearance. The patent lumen of the aneurysm should appear as a flow void, unless the flow is turbulent; if large enough, arterial pulsations from the patent lumen will result in ghosting artifact in the phase encoded direction (Saatci et al., 2003). Larger aneurysms can also show thin enhancement of the wall, and mild regional parenchymal edema (Olsen et al., 1987). Occasionally, cavernous aneurysms will enlarge medially into the sella, potentially mimicking a pituitary adenoma or intrasellar craniopharyngioma. In the absence of T1-weighted hyperintensity associated with a suprasellar mass, 3-D time of flight MR angiography is reliable in making the diagnosis of aneurysm (an exception being a larger aneurysm with slow/turbulent flow and resultant poor flow-related enhancement). As stated previously, non-aneurysmal lesions with T1-weighted hyperintensity can mimic flow-related enhancement on 3-D time of flight (but not phase contrast) MR angiography (Tsuruda et al., 1992; Ozsarlak et al., 2004). CT angiography is an indispensable tool in difficult cases. Diagnostic clues on MRI/MRA imaging, such as pulsation artifact, susceptibility, and flow-related enhancement, may be less apparent on lower field strength MRI units.

Chiasmatic/hypothalamic glioma and hamartomas of the tuber cinereum are most common in the pediatric age group. Chiasmatic/hypothalamic gliomas are most often pilocytic in histology, although more aggressive lesions may occur (Figure 3.34). Unlike adamantinimatous craniopharyngioma, they typically manifest as large, mostly solid, enhancing masses with small cystic/necrotic components; calcification is rare (Saleem et al., 2007). Hamartoma of the tuber cinereum is a congenital, non-neoplastic heterotopia. These lesions can be sessile or pedunculated, residing between the infundibulum anteriorly and the mammillary bodies posteriorly. They are similar in signal to gray matter, and do not show cyst formation,

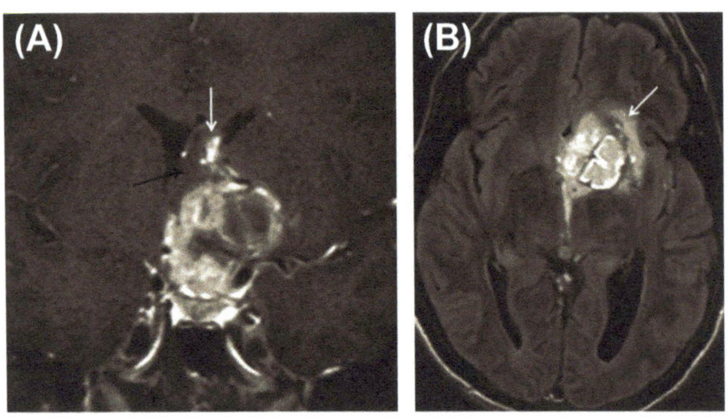

FIGURE 3.34 **A 39-year-old man with type I neurofibromatosis and glioblastoma multiforme of the optic chiasm. A,** Coronal, T1-weighted enhanced MR image shows a large, heterogeneously enhancing suprasellar mass, with extension along the ependyma of the left frontal horn (white arrow) and thickening of the septum pellucidum (black arrow); these latter features are most consistent with a glial neoplasm. **B,** Axial FLAIR image shows edema and/or infiltrative tumor (arrow) adjacent to the tumor.

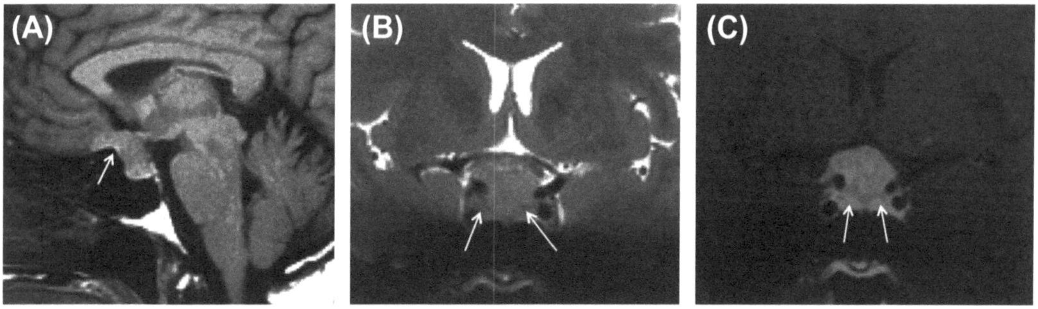

FIGURE 3.35 **A 51-year-old woman with planum sphenoidale/diaphragma sella meningioma. A,** Sagittal, T1-weighted MR image shows a dural-based mass along the planum sphenoidale/diaphragm sella, extending into the sella, that is isointense to parenchyma. There is "blistering" (superior convexity) (arrow) of the planum, which is characteristic of meningiomas in this location. **B,** Coronal, T2-weighted MR image enables distinction of the tumor from the compressed pituitary gland (arrows). The tumor is slightly hyperintense relative to parenchyma. **C,** Coronal, T1-weighted enhanced MR image shows homogeneous enhancement of the tumor, which can be distinguished from the compressed pituitary gland (arrows); the tumor partially surrounds the internal carotid arteries.

calcification, or enhancement; they should not be confused with either pathologic type of craniopharyngioma (Boyko et al., 1991).

Similar to meningiomas in other locations, suprasellar meningiomas arising from the planum sphenoidale/diaphragm sella (Figure 3.35) are typically isointense to parenchyma on T1-weighted images, iso- to hyopointense on T2-weighted images, and enhance intensely and uniformly. Calcification may be present. These dural-based masses can cause "blistering" (superior convexity) of the planum sphenoidale and/or hyperostosis (Kinjo et al., 1995). These adult tumors are generally not difficult to distinguish from papillary craniopharyngioma.

Non-neoplastic, mass-like enlargement of the infundibulum can be due to Langerhans cell histiocytosis, sarcoid, lymphocytic hypophysitis (Figure 3.36), and meningitis (Ahmadi et al., 1995; Hamilton et al., 2007; Nakata et al., 2010). Neoplasms that affect the infundibulum include germinoma, lymphoma, and metastasis. Primary stalk neoplasms are rare and include pituicytoma (Figure 3.37) and granular cell tumor; most of these tumors are intrasellar/suprasellar or suprasellar; a minority of pituicytomas will be purely intrasellar. Primary stalk tumors are typically isodense to hyperdense relative to parenchyma on CT imaging, isointense to the cortex on T1-weighted imaging, iso- to hyperintense on T2-weighted imaging, with homogeneous or heterogeneous enhancement. Approximately 75% cannot be separated from the pituitary gland, which helps in the radiologic differentiation from craniopharnygioma; unfortunately, these tumors can be indistinguishable from pituitary adenomas (Covington et al., 2011). The inability to distinguish primary stalk tumors from pituitary adenomas is important, because primary stalk tumors tend to be very vascular and prone to heavy bleeding during surgical resection. From a clinical perspective, diabetes insipidus, prolactinemia, and galactorrhea are rarely associated with primary stalk tumors.

Table 3.1 highlights the imaging characteristics of adamantinomatous and papillary craniopharyngioma and several potentially similar-appearing lesions.

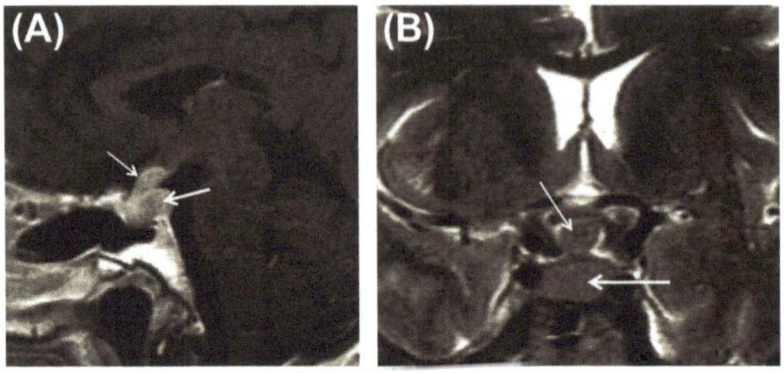

FIGURE 3.36 **A 56-year-old woman with lymphocytic hypophysitis. A,** Sagittal, T1-weighted enhanced MR image shows bulbous enlargement and diffuse enhancement of the infundibulum (thin arrow) and pituitary gland (thick arrow); involvement of both structures is the clue to the correct diagnosis. **B,** Coronal, T2-weighted MR image shows enlargement of the infundibulum (thin arrow) and pituitary gland (thick arrow) by soft tissue that is isointense relative to parenchyma.

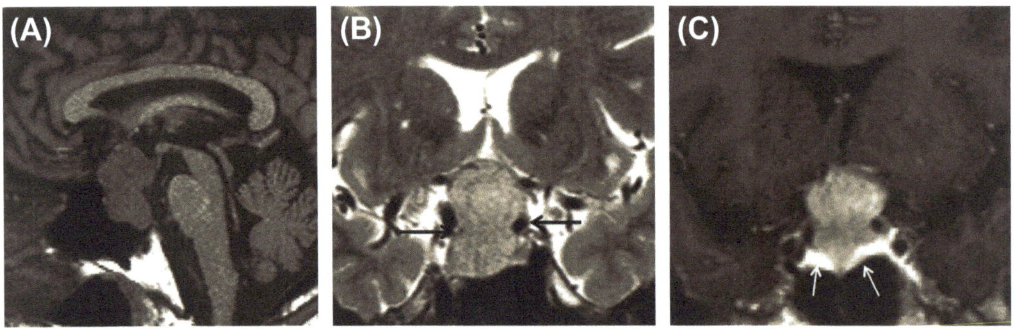

FIGURE 3.37 **A 56-year-old woman with pituicytoma. A,** Sagittal, T1-weighted MR image shows a large intrasellar and suprasellar mass that is mildly hypointense relative to parenchyma. **B,** Coronal, T2-weighted MR image shows constriction of the mass (arrows) at the diaphragma sella. The appearance is most consistent with a pituitary macroadenoma. **C,** Coronal, T1-weighted enhanced MR image shows diffuse enhancement of the mass; the pituitary gland is compressed and located at the inferior aspect of the sella (arrows); the gland enhances more avidly than the tumor, and can be identified as a separate structure, which is the clue to the correct diagnosis. CT imaging showed an isodense mass, without calcification (not shown).

VASCULAR PEDICLE NASOSEPTAL FLAP

A trans-sphenoidal endoscopic approach is being increasingly utilized for the resection of sellar/suprasellar lesions. The vascular pedicle nasoseptal flap has had an important role in the broader application of this approach; for large skull base defects, its use has led to a sharp decrease in the incidence of postoperative cerebrospinal fluid leaks (Hadad et al., 2006). It is important to become familiar with the expected MR imaging appearance of the nasoseptal flap, so that the flap is not confused with residual or recurrent tumor.

TABLE 3.1 Imaging Characteristics of Craniopharyngioma and Other Sellar Region Lesions

	Adamantinomatous Craniopharyngioma	Papillary Craniopharyngioma	Rathke Cleft Cyst	Pituitary Adenoma	Chordoid Glioma	Diaphragma Sella Meningioma	Aneurysm With Thrombus
Age	All ages; peaks in childhood (5–10 yrs); second peak in 6th decade	Almost exclusively in adults; peaks in 6th decade	All ages; peaks in 4th–6th decades	Rare in prepubescent children. All ages in adults	Adults	Adults	Adults; very uncommon in children
Location	Suprasellar; less likely intrasellar and suprasellar, or purely intrasellar	Suprasellar	Intrasellar; less likely intrasellar with suprasellar extension, or purely suprasellar	Intrasellar, or intrasellar with suprasellar extension	Anterior third ventricle	Diaphragma sella/planum sphenoidale	Suprasellar or parasellar; rarely intrasellar extension
Calcification	90%; frequent rim calcification	Very uncommon	Rare	Rare	Rare	Occasional; planum lesions cause blistering	Occasional; rim calcification
Composition	Cystic and solid	Mostly solid	Cystic	Mostly solid; internal cystic changes common	Mostly solid	Solid	Complex; blood products of variable age, flow void
Enhancement	Solid portions and cyst walls	Solid but heterogeneous	Rare	Solid but often heterogeneous	Solid, mostly homogenous	Homogeneous	Variable
Lobulation	Often multilobulated	Occasional lobulation	Occasional lobulation	When large, often lobulated	No lobulation	No lobulation	Occasional lobulation
Homogeneity	Most heterogeneous sellar/suprasellar mass	Relatively homogenous	Relatively homogenous	Variable	Homogenous	Homogenous	Variable; depends upon degree and age of thrombus
Classic Appearance	Heterogeneously enhancing, lobulated, cystic, and solid suprasellar mass with calcification	Solid, heterogeneously enhancing, suprasellar mass in adult	Noncalcified, non-enhancing, intrasellar, proteinaceous cyst, possibly with suprasellar extension	Enhancing intrasellar, or intrasellar and suprasellar mass, inseparable from pituitary gland	Homogeneously enhancing, third ventricular mass	Homogeneously enhancing, dural-based mass	Flow void, blood products of variable signal, blooming on T2* gradient echo imaging

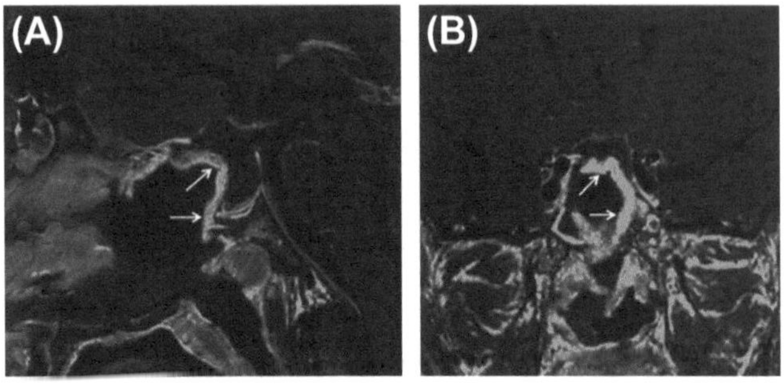

FIGURE 3.38 **A 33-year-old man status post endoscopic resection of an intrasellar and suprasellar adamantinomatous craniopharyngioma. A,** Sagittal, T1-weighted enhanced MR image obtained one day after surgery shows the typical C-shaped configuration (arrows) of the enhancing nasoseptal flap covering the skull base defect. **B,** Coronal, T1-weighted enhanced MR image also shows the C-shaped, enhancing nasoseptal flap (arrows).

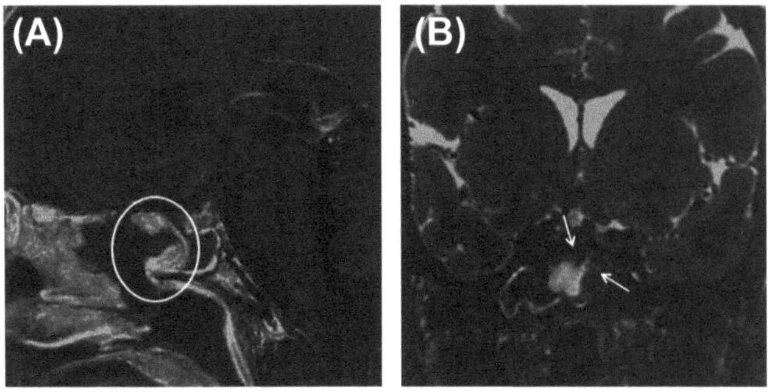

FIGURE 3.39 **A 48-year-old woman status post endoscopic resection of a suprasellar adamantinomatous craniopharyngioma. A,** Sagittal, T1-weighted enhanced MR image obtained one day after surgery shows the C-shaped, enhancing nasoseptal flap (oval). **B,** Coronal, T2-weighted MR image shows that the nasoseptal flap (arrows) is isointense relative to parenchyma.

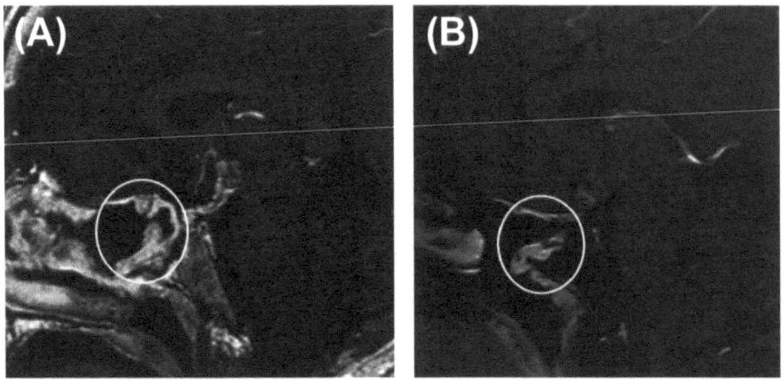

FIGURE 3.40 **A 26-year-old man status post endoscopic resection of a suprasellar adamantinomatous craniopharnyngioma. A,** Sagittal, T1-weighted enhanced MR image obtained one day after surgery shows the C-shaped, enhancing nasoseptal flap (oval). **B,** Sagittal, T1-weighted enhanced MR image obtained approximately 7 months after surgery shows interval contraction of the nasoseptal flap (oval).

Typically, the nasoseptal flap (Figure 3.38) has a C-shaped configuration within the operative defect, and is isointense on T1- and T2-weighted images (Figure 3.39) on both immediate and delayed postoperative MR imaging studies. In addition, most flaps enhance after contrast administration on both immediate and delayed studies. On delayed postoperative scans, some flaps become thinner (presumably due to flap contraction) (Figure 3.40), while others become thicker (presumably due to granulation tissue and/or increased mucosalization). Variations in flap enhancement are difficult to correlate with flap failure, particularly on delayed scans, because there is overlap in the appearance of an enhancing flap and granulation tissue. However, non-enhancement of the flap is concerning for vascular compromise and ultimate flap failure (Kang et al., 2009).

CONCLUSION

The radiographic appearance of craniopharyngiomas can demonstrate extreme heterogeneity, and although most commonly found in the suprasellar cistern, these tumors can occur in a variety of anatomical locations. Therefore, knowledge of the appearances of craniopharyngiomas on imaging studies, along with the complementary roles played by CT and MR imaging in the evaluation of intrasellar and suprasellar lesions, is pivotal for treating physicians. Additionally, recognition of the wide differential diagnosis of similar-appearing lesions, from Rathke cleft cysts to pituitary adenomas and aneurysms, and their radiographic distinction from craniopharyngiomas must be made as all of these have widely varying methods and goals of treatment.

References

Abrahams, J.J., Lidov, M., Artiles, C., 1989. MR imaging of intracranial fluid levels. AJR Am. J. Roentgenol. 153, 597–604.

Adamson, T.E., Wiestler, O.D., Kleihues, P., Yasargil, M.G., 1990. Correlation of clinical and pathological features in surgically treated craniopharyngiomas. J. Neurosurg. 73, 12–17.

Ahmadi, J., Destian, S., Apuzzo, M.L.J., Segall, H.D., Zee, C.S., 1992. Cystic fluid in craniopharyngiomas: MR imaging and quantitative analysis. Radiology 182, 783–785.

Ahmadi, J., Meyers, G.S., Segall, H.D., Sharma, O.P., Hinton, D.R., 1995. Lymphocytic adenohypophysitis: contrast-enhanced MR imaging in five cases. Radiology 195, 30–34.

Arriada-Mendicoa, N., Celis-Lopez, A., Higuera-Calleja, J., Corona-Vazquez, T., 2003. Imaging features of sellar cysticercosis. AJNR Am. J. Neuroradiol. 24, 1386–1389.

Baker, H.K., 1972. The angiographic delineation of sellar and parasellar masses. Radiology 104, 67–78.

Behari, S., Banerji, D., Mishra, A., Sharma, S., Chhabra, D.K., Jain, V.K., 2003. Intrinsic third ventricular craniopharyngiomas: report on six cases and review of the literature. Surg. Neurol. 60 (3), 245–252.

Bianco, A.M., Madeira, L.V., Rosemberg, S., Shibata, M.K., 2006. Cortical seeding of a craniopharyngioma after craniotomy: case report. Surg. Neurol. 66 (4), 437–440.

Bonneville, F., Cattin, F., Marsot-Dupuch, K., Dormont, D., Bonneville, J.F., Chiras, J., 2006. T1-signal hyperintensity in the sellar region: spectrum of findings. RadioGraphics 26, 93–113.

Bonneville, F., Chiras, J., Cattin, F., Bonneville, J.F., 2007. T2 hypointense signal of Rathke cleft cyst. AJNR Am. J. Neuroradiol. 28, 397.

Boyko, O.B., Curnes, J.T., Oakes, W.J., Burger, P.C., 1991. Hamartomas of the tuber cinereum: CT, MR, and pathologic findings. AJNR Am. J. Neuroradiol. 1991 (12), 309–314.

Bunin, G.R., Surawicz, T.S., Witman, P.A., Preston-Martin, S., Davis, F., Bruner, J.M., 1998. The descriptive epidemiology of craniopharyngioma. J. Neurosurg. 89, 547–551.

Byun, W.M., Kim, O.L., Kim, D.S., 2000. MR imaging findings of Rathke's cleft cysts: significance of intracystic nodules. AJNR Am. J. Neuroradiol. 21, 485–488.

Chaiban, J.T., Abdelmannan, D., Cohen, M., Selman, W.R., Arafah, B.M., 2011. Rathke cleft cyst apoplexy: a newly characterized distinct clinical entity. J. Neurosurg. 114, 318–324.

Choi, S.H., Kwon, B.J., Na, D.G., Kim, J.H., Han, M.H., Chang, K.H., 2007. Pituitary adenoma, craniopharyngioma, and Rathke cleft cyst involving both intrasellar and suprasellar regions: differentiation using MRI. Clin. Radiol. 62 (5), 453–462.

Covington, M.F., Chin, S.S., Osborn, A.G., 2011. Pituicytoma, spindle cell oncocytoma, and granular cell tumor: clarification and meta-analysis of the world literature since 1893. AJNR Am. J. Neuroradiol. 32, 2067–2072.

Crotty, T.B., Scheithauer, B.W., Young Jr., W.F., Davis, D.H., Shaw, E.G., Miller, G.M., Burger, P.C., 1995. Papillary craniopharyngioma; a clinicopathological study of 48 cases. J. Neurosurg. 83, 206–214.

Deutsch, H., Kothbauer, K., Persky, M., Epstein, F.J., Jallo, G.I., 2001. Infrasellar craniopharyngiomas: case report and review of the literature. Skull Base 11 (2), 121–128.

Donovan, J.L., Nesbit, G.M., 1996. Distinction of masses involving the sella and suprasellar space: specificity of imaging features. AJR Am. J. Roentgenol. 167, 597–603.

Effenterre, R.V., Boch, A.L., 2002. Craniopharyngioma in adults and children: a study of 122 surgical cases. J. Neurosurg. 97, 3–11.

Eldevik, O.P., Blaivas, M., Gabrielsen, T.O., Hald, J.K., Chandler, W.F., 1996. Craniopharyngioma: radiologic and histologic findings and recurrence. AJNR Am. J. Neuroradiol. 17, 1427–1439.

Fischer, E.G., Welch, K., Shillito Jr, J., Winston, K.R., Tarbell, N.J., 1990. Craniopharyngiomas in children: long term effects of conservative surgical procedures combined with radiation therapy. J. Neurosurg. 73, 534–540.

Fitz, C.R., Wortzman, G., Harwood-Nash, D.C., Holgate, R.C., Barry, J.F., Boldt, D.W., 1978. Computed tomography in craniopharyngiomas. Radiology 127, 687–691.

Ginat, D.T., Meyers, S.P., 2012. Intracranial lesions with high signal intensity on T1-weighted MR images; differential diagnosis. RadioGraphics 32, 499–516.

Glastonbury, C.M., Osborn, A.G., Salzman, K.L., 2011. Masses and malformations of the third ventricle: normal anatomic relationships and differential diagnoses. RadioGraphics 31, 1889–1905.

Gupta, K., Kuhn, M.J., Shevlin, D.W., Wacaser, L.E., 1999. Metastatic craniopharyngioma. AJNR Am. J. Neuroradiol. 20, 1059–1060.

Hadad, G., Bassagasteguy, L., Carrau, R.L., Mataza, J.C., Kassam, A., Snyderman, C.H., Mintz, A., 2006. A novel reconstructive technique after endoscopic expanded endonasal approaches: vascular pedicle nasoseptal flap. Laryngoscope 116, 1882–1886.

Hamilton, B.E., Salzman, K.L., Osborn, A.G., 2007. Anatomic and pathologic spectrum of pituitary infundibulum lesions. AJR Am. J. Roentgenol. 188, W-223–W232.

Harrrison, M.J., Morgello, S., Post, K.D., 1994. Epithelial cystic lesions of the sellar and parasellar region: a continuum of ectodermal derivatives? J. Neurosurg. 80, 1018–1025.

Harwood-Nash, D.C., 1994. Neuroimaging of childhood craniopharyngioma. Pediatr. Neurosurg. 21, 2–10.

Hood, M.N., Ho, V.B., Smirniotopoulos, J.G., Szumowski, J., 1999. Chemical shift: the artifact and clinical tool revisited. RadioGraphics 19, 357–371.

Ito, M., Jamshidi, J., Yamanaka, K., 2001. Does craniopharyngioma metastasize? Case report and review of the literature. Neurosurgery 48 (4), 933–936.

Johnsen, D.E., Woodruff, W.W., Allen, I.S., Cera, P.J., Funkhouser, G.R., Coleman, L.L., 1991. MR imaging of the sellar and juxtasellar regions. RadioGraphics 11, 727–758.

Kang, M.D., Escott, E., Thomas, A.J., Carrau, R.L., Snyderman, C.H., Kassam, A.B., Rothfus, W., 2009. The MR imaging appearance of the vascular pedicle nasoseptal flap. AJNR Am. J. Neuroradiol. 30, 781–786.

Kanungo, N., Just, N., Black, M., Mohr, G., Glikstein, R., Rochon, L., 1995. Nasopharyngeal craniopharyngioma in an unusual location. AJNR Am. J. Neuroradiol. 16, 1372–1374.

Karnaze, M.G., Sartor, K., Winthrop, J.D., Gado, M.H., Hodges 3rd, F.J., 1986. Suprasellar lesions: evaluation with MR imaging. Radiology 161, 77–82.

Kimura-Hayama, E.T., Higuera, J.A., Corona-Cedillo, R., Chávez-Macías, L., Perochena, A., Quiroz-Rojas, L.Y., Rodríguez-Carbajal, J., Criales, J.L., 2010. Neurocysticercosis: radiologic-pathologic correlation. RadioGraphics 30, 1705–1719.

Kinjo, T., Al-Mefty, O., Ciric, I., 1995. Diaphragma sella meningiomas. Neurosurgery 36 (6), 1082–1092.

Kucharczyk, W., Peck, W.W., Kelly, W.M., Norman, D., Newton, T.H., 1987. Rathke cleft cyst: CT, MR imaging, and pathologic features. Radiology 165, 491–495.

Kulkarni, V., Daniel, R.T., Pranatartiharan, R., 2000. Spontaneous intraventricular rupture of craniopharyngioma cyst. Surg. Neurol. 54 (3), 249–253.

Lee, B.C., Deck, M.D., 1985. Sellar and juxtasellar lesion detection with MR. Radiology 157, 143–147.

Megdiche-Bazarbachaa, H., Ben Hammouda, K., Aicha, A.B., Sebai, R., Belghith, L., Khaldi, M., Touibi, S., 2006. Intrasphenoidal Rathke cleft cyst. AJNR Am. J. Neuroradiol. 27, 1098–1100.

Miller, D.C., 1994. Pathology of craniopharyngiomas: clinical import of pathological findings. Pediatr Neurosurg. 1994 21 (Suppl. 1), 11–17.

Nakasu, Y., Nakasu, S., Nakajima, M., Itoh, R., Matsuda, M., 1999. Atypical Rathke's cleft cyst associated with ossification. AJNR Am. J. Neuroradiol. 20, 1287–1289.

Nakata, Y., Sato, N., Masumoto, T., Mori, H., Akai, H., Nobusawa, H., Adachi, Y., Oba, H., Ohtomo, K., 2010. Parasellar T2 dark sign on MR imaging in patients with lymphocytic hypophysitis. AJNR Am. J. Neuroradiol. 31, 1944–1950.

Olsen, W.L., Brant-Zawadzki, M., Hodes, J., Norman, D., Newton, T.H., 1987. Giant intracranial aneurysms: MR imaging. Radiology 163, 431–435.

Osborn, A.G., Preece, M.T., 2006. Intracranial cysts: radiologic-pathologic correlation and imaging approach. Radiology 239, 650–664.

Ozsarlak, O., Van Goethem, J., Maes, M., Parizel, P.M., 2004. MR angiography of the intracranial vessels: technical aspects and clinical applications. Neuroradiology 46, 955–972.

Petito, C.K., 1996. Craniopharyngioma: prognostic importance of histologic features. AJNR Am. J. Neuroradiol. 17, 1441–1442.

Plaza, M.J., Borja, M.J., Altman, N., Saigal, G., 2013. Conventional and advanced MRI features of pediatric intracranial tumors: posterior fossa and suprasellar tumors. AJR Am. J. Roentgenol. 200, 1115–1124.

Pomper, M.G., Passe, T.J., Burger, P.J., Scheithauer, B.W., Brat, D.J., 2001. Chordoid glioma: a neoplasm unique to the hypothalamus and anterior third ventricle. AJNR Am. J. Neuroradiol. 22, 464–469.

Prabhu, V.C., Brown, H.G., 2005. The pathogenesis of craniopharyngiomas. Childs Nerv. Syst. 21, 622–627.

Pusey, E., Kortman, K.E., Flannigan, B.D., Tsuruda, J., Bradley, W.G., 1987. MR of craniopharnyngiomas: tumor delineation and characterization. AJR Am. J. Roentgenol. 149, 83–388.

Saatci, I., Cekirge, H.S., Ciceri, E.F.M., Mawad, M.E., Pamuk, A.G., Besima, A., 2003. CT and MR imaging findings and their implications in the follow-up of patients with intracranial aneurysms treated with endosaccular occlusion with onyx. AJNR Am. J. Neuroradiol. 24, 567–578.

Saeki, N., Uchino, Y., Murai, H., Kubota, M., Isobe, K., Uno, T., Sunami, K., Yamaura, A., 2003. MR imaging study of edema-like change along the optic tract in patients with pituitary region tumors. AJNR Am. J. Neuroradiol. 24, 336–342.

Saleem, S.N., Said, A.H., Lee, D.H., 2007. Lesions of the hypothalamus: MR imaging diagnostic features. RadioGraphics 27, 1087–1108.

Sartoretti-Schefer, S., Wichmann, W., Aguzzi, A., Valvanis, A., 1997. MR differentiation of adamantinous and squamous-papillary craniopharyngioma. AJNR Am. J. Neuroradiol. 18, 77–87.

Sener, R.N., 1993. Giant craniopharyngioma extending to the anterior cranial fossa and nasopharynx. AJR Am. J. Roentgenol. 162, 441–442.

Shida, N., Nakasato, N., Mizoi, K., Kanaki, M., Yoshimoto, T., 1998. Symptomatic vessel narrowing caused by spontaneous rupture of craniopharyngioma cyst. Neurol. Med. Chir. (Tokyo) 38, 666–668.

Shin, J.L., Asa, S.L., Woodhouse, L.J., Smyth, H.S., Ezzat, S., 1999. Cystic lesions of the pituitary: clinicopathological features distinguishing craniopharyngioma, Rathke's cleft cyst, and arachnoid cyst. J. Clin. Endocrinol. Metab. 84 (11), 3972–3982.

Smirniotopoulos, J.G., Chiechi, M.V., 1995. Teratomas, dermoids, and epidermoids of the head and neck. Radiographics 15, 1437–1455.

Sorva, R., Jaaskinen, J., Heiskanen, O., 1987. Craniopharyngioma in children and adults: correlations between radiological and clinical manifestations. Acta. Neurochir. 89, 3–9.

Sumida, M., Uozumi, T., Mukada, K., 1994. Rathke cleft cysts: correlation of enhanced MR and surgical findings. AJNR Am. J. Neuroradiol. 15, 525–532.

Szeifert, G.T., Sipos, L., Horvfith, M., Sarker, M.H., Major, O., Salomváry, B., Czirják, S., Bálint, K., Slowik, F., Kolonics, L., 1993. Pathological characteristics of surgically removed craniopharyngiomas; analysis of 131 cases. Acta. Neurochir. 124, 139–143.

Tavangar, S.M., Larijani, B., Mahta, A., Hosseini, S.M.A., Mehrazine, M., Bandarian, F., 2004. Craniopharyngioma: a clinicopathological study of 141 cases. Endocr. Pathol. 15 (4), 339–344.

Trifanescu, R., Ansorge, O., Wass, J.A.H., Grossman, A., Karavitaki, N., 2012. Rathke's cleft cysts. Clin. Endocrinol. 76, 151–160.

Truwit, C.L., Barkovich, A.J., 1990. Pathogenesis of intracranial lipoma; an MR study in 42 patients. AJR Am.J. Roentgenol. 155, 855–864.

Tsuruda, J.S., Chew, W.M., Moseley, M.E., Norman, D., 1990. Diffusion-weighted MR imaging of the brain: value of differentiating between extraaxial cysts and epidermoid tumors. AJNR Am. J. Neuroradiolol. 11, 925–931.

Tsuruda, J., Saloner, D., Norman, D., 1992. Artifacts associated with MR neuroangiography. AJNR Am. J. Neuroradiol. 13, 1411–1422.
Wolfe, S.Q., Heros, R.C.A., 2010. Rathke cleft cyst to craniopharyngioma: is there a spectrum? J. Neurosurg. 112, 1322–1323.
Yousem, D.M., Arrington, J.A., Kumar, A.J., Bryan, R.N., 1990. Bright lesions on sellar/parasellar T1-weighted scans. Clin. Imaging 14, 99–105.

CHAPTER

4

Craniopharyngioma: Embryology, Pathology, and Molecular Aspects

Anthony T. Yachnis

Neuropathology Section, Department of Pathology, Immunology, and Laboratory Medicine, University of Florida College of Medicine, Gainesville, FL, USA

"An epithelial tumor developing in the sella turcica from fragments of undifferentiated epithelium developing from the craniopharyngeal duct." **DD Lewis, 1910**

DEFINITION AND EMBRYOGENESIS

Craniopharyngioma has been defined by the World Health Organization (WHO) as "a benign, partially cystic epithelial tumor of the sellar region, presumably derived from Rathke pouch epithelium" (Rushing et al., 2007). Despite a WHO Grade I designation, the tendency of craniopharyngiomas (especially the adamantinomatous type) to densely adhere to and invade surrounding structures such as the infundibular stalk, hypothalamus, and basal vessels creates significant clinical challenges that are discussed elsewhere in this book. In this chapter, an overview of the possible embryogenetic origins of this tumor is presented. This is followed by a discussion of the pathology of craniopharyngioma and a summary of the molecular pathogenesis as currently understood.

The adamantinomatous craniopharyngioma accounts for about 85–90% of all craniopharyngiomas, is most common in childhood, and has bimodal peaks of incidence between 5–10 years of age and 50–60 years (Larkin and Ansorge, 2013). This variant frequently shows evidence of Wnt pathway activation, which is typically manifest as nuclear β-catenin expression in clusters of tumor cells by immunohistochemistry. Histological and molecular genetic similarities between the adamantinomatous craniopharyngioma and tumors of the jaw, such as ameloblastoma and calcifying odontogenic cyst, including expression of enamel proteins by this variant of craniopharyngioma (Sekine et al., 2004), suggests an origin from odontogenic epithelium (Paulus et al., 1997; Song-Tao et al., 2014). In contrast, papillary craniopharyngiomas make up only 11–14% of tumors and occur almost exclusively in adults (Pekmezci et al., 2010). The papillary variant does not employ Wnt pathway activation, but shows histologic features

Craniopharyngiomas
http://dx.doi.org/10.1016/B978-0-12-416706-3.00004-0

reminiscent of Rathke cleft epithelium. Although rare, congenital/neonatal craniopharyngiomas comprise about 7% of all congenital brain tumors (Raisanen and Davis, 1993). Such tumors may become quite large (Arai et al., 2003; Chentli et al., 2012; do Prado Aguiar et al., 2013). "Giant" craniopharyngiomas may also arise in the non-neonatal period (Garg et al., 2013).

Adamantinomatous craniopharyngiomas are believed to arise from neoplastic transformation of embryonic rests that occur during development and involution of Rathke's pouch (Senthilvel et al., 2014). During development, the adenohypophysis is formed by an out pouching of ectodermal epithelium that forms the roof of the stomadeum ("Rathke's diverticulum"). This epithelium comes into contact with a downward evagination of neuroepithelium from the infundibular region of the third ventricular floor. The latter neuroepithelium gives rise to the neurohypophysis and infundibular stalk.

By the fifth gestational week in humans, Rathke's pouch has elongated and becomes constricted at the oral epithelium, forming a pharyngo-hypophyseal stalk/duct (Prabhu and Brown, 2005; Karavitaki et al., 2006; Senthilvel et al., 2014). This Rathke's pouch remnant becomes separated from the oral epithelium during weeks 6–8 (Larkin and Ansorge, 2013). Involution of Rathke's cleft occurs during the 7th week of gestation, with the pharyngo-hypophyseal duct persisting in about 33% of cases and extending from the floor of the sella to the vomer. Remnants of this duct may give rise to craniopharyngiomas (Nourbakhsh et al., 2010), as first suggested by Erdheim (1904). Also, the location of pharyngo-hypophyseal duct remnants helps to explain the suprasellar location of most craniopharyngiomas. Rare examples of intrasellar craniopharyngiomas have been described (Deutsch et al., 2001; Arndt et al., 2007; Nourbakhsh et al., 2010; Senthilvel et al., 2014). Craniopharyngiomas have also presented in infrasellar location (Falavigna and Kraemer, 2001), as clival lesions (Kawamata et al., 2002), and as sphenoid bone tumors (Cooper and Ransohoff, 1972). They may also arise in the third ventricle, pineal gland, Sylvian fissure, and cerebellopontine angle (Thapar and Kovacs, 1998).

While an "embryogenetic" theory currently is used to explain the origin of adamantinomatous craniopharyngiomas, a "metaplastic" theory of tumorigenesis has been suggested for the papillary variant. In the latter, the differentiated squamous epithelium found in papillary craniopharyngiomas is derived from metaplastic transformation of epithelium that forms part of the anterior pituitary gland or pituitary stalk (Larkin and Ansorge, 2013).

PATHOLOGY

Grossly, about 50% of all craniopharyngiomas are cystic, 15% are solid, and the rest contain both cystic and solid elements (Thapar and Kovacs, 1998). Tumors are usually lobulated suprasellar masses that have an irregular interface with surrounding tissue. The adamantinomatous form is usually densely adherent to the mesial wall of the third ventricle and hypothalamus and is intimately associated with the infundibular stalk, often distorting or disrupting this structure (Asa, 1997). They may also adhere to blood vessels and cranial nerves of the basal aspect (Scheithauer et al., 2010; Fernandez et al., 2012). Papillary craniopharyngiomas usually arise in suprasellar locations, often within the third ventricle, and are better demarcated from surrounding structures than the adamantinomatous variant.

On cut surface, the adamantinomatous variant typically has a variable cystic component that can impart a spongy character to the lesion (Rushing et al., 2007). Cysts can contain machine oil-like fluid that is composed of birefringent cholesterol-like material and desquamated keratinaceous debris. Release of this dense liquid material due to spontaneous cyst rupture or during surgery can cause chemical meningitis (Scheithauer et al., 2010). There are varying degrees of calcification that occasionally are manifest as focal bone formation. In contrast, the papillary craniopharyngioma is typically solid but may have minor cystic components that lack "machine oil" quality. Little calcification or other degenerative changes are associated with this variant.

The two variants of craniopharyngioma are histologically, and as will be discussed later in the chapter, molecularly distinct. The adamantinomatous type is composed of nests and trabeculae of epithelium that are usually embedded within gliotic adjacent brain tissue (Asa, 1997; Rushing et al., 2007; Scheithauer et al., 2010). The basal layer of the epithelium is composed of a compact row of tumor cell nuclei that is referred to as peripheral or basal "palisading," which segues into a loose arrangement of epithelial cells called "stellate reticulum" (Figures 4.1 and 4.2). Transitions of classic adamantinomatous epithelium to a rather

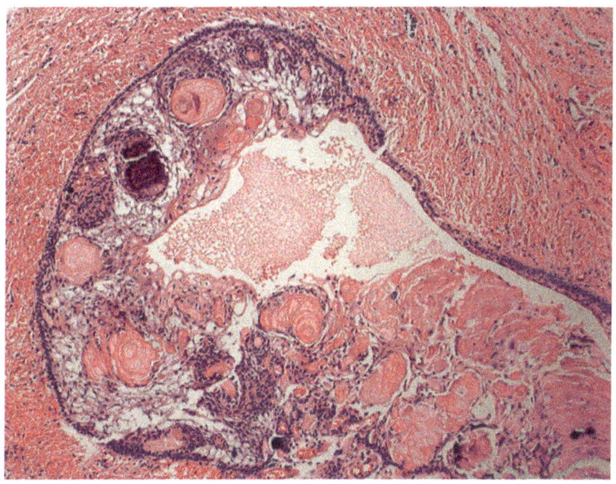

FIGURE 4.1 Craniopharyngioma, adamantinomatous type. This low-magnification view shows a sharp demarcation between the neoplastic epithelium and adjacent CNS tissue to which it is densely adherent.

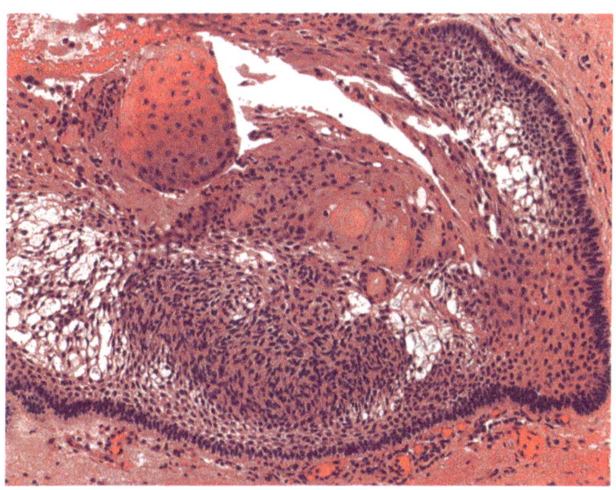

FIGURE 4.2 Craniopharyngioma, adamantinomatous type. The epithelium shows classic features of basal (peripheral) pallisading of tumor cell nuclei and loosely arranged epithelium (stellate reticulum).

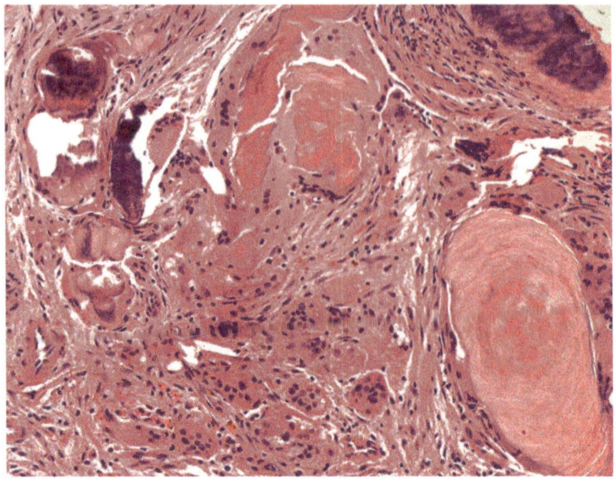

FIGURE 4.3 Craniopharyngioma, adamantinomatous type. Degenerative changes may include a foreign body giant cell reaction with multinucleated giant cells (center of image). Wet keratin (pink material at lower right) and calcifications (upper right and upper left) are common.

thin stratified squamous-like epithelium may occur, especially in areas of cyst degeneration. Mitotic activity is low and typically confined to the basal epithelial layer. Accumulations of eosinophilic "wet" keratin are a hallmark of craniopharyngioma and in some cases may dominate the histological picture. In fact, desquamation of wet keratin may incite a foreign body giant cell reaction with further degeneration leading to a marked xanthogranulomatous reaction with cholesterol clefts, and non-specific inflammatory changes (Figure 4.3). In such areas the epithelium may not be apparent.

Adamantinomatous craniopharyngiomas incite a striking gliotic reaction in the adjacent brain with an abundance of Rosenthal fibers (Figure 4.4), which are elongated

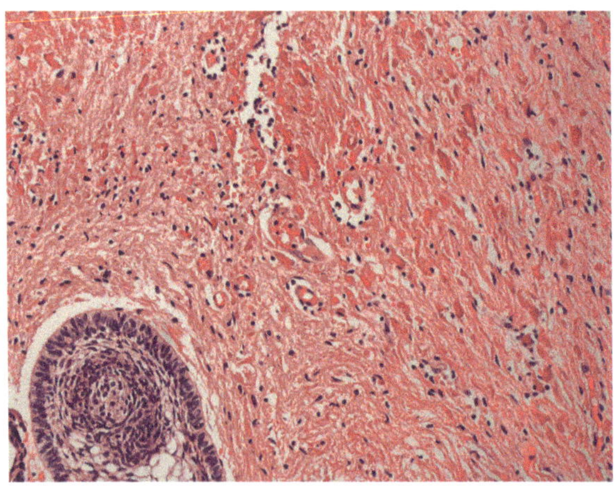

FIGURE 4.4 Craniopharyngioma, adamantinomatous type. Extensive piloid gliosis with Rosenthal fibers (elongated eosinophilic deposits) surrounds an island of adamantinomatous epithelium (lower left).

hypereosinophilic proteinaceous deposits composed of GFAP (glial fibrillary acidic protein) and αB-crystallin (Wisniewski and Goldman, 1998). Such "piloid gliosis" is a non-specific reaction of brain tissue comprising walls of cysts associated with tumors such as pilocytic astrocytomas and hemangioblastomas. It can also occur in the walls of syringomyelic cysts and pineal cysts. This reactive change of adjacent central nervous system (CNS) tissue in craniopharyngioma may mimic the appearance of a pilocytic astrocytoma, which also may arise as a suprasellar, hypothalamic, or optic pathway tumor of childhood. Thus, an important caveat in surgical neuropathology of suprasellar masses is that the amount of neoplastic epithelial elements, xanthogranulomatous reaction, and surrounding piloid gliosis may vary in a given biopsy or resection such that the classic adamantinomatous epithelium may represent a minority of the specimen or be entirely absent.

The papillary craniopharyngioma (Figures 4.5 and 4.6) has a distinct papillary architecture and is composed of low-grade or bland-appearing stratified squamous epithelium that is focally interrupted by cores of fibrovascular tissue (Crotty et al., 1995). This variant shows no basal nuclear pallisading or stellate reticulum of the epithelium, and there is no calcification, or xanthogranulomatous change. Inflammatory infiltrates may occur within the stroma of fibrovascular tissue cores (Figure 4.7). Occasional aggregates of keratinized cells are present but no wet keratin seen in the adamantinomatous variant or flaky "dry" keratin typical of epidermoid cysts is present. The occasional co-occurrence of this variant with Rathke cleft cyst epithelium has suggested a common origin of these two entities. In fact, goblet cells may be seen in up to 33% of papillary craniopharyngiomas and ciliated cells can be seen in about 4% of tumors (Crotty et al., 1995). The co-existence of both an adamantinomatous craniopharyngioma and the papillary variant in the same patient has been reported (Okada et al., 2012). In so-called "collision lesions" of the sella, multiple tumor types have occurred together such as craniopharyngioma, pituitary adenoma, and Rathke cleft cyst (Karavitaki et al., 2008).

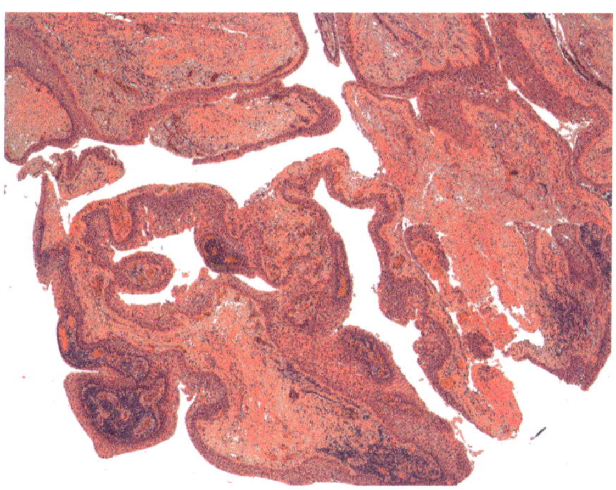

FIGURE 4.5 Craniopharyngioma, papillary type. At low magnification, papillary structures are composed of squamous epithelium that lines fibrovascular cores of tissue. There is no basal palisading, stellate reticulum, or wet keratin.

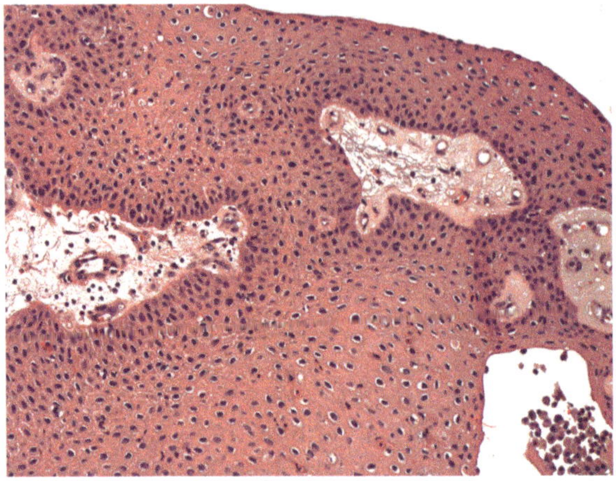

FIGURE 4.6 Craniopharyngioma, papillary type. Mature-appearing stratified squamous epithelium surrounds fibrovascular cores of tissue.

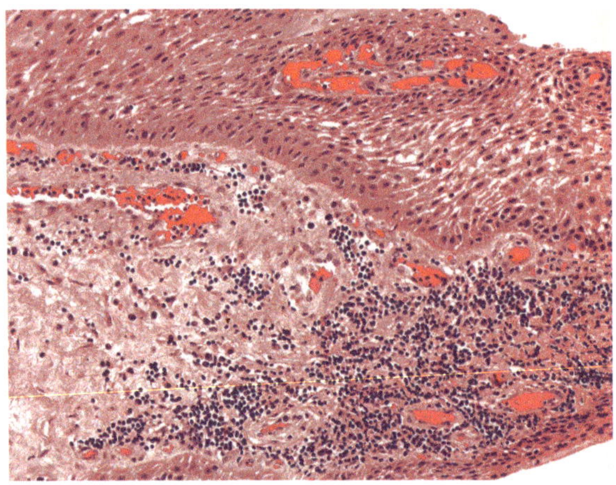

FIGURE 4.7 Craniopharyngioma, papillary type. A chronic inflammatory reaction with an abundance of mature lymphocytes may be found within the stroma of fibrovascular cores.

Although ancillary studies are not usually necessary to make the diagnosis of craniopharyngioma, they may be useful with small or limited samples. Both types of craniopharyngiomas are strongly immunoreactive for cytokeratins and epithelial membrane antigen. Craniopharyngioma tumors are negative for chromogranin, prolactin, ACTH, growth homone, and other antigens expressed by pituitary adenomas. Ki-67 (MIB-1) is most strongly expressed in the basal epithelium of the adamantinomatous type, while being more randomly distributed in the papillary type (Rushing et al., 2007; Scheithauer et al., 2010). However, a definite prognostic significance of Ki-67 labeling index has not been shown for either type of craniopharyngioma (Raghavan et al., 2000; Duo et al., 2003).

The occurrence of frank histological malignancy in craniopharyngiomas is exceedingly rare, but has been documented in case reports and small series (Akachi et al., 1987; Nelson et al., 1988; Suzuki et al., 1989; Plowman et al., 2004; Rodriguez et al., 2007; Boodgrid et al., 2009; Aquilina et al., 2010; Gao et al., 2011; Lauriola et al., 2011). Both de novo malignancy and malignant transformation have been reported, the latter often associated with prior radiation therapy (Virik et al., 1999; Boodgrid et al., 2009; Aquilina et al., 2010; Ishida et al., 2010; Ujifuku et al., 2010; Gao et al., 2011). The adamantinomatous variant has been most frequently associated with malignant transformation and the malignant histology is most often a squamous cell carcinoma. Other cases have been interpreted as an odontogenic ghost cell carcinoma (Rodriguez et al., 2007), myoepithelial carcinoma (Rodriguez et al., 2007), and ameloblastic carcinoma (Gao et al., 2011). Specific criteria for malignancy in craniopharyngioma have not been defined but high mitotic activity, elevated Ki-67 (MIB-1) labeling index, cellular atypia, hyperchromatic nuclei, vascular invasion, infiltrative growth, and coagulative necrosis have been suggested (Rodriguez et al., 2007; Aquilina et al., 2010; Lauriola et al., 2011).

The main differential diagnosis in children is the pilocytic astrocytoma, in which the presence of abundant Rosenthal fibers can mimic the reactive gliotic wall of a craniopharyngioma. Langerhans cell histiocytosis may present as a suprasellar hypothalamic lesion, especially in children with hyperostotic bone lesions and diabetes insipidus. Other suprasellar neoplasms include the pituitary adenoma, but such tumors typically show expansion of the sella tursica by imaging studies, the pituicytoma (a tumor of posterior pituitary glial cells) and granular cell tumors. In adults, a Rathke cleft cyst should be considered and rarely, a dermoid or epidermoid cyst may arise in the suprasellar region. Arachnoid cysts also occur in this region (Shin et al., 1999). Adult tumors presenting in the third ventricle include the chordoid glioma, choroid plexus papilloma, ependymoma, or a metastasis. The floor of the third ventricle is a typical location for neurosarcoidosis.

MOLECULAR GENETICS

Recent advances in the molecular classification of craniopharyngiomas have provided further insights into the possible origins of this tumor. Its neoplastic nature is supported by studies confirming clonality (Sarubi et al., 2001).

The discovery of mutations in the β-catenin gene (CTNNB1 on chromosome 3) in adamantinomatous craniopharyngioma (Sekine et al., 2002; Kato et al., 2004; Buslei et al., 2005; Oikonomou et al., 2005; Campanini et al., 2010; Cao et al., 2010) and demonstration of Wnt pathway activation (Holsken et al., 2009) were major advances in understanding the molecular pathology of this tumor. CTNNB1 mutations had been previously identified in several cancers, such as colorectal (Polakis, 2012) and hepatocellular (de La Coste et al., 1998) carcinomas, and in a molecular subtype of medulloblastomas (Jones et al., 2012).

The canonical Wnt/β-catenin pathway plays a crucial role in cell proliferation, differentiation, and migration, and in establishing the dorsoventral axis of the neural tube during vertebrate embryogenesis (Hussain et al., 2013). The Wnt pathway is activated when Wnt ligand binds to a cell surface receptor complex that is composed of Frizzled (Fz) and low-density lipoprotein receptor-related protein (LRP), which also is bound to Disheveled

(DSH) and axin on the cytoplasmic side of the cell membrane (Hussain et al., 2013; Larkin et al., 2013). When Wnt is bound to this receptor complex, β-catenin exists in a non-phosphorylated state, accumulates in the cytoplasm, and is translocated to the nucleus where it promotes cell growth and motility. In the absence of Wnt, axin is released from the cell surface receptor complex and forms a cytoplasmic complex with glycogen synthase kinase-3β (GSK-3β) and the adenomatous polyposis coli protein (APC). This axin/GSK-3β-APC complex functions to phosphorylate β-catenin, thereby targeting the latter for ubiquitin-mediated proteosomal degradation, such that in the absence of Wnt activation, β-catenin does not accumulate in the nucleus. Thus, the demonstration of nuclear localization of β-catenin by immunohistochemical studies supports Wnt pathway activation. However, in adamantinomatous craniopharyngiomas, nuclear localization of β-catenin does not occur in all cells of the tumor but only in isolated cell nests (Hofmann et al., 2006) that are growing slowly and have been suggested to share some of the characteristics of pituitary stem cells (Andoniadou et al., 2012; Larkin et al., 2013). Such cells have also been identified at the invading edges of craniopharyngiomas (Larkin et al., 2013).

Reports of Wnt pathway activation in ameloblastoma (Tanahashi et al., 2008) and calcifying odontogenic tumor (Hassanein et al., 2008) also occur providing support for a relationship between these tumors. Molecular analysis using comparative genomic hybridization has revealed random gains or deletions in several chromosomes (1, 2, 3, 6, 7, 9, 12, 14, 19, 21, and 22) (Rienstein et al., 2003; Hussain et al., 2013) or no apparent copy number changes in other analyses (Bhattacharjee et al., 1997; Rickert and Paulus, 2003). It has been suggested that the Wnt pathway might be targeted by novel therapeutic approaches in recurrent tumors, surgically unresectable cases, or even as frontline therapies in the future (Hussain et al., 2013).

The molecular pathways of tumorigenesis for papillary craniopharyngioma are less well understood than those for the adamantinomatous variant. However, the recent finding of BRAF V600E mutations in the majority of papillary craniopharyngiomas (Larkin et al., 2014) adds this tumor to the growing list of human neoplasia that harbor this mutation. This finding suggests the possibility of targeted BRAF-inhibitor therapy for patients with this subtype.

References

Akachi, K., Takahashi, H., Ishijima, B., Nakamura, Y., Oda, M., Takizawa, T., Iwamoto, M., Kuriyama, G., Shizuki, K., 1987. Malignant changes in a craniopharyngioma. No Shinkei Geka 15 (8), 843–848.

Andoniadou, C.L., Gaston-Massuet, C., Reddy, R., Schneider, R.P., Blasco, M.A., Le Tissier, P., Jacques, T.S., Pevny, L.H., Dattani, M.T., Martinez-Barbera, J.P., 2012. Identification of novel pathways involved in the pathogenesis of human adamantinomatous craniopharyngioma. Acta Neuropathol. 124 (2), 259–271.

Aquilina, K., Merchant, T.E., Rodriguez-Galindo, C., Ellison, D.W., Sanford, R.A., Boop, F.A., 2010. Malignant transformation of irradiated craniopharyngioma in children: report of 2 cases. J. Neurosurg. Pediatr. 5 (2), 155–161.

Arai, T., Ohno, K., Takada, Y., Aoyagi, M., Hirakawa, K., 2003. Neonatal craniopharyngioma and inference of tumor inception time: case report and review of the literature. Surg. Neurol. 60 (3), 254–259.

Arndt, S., Wiech, T., Mader, I., Maier, W., 2007. Entire infrasellar craniopharyngioma simulating clival chordoma. Otolaryngol. Head Neck Surg. 137 (6), 981–983.

Asa, S., 1997. Craniopharyngioma. In: Asa, S. (Ed.), Atlas of tumor pathology: tumors of the pituitary gland. Fascicle, vol 22. Armed Forces Institute of Pathology, Washington, DC, pp. 167–172.

Bhattacharjee, M.B., Armstrong, D.D., Vogel, H., Cooley, L.D., 1997. Cytogenetic analysis of 120 primary pediatric brain tumors and literature review. Cancer Genet. Cytogenet. 97 (1), 39–53.

Boongird, A., Laothamatas, J., Larbcharoensub, N., Phudhichareonrat, S., 2009. Malignant craniopharyngioma; case report and review of the literature. Neuropathology 29 (5), 591–596.

Buslei, R., Nolde, M., Hofmann, B., Meissner, S., Eyupoglu, I.Y., Siebzehnrübl, F., Hahnen, E., Kreutzer, J., Fahlbusch, R., 2005. Common mutations of beta-catenin in adamantinomatous craniopharyngiomas but not in other tumours originating from the sellar region. Acta Neuropathol. 109 (6), 589–597.

Campanini, M.L., Colli, L.M., Paixao, B.M., Cabral, T.P., Amaral, F.C., Machado, H.R., Neder, L.S., Saggioro, F., Moreira, A.C., Antonini, S.R., de Castro, M., 2010. CTNNB1 gene mutations, pituitary transcription factors, and MicroRNA expression involvement in the pathogenesis of adamantinomatous craniopharyngiomas. Horm. Cancer 1 (4), 187–196.

Cao, J., Lin, J.P., Yang, L.X., Chen, K., Huang, Z.S., 2010. Expression of aberrant beta-catenin and impaired p63 in craniopharyngiomas. Br. J. Neurosurg. 24 (3), 249–256.

Chentli, F., Belhimer, F., Kessaci, F., Mansouri, B., 2010. Congenital craniopharyngioma: a case report and literature review. J. Pediatr. Endocrinol. Metab. 25 (11–12), 1181–1183.

Cooper, P.R., Ransohoff, J., 1972. Craniopharyngioma originating in the sphenoid bone. Case report. J. Neurosurg. 36 (1), 102–106.

Crotty, T.B., Scheithauer, B.W., Young Jr., W.F., Davis, D.H., Shaw, E.G., Miller, G.M., Burger, P.C., 1995. Papillary craniopharyngioma: a clinicopathological study of 48 cases. J. Neurosurg. 83 (2), 206–214.

de La Coste, A., Romagnolo, B., Billuart, P., Renard, C.A., Buendia, M.A., Soubrane, O., Fabre, M., Chelly, J., Beldjord, C., Kahn, A., Perret, C., 1998. Somatic mutations of the beta-catenin gene are frequent in mouse and human hepatocellular carcinomas. Proc. Natl. Acad. Sci. U.S.A. 95 (15), 8847–8851.

Deutsch, H., Kothbauer, K., 2001. Infrasellar craniopharyngiomas: case report and review of the literature. Skull Base 11 (2), 121–128.

Do Prado Aguiar, U., Araujo, J.L., Veiga, J.C., Toita, M.H., de Aguiar, G.B., 2013. Congenital giant craniopharyngioma. Childs Nerv. Syst. 29 (1), 153–157.

Duo, D., Gasverde, S., Benech, F., Zenga, F., Giordana, M.T., 2003. MIB-1 immunoreactivity in craniopharyngiomas: a clinico-pathological analysis. Clin. Neuropathol. 22 (5), 229–234.

Erdheim, J., 1904. Ueber Hyphohysengangsgeshwulste und Hirnscholesteatome. Akademie der Wissenchaften. Mathematisch-naturwissen-schaftliche Classe 113 (5), 537–726.

Falavigna, A., Kraemer, J.L., 2001. Infrasellar craniopharyngioma: Case report. Arq. Neuropsiquiatr. 59 (2), 424–430.

Fernandez-Miranda, J.C., Gardner, P.A., Snyderman, C.H., Devaney, K.O., Strojan, P., Suárez, C., Genden, E.M., Rinaldo, A., Ferlito, A., 2012. Craniopharyngioma: a pathologic, clinical, and surgical review. Head Neck 34 (7), 1036–1044.

Garg, K., Chandra, P.S., Singh, P.K., Sharma, B.S., 2013. Giant craniopharyngioma: can it grow bigger than this? Pediat. Neurosurg. 49 (2), 124–125.

Gao, S., Shi, X., Wang, Y., Qian, H., Liu, C., 2011. Malignant transformation of craniopharyngioma: case report and review of the literature. J. Neurooncol. 103 (3), 719–725.

Hassanein, A.M., Glanz, S.M., Kessler, H.P., Eskin, T.A., Liu, C., 2003. beta-Catenin is expressed aberrantly in tumors expressing shadow cells. Pilomatricoma, craniopharyngioma, and calcifying odontogenic cyst. Am. J. Clin. Pathol. 120 (5), 732–736.

Hofmann, B.M., Kreutzer, J., Saeger, W., Buchfelder, M., Blümcke, I., Fahlbusch, R., Buslei, R., 2006. Nuclear b-catenin accumulation as reliable marker for the differentiation between cystic craniopharyngiomas and Rathke cleft cysts: a clinico-pathologic approach. Am. J. Surg. Pathol. 30 (12), 1595–1603.

Holsken, A., Kreutzer, J., Hofmann, BM, Hans, V., Oppel, F., Buchfelder, M., Fahlbusch, R., Blümcke, I., Buslei, R., 2009. Target gene activation of the Wnt signaling pathway in nuclear b-catenin accumulating cells of adamantinomatous craniopharyngiomas. Brain Pathol. 19 (3), 357–364.

Husain, B.A., Eloy, J.A., Carmel, P.W., Liu, J.K., 2013. Molecular oncogenesis of craniopharyngioma: current and future strategies for the development of targeted therapies: a review. J. Neurosurg. 119 (1), 106–112.

Ishida, M., Hotta, M., Tsukamura, A., Taga, T., Kato, H., Ohta, S., Takeuchi, Y., Nakasu, S., Okabe, H., 2010. Malignant transformation in craniopharyngioma after radiation therapy: a case report and review of the literature. Clin. Neuropathol. 29 (1), 2–8.

Jones, D.T., Jäger, N., Kool, M., Zichner, T., Hutter, B., Sultan, M., Cho, Y.J., Pugh, T.J., Hovestadt, V., Stütz, A.M., Rausch, T., Warnatz, H.J., Ryzhova, M., Bender, S., Sturm, D., Pleier, S., Cin, H., Pfaff, E., Sieber, L., Wittmann, A., Remke, M., Witt, H., Hutter, S., Tzaridis, T., Weischenfeldt, J., Raeder, B., Avci, M., Amstislavskiy, V., Zapatka, M., Weber, U.D., Wang, Q., Lasitschka, B., Bartholomae, C.C., Schmidt, M., von Kalle, C., Ast, V., Lawerenz, C., Eils, J., Kabbe, R., Benes, V., van Sluis, P., Koster, J., Volckmann, R., Shih, D., Betts, M.J., Russell, R.B., Coco, S., Tonini, G.P., Schüller, U., Hans, V., Graf, N., Kim, Y.J., Monoranu, C., Roggendorf, W., Unterberg, A., Herold-Mende, C., Milde, T., Kulozik, A.E., von Deimling, A., Witt, O., Maass, E., Rössler, J., Ebinger, M., Schuhmann, M.U., Frühwald, M.C., Hasselblatt, M., Jabado, N., Rutkowski, S., von Bueren, A.O., Williamson, D., Clifford, S.C., McCabe, M.G., Collins, V.P., Wolf, S., Wiemann, S., Lehrach, H., Brors, B., Scheurlen, W., Felsberg, J., Reifenberger, G., Northcott, P.A., Taylor, M.D., Meyerson, M., Pomeroy, S.L., Yaspo, M.L., Korbel, J.O., Korshunov, A., Eils, R., Pfister, S.M., Lichter, P., 2012. Dissecting the genomic complexity underlying medulloblastoma. Nature 488 (7409), 100–105.

Karavitaki, N., Cudlip, S., Adams, C.B., Wass, J.A., 2006. Craniopharyngiomas. Endocr. Rev. 27 (4), 371–397.

Karavitaki, N., Scheithauer, B.W., Watt, J., Ansorge, O., Moschopoulos, M., Llaguno, A.V., Wass, J.A., 2008. Collision lesions of the sella: co-existence of craniopharyngyioma with gonadotroph adenoma and of Rathke's cleft cyst with corticotroph adenoma. Pituitary 11 (3), 317–323.

Kato, K., Nakatani, Y., Kanno, H., Inayama, Y., Ijiri, R., Nagahara, N., Miyake, T., Tanaka, M., Ito, Y., Aida, N., Tachibana, K., Sekido, K., Tanaka, Y., 2004. Possible linkage between specific histological structures and aberrant reactivation of the Wnt pathway in adamantinomatous craniopharyngioma. J. Pathol. 203 (3), 814–821.

Kawamata, T., Kubo, O., Kamikawa, S., Hori, T., 2002. Ectopic clival craniopharyngioma. Acta Neurochir. 144 (11), 1221–1224.

Larkin, S.J., Ansorge, O., 2013. Pathology and pathogenesis of cranyopharyngiomas. Pituitary 16 (1), 9–17.

Larkin, S.J., Preda, V., Karavitaki, N., Grossman, A., Ansorge, O., 2014. BRAF V600E mutations are characteristic for papillary craniopharyngioma and may coexist with CTNNB1-mutated adamantinomatous craniopharyngioma. Acta. Neuropathol. http://dx.doi.org/10.1007/s00401–014–1270–6.

Lauriola, L., Doglietto, F., Novello, M., Signorelli, F., Montano, N., Pallini, R., Maira, G., 2011. *De novo* malignant craniopharyngioma: case report and literature review. J. Neurooncol. 103 (2), 381–386.

Lewis, D.D., 1910. A contribution to the subject of tumors of the hypophysis. J. Am. Med. Assoc. 55, 1002–1008.

Nelson, G.A., Bastian, F.O., Schlitt, M., White, R.L., 1988. Malignant transformation in craniopharyngioma. Neurosurgery 22 (2), 427–429.

Nourbakhsh, A., Brown, B., Vannemreddy, P., Lian, T., Nanda, A., Guthikonda, B., 2010. Extracranial infrasellar ectopic craniopharyngioma: A case report and review of the literature. Skull Base 20 (6), 475–480.

Oikonomou, E., Barreto, D.C., Soares, B., De Marco, L., Buchfelder, M., Adams, E.F., 2005. Beta-catenin mutations in craniopharyngiomas and pituitary adenomas. J. Neurooncol. 73 (3), 205–209.

Okada, T., Fujistu, K., Ichikawa, T., Mukaihara, S., Miyahara, K., Kaku, S., Uryuu, Y., Niino, H., Yagishita, S., Shiina, T., 2012. Coexistence of adamantinomatous and squamous-papillary type of craniopharyngioma: Case report and discussion of etiology and pathology. Neuropathology 32 (2), 171–173.

Paulus, W., Stockel, C., Krauss, J., Sorensen, N., Roggendorf, W., 1997. Odontogenic classification of craniopharyngiomas: a clinicopathological study of 54 cases. Histopathology 30 (2), 172–176.

Pekmezci, M., Louie, J., Gupta, N., Bloomer, M.M., Tihan, T., 2010. Clinicopathological characteristics of adamantinomatous and papillary craniopharyngiomas: University of California, San Francisco experience 1985–2005. Neurosurgery 67 (3), 1341–1349.

Plowman, P.N., Besser, G.M., Shipley, J., Summersgill, B., Geddes, J., Afshar, F., 2004. Dramatic response of malignant craniopharyngioma to cis-platin-based chemotherapy. Should craniopharyngioma be considered as a suprasellar 'germ cell' tumour? Br. J. Neurosurg. 18 (5), 500–505.

Polakis, P., 2012. Wnt signaling in cancer. Cold Spring Harb. Perspect. Biol. 4 (5), 1–13.

Prabhu, V.C., Brown, H.G., 2005. The pathogenesis of craniopharyngiomas. Childs Nerv. Syst. 21 (8–9), 622–627.

Raghavan, R., Dickey, W.T., Margraf, L.R., White, C.L., Coimbra, C., Hynan, L.S., Rushing, E.J., 2000. Proliferative activity in craniopharyngiomas: clinicopathological correlations in adults and children. Surg. Neurol. 54 (3), 241–247.

Raisanen, J.M., Davis, R.L., 1993. Congenital brain tumors. Pathology 2 (1), 103–116.

Rickert, C.H., Paulus, W., 2003. Lack of chromosomal imbalances in adamantinomatous and papillary craniopharyngiomas. J. Neurol. Neurosurg. Psychiatr. 74 (2), 260–261.

Rienstein, S., Adams, E.F., Pilzer, D., Goldring, A.A., Goldman, B., Friedman, E., 2003. Comparative genomic hybridization analysis of craniopharyngiomas. J. Neurosurg. 98 (1), 162–164.
Rodriguez, F.J., Scheithauer, B.W., Tsunoda, S., Kovacs, K., Vidal, S., Piepgras, D.G., 2007. The spectrum of malignancy in craniopharyngioma. Am. J. Surg. Pathol. 31 (7), 1020–1028.
Rushing, E.J., Giangaspero, F., Paulus, W., Burger, P.C., 2007. Craniopharyngioma. In: Louis, D.N., Ohgaki, H., Wiestler, O.D., Cavenee, W.K. (Eds.), Pathology and genetics. WHO Classification of Tumours of the Central Nervous System, Lyon: IARC, pp. 244–246.
Sarubi, J.C., Bei, H., Adams, E.F., Boson, W.L., Friedman, E., Brandão, K., Kalapothakis, E., Miranda, D., Valle, F.L., Sarquis, M.S., De Marco, L., 2001. Clonal composition of human adamantinomatous craniopharyngiomas and somatic mutation analyses of the patched (PTCH), Gsalpha and Gi2alpha genes. Neurosci. Lett. 310 (1), 5–8.
Scheithauer, B.W., Kovacs, K., Horvath, E., Silva, A.I., Lloyd, R.V., 2010. Pathology of the pituitary and sellar region. In: Perry, A., Brat, D.J. (Eds.), Practical Surgical Neuropathology: A Diagnostic Approach. Elsevier, Philadelphia, PA, pp. 371–416.
Sekine, S., Shibata, T., Kokubu, A., Morishita, Y., Noguchi, M., Nakanishi, Y., Sakamoto, M., Hirohashi, S., 2002. Craniopharyngiomas of adamantinomatous type harbor beta-catenin gene mutations. Am. J. Pathol. 161 (6), 1997–2001.
Sekine, S., Takata, T., Shibata, T., Mori, M., Morishita, Y., Noguchi, M., Uchida, T., Kanai, Y., Hirohashi, S., 2004. Expression of enamel proteins and LEF1 in adamantinomatous craniopharyngioma: evidence for its odontogenic epithelial differentiation. Histopathology 45 (6), 573–579.
Senthilvel, H.N.P., Krishnan, S.S., Vasudevan, M.C., 2014. Extracranial infrasellar craniopharyngioma. Neurol. India 62 (1), 100–103.
Shin, J.L., Asa, S.L., Woodhouse, L.J., Smyth, H.S., Ezzat, S., 1999. Cystic lesions of the pituitary: clinicopathological features distinguishing craniopharyngioma, Rathke's cleft cyst, and arachnoid cyst. J. Clin. Endocrinol. Metab. 84 (11), 3972–3982.
Song-tao, Q., Xiao-rong, Y., Jun, P., Yong-Jian, D., Jin, L., Guang-Long, H., Yun-Tao, L., Jian, R., Xiang-Zhao, L., Jia-Ming, X., 2014. Does the calcification of adamantinomatous craniopharyngioma resemble the calcium deposition of osteogenesis/odontogenesis? Histopathology 64 (3), 336–347.
Suzuki, F., Konuma I,Matsumoto, M., Aoki, M., Hayakawa, I., 1989. Craniopharyngioma with malignant transformation – a report of two cases. Gan No Rinsho 35 (6), 723–728.
Tanahashi, J., Daa, T., Yada, N., Kashima, K., Kondoh, Y., Yokohama, S., 2008. Mutational analysis of Wnt signaling molecules in ameloblastoma with aberrant nuclear expression of beta-catenin. J. Oral. Pathol. Med. 37 (9), 565–570.
Thapar, K., Kovacs, K., 1998. Neoplasms of the sellar region. In: Bigner, D.D., McLendon, R.E., Bruner, J.M. (Eds.), Russell & Rubinstein's Pathology of Tumors of the Nervous System, Sixth. ed. Oxford University Press, London, UK, pp. 561–677.
Ujifuku, K., Matsuo, T., Takeshita, T., Hayashi, Y., Hayashi, K., Kitagawa, N., Hayashi, T., Suyama, K., Nagata, I., 2010. Malignant transformation of craniopharyngioma associated with moyamoya syndrome. Neurol. Med. Chir. (Tokyo) 50 (7), 599–603.
Virik, K., Turner, J., Garrick, R., Sheehy, J.P., 1999. Malignant transformation of craniopharyngioma. J. Clin. Neurosci. 6 (6), 527–530.
Wisniewski, T., Goldman, J.E., 1998. Alpha B-cyrstallin is associated with intermediate filaments in astrocytoma cells. Neurochem. Res. 23 (3), 385–392.

SECTION II

MEDICAL EVALUATION

CHAPTER

5

Craniopharyngioma: Neuroendocrine Evaluation and Management

Nicholas A. Tritos[*,†], *Anne Klibanski*[*,†]

[*]Neuroendocrine Unit, Massachusetts General Hospital, Boston, MA, USA;

[†]Harvard Medical School, Boston, MA, USA

"The first patient to have ACTH in support of total removal of a craniopharyngioma is now 18 years postoperative and has a responsible position as an advertising agent with a television station, is a college graduate, and a charming, normal person." ***DD Matson and Crigler JF Jr, 1969***

INTRODUCTION

Craniopharyngiomas are rare, generally benign tumors arising from remnants of the craniopharyngeal duct (Goldberg and Eshbaugh, 1960; Bunin et al., 1998). So named by Cushing, craniopharyngiomas have long been recognized as generally associated with substantial neuroendocrine dysfunction (Cushing, 1932). The central location of these tumors frequently leads to hypopituitarism and hypothalamic dysfunction, occurring as a result of disruption of critical hypothalamic structures involved in neuroendocrine regulation, along with damage to the hypophyseal stalk and the pars distalis. Aggressive attempts at tumor removal at the time of surgery and long-term effects of radiation therapy may lead to additional neuroendocrine deficits (De Vile et al., 1996; Lustig et al., 2003).

The purpose of the present chapter is to summarize data on the prevalence of neuroendocrine dysfunction in patients with craniopharyngiomas, discuss clinical features, and review pertinent aspects of the diagnosis and neuroendocrine management of these patients.

PREVALENCE OF NEUROENDOCRINE DYSFUNCTION

Hypopituitarism is highly prevalent in patients with craniopharyngiomas, being present in approximately 85% of patients at the time of diagnosis (Van Effenterre and Boch, 2002). As the age at presentation of patients with these tumors shows a bimodal distribution,

Craniopharyngiomas
http://dx.doi.org/10.1016/B978-0-12-416706-3.00005-2

with peaks occurring in childhood/adolescence and older middle age/elderly, several case series report data from children and adult patients together.

At diagnosis, growth hormone (GH) deficiency may represent the most common pituitary hormone deficiency and has been reported in 35–100% of patients (Thomsett et al., 1980; Baskin and Wilson, 1986; Hetelekidis et al., 1993; Paja et al., 1995; De Vile et al., 1996; Honegger et al., 1999; Shin et al., 1999; Karavitaki et al., 2005). Gonadotropin deficiencies [luteinizing hormone (LH) and follicle stimulating hormone (FSH)] are also quite common, affecting 38–91% of patients at presentation (Thomsett et al., 1980; Baskin and Wilson, 1986; Hetelekidis et al., 1993; Paja et al., 1995; DeVile et al., 1996; Honegger et al., 1999; Shin et al., 1999; Karavitaki et al., 2005). Corticotropin (ACTH) deficiency has been reported in 21–68% of patients, and thyrotropin (TSH) deficiency may affect 20–42% of patients at the time of presentation (Thomsett et al., 1980; Baskin and Wilson, 1986; Hetelekidis et al., 1993; Paja et al., 1995; DeVile et al., 1996; Honegger et al., 1999; Shin et al., 1999; Karavitaki et al., 2005). Mild hyperprolactinemia (< 150 ng/ml) has been reported in up to 55% of patients, occurring as a result of "stalk effect" (disruption of inhibitory dopamine outflow from the hypothalamus to pituitary lactotrophs) (Thomsett et al., 1980; Baskin and Wilson, 1986; Hetelekidis et al., 1993; Paja et al., 1995; DeVile et al., 1996; Honegger et al., 1999; Shin et al., 1999; Karavitaki et al., 2005). Diabetes insipidus (DI) has been reported in 6–38% of patients at the time of diagnosis (Thomsett et al., 1980; Baskin and Wilson, 1986; Hetelekidis et al., 1993; Paja et al., 1995; DeVile et al., 1996; Honegger et al., 1999; Shin et al., 1999; Karavitaki et al., 2005). It may be noted that these data were collected retrospectively and may involve use of different diagnostic criteria, which may partly explain the observed variations in prevalence.

Additional pituitary hormone deficiencies may occur as a result of surgery or radiation therapy. In particular, DI may occur in up to 80% of children and 63% of adults postoperatively (Pratheesh et al., 2013). The syndrome of inappropriate antidiuretic hormone secretion (SIADH) and precocious puberty may also occur in these patients (the latter obviously in children) (Zachmann and Illig, 1979; Cabezudo et al., 1981). Based on available data, it appears that pituitary hormone deficiencies resolve rarely, if at all, after surgical decompression (Thomsett et al., 1980; Paja et al., 1995; Honegger et al., 1999). In fact, aggressive attempts at complete tumor resection may be associated with more severe neuroendocrine dysfunction (De Vile et al., 1996).

In addition to pituitary hormone deficiencies, patients with craniopharyngiomas may experience symptoms of hypothalamic dysfunction, including obesity, reported in up to 61% of operated patients (Hoffman et al., 1992; Hetelekidis et al., 1993; Curtis et al., 1994; Duff et al., 2000; Karavitaki et al., 2005). In this population, obesity may occur as a result of hyperphagia induced by destruction of the hypothalamic pathways mediating satiety, but also as a result of decreased energy expenditure, associated with decreased sympathetic tone and diminished physical activity (Skorzewska et al., 1989; Roth et al., 2007). In addition, deficient thirst (adipsia or hypodipsia) with DI may occur in ~14% of patients (as reported in one study of children with craniopharyngiomas) and can be exceedingly difficult to treat (DeVile et al., 1996). Temperature dysregulation and abnormalities in sleep wakefulness (daytime excessive somnolence or insomnia) may also occur (Lipton et al., 1981; Palm et al., 1992; Muller et al., 2002). In addition to overzealous attempts at surgical resection, younger age at the time of presentation, larger tumor size, suprasellar extension, and higher radiation doses to the hypothalamus have been associated with greater risks of hypothalamic dysfunction (De Vile et al., 1996; Lustig et al., 2003; Poretti et al., 2004).

CLINICAL FEATURES AND FINDINGS

In children, GH deficiency leads to decreased linear growth (Toogood and Stewart, 2008). Decreased muscle development and bone mineral accrual may also occur. In addition, hypoglycemia may be present in young children with GH deficiency. It may be noted that linear growth has been reported to occur in some GH-deficient children without a clear-cut explanation of underlying mechanisms. In adults, the GH deficiency syndrome may include abnormal body composition (increased central adiposity, decreased muscle and bone mineral content), decreased exercise capacity, dyslipidemia, insulin resistance, increased cardiometabolic risk, and poor quality of life (QoL) (Toogood and Stewart, 2008).

Gonadotropin deficiency leads to lack of pubertal maturation in children. It may be noted that precocious puberty has occasionally been reported in children post-operatively (Zachmann and Illig, 1979; Cabezudo et al., 1981). In adults, gonadotropin deficiency leads to central hypogonadism, including oligomenorrhea or amenorrhea in women, and low libido/erectile dysfunction and gynecomastia in men, as well as infertility and low bone mineral density in adults of both genders. Men may also develop increased body adiposity and anemia (Toogood and Stewart, 2008).

Corticotropin deficiency results in central hypoadrenalism, which may present with chronic symptoms and findings, including decreased stamina, weight loss, headache, nausea, orthostatic dizziness/hypotension, joint aches, and hyponatremia (Toogood and Stewart, 2008). Acute adrenal insufficiency may occur, particularly during intercurrent physical illness, major surgery or injury, leading to prostration, vomiting, dehydration, hypotension, shock, severe hyponatremia, and death. Notably absent in these patients are skin/mucosal hyperpigmentation and hyperkalemia, reflecting lack of ACTH and preserved aldosterone secretion, respectively.

Thyrotropin deficiency results in central hypothyroidism, which is clinically indistinguishable from hypothyroidism of other causes, with lack of goiter being the notable exception (Toogood and Stewart, 2008). These patients may experience typical hypothyroid symptoms, including fatigue, weight gain, lack of growth in childhood, constipation, dry skin, myxedema, slow mentation, dysthymia, and cold intolerance. Hyponatremia and dyslipidemia may also occur.

Hyperprolactinemia may lead to central hypogonadism and infertility in patients of both genders as well as galactorrhea in women and gynecomastia in men (Klibanski, 2010). In patients with craniopharyngiomas, mild hyperprolactinemia is unlikely to be a major factor involved in the pathogenesis of central hypogonadism, as most of these patients often have substantial structural damage to the hypothalamic–pituitary axis. However, it should be assessed and may occur during follow-up as a result of radiation therapy.

As already noted, central DI may occur in a subset of patients with craniopharyngiomas, and may result in hyposthenuric polyuria, hypernatremia, and hyperosmolar dehydration (Toogood and Stewart, 2008). Of note, among patients with an intact thirst mechanism, hypernatremia and dehydration are infrequent unless access to water is limited or sensorium is compromised. In contrast, patients with deficient thirst and DI may experience wide swings in serum sodium and volume status, ranging from hyponatremic hypervolemia to hypernatremic dehydration.

Excessive weight gain and obesity are more frequently noted during follow-up of patients with treated craniopharyngiomas than at presentation. Earlier data have identified the presence of hyperphagia in some of these patients (Skorzewska et al., 1989). More recently, reports of decreased sympathetic tone and energy expenditure have been published (Coutant et al., 2003; Roth et al., 2007; Holmer et al., 2010). In addition, physical activity is often decreased in these patients, further contributing to positive energy balance and weight gain (Roth et al., 2007). Hypothalamic damage appears to have a central role in the pathogenesis of obesity in these patients, who may exhibit increased parasympathetic vagal output leading to hyperinsulinism, leptin resistance, decreased postprandial (orexigenic) ghrelin suppression, and (anorexigenic) peptide YY secretion (Lustig et al., 1999; Lustig, 2008; Holmer et al., 2010; Roth et al., 2011). Other factors that may be involved in the pathogenesis of excess adiposity in these patients include excess glucocorticoid replacement, insufficient thyroid hormone replacement, growth hormone deficiency, and lack of appropriate testosterone replacement in men (Filipsson et al., 2006; Koulouri et al., 2011).

Temperature dysregulation and abnormal sleep-wakefulness patterns (including severe daytime hypersomnolence and insomnia) may also be present in some patients as a result of hypothalamic damage (Lipton et al., 1981; Palm et al., 1992; Muller et al., 2002).

DIAGNOSIS

All patients with craniopharyngiomas should have a neuroendocrine assessment at the time of presentation (Table 5.1). In addition, these patients require lifelong periodic follow-up assessment and management of neuroendocrine deficits, which may occur as a result of tumor progression or recurrence, surgery, and radiation therapy (Toogood and Stewart, 2008).

The detection and management of central hypoadrenalism as well as disorders of sodium and water homeostasis represent the highest neuroendocrine priorities in terms of potential morbidity and mortality. In patients with hemodynamic instability, treatment for suspected central hypoadrenalism should be initiated without awaiting the results of diagnostic testing.

Morning (or randomly drawn) serum cortisol levels ≥ 18 mcg/dl assure adrenocortical sufficiency (albeit with low diagnostic sensitivity). Low (< 3 mcg/dl) morning serum cortisol levels are diagnostic of hypoadrenalism. Intermediate (3–17 mcg/dl) morning cortisol levels are indeterminate and require stimulation testing. In hemodynamically stable patients, evaluation of the pituitary–adrenal axis is traditionally performed using the insulin tolerance test (ITT), which additionally provides a robust assessment of GH secretion (Toogood and Stewart, 2008). However, this test requires the induction of severe hypoglycemia (< 45 mg/dl), which carries some risk (precipitation of myocardial ischemia and seizures) and is therefore contraindicated in older patients, as well as those with cardiovascular disease or seizures. The metyrapone test is also useful in the evaluation of the integrity of the pituitary–adrenal axis, but is seldom performed in the US, as it carries some risk of inducing acute adrenal insufficiency (of particular concern if the test is performed in an outpatient) and requires the oral administration of metyrapone, which is not widely available in the US. Another diagnostic test of adrenal function is the 60-minute cosyntropin stimulation test,

TABLE 5.1 Laboratory Assessment of Neuroendocrine Function

Pituitary function	Test	Interpretation	Comments
Adrenal axis	Early morning serum cortisol and plasma ACTH levels	Morning serum cortisol < 3 mcg/dl is diagnostic of hypoadrenalism; absence of elevated plasma ACTH confirms the presence of corticotroph dysfunction Morning serum cortisol 3–17 mcg/dl requires stimulation testing	Serum cortisol ≥ 18 mcg/dl assures sufficient cortisol secretion with high specificity but low sensitivity
	Insulin tolerance test	Peak serum cortisol < 18 mcg/dl is diagnostic of hypoadrenalism	"Gold standard test"; can be unpleasant and carries some risk; contraindicated in the elderly, patients with seizures or coronary artery disease
	Metyrapone test	Low (morning) serum 11-deoxycortisol (< 7 mcg/dl) with low (morning) serum cortisol (< 5 mcg/dl) is diagnostic of hypoadrenalism	May potentially precipitate adrenal insufficiency; limited metyrapone availability in the US
	Cosyntropin stimulation test	Peak serum cortisol < 18 mcg/dl is diagnostic of hypoadrenalism	Directly evaluates adrenal response; indirect assessment of corticotroph function; can be falsely reassuring in patients with central hypoadrenalism of recent onset
Thyroid axis	TSH, free T_4	Low free T4 (cutpoint is assay-dependent) without elevated TSH is diagnostic of central hypothyroidism	TSH levels are often inappropriately "normal" in patients with central hypothyroidism
Gonadal axis	FSH, LH, early morning (total and free) testosterone and sex hormone binding globulin (SHBG) (men) FSH, LH, estradiol, and menstrual history (women)	Low testosterone (generally < 250–300 ng/dl) without elevated gonadotropin (LH) is diagnostic of central hypogonadism in men Oligomenorrhea/amenorrhea with low estradiol (cutpoint is assay-dependent) in the absence of elevated gonadotropin is diagnostic of central hypogonadism in women	In men, a minimum of two early morning testosterone levels should be obtained In women, estradiol levels can be measured, but add little to the diagnosis if oligomenorrhea is present

(Continued)

TABLE 5.1 Laboratory Assessment of Neuroendocrine Function—cont'd

Pituitary function	Test	Interpretation	Comments
Growth hormone	GH stimulation testing	Peak GH < 3 ng/ml is diagnostic of GH deficiency after insulin or glucagon administration; varying (BMI-dependent) cutpoints recommended for GHRH-arginine testing	Stimuli used include insulin, glucagon, GHRH and arginine, or arginine alone (the latter having reduced diagnostic accuracy in adults)
Prolactin	Serum prolactin	Prolactin levels > 150–200 ng/ml generally occur in patients with prolactin-secreting adenomas	Serum prolactin levels < 150 ng/ml in patients with larger (> 1 cm) sellar lesions generally indicate the presence of "stalk effect"
Antidiuretic hormone	(Morning) serum sodium and osmolality; urine osmolality Water deprivation testing	Hyposthenuria (urine osmolality < 700 mOsm/kg) in the presence of hypernatremia/hyperosmolality is diagnostic of diabetes insipidus	Renal response (> 50% increase in urine osmolality) to desmopressin confirms the diagnosis of central diabetes insipidus

Abbreviations: ACTH: corticotropin; GH: growth hormone; GHRH: growth hormone releasing hormone; FSH: follicle stimulating hormone; LH: luteinizing hormone; SHBG: sex hormone binding globulin; TSH: thyrotropin; T_4: thyroxine.

which directly assesses adrenocortical cortisol output in response to cosyntropin administration. As this test does not directly evaluate pituitary function, it can often be falsely reassuring in patients with central hypoadrenalism of recent onset (including patients undergoing pituitary surgery, in whom it should be deferred for approximately 6 weeks post-operatively). In patients with hypoadrenalism, the detection of ACTH levels that are inappropriately "normal" or low establishes the presence of corticotroph dysfunction as the cause of adrenal insufficiency.

Assessment of the pituitary–thyroid axis requires evaluation of both serum TSH and free thyroxine (T_4) levels (as serum TSH levels may often be inappropriately "normal" in patients with central hypothyroidism) (Toogood and Stewart, 2008). As some free T_4 assays lack sufficient accuracy, borderline low test results should be confirmed (by retesting) before they are accepted as valid. Similarly, assessment of the pituitary–gonadal axis requires evaluation of morning serum (total and/or free) testosterone levels and serum gonadotropins in men. In women, obtaining a menstrual history is critical in the assessment of gonadal function. Inappropriately low or "normal" serum gonadotropin levels in women with amenorrhea or those of menopausal age indicate the presence of gonadotropin deficiency.

Evaluation of GH secretion rests upon performing appropriate stimulation testing, since random serum GH levels are often undetectable in healthy adults and serum insulin-like growth factor 1 (IGF-1) levels are often within the normal range in GH-deficient adults (Ho, 2007). In addition to insulin-induced hypoglycemia, agents used to stimulate GH secretion include glucagon, the combination of growth hormone releasing hormone (GHRH) and arginine, or arginine alone (albeit with lower diagnostic accuracy in adults tested with arginine alone) (Biller et al., 2002). Evaluation of GH secretion is advisable only after other pituitary hormones have been assessed and respective deficits replaced (Toogood and Stewart, 2008).

In patients with hypernatremia (> 145 mmol/l) and hyperosmolality (> 295 mOsm/kg), the presence of inappropriately dilute urine (< 700 mOsm/kg) establishes the diagnosis of DI, provided that medications interfering with renal concentrating mechanisms (including diuretics or mannitol) have not been administered. However, in eunatremic patients, a water deprivation test is generally needed in order to establish the diagnosis of DI and this may also help to distinguish between central DI [caused by antidiuretic hormone (ADH) deficiency] and nephrogenic DI by assessing the ability of the kidneys to respond to exogenous desmopressin by concentrating urine (Toogood and Stewart, 2008). Assessment of thirst is generally performed by history, but can also be recorded on a visual analog scale (generally used in research settings).

MANAGEMENT

The prompt institution of glucocorticoid replacement is the highest priority in the neuroendocrine management of these patients (Table 5.2) and should always be administered before thyroid hormone replacement in order to avoid precipitating an acute adrenal crisis

TABLE 5.2 Replacement Therapies for Hypopituitarism

Replacement therapy	Medication	Comments
Adrenal axis	Prednisone	Generally administered in a single morning oral dose; adequacy of replacement assessed based on clinical criteria
	Hydrocortisone	Generally administered orally in divided doses (2–3 daily); adequacy of replacement assessed based on clinical criteria
Thyroid axis	Levothyroxine	Dose titrated to free thyroxine levels in the upper half of normal range
Gonadal axis	Testosterone (men)	Forms include transdermal gels, patches, intramuscular injections or subcutaneously implanted pellets; dose titrated to normal testosterone levels
	Combination oral contraceptive (OCP) or estradiol/progestin combination (women)	Progestin administration is essential in women with intact uterus
Growth hormone	Somatropin (recombinant growth hormone)	Dose titrated to IGF-1 levels between 0–1 SDS
Prolactin	NA	
Antidiuretic hormone	Desmopressin	Forms include nasal spray, oral tablets or subcutaneous injection; administered in 1–2 daily doses; dose titrated to urine output and normal serum sodium levels

Abbreviations: IGF-1: insulin-like growth factor 1; NA: not needed; OCP: oral contraceptive; SDS: standard deviation score.

(Toogood and Stewart, 2008). Stress dose glucocorticoid coverage (hydrocortisone in doses up to 100 mg intravenously every 8 hr, or equivalent) should be urgently provided to hemodynamically unstable and/or acutely ill patients with known or suspected central hypoadrenalism (without awaiting diagnostic confirmation). In stable outpatients, glucocorticoid replacement doses in adults generally include prednisone (3–5 mg by mouth daily, generally administered in a single morning dose) or hydrocortisone (15–25 mg by mouth daily, divided in 2–3 doses). Glucocorticoid excess should be avoided, as it is associated with central adiposity, dyslipidemia, and increased cardiovascular mortality (Filipsson et al., 2006). All patients with central hypoadrenalism should be instructed in the use of "sick day" (stress dose) glucocorticoid administration (equal to 2–3 times daily maintenance dose) in the case of intercurrent illness, inform all physicians of their need for increased glucocorticoid replacement prior to elective surgery and advise the patients to wear a medical identification bracelet or necklace.

Patients with central hypothyroidism are treated with levothyroxine in doses sufficient to maintain free T_4 levels in the upper half of the reference range. Serum TSH levels should not be relied upon in these patients to gauge thyroid hormone replacement dosing (Toogood and Stewart, 2008).

Sex steroid replacement should be considered in men and women of premenopausal age, if not contraindicated (Toogood and Stewart, 2008). In men, testosterone replacement is available in the form of transdermal gels or patches (applied daily), intramuscular injections (administered every 2–3 weeks) and subcutaneous pellets (inserted every 3–6 months). In women, sex steroid replacement options include an estrogen-containing oral contraceptive, transdermal estrogen-containing patches, or creams together with oral cyclic or continuous progestin (progestin required only in women who have not had a hysterectomy). If fertility is of interest, gonadotropin administration is needed in patients of both genders.

Growth hormone replacement improves the growth of pediatric patients with GH deficiency (Toogood and Stewart, 2008). Growth hormone replacement improves linear growth to the same extent as in other GH-deficient children, but does not prevent weight gain (Geffner et al., 2004). It may be noted that growth in the absence of GH has been reported in some cases, but the underlying pathophysiology remains incompletely understood (Bucher et al., 1983; DeVile et al., 1996). Growth hormone replacement should also be considered in adult patients with documented GH deficiency and no contraindications, and this may improve exercise capacity, QoL, body composition (including decrease in body fat and increase in muscle and bone mineral density), and dyslipidemia (Ho, 2007). Adult patients with craniopharyngiomas appear to derive comparable benefit from GH replacement in comparison with other hypopituitary patients (Yuen et al., 2013). Available data from retrospective series suggest that GH replacement does not appear to increase the risk of progression or recurrence of craniopharyngiomas (Muller et al., 2010; Rohrer et al., 2010). Nevertheless, good clinical practice dictates that the underlying tumor is in remission before the initiation of GH replacement, and that GH-replaced patients follow age-appropriate recommendations for screening tests for malignancies. In addition to clinical evaluation, serum IGF-1 levels should be used to titrate GH dosing, with a goal of maintaining IGF-1 standard deviation score (SDS) between 0 to 1 (Ho, 2007). Glycemia should be monitored on GH replacement. In particular, obese patients are at greater risk of developing diabetes mellitus during GH replacement.

Desmopressin is used as replacement therapy in patients with central DI, and is administered as nasal spray or oral tablet (chronically), or subcutaneous injection acutely (generally in 1–2 daily doses) (Toogood and Stewart, 2008). Patients should be advised to allow for the effect of the medication to wear off between doses to minimize the possibility of excess water retention, leading to hyponatremia. Patients with an intact thirst mechanism should also be instructed to drink to thirst only (avoiding habitual or compulsive water drinking) in order to avoid hyponatremia. Serum sodium levels should be periodically monitored in patients receiving desmopressin therapy. The management of patients with deficient thirst is very challenging, and generally requires meticulous monitoring of fluid intake, urine output, body weight, and serum sodium levels to guide fluid administration and desmopressin therapy (Mavrakis and Tritos, 2008).

The management of obesity in patients with craniopharyngiomas can be quite problematic. Medical therapies aimed at ameliorating hyperinsulinism (such as octreotide, or the combination of metformin and diazoxide) have had only modest benefits with regards to weight control thus far (Lustig et al., 2006; Lustig, 2008; Hamilton et al., 2011). Bariatric surgery, including Roux-en-Y gastric bypass surgery, sleeve gastrectomy and laparoscopic adjustable gastric band, is indicated in adults with body mass index (BMI) exceeding 40 kg/m^2 or those with BMI exceeding 35 kg/m^2 in the presence of serious comorbidities (such as diabetes mellitus or sleep apnea) (Pories et al., 1995; Runkel et al., 2011). In adolescents, more conservative recommendations have been made regarding appropriate candidates for bariatric surgery, but the exact role of surgery is being debated (August et al., 2008; Pratt et al., 2009). The success of bariatric surgery in inducing significant weight loss in patients with craniopharyngiomas has been recently documented in a review of 21 cases (Bretault et al., 2013).

Stimulant (such as methylphenidate or modafinil) or melatonin therapy can improve alertness in patients with daytime somnolence as a result of hypothalamic dysfunction (Muller et al., 2002, 2006). In addition, patients with sleep apnea may benefit from appropriate therapy, including nocturnal continuous positive air pressure (CPAP) administration.

Patients with craniopharyngiomas have increased total mortality (standardized mortality ratio ranging between 2.88 and 9.28 in comparison to the general population), as well as cardiovascular (3–19-fold increase) and cerebrovascular mortality (Karavitaki et al., 2006; Karavitaki and Wass, 2008; Erfurth et al., 2013). Central hypoadrenalism or severe electrolyte disturbances (hyponatremia or hypernatremia) may also contribute to excess mortality. Optimizing replacement therapies for pituitary hormone deficiencies and treating obesity aggressively may help mitigate the excess mortality risk.

SUMMARY – FUTURE DIRECTIONS

Patients with craniopharyngiomas often have one or several pituitary hormone deficiencies and/or additional evidence of hypothalamic dysfunction, occurring as a result of the underlying tumor, surgery, and radiation therapy. These patients require lifelong periodic evaluation including testing to detect and manage neuroendocrine dysfunction. Optimizing pituitary hormone replacement therapies and improving weight control may help improve the overall outlook and mitigate the excess mortality associated with this frequently devastating condition.

References

August, G.P., Caprio, S., Fennoy, I., Freemark, M., Kaufman, F.R., Lustig, R.H., Silverstein, J.H., Speiser, P.W., Styne, D.M., Montori, V.M., 2008. Prevention and treatment of pediatric obesity: an endocrine society clinical practice guideline based on expert opinion. J. Clin. Endocrinol. Metab. 93, 4576–4599.

Baskin, D.S., Wilson, C.B., 1986. Surgical management of craniopharyngiomas. A review of 74 cases. J. Neurosurg. 65, 22–27.

Biller, B.M., Samuels, M.H., Zagar, A., Cook, D.M., Arafah, B.M., Bonert, V., Stavrou, S., Kleinberg, D.L., Chipman, J.J., Hartman, M.L., 2002. Sensitivity and specificity of six tests for the diagnosis of adult GH deficiency. J. Clin. Endocrinol. Metab. 87, 2067–2079.

Bretault, M., Boillot, A., Muzard, L., Poitou, C., Oppert, J.M., Barsamian, C., Gatta, B., Muller, H., Weismann, D., Rottembourg, D., Inge, T., Veyrie, N., Carette, C., Czernichow, S., 2013. Clinical review: Bariatric surgery following treatment for craniopharyngioma: a systematic review and individual-level data meta-analysis. J. Clin. Endocrinol. Metab. 98, 2239–2246.

Bucher, H., Zapf, J., Torresani, T., Prader, A., Froesch, E.R., Illig, R., 1983. Insulin-like growth factors I and II, prolactin, and insulin in 19 growth hormone-deficient children with excessive, normal, or decreased longitudinal growth after operation for craniopharyngioma. N. Engl. J. Med. 309, 1142–1146.

Bunin, G.R., Surawicz, T.S., Witman, P.A., Preston-Martin, S., Davis, F., Bruner, J.M., 1998. The descriptive epidemiology of craniopharyngioma. J. Neurosurg. 89, 547–551.

Cabezudo, J.M., Perez, C., Vaquero, J., Garcia-De-Sola, R., Bravo, G., 1981. Pubertas praecox in craniopharyngioma. Case report. J. Neurosurg. 55, 127–131.

Coutant, R., Maurey, H., Rouleau, S., Mathieu, E., Mercier, P., Limal, J.M., Le Bouil, A., 2003. Defect in epinephrine production in children with craniopharyngioma: functional or organic origin? J. Clin. Endocrinol. Metab. 88, 5969–5975.

Curtis, J., Daneman, D., Hoffman, H.J., Ehrlich, R.M., 1994. The endocrine outcome after surgical removal of craniopharyngiomas. Pediatr. Neurosurg. 21 (Suppl. 1), 24–27.

Cushing, H., 1932. The craniopharyngioma. *Intracranial tumors*. London, Bailliere, Tindall and Cox.

De Vile, C.J., Grant, D.B., Kendall, B.E., Neville, B.G., Stanhope, R., Watkins, K.E., Hayward, R.D., 1996. Management of childhood craniopharyngioma: can the morbidity of radical surgery be predicted? J. Neurosurg. 85, 73–81.

Devile, C.J., Grant, D.B., Hayward, R.D., Stanhope, R., 1996. Growth and endocrine sequelae of craniopharyngioma. Arch. Dis. Child. 75, 108–114.

Duff, J., Meyer, F.B., Ilstrup, D.M., Laws Jr., E.R., Schleck, C.D., Scheithauer, B.W., 2000. Long-term outcomes for surgically resected craniopharyngiomas. Neurosurgery 46, 291–302 discussion 302–5.

Erfurth, E.M., Holmer, H., Fjalldal, S.B., 2013. Mortality and morbidity in adult craniopharyngioma. Pituitary 16, 46–55.

Filipsson, H., Monson, J.P., Koltowska-Haggstrom, M., Mattsson, A., Johannsson, G., 2006. The impact of glucocorticoid replacement regimens on metabolic outcome and comorbidity in hypopituitary patients. J. Clin. Endocrinol. Metab. 91, 3954–3961.

Geffner, M., Lundberg, M., Koltowska-Haggstrom, M., Abs, R., Verhelst, J., Erfurth, E.M., Kendall-Taylor, P., Price, D.A., Jonsson, P., Bakker, B., 2004. Changes in height, weight, and body mass index in children with craniopharyngioma after three years of growth hormone therapy: analysis of KIGS (Pfizer International Growth Database). J. Clin. Endocrinol. Metab. 89, 5435–5440.

Goldberg, G.M., Eshbaugh, D.E., 1960. Squamous cell nests of the pituitary gland as related to the origin of craniopharyngiomas. A study of their presence in the newborn and infants up to age four. Arch. Pathol. 70, 293–299.

Hamilton, J.K., Conwell, L.S., Syme, C., Ahmet, A., Jeffery, A., Daneman, D., 2011. Hypothalamic Obesity following Craniopharyngioma Surgery: Results of a Pilot Trial of Combined Diazoxide and Metformin Therapy. Int. J. Pediatr. Endocrinol. 2011, 417949.

Hetelekidis, S., Barnes, P.D., Tao, M.L., Fischer, E.G., Schneider, L., Scott, R.M., Tarbell, N.J., 1993. 20-year experience in childhood craniopharyngioma. Int. J. Radiat. Oncol. Biol. Phys. 27, 189–195.

Ho, K.K., 2007. Consensus guidelines for the diagnosis and treatment of adults with GH deficiency II: a statement of the GH Research Society in association with the European Society for Pediatric Endocrinology, Lawson Wilkins Society, European Society of Endocrinology, Japan Endocrine Society, and Endocrine Society of Australia. Eur. J. Endocrinol. 157, 695–700.

Hoffman, H.J., De Silva, M., Humphreys, R.P., Drake, J.M., Smith, M.L., Blaser, S.I., 1992. Aggressive surgical management of craniopharyngiomas in children. J. Neurosurg. 76, 47–52.

Holmer, H., Pozarek, G., Wirfalt, E., Popovic, V., Ekman, B., Bjork, J., Erfurth, E.M., 2010. Reduced energy expenditure and impaired feeding-related signals but not high energy intake reinforces hypothalamic obesity in adults with childhood onset craniopharyngioma. J. Clin. Endocrinol. Metab. 95, 5395–5402.

Honegger, J., Buchfelder, M., Fahlbusch, R., 1999. Surgical treatment of craniopharyngiomas: endocrinological results. J. Neurosurg. 90, 251–257.

Karavitaki, N., Brufani, C., Warner, J.T., Adams, C.B., Richards, P., Ansorge, O., Shine, B., Turner, H.E., Wass, J.A., 2005. Craniopharyngiomas in children and adults: systematic analysis of 121 cases with long-term follow-up. Clin. Endocrinol. (Oxf) 62, 397–409.

Karavitaki, N., Cudlip, S., Adams, C.B., Wass, J.A., 2006. Craniopharyngiomas. Endocr. Rev. 27, 371–397.

Karavitaki, N., Wass, J.A., 2008. Craniopharyngiomas. Endocrinol. Metab. Clin. North. Am. 37, 173–193 ix–x.

Klibanski, A., 2010. Clinical practice. Prolactinomas N. Engl. J. Med. 362, 1219–1226.

Koulouri, O., Auldin, M.A., Agarwal, R., Kieffer, V., Robertson, C., Falconer Smith, J., Levy, M.J., Howlett, T.A., 2011. Diagnosis and treatment of hypothyroidism in TSH deficiency compared to primary thyroid disease: pituitary patients are at risk of under-replacement with levothyroxine. Clin. Endocrinol. (Oxf) 74, 744–749.

Lipton, J.M., Rosenstein, J., Sklar, F.H., 1981. Thermoregulatory disorders after removal of a craniopharyngioma from the third cerebral ventricle. Brain Res. Bull. 7, 369–373.

Lustig, R.H., Rose, S.R., Burghen, G.A., Velasquez-Mieyer, P., Broome, D.C., Smith, K., Li, H., Hudson, M.M., Heideman, R.L., Kun, L.E., 1999. Hypothalamic obesity caused by cranial insult in children: altered glucose and insulin dynamics and reversal by a somatostatin agonist. J. Pediatr. 135, 162–168.

Lustig, R.H., Post, S.R., Srivannaboon, K., Rose, S.R., Danish, R.K., Burghen, G.A., Xiong, X., Wu, S., Merchant, T.E., 2003. Risk factors for the development of obesity in children surviving brain tumors. J. Clin. Endocrinol. Metab. 88, 611–616.

Lustig, R.H., Greenway, F., Velasquez-Mieyer, P., Heimburger, D., Schumacher, D., Smith, D., Smith, W., Soler, N., Warsi, G., Berg, W., Maloney, J., Benedetto, J., Zhu, W., Hohneker, J., 2006. A multicenter, randomized, double-blind, placebo-controlled, dose-finding trial of a long-acting formulation of octreotide in promoting weight loss in obese adults with insulin hypersecretion. Int. J. Obes. (Lond) 30, 331–341.

Lustig, R.H., 2008. Hypothalamic obesity: causes, consequences, treatment. Pediatr. Endocrinol. Rev. 6, 220–227.

Matson, D.D., Crigler Jr, J.F., 1969. Management of craniopharyngioma in childhood. J. Neurosurg. 30, 377–399.

Mavrakis, A.N., Tritos, N.A., 2008. Diabetes insipidus with deficient thirst: report of a patient and review of the literature. Am. J. Kidney. Dis. 51, 851–859.

Muller, H.L., Gebhardt, U., Schroder, S., Pohl, F., Kortmann, R.D., Faldum, A., Zwiener, I., Warmuth-Metz, M., Pietsch, T., Calaminus, G., Kolb, R., Wiegand, C., Sorensen, N., 2010. Analyses of treatment variables for patients with childhood craniopharyngioma – results of the multicenter prospective trial KRANIOPHARYNGEOM 2000 after three years of follow-up. Horm. Res. Paediatr. 73, 175–180.

Muller, H.L., Handwerker, G., Wollny, B., Faldum, A., Sorensen, N., 2002. Melatonin secretion and increased daytime sleepiness in childhood craniopharyngioma patients. J. Clin. Endocrinol. Metab. 87, 3993–3996.

Muller, H.L., Muller-Stover, S., Gebhardt, U., Kolb, R., Sorensen, N., Handwerker, G., 2006. Secondary narcolepsy may be a causative factor of increased daytime sleepiness in obese childhood craniopharyngioma patients. J. Pediatr. Endocrinol. Metab. 19 (Suppl. 1), 423–429.

Paja, M., Lucas, T., Garcia-Uria, J., Salame, F., Barcelo, B., Estrada, J., 1995. Hypothalamic-pituitary dysfunction in patients with craniopharyngioma. Clin. Endocrinol. (Oxf) 42, 467–473.

Palm, L., Nordin, V., Elmqvist, D., Blennow, G., Persson, E., Westgren, U., 1992. Sleep and wakefulness after treatment for craniopharyngioma in childhood; influence on the quality and maturation of sleep. Neuropediatrics 23, 39–45.

Poretti, A., Grotzer, M.A., Ribi, K., Schonle, E., Boltshauser, E., 2004. Outcome of craniopharyngioma in children: long-term complications and quality of life. Dev. Med. Child. Neurol. 46, 220–229.

Pories, W.J., Swanson, M.S., Macdonald, K.G., Long, S.B., Morris, P.G., Brown, B.M., Barakat, H.A., Deramon, R.A., Israel, G., Dolezal, J.M., et al., 1995. Who would have thought it? An operation proves to be the most effective therapy for adult-onset diabetes mellitus. Ann. Surg. 222, 339–350 discussion 350–352.

Pratheesh, R., Swallow, D., Rajaratnam, S., Jacob, K., Chacko, G., Joseph, M., Chacko, A., 2013. Incidence, predictors, and early post-operative course of diabetes insipidus in pediatric craniopharyngioma: a comparison with adults. Childs. Nerv. Syst. 29, 941–949.

Pratt, J.S., Lenders, C.M., Dionne, E.A., Hoppin, A.G., Hsu, G.L., Inge, T.H., Lawlor, D.F., Marino, M.F., Meyers, A.F., Rosenblum, J.L., Sanchez, V.M., 2009. Best practice updates for pediatric/adolescent weight loss surgery. Obesity (Silver Spring) 17, 901–910.

Rohrer, T.R., Langer, T., Grabenbauer, G.G., Buchfelder, M., Glowatzki, M., Dorr, H.G., 2010. Growth hormone therapy and the risk of tumor recurrence after brain tumor treatment in children. J. Pediatr. Endocrinol. Metab. 23, 935–942.

Roth, C.L., Gebhardt, U., Muller, H.L., 2011. Appetite-regulating hormone changes in patients with craniopharyngioma. Obesity (Silver Spring) 19, 36–42.

Roth, C.L., Hunneman, D.H., Gebhardt, U., Stoffel-Wagner, B., Reinehr, T., Muller, H.L., 2007. Reduced sympathetic metabolites in urine of obese patients with craniopharyngioma. Pediatr. Res. 61, 496–501.

Runkel, N., Colombo-Benkmann, M., Huttl, T.P., Tigges, H., Mann, O., Sauerland, S., 2011. Bariatric surgery. Dtsch. Arztebl. Int. 108, 341–346.

Shin, J.L., Asa, S.L., Woodhouse, L.J., Smyth, H.S., Ezzat, S., 1999. Cystic lesions of the pituitary: clinicopathological features distinguishing craniopharyngioma, Rathke's cleft cyst, and arachnoid cyst. J. Clin. Endocrinol. Metab. 84, 3972–3982.

Skorzewska, A., Lal, S., Waserman, J., Guyda, H., 1989. Abnormal food-seeking behavior after surgery for craniopharyngioma. Neuropsychobiology 21, 17–20.

Thomsett, M.J., Conte, F.A., Kaplan, S.L., Grumbach, M.M., 1980. Endocrine and neurologic outcome in childhood craniopharyngioma: Review of effect of treatment in 42 patients. J. Pediatr. 97, 728–735.

Toogood, A.A., Stewart, P.M., 2008. Hypopituitarism: clinical features, diagnosis, and management. Endocrinol. Metab. Clin. North. Am. 37, 235–261 x.

Van Effenterre, R., Boch, A.L., 2002. Craniopharyngioma in adults and children: a study of 122 surgical cases. J. Neurosurg. 97, 3–11.

Yuen, K.C., Koltowska-Haggstrom, M., Cook, D.M., Fox, J.L., Jonsson, P.J., Geffner, M., Abs, R., 2013. Clinical characteristics and effects of GH replacement in adults with childhood-onset craniopharyngioma compared to adults with other causes of childhood-onset hypothalamic-pituitary dysfunction. Eur. J. Endocrinol.

Zachmann, M., Illig, R., 1979. Precocious puberty after surgery for craniopharyngioma. J. Pediatr. 95, 86–88.

CHAPTER

6

Neuro-Ophthalmic Manifestations of Craniopharyngiomas

Robert C. Sergott

Wills Eye Hospital and Thomas Jefferson University, Philadelphia, PA, USA

"Owing to their intimate relationship to the optic tracts, it is most surprising that any of these patients fail to show hemianopia." **Walter Dandy, 1945**

INTRODUCTION AND HISTORICAL BACKGROUND

The term "craniopharyngioma", used to describe this tumor's embryonic origin, and the description "chiasmal syndrome", used to define the visual loss associated with this lesion, share not only a common anatomical location at the base of the skull, but also a common medical legacy, since both identities were devised by Harvey Cushing, the world famous neurosurgeon (Cushing, 1929, 1932).

In this chapter, we will describe the neuro-ophthalmological manifestations of craniopharyngiomas. With the benefit of retrospective analysis, Cushing's choice of "chiasmal syndrome" as a descriptive term has proven to be much more accurate than his selection of "craniopharyngioma." The latter is somewhat misleading, since these tumors arise from the origins of the buccal mucosa or Rathke's pouch, not the pharynx. However, the term does have value in that it directs attention to the anatomical location of the tumor and hence its clinical manifestations.

However, Cushing could not be more accurate in his choice of the term "chiasmal syndrome" to localize the compression of the partial decussation of the intracranial optic nerves just superior to the pituitary gland and just inferior to the third ventricle (Cushing, 1929). To return to the embryological origin of these lesions, we must recall that the pituitary gland arises from the union of two entities – an ectodermal process of the diencephalon and Rathke's pouch, the buccal mucosa (Erdenheim, 1904).

Craniopharyngiomas
http://dx.doi.org/10.1016/B978-0-12-416706-3.00006-4

PATHOPHYSIOLOGY OF THE VISUAL SYMPTOMS

Children and adults with craniopharyngiomas will frequently present with loss of vision. While Cushing's chiasmal syndrome is most often remembered as producing bitemporal heminanopic visual field loss, these patients invariably report decreased central vision. The anatomy of the optic nerves and chiasm explains the central loss of vision, since 80% of the fibers comprising these two structures originate in the macula, the area of the retina responsible for central visual acuity. Therefore, the loss of visual acuity will often steer the patients to ophthalmologists for their initial evaluations, based upon the assumption that their acquired poor vision must be based upon a problem with the eye, not the central nervous system.

In the era before computerized tomographic (CT) and magnetic resonance imaging (MRI), the most fortunate patients developed visual symptoms early in their course, because the bitemporal field defects or a central scotoma in one eye and temporal defect in the opposite eye (the so-called "junctional syndrome" of Cushing) quickly directed the neuro-ophthalmologist and neurosurgeon to detect the pathology precisely in the area of the chiasm. Once the neuro-ophthalmological localization was established, clinicians knew that chiasmal syndromes are caused by mass lesions in 95% of patients. Craniopharyngioma is merely one of the mass lesions in this area. Non-compressive lesions of the chiasm do exist – such as multiple sclerosis, sarcoidosis, and trauma – but these entities always have to be a diagnosis of exclusion.

Less fortunate patients developed little or no visual loss, and their initial symptoms could be caused by extension of a craniopharyngioma to the thalamus, cerebral peduncles, and floor of the third ventricle. To involve these structures, the tumor grew in virtual silence to considerable dimensions, and frequently became not only a vision-threatening problem, but also a life-threatening one as well. Today, modern neuro-imaging techniques allow a much more prompt diagnosis and surgical intervention, as so vividly illustrated in Dr. David Friedman's chapter in this volume. In fact, it is difficult to find a CT or MRI scan of a lesion with such widespread involvement as was seen during the age of skull X-rays and pneumo-encephalography. The extent of these lesions in the 1930s was actually best recorded by medical illustrators, as shown in Figure 6.1.

Visual Acuity, Visual Fields, Color Vision, and Pupils

Whenever a patient has visual acuity less than 20/20 with correction of the appropriate refractive error (refraction is prescribing the correct glasses) and there is no explanation for the loss of vision within the eye, such as a corneal problem, cataract, or disease of the macula or intraocular optic nerve, then clinicians must search for possible involvement of the intracranial afferent visual system.

Visual field testing is the most cost-effective, safe, and painless method for identifying the cause of visual loss when the ocular examination is normal. Many methods and approaches to perimetry, the term used to describe visual field testing, are available, and the testing must be individualized to consider the age, cognitive function, and overall medical condition of the patient.

Confrontation visual field testing should be performed on every patient undergoing an ophthalmic examination. While confrontation testing does not replace more advanced

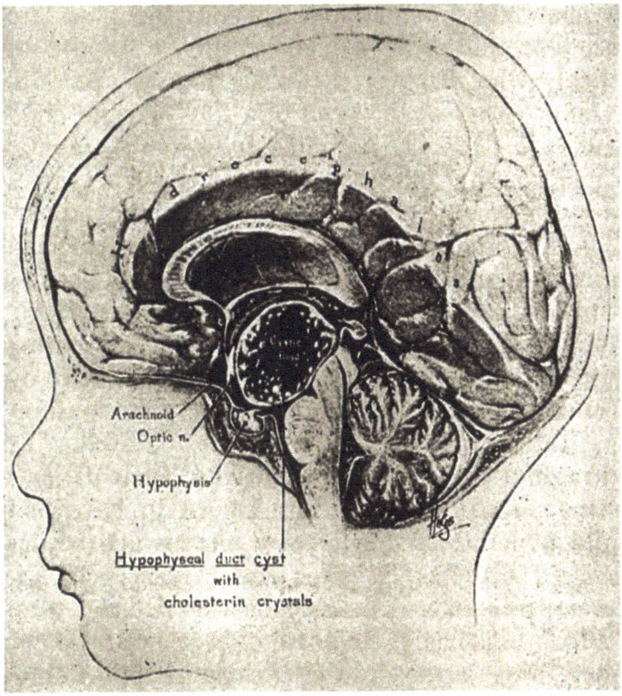

FIGURE 6.1 Mass lesion originating in the hypophyseal duct. In the era before CT and MRI scanning, these craniopharyngiomas grew to very large dimensions, such as this case, where the tumor compresses the brainstem and the intracranial optic nerve. *[W.E. Dandy, Practice of Surgery, edited by D.D. Lewis, volume 12, Hagerstown, Md. W. F. Prior Company, 1936.] Picture in Walsh and Hoyt, Clinical Neuro-Ophthalmology 1969, C.V. Mosby.*

methods of perimetry, it provides both the patient and examiner with information about the basic principles of fields examination: (Cushing, 1932) maintaining steady fixation on a target without moving the eyes to the test object in the peripheral visual field and (Cushing, 1929) making quick, accurate responses following presentation of the stimulus. In some cases, confrontation testing may provide the most reliable information about the patient's peripheral visual fields.

The testing algorithm is as follows:

1. The examiner requests that the patient cover his left eye with the palm of his left hand and fix the central vision of his right eye on the examiner's nose.
2. The examiner then presents one, two, or five fingers statically (that is, no moving of the fingers from non-seeing areas to seeing areas or wiggling of fingers) in each quadrant of the visual field.
3. One, two, or five fingers are presented since it is too difficult to determine if three or four are being presented.
4. If the patient fails to identify the statically presented fingers, then the examiner should move the fingers (changing the test from static to kinetic perimetry) to determine when the patient reports seeing the fingers.
5. Some neuro-ophthalmologists recommend testing the visual field with red targets, such as the red caps from bottles of eye drops for dilating the pupil. We have found that

this method is too subjective and rarely provides data that alter the approach to the diagnostic evaluation.

We advocate confrontation testing for all patients before they undergo so-called "formal perimetry" with either kinetic Goldmann testing or static testing with a variety of devices. Goldmann field testing requires a skilled technician, but has the distinct advantage of human-to-human interaction so that central fixation can be monitored and the validity of the patient's responses may be graded.

In contrast, automated, software program directed visual field testing does not require a skilled technician and depends upon the software assessing the reliability of the patient's test-taking performance. Because of multiple patient-related issues, ranging from alertness to cognitive function to intentional poor performance, automated perimetry has not realized the hope that "machine-driven" perimetry would always be superior to testing performed on humans by other humans. Because of the psycho-physical nature of automated visual field testing, the devices have very elegant software programs to assess the patient's fixation, false-negative and false-positive errors, but unfortunately at the end of the day poor human performance, whether intentional or unintentional, will defeat the intelligence of the software programs and provide confusing, usually contradictory, results when taken in context with the rest of the patient's clinical examination (see Figure 6.2).

The variability and "learning curve" effect of automated perimetry was demonstrated impeccably by the serial visual field analysis in the prospective, multicenter ocular hypertension trial (Keltner et al., 2000). In this study, over 80% of visual field abnormalities observed on the first visual field test with good reliability parameters resolved with repeated testing. Therefore, automated visual fields, while quite helpful in many cases for both the initial diagnosis and detecting change over consecutive examinations, must be interpreted with caution and integrated into other observations and testing in the neuro-ophthalmic examination. On occasion, the bitemporal nature of the visual field defects may be difficult to determine and only with serial analysis will the temporal defects respecting the vertical meridian of the field become apparent (Figure 6.3).

The Amsler grid is a very effective, simple method to assess the central visual field. Since in most cases of visual field defects, what occurs in the peripheral field also takes place in the central field, we can use the Amsler grid to screen patients for central defects and bitemporal defects. The grid is essentially a piece of graph paper and may be colored either black or red. It is most often used to monitor macular function, but since 80% of the fibers comprising the optic nerves, chiasm, and optic tract arise from the macula, the grid is also very effective for detecting scotomas from these anatomic locations.

Patients with optic nerve, chiasmal, and optic tract compression will also lose color vision. The assessment of color vision is a highly reliable method to distinguish loss of vision due to optic nerve, chiasmal, and tract lesions from many forms of intraocular pathology, or from most pathology located posterior to the lateral geniculate body.

Moreover, because approximately only 1% of women and 8% of men are congenitally color blind, the development of acquired loss of color blindness mandates neuro-ophthalmic evaluation. Testing color vision clinically is easily done with the Ishihara pseudo-isochromatic color plates. However, testing color vision in clinical trials for regulatory purposes is much

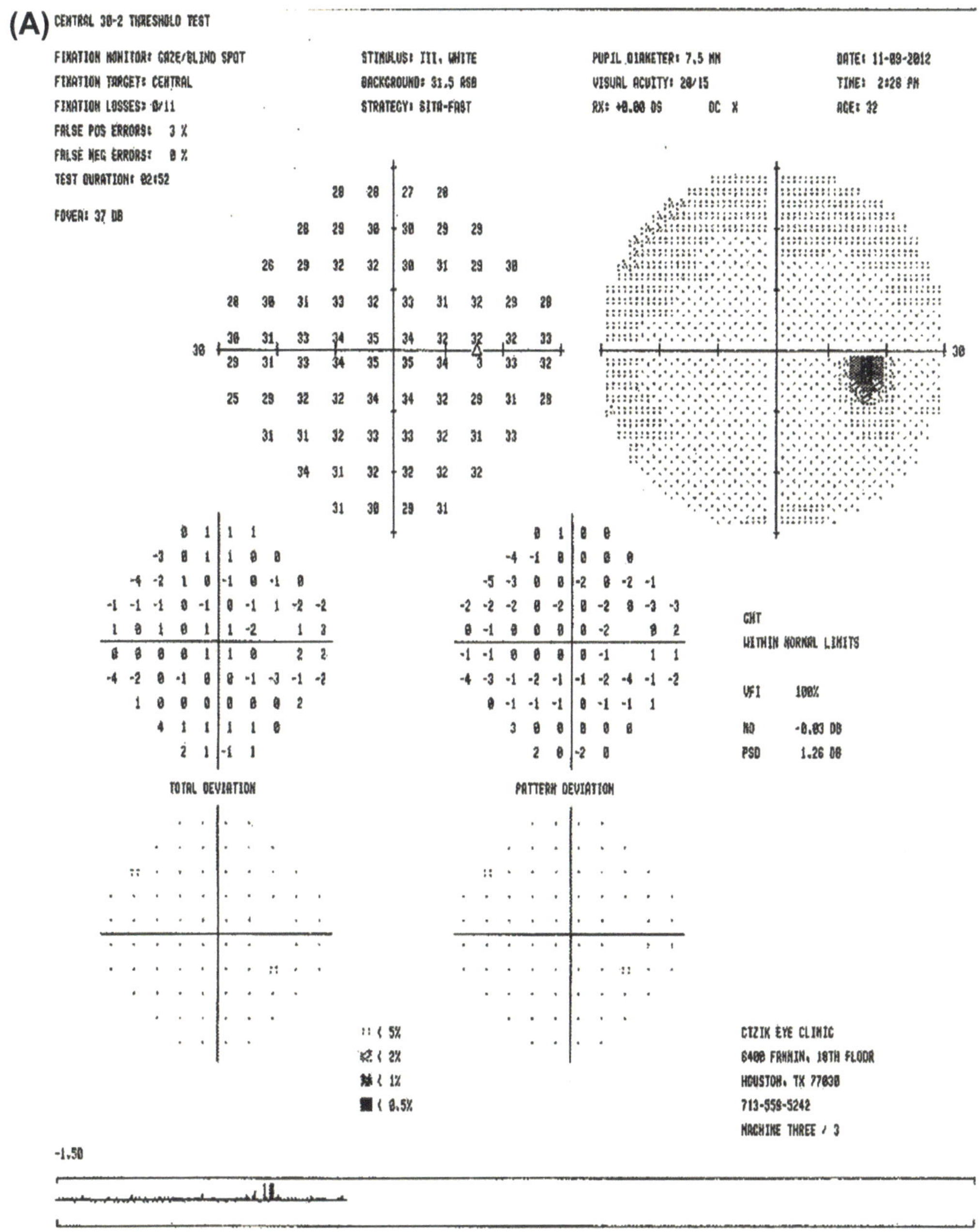

FIGURE 6.2 **A,** Patient with excellent visual field performance. Note the lack of fixation losses and false-negative errors and low false-positive errors. This is a normal automated perimetry test using a program interrogating the central 24 degrees of the visual field of the right eye.

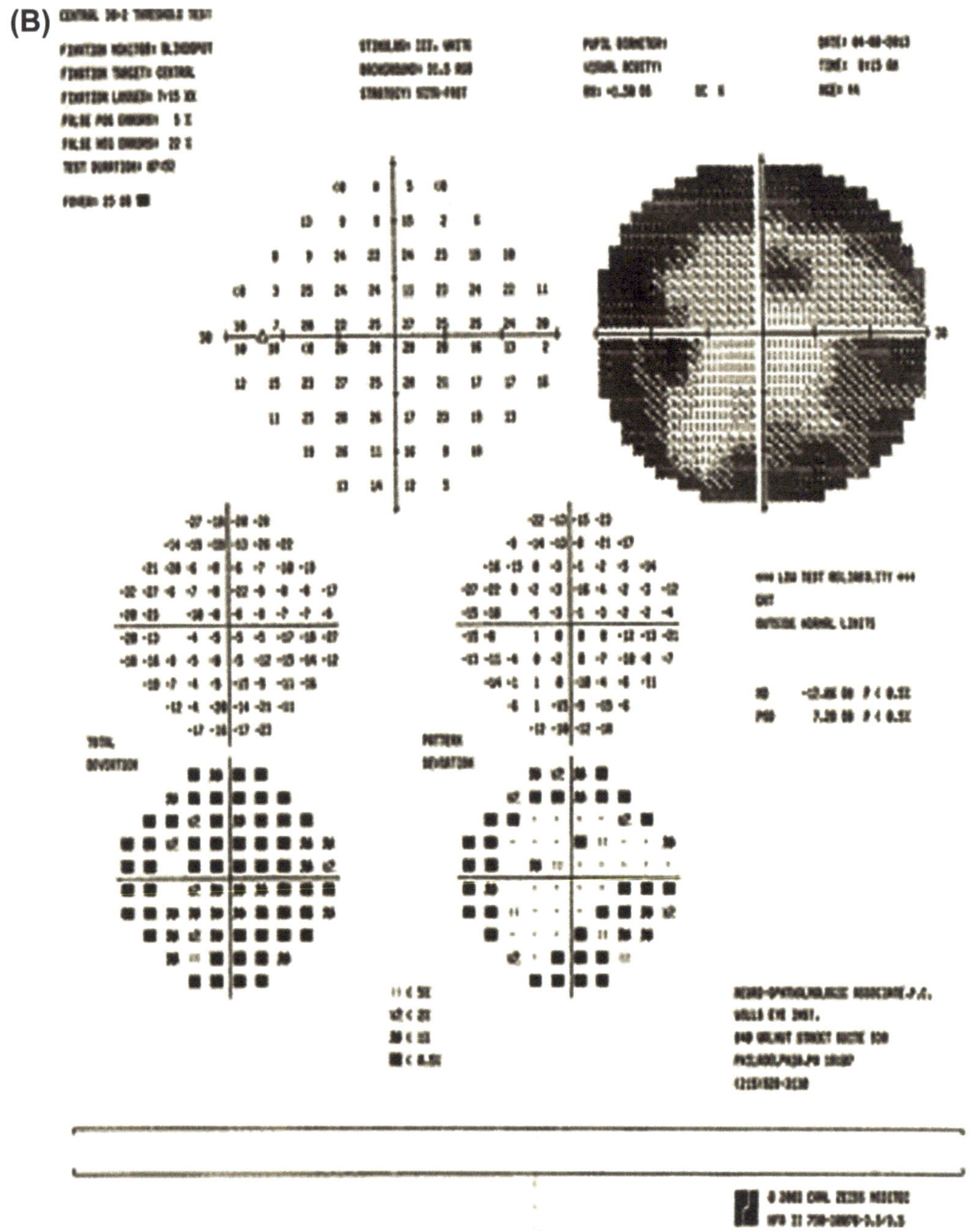

FIGURE 6.2 **B,** Poor visual field performance. The combination of high false-negative errors, fixation losses and long testing time frequently produces a visual field that with an artifact of concentric constriction.

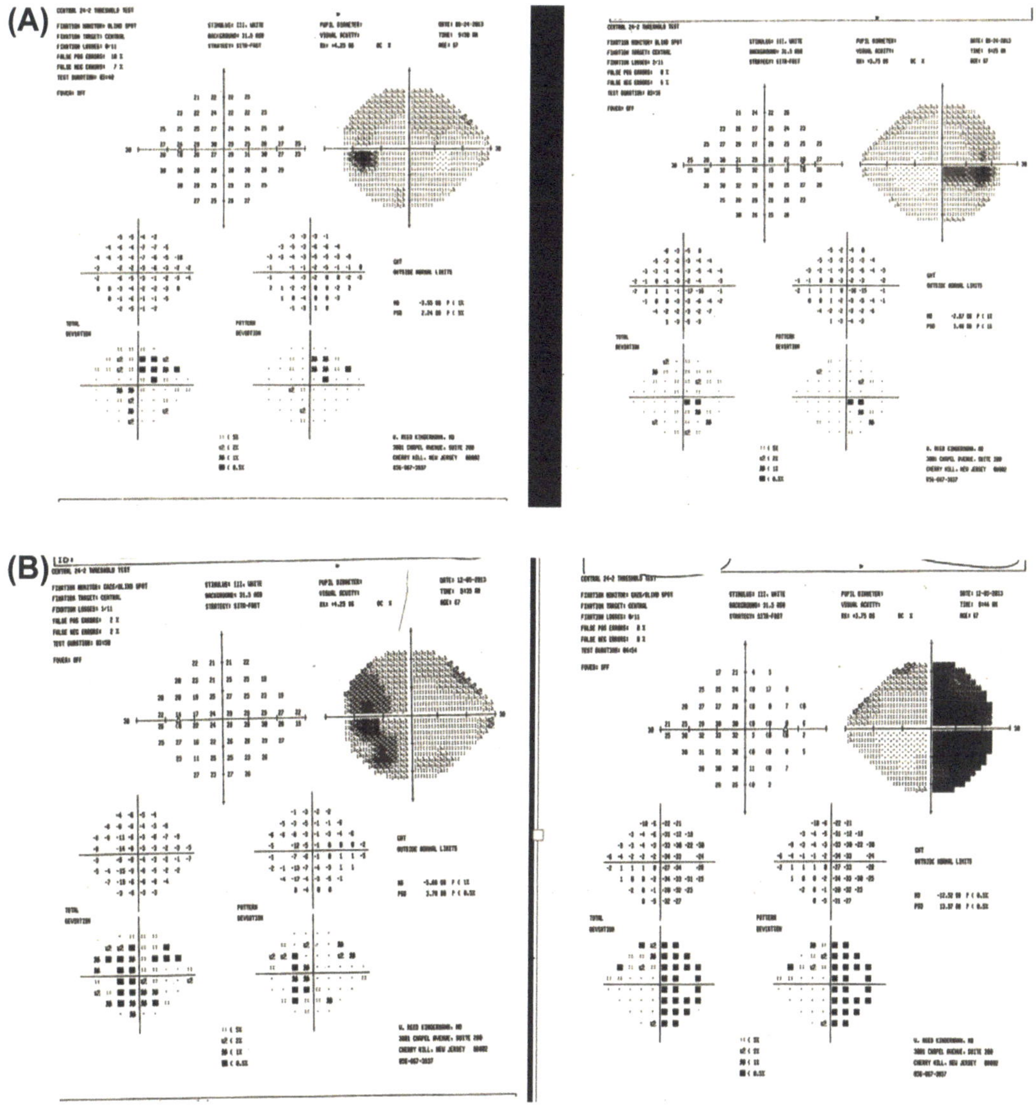

FIGURE 6.3 **A,** Subtle bitemporal heminanopic defect that progressed within two months to a much more recognizable bitemporal defect in **B**. The cystic craniopharyngioma was detected with MRI shown in **C**.

more difficult, because of the difficulty and variability of the Farnsworth-Munsell 100 hue and the Roth 28 examinations.

The fibers controlling the reactivity of the pupils to direct light stimulation also travel within the optic nerves, chiasm, and optic tract until they exit the afferent visual system on

(C)

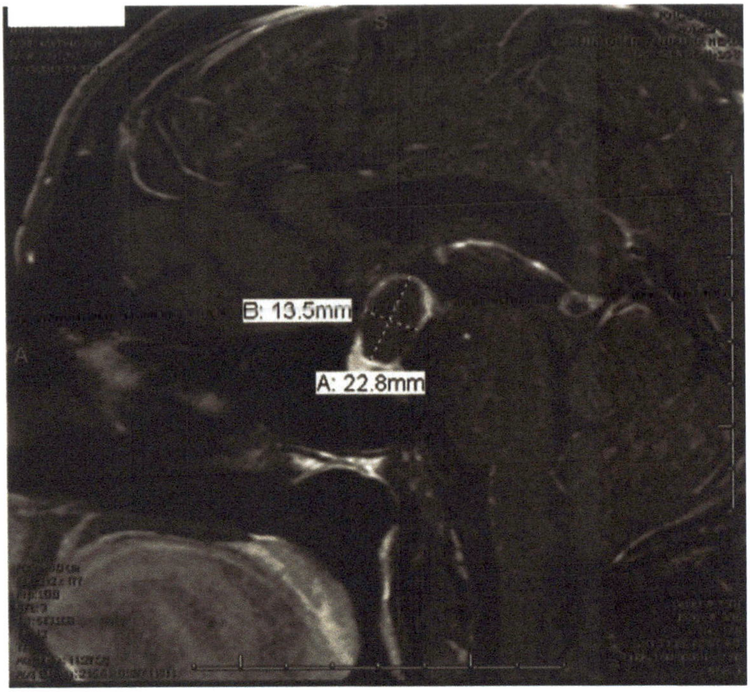

FIGURE 6.3 C, Cystic suprasellar mass with an enhancing wall. It exerts a severe mass effect on the optic chiasm, with edema seen in the left optic tract. The mass has a broad base oriented towards the sella. There is also a small lesion in the left posterior sella, with presumably proteinaceous contents. The differential diagnoses for these lesions are craniopharyngioma and Rathke's cleft cyst; given the enhancing wall, craniopharyngioma is favored over Rathke's cleft cyst. A cystic macroadenoma could have a similar appearance, but is less likely.

route to the midbrain as the retino-tectal fibers. Here, they interact with nuclei of the oculomotor nerve to provide input into the efferent limb of the pupillary reflex.

Therefore, lesions compressing the intracranial optic nerve, chiasm, and tract will demonstrate sluggish pupillary responses to direct light stimulation. When the involvement of the pupillary fibers and the afferent fibers is asymmetric, a subsequent asymmetry of the pupillary reaction will be seen, and on the side with the greater involvement, a Marcus Gunn afferent pupillary defect (APD) will be observed. The Marcus Gunn pupil is one of the classic physical examination findings in neuro-ophthalmology; however, it is not specific to chiasmal compression, and may be observed whenever there is a highly asymmetric lesion of the afferent visual system, including some large, unilateral retinal lesions.

Optic Disc Pallor and Optical Coherence Tomography

Pallor of the optic disc invariably develops following any pathological process affecting the optic nerve, chiasm, and optic tract. Many studies have been undertaken to determine whether the presence of optic disc pallor can predict recovery of visual function after resection of craniopharyngiomas. No definitive conclusions can be made about the predictive value of pallor, probably because of the subjective nature of this assessment.

Spectral domain optical coherence tomography (SD-OCT) offers greater promise for predicting visual outcome after surgery. SD-OCT uses confocal laser imaging and inferometry to quantify the number of unmyelinated axons in each optic nerve (Figure 6.4). Likewise, SD-OCT also can measure the thickness of all the layers of the retina. These structural parameters are complimentary to visual acuity, visual field, and color vision testing and do not replace these functional metrics. A report about time domain OCT has supported this concept. SD-OCT is much more sensitive and reproducible than time domain OCT, and therefore may provide even more accurate metrics for predicting visual acuity and visual field recovery post-operatively (Danesh-Meyer et al., 2006).

Anatomical Basis for Neuro-Ophthalmic Findings

The optic chiasm sits 12–14 millimeters above the sella turcica. Therefore, any lesion in and around the areas of the sella turcica, pituitary, or pituitary stalk must reach at least these dimensions to cause visual dysfunction (Figures 6.5, 6.6, 6.7). This structural relationship explains why pituitary microadenomas can never produce loss of visual acuity or visual field loss.

While craniopharyngiomas may remain dormant for many years, they often enlarge with both solid and cystic components to reach the afferent visual system. The symptoms then depend upon the size and the path of the enlargement. Once again, drawings from medical artists beautifully illustrate how these lesions compress the afferent visual system.

Optic Tract Syndrome

Although optic tract syndromes are exceedingly rare, craniopharyngiomas are one of the leading etiologies of this condition. Rather than a bitemporal visual field defect, these patients develop incongruous homonymous heminanopsias with loss of central vision (Savino et al., 1978; Newman & Miller, 1983). Homonymous hemianopsias produced by lesions in the parietal, temporal, and occipital lobes are usually very congruous and do not produce loss of central vision except in the case of large bilateral occipital lesions.

In addition, such patients will have afferent pupillary defects, since the compression occurs before the pupillary fibers leave the tract for the midbrain. Optic disc pallor will also develop as in chiasmal syndromes.

Ocular Motility Defects and Double Vision with Craniopharyngiomas

Double vision and ocular motility abnormalities are very, very rare neuro-ophthalmic manifestations of chiasmal syndromes, including craniopharyngiomas. A patient who reports double vision and has less than 20/20 vision should undergo visual field testing looking for a bitemporal defect.

Double vision with chiasmal lesions has almost as long a history as Cushing's description of the afferent visual system abnormalities in chiasmal syndrome, beginning with Kubie and

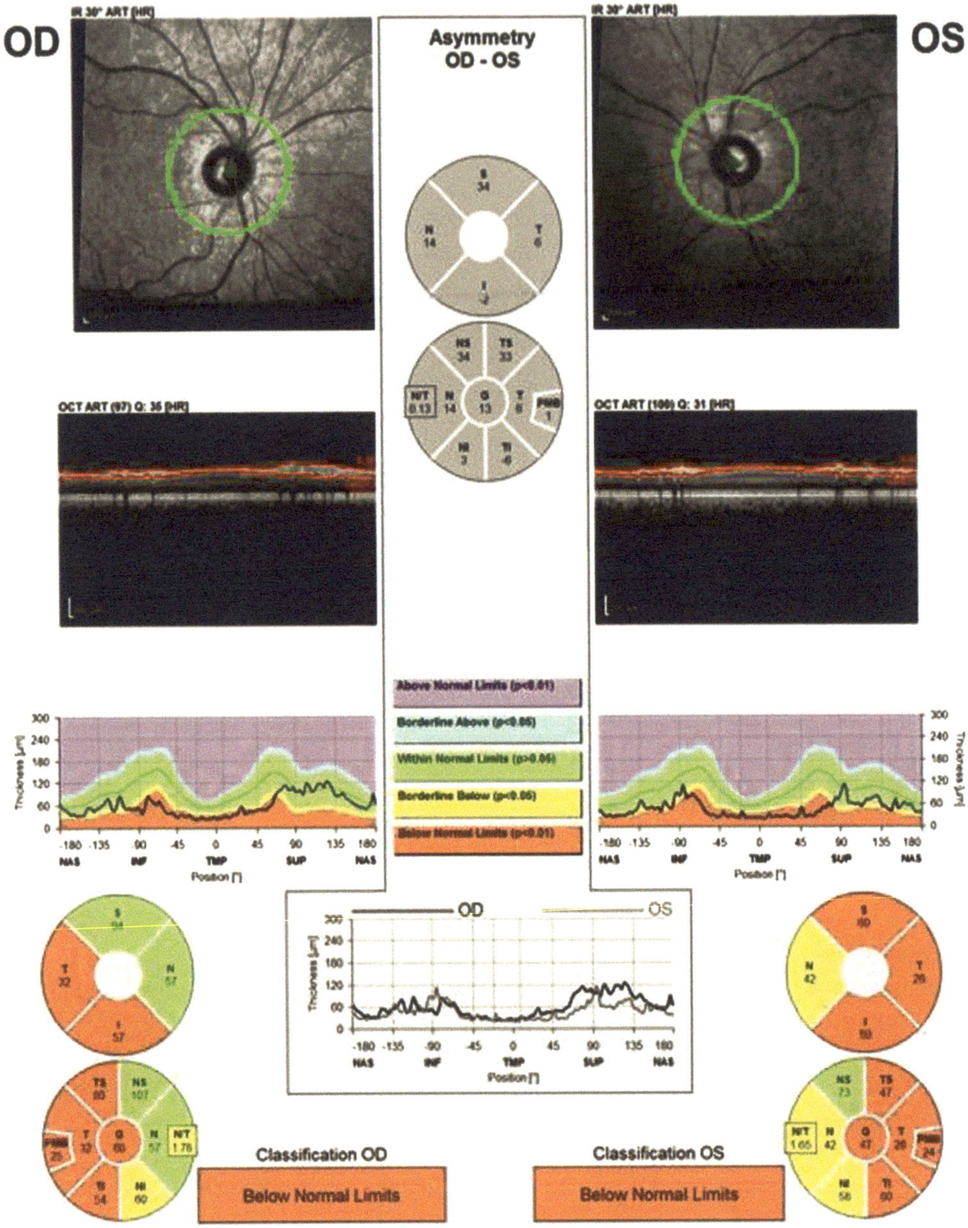

FIGURE 6.4 Spectral domain optical coherence tomogram (SD-OCT) of patient with bilateral axon loss due to chiasmal compression from the pituitary adenoma. The upper image illustrates the area imaged around the optic nerve in each eye, and the middle image shows how the SD-OCT isolates the retinal nerve fiber layer. The colored circular maps indicate that the patient has a nerve fiber layer thickness that is two standard deviations less than expected from age- and gender-matched data. When reduced retinal nerve fiber layer thickness is present pre-operatively, patients seem to be less likely to recover vision after surgical removal of the mass lesion.

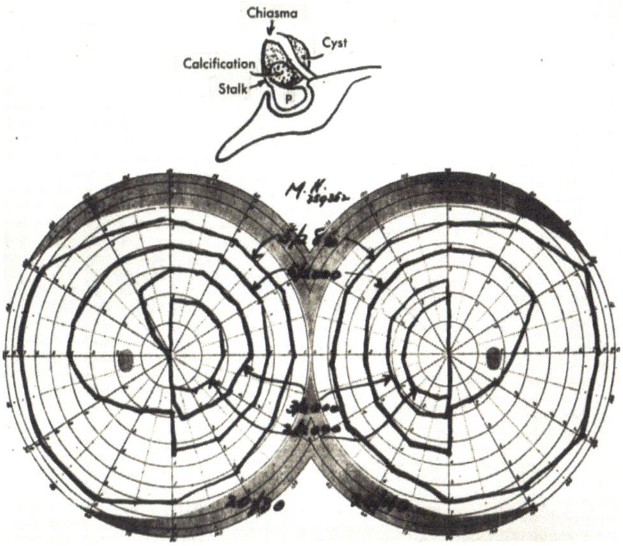

FIGURE 6.5 Classic compression of the chiasm by a craniopharyngioma. The visual fields were performed with the traditional tangent screen method. Notice that the patient's central vision is decreased to 20/30 in the right eye and 20/40 in the left. *[From Bronson Ray: Surgical lesions of the optic nerves and chiasm in infants and children. Neuro-Ophthalmology CV Mosby.]*

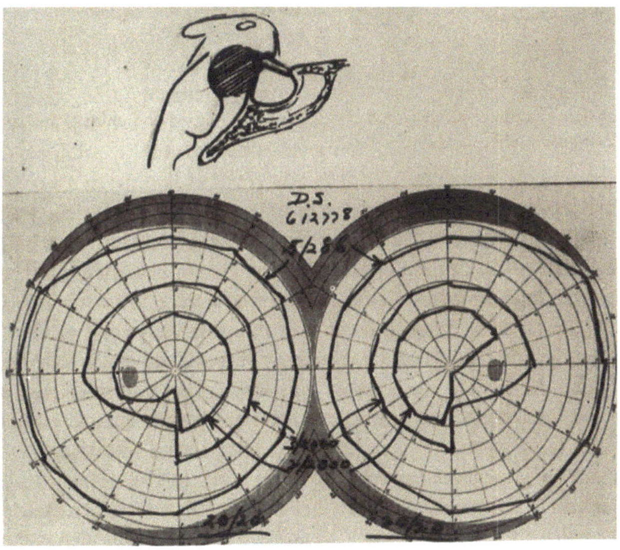

FIGURE 6.6 Illustration of posterior growth of craniopharyngioma with compression of the posterior chiasm. Note how the field defect involves the inferior field of each eye in a bitemporal pattern. *[From Bronson Ray: Surgical lesions of the optic nerves and chiasm in infants and children. Neuro-Ophthalmology CV Mosby.]*

Beckman in 1929 (Kubie & Beckmann, 1929). Nachtigaller and Hoyt explained this phenomenon in 1972, writing in the German literature (Nactigaller & Hoyt, 1970). The separation and vertical slip of the intact nasal hemifields develops with small changes in the alignment of the eyes. An exotropia ensues, producing double vision with a central vertical zone. Kirkham then labeled this phenomenon as a "hemifield slide" (Kirkham, 1972).

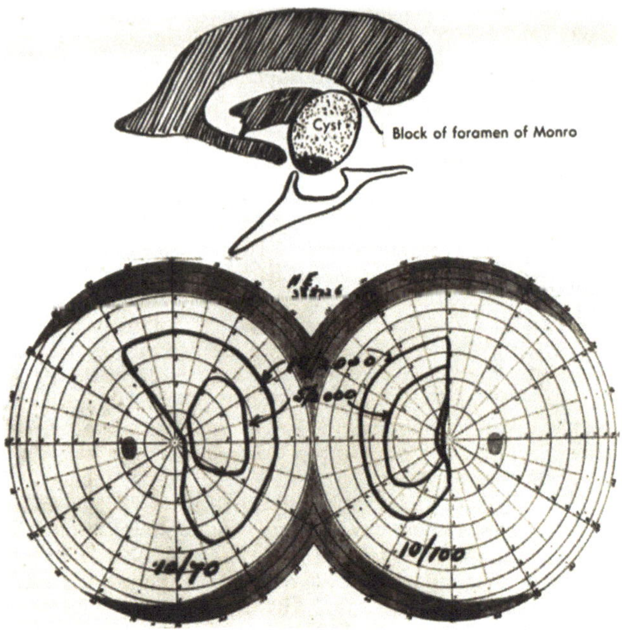

FIGURE 6.7 This drawing illustrates another path of growth for a craniopharyngioma, with extension upward to the foramen of Monro. This lesion has produced a bitemporal hemianopia and also may produce papilledema due to obstructive hydrocephalus. *[From Bronson Ray: Surgical lesions of the optic nerves and chiasm in infants and children. Neuro-Ophthalmology CV Mosby.]*

Borchert, Lessell, and Hoyt reported the hemifield slide double vision developing with heteronymous altitudinal defects. The patients they observed developed loss of binocular fusion and transient overlap of the intact visual fields (Borchert et al., 1996). These cases imply that the overlap of the preserved fields and not a specific bitemporal defect creates the double vision.

The experience with children and craniopharyngiomas vividly demonstrates why clinicians must be aware of the phenomenon of double vision with lesions producing visual field loss and hemifield slide. In a comprehensive clinical review of 45 patients with craniopharyngioma with special attention to the presenting symptoms, more than half were first referred for ophthalmic evaluation (Kennedy & Smith, 1975). Over 50% of the children presented with increased intracranial pressure and papilledema, and one-third had optic atrophy. Most importantly, one-third presented with strabismus syndrome and intermittent double vision. Only one patient had a cranial nerve palsy that produced strabismus.

SUMMARY

Neuro-ophthalmic involvement of the afferent visual system remains one of the most common ways for craniopharyngiomas to come to clinical attention. Deficits in visual acuity, color vision, and visual fields are much more common than reports of double vision. Visual field testing remains the cornerstone for localizing a patient's loss of vision at the intracranial optic nerve, chiasm, and optic tract. However, modern neuro-imaging has enabled much more rapid diagnoses, with much less pain and potential morbidity for the patient. Optical coherence tomography offers great promise for defining the mechanisms of permanent visual loss and the hopes for monitoring various therapeutic attempts with regenerative medicine strategies.

References

Borchert, M.S., Lessell, S., Hoyt, W.F., 1996. Hemifield slide diplopia from altitudinal visual field defects. J. Neuro-ophthalmol. 16, 107–109.

Cushing, H., 1929. The chiasmal syndrome of primary optic atrophy and bitemporal field defects in adult patients with a normal sella turcica. XIII Concilium Ophthalmologicum Hollandia, 97.

Cushing, H., 1932. Intracranial Tumors.

Danesh-Meyer, H.V., Carroll, S.C., Foroozan, R., Savino, P.J., Fan, J., Jiang, Y., Hoorn, S.V., 2006. Relationship between retinal nerve fiber layer and visual field sensitivity as measured by optical coherence tomography in chiasmal compression. Invest. Ophthalmol. Vis. Sci. 47, 4827–4835.

Dandy, Walter E., 1945. Surgery of the Brain. W. F. Prior Company, Inc, Hagerstown. Print, p 576.

Erdenheim, J., 1904. Ueber hypophysenganggeechwzungulste und hirncholesteatome, Sitzungsb. d. k. Acad d. Wissench 113, 537.

Keltner, J.L., Johnson, C.A., Quigg, J.M., et al., 2000. Confirmation of visual field abnormalities in the Ocular Hypertension Treatment Study. Arch. Ophthalmol. 118, 1187–1194.

Kennedy, H.B., Smith, R.J., 1975. Eye signs in craniopharyngioma. Br. J. Ophthalmol. 12, 689–695.

Kirkham, T.H., 1972. The ocular symptomatology of pituitary tumours. Proc. R. Soc. Med. 65, 517.

Kubie, L.S., Beckmann, J.W., 1929. Diplopia without extra-ocular palsies caused by heteronymous defects in the visual fields associated with defective macular vision. Brain 52, 317.

Nactigaller, V.H., Hoyt, W.F., 1970. Storungen des Seheindruckes bei bitemporaler Hemanopsie and Versschiebung der Sehachsen. Klin. Monatsbl. Augenheilkd. 156, 821–836.

Newman, S.A., Miller, N.R., 1983. Optic tract syndrome: neuro-ophthalmologic considerations. Arch. Ophthalmol. 101, 1241–1250.

Savino, P.J., Paris, M., Schatz, N.J., Orr, L.S., Corbett, J.J., 1978. Optic tract syndrome. Arch. Ophthalmol. 96, 656–663.

SECTION III

SURGICAL APPROACHES

CHAPTER

7

Surgical Approaches

Introduction and Outcomes

Paolo Cappabianca, Luigi Maria Cavallo*, Domenico Solari*, Alberto Di Somma*, Maria Laura Del Basso De Caro*[†]

[*]Department of Neurosciences and Reproductive and Odontostomatological Sciences, Division of Neurosurgery, Università degli Studi di Napoli Federico II, Naples, Italy; [†]Department of Advanced Biomedical Sciences, Division of Pathology, Università degli Studi di Napoli Federico II, Naples, Italy

"The most forbidding of the intracranial tumors." **Harvey Cushing, 1932**

INTRODUCTION

Craniopharyngiomas are disembryogenetic tumors arising from the squamous epithelial remnants of Rathke's pouch and, for this reason, can arise from its whole pathway, from the rhinopharynx to the hypothalamus (Jane and Laws, 2006; Karavitaki, 2014). They tend to involve a great number of vital neurovascular structures, including the optic nerves, internal carotid arteries (ICAs), the third ventricle – above all of its floor – the hypothalamus, and the pituitary gland, causing a variety of symptoms.

Common clinical presentations include visual dysfunction, with symptoms of chiasmatic and/or retrochiasmatic compression, hypothalamic dysfunction, such as behavioral changes, alterations of eating patterns, apathy, or even stupor, and finally pituitary dysfunction, often presenting as panhypopituitarism (Karavitaki, 2014).

These lesions account for 1.2 to 4.6% of all intracranial tumors (Central Brain Tumor Registry of the United States) and exhibit a bimodal distribution, with one peak occurring during childhood (5–14 years of age) and another in late adulthood (50–74 years of age) (Bunin et al., 1998).

Description of a craniopharyngioma was first presented by the German pathologist, Friedrich Albert von Zenker (Zenker, 1857), who in 1857 depicted a cystic suprasellar mass containing

Craniopharyngiomas
http://dx.doi.org/10.1016/B978-0-12-416706-3.00007-6

cholesterol crystals and squamous epithelium. In 1904, Jakob Erdheim accurately defined the histopathological features of a craniopharyngioma (Erdheim, 1904); according also to previous reports by Mott and Barret (Mott and Barret, 1899), he confirmed that these tumors arise from squamous cell rests originating from a partially involuted hypophyseal-pharyngeal duct.

Rupert Boyce and Cecil Beadles (Boyce and Beadles, 1893) described a 35-year-old blind patient who became comatose and died as a result of a large, partially ossified, cystic lesion — suspected to be a craniopharyngioma — causing brainstem, optic chiasm, and optic tract compression. Subsequently, Babinski (Babinski, 1900) and Frohlich (Frohlich, 1901) reported similar clinical signs in patients with cystic pituitary masses without acromegaly.

From a neuropathological standpoint, two subtypes of craniopharyngioma have been recognized, namely adamantinomatous and papillary. The adamantinomatous form occurs in children (5–10 years) and adults (50–60 years), while the papillary form is seen almost exclusively in adults; generally, the adamantinomatous form is the more common (ratio: 9/1) (Yasargil et al., 1990; Paulus et al., 1997). Regarding macroscopic features, the adamantinomatous subtype shows an irregular interface, adhesions to surrounding structures, and cystic contents have dark "motor oil" fluid, with cholesterol crystals inside; calcification may occur in the majority of cases. In contrast, the papillary form shows no adherence to surrounding structures and/or calcifications, while the cystic contents are often clear (Crotty et al., 1995). The two distinct craniopharyngioma types have different biological behaviors, and immunohistochemical examinations appear to be relevant in order to analyze this issue; as a matter of fact, the adamantinomatous subtype demonstrates positivity for CK7, CK8, CK14 (Kurosaki et al., 2001; Tateyama et al., 2001; Xin et al., 2002), and beta-catenin (Sekine et al., 2002; Hofmann et al., 2006; Holsken et al., 2013). In particular, clusters of cells with nuclear beta-catenin are predominantly represented in invasive tumors. This pattern is suggestive of an involvement of the beta-catenin signaling in the migratory behavior of these tumors; the cellular clusters with nuclear beta-catenin may coordinate the infiltration of the tumor into surrounding tissues, thus explaining the greater aggressiveness of the adamantinomatous tumor histotype (Hussain et al., 2013; Larkin and Ansorge, 2013).

Craniopharyngiomas involve the sella and parasellar areas, but in contrast to pituitary tumors, they often adhere to the neurovascular structures of the suprasellar space, such as perforating vessels from the anterior and posterior cerebral arteries and/or ICAs, the optic chiasm and pathways, the hypothalamus, and third ventricular regions. These close anatomical relationships represent a key aspect to be considered during surgical maneuvers for tumor removal. Above all, the relationship with the stalk and the infundibulum area should be noted, since surgical damage here could lead to diabetes insipidus and hypopituitarism. The relationship with the hypothalamus and third ventricle floor is also of great importance, since injury to these structures could cause physical and mental growth retardation.

Furthermore, craniopharyngiomas can recur even after radical resection, and surgical removal of recurrent craniopharyngioma is even more troublesome due to scar formation and new adhesions (Minamida et al., 2005; Cavallo et al., 2009).

The first successful surgical resection of a craniopharyngioma was performed by A. E. Halstead (Halstead, 1910), and subsequently, Lewis (Lewis, 1910), Cushing (Cushing, 1932), and Schloffer (Schloffer, 1907) attempted to remove craniopharyngiomas using either transcranial or transnasal approaches. As a general rule, the choice of corridor to access such lesions is primarily along the vertical axis.

Historically, different neurosurgical pathways have been used to access the areas these tumors may extend within (Ciric and Cozzens, 1980; Laws, 1980; Yasargil et al., 1990; Honegger et al., 1992; Fahlbusch et al., 2000; Samii and Samii, 2000; Maira et al., 2004; Aryan et al., 2005; Shi et al., 2006; Zhang et al., 2008; Jung et al., 2009; Jiang et al., 2010; Liu et al., 2010).

Over the years, several authors have defined classifications for craniopharyngiomas in terms of their growth path and the surgical route used, all of which share the principle of subdividing lesions along the length of extension in the primary vertical axis, as related to the optic chiasm, diaphragma sellae, third ventricle, or more recently to the infundibulum (Yaşargil, 1984; Samii and Samii, 2000; Steno et al., 2004; Kassam et al., 2008a; Pascual et al., 2011).

Yasargil divided craniopharyngiomas into (Yasargil et al., 1990):

a) purely intrasellar-infradiaphragmatic,
b) intra- and suprasellar, infra- and supradiaphragmatic,
c) supradiaphragmatic, parachiasmatic, extra-ventricular,
d) intra and extra-ventricular,
e) paraventricular,
f) purely intraventricular.

On the other hand, Samii et al. classified craniopharyngiomas into grades based on their vertical projections: grade I (intrasellar or infradiaphragmatic), grade II (cisternal with or without an intrasellar component), grade III (lower half of the third ventricle), grade IV (upper half of the third ventricle), and grade V (reaching the septum pellucidum or lateral ventricles) (Samii and Tatagiba, 1997). More recently, Kassam et al (Kassam et al., 2008a). proposed another classification useful during endonasal approaches, which is based on the relation of the craniopharyngioma with the infundibulum, so we can have type 1, preinfundibular; type 2, transinfundibular; type 3, post- or retro-infundibular (further subdivision is based on rostral or caudal extension, whether it is to the anterior third ventricular [infundibular recess, hypothalamic], and interpeduncular fossa); and type 4, isolated third ventricular.

Many different routes (i.e., pterional, subfrontal, supraorbital, and transventricular) have been adopted to remove craniopharyngiomas, evolving through the decades in attempts to achieve better outcomes with lower morbidity and mortality rates.

Surgical resection via a fronto-temporal approach, which is widely used, provides the shortest route to the suprasellar space, even if the visualization of the contralateral optic nerve and carotid artery may be reached at the end of tumor removal. This route has been validated throughout decades as the standard technique for managing these lesions, and its effectiveness has made it accepted worldwide in routine neurosurgical practice (Yasargil et al., 1990; Samii and Samii, 2000). Variations of the traditional pterional or frontal interhemispheric approaches have been used for lesions with hypothalamic extension. Over the last few decades, the evolution of surgical techniques has led to a progressive reduction of the invasiveness of the neurosurgical approaches and, according to the keyhole concept, the supraorbital approach has been defined as a valid alternative to the conventional transcranial routes. It allows wide and bilateral exposure, offering equal possibilities with lower approach-related morbidity, thanks to minimal brain retraction (Reisch and Perneczky, 2005; Fatemi et al., 2009).

On the other hand, the transsphenoidal approach was introduced according to the indications defined by Guiot and Derome in the early 1960s (Guiot and Derome, 1972), being initially proposed only for infradiaphragmatic lesions, with enlarged sella, that preferably had already developed panhypopitutarism. It was Weiss in 1987 (Weiss, 1987) that termed and originally described the extended transsphenoidal approach, intending a transsphenoidal approach with removal of additional bone along the tuberculum sellae and the posterior planum sphenoidale, between the optic canals, with subsequent opening of the dura mater above the diaphragma sellae. This route allows midline access and visibility to the suprasellar space while obviating brain retraction, and makes it possible to transsphenoidally treat small midline suprasellar lesions that had been traditionally approached transcranially, namely tuberculum sellae and sphenoid planum meningiomas, and craniopharyngiomas. Initially, such operations were done with the aid of the microscope (Weiss, 1987; Honegger et al., 1992; Fahlbusch et al., 1999; Fahlbusch et al., 2000; Maira et al., 2004; Kitano and Taneda, 2008; Hofmann et al., 2012). Later, endoscopy has caused a renewal of interest in anatomical studies, which are essential for the comprehension of the approach itself, and has contributed to the more contemporary knowledge of the possibilities of the transsphenoidal approach (de Divitiis et al., 2002; Frank and Pasquini, 2002; Cappabianca et al., 2003; Cavallo et al., 2005; Kassam et al., 2005a, 2005b, 2008b; Cavallo et al., 2007a; de Notaris et al., 2012). The wider and panoramic view offered by the endoscope, and the rapid growth of neuroradiological diagnostic techniques together with intraoperative neuronavigation systems, have increased the versatility of the transsphenoidal approach, thus allowing the extension towards different areas of the skull base; and, because of craniopharyngiomas are often midline tumors, the endonasal route provides the advantage of accessing the tumor upon dural opening, without brain or optic nerve retraction and with a direct view through a straight surgical route. The endoscopic endonasal approach has allowed some of the limits of the microsurgical transsphenoidal route to the sella to be overcome, permitting the management of different purely supra- and retrosellar cystic/solid craniopharyngiomas, regardless of the sellar size or the pituitary function. The relationship of the craniopharyngioma with the diaphragma sellae is essential when deciding on a transsphenoidal approach. Infradiaphragmatic location with sellar involvement is observed in approximately one-third of craniopharyngioma cases. They are traditionally considered suitable for a transsphenoidal procedure. An enlarged pituitary fossa facilitates transsphenoidal removal. However, sellar enlargement is not a prerequisite for transsphenoidal surgery. Generally, craniopharyngiomas amenable to endonasal treatment should have precise features, i.e., median lesions, without a solid parasellar component or encasement of the main neurovascular structures. The transsphenoidal approach can avoid transcranial surgery with its inherent risks. However, it is associated with a relatively high risk of postoperative CSF leak and meningitis. The effectiveness of this endoscopic endonasal technique for the treatment of such featured craniopharyngiomas has been validated in recently published surgical series (Frank et al., 2006; de Divitiis et al., 2007; Leng et al., 2012; Koutourousiou et al., 2013).

Several other surgical techniques can be used for the management of craniopharyngiomas. Indeed, cyst drainage can be realized via a trascranial burr-hole approach with catetherization of the cyst connected to an Ommaya reservoir or with transsphenoidal insertion of the catether into the cyst for cyst content drainage (Spaziante et al., 1989; Spaziante and de Divitiis, 1997); wide marsupialization of the cysts into CSF spaces (cysto-ventriculo-cisternostomy) with neuroendoscopic techniques (Delitala et al., 2004) can be used as an alternative, in order to ensure mass effect control, and diversion of the cyst's fluid. These techniques could be implemented with other therapeutic modalities, such as radiotherapy, to achieve longer-term tumor control. In addition, stereotactic aspiration with the instillation of bleomycin or interferon alpha (Backlund et al., 1989; Liu et al., 2012) resulted in an effective, minimally invasive treatment route (Hasegawa et al., 2004; Hukin et al., 2007; Julow et al., 2007; Derrey et al., 2008). On the other hand, intracavitary irradiation has been proposed for the treatment of cystic components of craniopharyngiomas.

The use of radiation treatment is usually reserved for residual or recurrent craniopharyngiomas, but when necessary, fractionated stereotactic radiotherapy can be effective as an initial treatment; after establishment of a tissue diagnosis, solid papillary craniopharyngiomas may be the most suitable for radiotherapy if surgical resection is not feasible (Chiou et al., 2001; Schulz-Ertner et al., 2002; Varlotto et al., 2002; Jackson et al., 2003; Combs et al., 2007; Minniti et al., 2009; Aggarwal et al., 2013; Iannalfi et al., 2013). However, the detrimental effects of such treatment on visual and pituitary function, especially in younger patients, should not be underestimated (Garnett et al., 2007). Concerning post-operative irradiation, it has been shown that after subtotal resection this leads to an improvement in the prognosis of the patient with craniopharyngiomas (Hoogenhout et al., 1984; Komotar et al., 2012). However, post-operative irradiation should not be performed in all cases. In cases of small residual tumors with calcified fragments and/or dense adherence to neurovascular vital structures that are not growing during follow-up, a watchful waiting strategy with close neuroradiological follow-up can be seen as a preferred approach. On the contrary, in case of large, rapidly growing, residual tumors an early second surgical procedure may be recommended. Additionally, after transnasal approaches, it is preferable to wait for a few months before performing radiotherapy, in order to allow the integration of the reconstruction materials.

Given that radical tumor removal at first attempt, when possible, is the preferred surgical strategy for these difficult neoplasms, when dealing with pediatric patients it may be preferred to accept the risk of a lower radical surgical resection – above all when hypothalamus is involved – in order to allow adequate psychic and motor development and reduce the risk of hypothalamic injuries (Sainte-Rose et al., 2005; Cohen et al., 2013).

OUTCOMES

The ideal treatment of craniopharyngiomas remains a challenge for neurosurgeons, with surgical management actually being considered as the primary choice. Craniopharyngiomas grow in a deep-seated area of the brain, involving several neurovascular structures, above all the hypothalamus, that are of paramount importance for vegetative, emotional, and endocrine function and for maintaining worthwhile life. The outcome of primary surgery for craniopharyngiomas is affected by different factors such as age, clinical conditions, and previous treatment. In the pertinent literature, rates of gross total resection range widely between 10% and 90% with an average of 58% (Fischer et al., 1990; Yasargil et al., 1990; Hoffman et al., 1992; Fahlbusch et al., 1999; Samii and Samii, 2000; Van Effenterre and Boch, 2002; Albright et al., 2005; Lena et al., 2005; Di Rocco et al., 2006; Lin et al., 2008; Hofmann et al., 2012; Kunihiro et al., 2014). Differently from other brain tumors, it has been emphasized that the surgical treatment of craniopharyngiomas is overburdened by a high peri-operative mortality rate, which ranges between 1.1% and 10% in the early post-operative period (Hoogenhout et al., 1984; Baskin and Wilson, 1986; Fischer et al., 1990; Symon et al., 1991; Hoffman et al., 1992; Mark et al., 1995; Fisher et al., 1998; Fahlbusch et al., 1999; Duff et al., 2000; Van Effenterre and Boch, 2002; Kalapurakal et al., 2003; Albright et al., 2005; Caldarelli et al., 2005; Chakrabarti et al., 2005; Lena et al., 2005; Mottolese et al., 2005; Dhellemmes and Vinchon, 2006; Di Rocco et al., 2006). These rates are influenced by the anatomical location of these lesions, and the infiltrative relationship with the hypothalamus and other vital neurovascular structures. Moreover, the surgical outcome is undoubtedly related to whether patients are operated on as a primary treatment or whether they had undergone previous treatments (Yaşargil, 1984; Yasargil et al., 1990; Minamida et al., 2005; Cavallo et al., 2009). In contrast, the tumor size appears to have no prognostic significance in recently reported series (Yaşargil, 1984; Hofmann et al., 2012; Leng et al., 2012; Koutourousiou et al., 2013; Mortini et al., 2013). Compressing the optic chiasm and nerves from below, craniopharyngiomas usually present with visual disturbances in the adult population, with the predominant defect being bilateral quadrantopia or bilateral hemianopia. In particular, the optic chiasm and nerves may be injured at the exit of the optic canal at the level of the falciform ligament, when the lesion extends upward and anteriorly, or by the anterior cerebral arteries if tumor displaces the chiasm by pushing it from its inferior aspect (Table 7.1).

TABLE 7.1 Patient and Tumor Characteristics in Open Transcranial, Transsphenoidal Microscopic, and Endoscopic Endonasal Craniopharyngioma Resection

	OT	TM	EE	Statistic Signif.
PRESENTING SYMPTOMS				
Visual disturbance	53.0 (%)	51.9 (%)	75.8 (%)	OT vs. EE ($P < 0.003$) TM vs. EE ($P < 0.003$)
Headache	52.6 (%)	39.7 (%)	35.5 (%)	EE vs. OT ($P = 0.024$)
Diabetes insipidus	12.2 (%)	22.2 (%)	32.3 (%)	OT vs. TM ($P < 0.003$) TM vs. EE ($P = 0.018$) EE vs. OT ($P < 0.003$)
Hypopituitarism	28.4 (%)	39.1 (%)	55.8 (%)	OT vs. TM ($P < 0.003$) TM vs. EE ($P = 0.018$) EE vs. OT ($P < 0.003$)
TUMOR CHARACTERISTICS				
Mixed solid & cystic	53.9 (%)	76.0 (%)	58.3 (%)	OT vs. TM ($P < 0.003$) TM vs. EE ($P = 0.033$)
Intraventricular growth	17.9 (%)	0.0 (%)	32.9 (%)	EE vs. OT ($P = 0.006$)
PLANNED ADJUVANT THERAPY				
Post-operative RT	27.3 (%)	2.2 (%)	37.5 (%)	OT vs. TM ($P < 0.003$) TM vs. EE ($P < 0.003$)

OT: open transcranial; TM: transsphenoidal microscopic; EE: endoscopic endonasal; RT: radiotherapy.

(Modified from Ricardo J. Komotar et. al.: Endoscopic endonasal compared with microscopic transsphenoidal and open transcranial resection of craniopharyngiomas. World Neurosurg 77:329–341, 2012.)

With regards to visual outcome, it has been shown that there was a greater rate of improved visual outcome in the endoscopic endonasal cohort than in the conventional transcranial cohort. The pertinent literature has shown that visual outcome can vary among different surgical procedures, i.e., transcranial or transnasal (microscopic or endoscopic) (Table 7.2). Visual improvement occurred in 60% of patients after transcranial surgery and in 75% after transsphenoidal surgery (Fahlbusch et al., 1999; Maira et al., 2004; Chakrabarti et al., 2005); in the endoscopic endonasal series, a 93% rate of visual improvement has been reported (Koutourousiou et al., 2013).

TABLE 7.2 Operative Outcomes and Complications in Transcranial, Transsphenoidal Microscopic, and Endoscopic Endonasal Resection Studies

	OT	TM	EE	Statistic Signif.
EXTENT OF RESECTION				
Gross total	48.3 (%)	69.1 (%)	66.9 (%)	OT vs. TM ($P < 0.003$) EE vs. OT ($P < 0.003$)
Subtotal	36.4 (%)	23.9 (%)	24.6 (%)	OT vs. TM ($P = 0.003$) EE vs. OT ($P = 0.012$)
COMPLICATIONS				
Seizure	8.5 (%)	0.0 (%)	0.0 (%)	OT vs. TM ($P < 0.003$) EE vs. OT ($P < 0.001$)
Wound/bone flap Infection	2.2 (%)	0.0 (%)	0.0 (%)	OT vs. TM ($P < 0.036$)
CSF leak	2.6 (%)	9.0 (%)	18.4 (%)	OT vs. TM ($P < 0.003$) TM vs. EE ($P = 0.024$) EE vs. OT ($P < 0.003$)
Permanent DI	54.8 (%)	31.7 (%)	27.7 (%)	OT vs. TM ($P < 0.003$) EE vs. OT ($P < 0.003$)
Hypopituitarism	48.1 (%)	12.8 (%)	47.1 (%)	OT vs. TM ($P < 0.003$) TM vs. EE ($P < 0.003$)
Hydrocephalus	10.1 (%)	0.0 (%)	15.8 (%)	NS
POST-OPERATIVE VISUAL OUTCOME				
Improved	33.1 (%)	44.0 (%)	56.2 (%)	OT vs. TM ($P = 0.003$) EE vs. OT ($P < 0.003$)
Stable	37.1 (%)	15.4 (%)	10.7 (%)	OT vs. TM ($P < 0.003$) EE vs. OT ($P < 0.003$)
Deteriorated	11.3 (%)	5.3 (%)	1.7 (%)	EE vs. OT ($P < 0.003$)
Recurrence	28.2 (%)	10.9 (%)	18.4 (%)	OT vs. TM ($P < 0.003$)

OT: open transcranial; TM: transsphenoidal microscopic; EE: endoscopic endonasal; DI: diabetes insipidus; NS: not significant.
(Modified from Ricardo J. Komotar et. al.: Endoscopic endonasal compared with microscopic transsphenoidal and open transcranial resection of craniopharyngiomas. World Neurosurg 77:329–341, 2012.)

With regards to the endocrinological outcome, rates of new endocrinopathy after transcranial surgeries range from 24% to 66% for panhypopituitarism and from 43% to 79% for diabetes insipidus (Fahlbusch et al., 1999; Duff et al., 2000; Garnett et al., 2007; Campbell et al., 2010; Hofmann et al., 2012; Mortini et al., 2013; Karavitaki, 2014; Kunihiro et al., 2014); in transsphenoidal series, up to 67% of patients demonstrated panhypopituitarism and up to 48% exhibited permanent diabetes insipidus (Laws, 1980; Kitano and Taneda, 2008; Campbell et al., 2010; Leng et al., 2012; Koutourousiou et al., 2013).

Historically, surgical treatment of craniopharyngiomas was performed by different transcranial approaches (i.e., pterional, subfrontal, supraorbital, and transventricular) (Laws, 1980; Yasargil et al., 1990; Honegger et al., 1992; Fahlbusch et al., 2000; Samii and Samii, 2000; Maira et al., 2004; Aryan et al., 2005; Shi et al., 2006; Zhang et al., 2008; Jung et al., 2009; Jiang et al., 2010; Liu et al., 2010), whereas transsphenoidal approaches, which were initially performed only in case of infradiaphragmatic lesions, have been considered also for supradiaphragmatic craniopharyngiomas in the last decade, either with the microscope or with the endoscope (Fahlbusch et al., 2000; Maira et al., 2004; Frank et al., 2006; de Divitiis et al., 2007; Gardner et al., 2008a, 2008b; Kitano and Taneda, 2008; Cavallo et al., 2009; Fatemi et al., 2009; Jane et al., 2010; Leng et al., 2012; Cavallo et al., 2013; Koutourousiou et al., 2013). However, it must be emphasized that neurosurgical procedures are most effective when performed as the result of a multidisciplinary team management (Duff et al., 2000; Cappabianca et al., 2008; Jane et al., 2010; Kassam et al., 2011; Komotar et al., 2012; Leng et al., 2012; Karavitaki, 2014). During the past few decades, there has been a pronounced increase in the frequency of the minimally invasive surgical approaches. In the early 1990s, the treatment strategy was extensive resection of tumors, and disease recurrence and/or regrowth were treated by means of secondary surgical procedure, radiation, or a combination of both. Since then, the treatment approach has shifted toward more conservative management, with the goal of reducing surgery-related morbidity and mortality.

Surgical outcomes, complications, and recurrence rates can vary between different approaches, and it is necessary to gain a more comprehensive view of the benefits and limitations of the various approaches used to remove a craniopharyngioma (Komotar et al., 2012) (Table 7.2). Any approach to the surgical management of craniopharyngiomas has pros, complications, and disadvantages.

Transcranial and endoscopic endonasal surgery series can be difficult to compare: as a matter of fact, transcranial series have a large number of patients and long follow-up; on the other hand, endoscopic endonasal transsphenoidal series are small in number, with short follow-up. There are several biases which hinder this comparison, such as homogeneity of tumor characteristics (size, location, neurovascular adhesions), and extent of surgical resection (Tables 7.3–7.5).

Overall, complication rates have been shown to be lower in the transsphenoidal group, either microsurgical or endoscopic, than in the transcranial one. Permanent diabetes insipidus, seizures, and wound infections were considered to be more frequent after open transcranial approaches (Komotar et al., 2012). On the other hand, the major challenge in the transsphenoidal route still remains the post-surgical cranial base repair. The rate of postoperative CSF leak in both endoscopic and microscopic transsphenoidal surgery has been reduced thanks to the development of specific paradigms for skull base reconstruction and

TABLE 7.3 Most Representative Surgical Series of Transcranial Approaches to Craniopharyngiomas (At Least Ten Patients Reported)

Author	Year	N° of patients	Extent of resection				Recurrence (%)	
			Total (%)		Subtotal (%)			
Maira et al.	1995	22	20	(90.9%)	2	(9.1%)	–	–
de Vile et al.	1995	75	29	(38.7%)	41	(54.7%)	31	(41.3%)
Zuccaro et al.	1996	48	13	(27.1%)	28	(58.3%)	–	–
Rajan et al.	1997	188	4	(2.1%)	35	(18.6%)	–	–
Villani et al.	1997	27	17	(63.0%)	9	(33.3%)	6	(22.2%)
Bulow et al.	1998	60	30	(50.0%)	30	(50.0%)	20	(33.3%)
Fisher et al.	1998	30	8	(26.7%)	22	(73.3%)	7	(23.3%)
Khafaga et al.	1998	44	17	(38.6%)	17	(38.6%)	–	–
Fahlbusch et al.	1999	94	43	(45.7%)	29	(30.9%)	–	–
Honneger et al.	1999	92	–	–	–	–	–	–
Gsponer et al.	1999	18	–	–	–	–	–	–
Duff et al.	2000	121	69	(57.0%)	–	–	29	(24.0%)
Kim et al.	2001	36	36	(100.0%)	0	(0%)	14	(38.9%)
Merchant et al.	2002	30	8	(26.7%)	11	(36.7%)	11	(36.7%)
van Effenterre et al.	2002	122	72	(59.0%)	35	(28.7%)	29	(23.8%)
Barua et al.	2003	61	10	(16.4%)	51	(83.6%)	22	(36.1%)
Chen et al.	2003	36	7	(19.4%)	25	(69.4%)	15	(41.7%)
Kalapurakal et al.	2003	25	19	(76.0%)	6	(24.0%)	12	(48.0%)
Larijani et al.	2004	93	5	(5.4%)	88	(94.6%)	15	(16.1%)
Stripp et al.	2004	75	44	(58.7%)	27	(36.0%)	–	–
Chakrabarti et al.	2005	18	11	(61.1%)	7	(38.9%)	4	(22.2%)
Albright et al.	2005	27	18	(66.7%)	7	(25.9%)	6	(22.2%)
Caldarelli et al.	2005	52	40	(76.9%)	9	(17.3%)	–	–
Ersahin et al.	2005	87	37	(42.5%)	39	(44.8%)	16	(18.4%)
Hukin et al.	2005	29	11	(37.9%)	4	(13.8%)	–	–
Karavitaki et al.	2005	74	11	(14.9%)	63	(85.1%)	–	–
Lena et al.	2005	47	27	(57.4%)	14	(29.8%)	7	(14.9%)
Minamida et al.	2005	37	26	(70.3%)	7	(18.9%)	11	(29.7%)
Moon et al.	2005	50	19	(38.0%)	22	(44.0%)	–	–

(Continued)

TABLE 7.3 Most Representative Surgical Series of Transcranial Approaches to Craniopharyngiomas (At Least Ten Patients Reported)—cont'd

Author	Year	N° of patients	Extent of resection				Recurrence (%)	
			Total (%)		Subtotal (%)			
Mottolese et al.	2005	60	27	(45.0%)	9	(15.0%)	–	–
Pierre-Kahn et al.	2005	14	9	(64.3%)	5	(35.7%)	–	–
Sainte-Rose et al.	2005	66	33	(50.0%)	24	(36.4%)	–	–
Sosa et al.	2005	35	29	(82.9%)	6	(17.1%)	12	(34.3%)
Thompson et al.	2005	48	16	(33.3%)	32	(66.7%)	–	–
Tomita et al.	2005	54	43	(79.6%)	11	(20.4%)	24	(44.4%)
Zuccaro.	2005	153	88	(57.5%)	65	(42.5%)	–	–
Gupta et al.	2006	116	19	(16.4%)	53	(45.7%)	15	(12.9%)
Shi et al.	2006	284	237	(83.5%)	34	(12.0%)	67	(23.6%)
Tena-Suck et al.	2006	47	17	(36.2%)	30	(63.8%)	–	–
Puget et al.	2007	125	38	(30.4%)	40	(32.0%)	35	(28.0%)
Elliott et al.	2009	19	18	(94.7%)	1	(5.3%)	6	(31.6%)
Golshani et al.	2009	10	10	(100.0%)	0	(0.0%)	2	(20.0%)
Jung et al.	2009	41	–	–	–	–	10	(24.4%)
Schubert et al.	2009	17	3	(17.6%)	11	(64.7%)	–	–
Elliott et al.	2010	86	75	(87.2%)	11	(12.8%)	18	(20.9%)

the appropriate use of suitable autologous, heterologous, and synthetic materials (Cappabianca et al., 2001, 2002, 2010; Kelly et al., 2001; Hadad et al., 2006; Esposito et al., 2007; Cavallo et al., 2007b; Leng et al., 2008; Kassam et al., 2008c). However, the expansion of endonasal approaches to different areas of the skull base for the removal of several lesions, such as craniopharyngiomas, has led to the re-emergence of the post-operative CSF leak as a major issue for this kind of surgery (Kassam et al., 2008c; Cavallo and Esposito, 2010; Malik et al., 2012; Cappabianca et al., 2013).

Furthermore, radiation therapy is another key topic that may influence the outcome of patients with craniopharyngiomas. Several authors have suggested adjuvant radiotherapy in all incomplete tumor removal cases, advocating the fractionated technique as the most suitable radiotherapy treatment for craniopharyngiomas (Schulz-Ertner et al., 2002; Varlotto et al., 2002; Combs et al., 2007; Minniti et al., 2007). However, during the past decade, several publications on treatment with stereotactic radiosurgery have reported favorable control rates at five years post-treatment (Chiou et al., 2001; Jackson et al., 2003; Aggarwal et al., 2013; Iannalfi et al., 2013). In conclusion, despite improvements in surgery,

TABLE 7.4 Most Representative Surgical Series of Transspenoidal Microscopic Approaches to Craniopharyngiomas (At Least Ten Patients Reported)

Author	Year	N° of patients	Extent of resection				Recurrence (%)	
			Total (%)		Subtotal (%)			
Maira et al.	1995	35	23	(65.7%)	4	(11.4%)	–	–
Fahlbusch et al.	1999	35	30	(85.7%)	4	(11.4%)	–	–
Honneger et al.	1999	35	–	–	–	–	–	–
Abe et al.	1999	11	3	(27.3%)	8	(72.7%)	0	(0.0%)
Couldwell et al.	2004	27	20	(74.1%)	–	–	4	(14.8%)
Maira et al.	2004	57	36	(63.2%)	–	–	8	(14.0%)
Karavitaki et al.	2005	26	8	(30.8%)	18	(69.2%)	–	–
Chakrabarti et al.	2005	68	61	(89.7%)	7	(10.3%)	7	(10.3%)
Dusick et al.	2008	18	5	(27.8%)	8	(44.4%)	1	(5.6%)

TABLE 7.5 Most Representative Surgical Series of Endoscopic Endonasal Approaches to Craniopharyngiomas (At Least Ten Patients Reported)

Author	Year	N° of patients	Extent of resection				Recurrence (%)	
			Total (%)		Subtotal (%)			
Frank et al.	2006	10	7	(70.0%)	1	(10.0%)	–	–
de Divitiis et al.	2007	10	7	(70.0%)	2	(20.0%)	–	–
Cavallo et al.	2009	22	17	(77.3%)	4	(18.2%)	4	(18.2%)
Fatemi et al.	2009	18	11	(61.1%)	6	(33.3%)	–	–
Jane et al.	2010	12	10	(83.3%)	2	(16.7%)	6	(50.0%)
Leng et al.	2011	23	17	(73.9%)	6	(26.1%)	6	(26.1%)
Koutourousiou et al.	2013	64	24	(37.5%)	22	(34.4%)	22	(34.4%)

radiotherapy remains part of the multidisciplinary management of patients with incompletely resected and recurrent craniopharyngiomas.

In consideration of these data, the management of craniopharyngioma patients requires interdisciplinary cooperation of the cogent disciplines and should be reserved for specialized centers. Total removal is the ultimate aim of the surgical treatment, with lower morbidity and mortality: nowadays, preservation of the quality of life and neurocognitive function as long-term survival maintenance are important aspects to be considered. In particular, apart from pre- or post-operative neurological disorders, hypothalamic obesity can lead to a significant decline in the quality of life and should be taken into consideration in the follow-up of patients with craniopharyngiomas.

In conclusion, craniopharyngiomas remain a challenging disease requiring patience, flexibility, surgical insight, and diligent post-operative management. National and international prospective co-operative trials are warranted to provide robust data to define a cogent multidisciplinary risk-based management strategy.

References

Aggarwal, A., Fersht, N., Brada, M., 2013. Radiotherapy for craniopharyngioma. Pituitary 16, 26–33.

Albright, A.L., Hadjipanayis, C.G., Lunsford, L.D., Kondziolka, D., Pollack, I.F., Adelson, P.D., 2005. Individualized treatment of pediatric craniopharyngiomas. Childs Nerv. Syst. 21, 649–654.

Aryan, H.E., Ozgur, B.M., Jandial, R., Levy, M.L., 2005. Subfrontal transbasal approach and technique for resection of craniopharyngioma. Neurosurg. Focus 18, E10.

Babinski, J., 1900. Tumeur du corps pituitaire sans acromé galie et avec arrêt de dé veloppement des organes genitaux. Revue. Neurol. Paris.

Backlund, E.O., Axelsson, B., Bergstrand, C.G., Eriksson, A.L., Noren, G., Ribbesjo, E., Rahn, T., Schnell, P.O., Tallstedt, L., Saaf, M., et al., 1989. Treatment of craniopharyngiomas – the stereotactic approach in a 10 to 23 year perspective. I. Surgical, radiological, and ophthalmological aspects. Acta. Neurochir. (Wien) 99, 11–19.

Baskin, D.S., Wilson, C.B., 1986. Surgical management of craniopharyngiomas. A review of 74 cases. J. Neurosurg. 65, 22–27.

Boyce, R., Beadles, C.F., 1893. A further contribution to the study of the pathology of the hypophysis cerebri. J. Pathol. 1, 359–383.

Bunin, G.R., Surawicz, T.S., Witman, P.A., Preston-Martin, S., Davis, F., Bruner, J.M., 1998. The descriptive epidemiology of craniopharyngioma. J. Neurosurg. 89, 547–551.

Caldarelli, M., Massimi, L., Tamburrini, G., Cappa, M., Di Rocco, C., 2005. Long-term results of the surgical treatment of craniopharyngioma: the experience at the Policlinico Gemelli, Catholic University, Rome. Childs Nerv. Syst. 21, 747–757.

Campbell, P.G., Mcgettigan, B., Luginbuhl, A., Yadla, S., Rosen, M., Evans, J.J., 2010. Endocrinological and ophthalmological consequences of an initial endonasal endoscopic approach for resection of craniopharyngiomas. Neurosurg. Focus 28, E8.

Cappabianca, P., Cavallo, L.M., Mariniello, G., De Divitiis, O., Romero, A.D., De Divitiis, E., 2001. Easy sellar reconstruction in endoscopic endonasal transsphenoidal surgery with polyester-silicone dural substitute and fibrin glue: technical note. Neurosurgery 49, 473–475 discussion 475–476.

Cappabianca, P., Cavallo, L.M., De Divitiis, E., 2002. Collagen sponge repair of small cerebrospinal fluid leaks obviates tissue grafts and cerebrospinal fluid diversion after pituitary surgery. Neurosurgery 50, 1173–1174 author reply 1174.

Cappabianca, P., Frank, G., Pasquini, E., De Divitiis, O., Calbucci, F., 2003. Extended endoscopic endonasal transsphenoidal approaches to the suprasellar region, planum sphenoidale and clivus. In: De Divitiis, E., Cappabianca, P. (Eds.), Endoscopic endonasal transsphenoidal surgery. Springer, Wien – New York.

Cappabianca, P., Cavallo, L.M., Esposito, F., De Divitiis, E., 2008. Craniopharyngiomas. J. Neurosurg. 109, 1–3.

Cappabianca, P., Esposito, F., Magro, F., Cavallo, L.M., Solari, D., Stella, L., De Divitiis, O., 2010. Natura abhorret a vacuo – use of fibrin glue as a filler and sealant in neurosurgical "dead spaces". Technical note. Acta. Neurochir. (Wien) 152, 897–904.

Cappabianca, P., Di Somma, A., De Notaris, M., 2013. Rerum magistra experientia est: The evolution of modern endoscopic endonasal skull base surgery and reconstruction techniques. World Neurosurg, 1878–8750 (Electronic). http://dx.doi.org/10.1016/j.wneu.2013.03.063.

Cavallo, L.M., De Divitiis, O., Aydin, S., Messina, A., Esposito, F., Iaconetta, G., Talat, K., Cappabianca, P., Tschabitscher, M., 2007a. Extended endoscopic endonasal transsphenoidal approach to the suprasellar area: anatomic considerations – part 1. Neurosurgery 61. ONS-24-ONS-34.

Cavallo, L.M., Esposito, F., 2010. Endoscopic anterior approaches and the cerebrospinal fluid (csf) leak effect: change one thing, change everything. World Neurosurg. 74, 566–567.

Cavallo, L.M., Messina, A., Cappabianca, P., Esposito, F., De Divitiis, E., Gardner, P., Tschabitscher, M., 2005. Endoscopic endonasal surgery of the midline skull base: anatomical study and clinical considerations. Neurosurg. Focus 19, E2.

Cavallo, L.M., Messina, A., Esposito, F., De Divitiis, O., Dal Fabbro, M., De Divitiis, E., Cappabianca, P., 2007b. Skull base reconstruction in the extended endoscopic transsphenoidal approach for suprasellar lesions. J. Neurosurg. 107, 713–720.

Cavallo, L.M., Prevedello, D.M., Solari, D., Gardner, P.A., Esposito, F., Snyderman, C.H., Carrau, R.L., Kassam, A.B., Cappabianca, P., 2009. Extended endoscopic endonasal transsphenoidal approach for residual or recurrent craniopharyngiomas. J. Neurosurg. 111, 578–589.

Cavallo, L.M., Solari, D., Esposito, F., Cappabianca, P., 2013. The endoscopic endonasal approach for the management of craniopharyngiomas involving the third ventricle. Neurosurg. Rev. 36, 27–37 discussion 38.

Chakrabarti, I., Amar, A.P., Couldwell, W., Weiss, M.H., 2005. Long-term neurological, visual, and endocrine outcomes following transnasal resection of craniopharyngioma. J. Neurosurg. 102, 650–657.

Chiou, S.M., Lunsford, L.D., Niranjan, A., Kondziolka, D., Flickinger, J.C., 2001. Stereotactic radiosurgery of residual or recurrent craniopharyngioma, after surgery, with or without radiation therapy. Neuro. Oncol. 3, 159–166.

Ciric, I.S., Cozzens, J.W., 1980. Craniopharyngiomas: transsphenoidal method of approach – for the virtuoso only? Clin. Neurosurg. 27, 169–187.

Cohen, M., Bartels, U., Branson, H., Kulkarni, A.V., Hamilton, J., 2013. Trends in treatment and outcomes of pediatric craniopharyngioma, 1975–2011. Neuro. Oncol. 15, 767–774.

Combs, S.E., Thilmann, C., Huber, P.E., Hoess, A., Debus, J., Schulz-Ertner, D., 2007. Achievement of long-term local control in patients with craniopharyngiomas using high precision stereotactic radiotherapy. Cancer 109, 2308–2314.

Crotty, T.B., Scheithauer, B.W., Young Jr., W.F., Davis, D.H., Shaw, E.G., Miller, G.M., Burger, P.C., 1995. Papillary craniopharyngioma: a clinicopathological study of 48 cases. J. Neurosurg. 83, 206–214.

Cushing, H., 1932. Intracranial Tumors. Charles C. Thomas, Baltimore.

Cushing, H., 1932. Intracranial tumors. Notes upon a series of two thousand cases with surgical mortality percentages pertaining thereto. Thomas, Springfield, IL.

De Divitiis, E., Cappabianca, P., Cavallo, L.M., 2002. Endoscopic transsphenoidal approach: adaptability of the procedure to different sellar lesions. Neurosurgery 51, 699–705 discussion 705–707.

De Divitiis, E., Cappabianca, P., Cavallo, L.M., Esposito, F., De Divitiis, O., Messina, A., 2007. Extended endoscopic transsphenoidal approach for extrasellar craniopharyngiomas. Neurosurgery 61, 219–227 discussion 228.

De Notaris, M., Solari, D., Cavallo, L.M., D'enza, A.I., Ensenat, J., Berenguer, J., Ferrer, E., Prats-Galino, A., Cappabianca, P., 2012. The "suprasellar notch," or the tuberculum sellae as seen from below: definition, features, and clinical implications from an endoscopic endonasal perspective. J. Neurosurg. 116, 622–629.

Delitala, A., Brunori, A., Chiappetta, F., 2004. Purely neuroendoscopic transventricular management of cystic craniopharyngiomas. Childs Nerv. Syst. 20, 858–862.

Derrey, S., Blond, S., Reyns, N., Touzet, G., Carpentier, P., Gauthier, H., Dhellemmes, P., 2008. Management of cystic craniopharyngiomas with stereotactic endocavitary irradiation using colloidal 186Re: a retrospective study of 48 consecutive patients. Neurosurgery 63, 1045–1052 discussion 1052–1053.

Dhellemmes, P., Vinchon, M., 2006. Radical resection for craniopharyngiomas in children: surgical technique and clinical results. J. Pediatr. Endocrinol. Metab. 19 (Suppl. 1), 329–335.

Di Rocco, C., Caldarelli, M., Tamburrini, G., Massimi, L., 2006. Surgical management of craniopharyngiomas – experience with a pediatric series. J. Pediatr. Endocrinol. Metab. 19 (Suppl. 1), 355–366.

Duff, J., Meyer, F.B., Ilstrup, D.M., Laws Jr., E.R., Schleck, C.D., Scheithauer, B.W., 2000. Long-term outcomes for surgically resected craniopharyngiomas. Neurosurgery 46, 291–302 discussion 302–305.

Erdheim, J., 1904. Uber hypophysenganggeschwwuste und hirncholesteatome. Gerold, Wien.

Esposito, F., Dusick, J.R., Fatemi, N., Kelly, D.F., 2007. Graded repair of cranial base defects and cerebrospinal fluid leaks in transsphenoidal surgery. Neurosurgery 60, 295–303 discussion 303–304.

Fahlbusch, R., Honegger, J., Paulus, W., Huk, W., Buchfelder, M., 1999. Surgical treatment of craniopharyngiomas: experience with 168 patients. J. Neurosurg. 90, 237–250.

Fahlbusch, R., Honneger, J., Buchfelder, M., 2000. Transsphenoidal microsurgery for craniopharyngiomas. In: Schmidek, H.H. (Ed.), Shmidek and Sweet Operative neurosurgical techniques. Indications, methods, and results. W. B. Saunders, Philadelphia.

Fatemi, N., Dusick, J.R., De Paiva Neto, M.A., Malkasian, D., Kelly, D.F., 2009. Endonasal versus supraorbital keyhole removal of craniopharyngiomas and tuberculum sellae meningiomas. Neurosurgery 64, 269–284 discussion 284–286.

Fischer, E.G., Welch, K., Shillito Jr., J., Winston, K.R., Tarbell, N.J., 1990. Craniopharyngiomas in children. Long-term effects of conservative surgical procedures combined with radiation therapy. J. Neurosurg. 73, 534–540.

Fisher, P.G., Jenab, J., Gopldthwaite, P.T., Tihan, T., Wharam, M.D., Foer, D.R., Burger, P.C., 1998. Outcomes and failure patterns in childhood craniopharyngiomas. Childs Nerv. Syst. 14, 558–563.

Frank, G., Pasquini, E., 2002. Endoscopic endonasal approaches to the cavernous sinus: surgical approaches. Neurosurgery 50, 675.

Frank, G., Pasquini, E., Doglietto, F., Mazzatenta, D., Sciaretta, V., Farneti, G., Calbucci, F., 2006. The endoscopic extended transsphenoidal approach for craniopharyngiomas. Neurosurgery 59 (Suppl. 1), ONS75–ONS83.

Frohlich, A., 1901. Ein fall von tumor der hypophysis cerebri ohne akromegalie. Alfred Hölder, Wien.

Gardner, P.A., Kassam, A.B., Snyderman, C.H., Carrau, R.L., Mintz, A.H., Grahovac, S., Stefko, S., 2008a. Outcomes following endoscopic, expanded endonasal resection of suprasellar craniopharyngiomas: a case series. J. Neurosurg. 109, 6–16.

Gardner, P.A., Prevedello, D.M., Kassam, A.B., Snyderman, C.H., Carrau, R.L., Mintz, A.H., 2008b. The evolution of the endonasal approach for craniopharyngiomas. J. Neurosurg. 108, 1043–1047.

Garnett, M.R., Puget, S., Grill, J., Sainte-Rose, C., 2007. Craniopharyngioma. Orphanet. J. Rare. Dis. 2, 18.

Guiot, G., Derome, P., 1972. Indications for trans-sphenoid approach in neurosurgery. 521 cases. Ann. Med. Interne. (Paris) 123, 703–712.

Hadad, G., Bassagasteguy, L., Carrau, R.L., Mataza, J.C., Kassam, A., Snyderman, C.H., Mintz, A., 2006. A novel reconstructive technique after endoscopic expanded endonasal approaches: vascular pedicle nasoseptal flap. Laryngoscope 116, 1882–1886.

Halstead, A.E., 1910. Remarks on the operative treatment of 256 tumors of the hypophysis. Surg. Gynecol. Obstet. 10, 494–502.

Hasegawa, T., Kondziolka, D., Hadjipanayis, C.G., Lunsford, L.D., 2004. Management of cystic craniopharyngiomas with phosphorus-32 intracavitary irradiation. Neurosurgery 54, 813–820 discussion 820–822.

Hoffman, H.J., De Silva, M., Humphreys, R.P., Drake, J.M., Smith, M.L., Blaser, S.I., 1992. Aggressive surgical management of craniopharyngiomas in children. J. Neurosurg. 76, 47–52.

Hofmann, B.M., Kreutzer, J., Saeger, W., Buchfelder, M., Blumcke, I., Fahlbusch, R., Buslei, R., 2006. Nuclear beta-catenin accumulation as reliable marker for the differentiation between cystic craniopharyngiomas and rathke cleft cysts: a clinico-pathologic approach. Am. J. Surg. Pathol. 30, 1595–1603.

Hofmann, B.M., Hollig, A., Strauss, C., Buslei, R., Buchfelder, M., Fahlbusch, R., 2012. Results after treatment of craniopharyngiomas: further experiences with 73 patients since 1997. J. Neurosurg. 116, 373–384.

Holsken, A., Stache, C., Schlaffer, S.M., Flitsch, J., Fahlbusch, R., Buchfelder, M., Buslei, R., 2013. Adamantinomatous craniopharyngiomas express tumor stem cell markers in cells with activated Wnt signaling: further evidence for the existence of a tumor stem cell niche? Pituitary.

Honegger, J., Buchfelder, M., Fahlbusch, R., Daubler, B., Dorr, H.G., 1992. Transsphenoidal microsurgery for craniopharyngioma. Surg. Neurol. 37, 189–196.

Hoogenhout, J., Otten, B.J., Kazem, I., Stoelinga, G.B., Walder, A.H., 1984. Surgery and radiation therapy in the management of craniopharyngiomas. Int. J. Radiat. Oncol. Biol. Phys. 10, 2293–2297.

Hukin, J., Steinbok, P., Lafay-Cousin, L., Hendson, G., Strother, D., Mercier, C., Samson, Y., Howes, W., Bouffet, E., 2007. Intracystic bleomycin therapy for craniopharyngioma in children: the Canadian experience. Cancer 109, 2124–2131.

Hussain, I., Eloy, J.A., Carmel, P.W., Liu, J.K., 2013. Molecular oncogenesis of craniopharyngioma: current and future strategies for the development of targeted therapies. J. Neurosurg. 119, 106–112.

Iannalfi, A., Fragkandrea, I., Brock, J., Saran, F., 2013. Radiotherapy in craniopharyngiomas. Clin. Oncol. (R. Coll. Radiol.) 25, 654–667.

Jackson, A.S., St George, E.J., Hayward, R.J., Plowman, P.N., 2003. Stereotactic radiosurgery. XVII: Recurrent intrasellar craniopharyngioma. Br. J. Neurosurg. 17, 138–143.

Jane Jr., J.A., Laws, E.R., 2006. Craniopharyngioma. Pituitary 9, 323–326.

Jane Jr., J.A., Prevedello, D.M., Alden, T.D., Laws Jr., E.R., 2010. The transsphenoidal resection of pediatric craniopharyngiomas: a case series. J. Neurosurg. Pediatr. 5, 49–60.

Jiang, Z.L., Ren, X.H., Chu, J.S., Lin, S., Zhang, M.Z., 2010. Microsurgical treatment of adult craniopharyngiomas in 156 cases. Zhonghua Yi Xue Za Zhi 90, 291–294.

Julow, J., Backlund, E.O., Lanyi, F., Hajda, M., Balint, K., Nyary, I., Szeifert, G.T., 2007. Long-term results and late complications after intracavitary yttrium-90 colloid irradiation of recurrent cystic craniopharyngiomas. Neurosurgery 61, 288–295 discussion 295–296.

Jung, T.Y., Jung, S., Choi, J.E., Moon, K.S., Kim, I.Y., Kang, S.S., 2009. Adult craniopharyngiomas: surgical results with a special focus on endocrinological outcomes and recurrence according to pituitary stalk preservation. J. Neurosurg. 111, 572–577.

Kalapurakal, J.A., Goldman, S., Hsieh, Y.C., Tomita, T., Marymont, M.H., 2003. Clinical outcome in children with craniopharyngioma treated with primary surgery and radiotherapy deferred until relapse. Med. Pediatr. Oncol. 40, 214–218.

Karavitaki, N., 2014. Management of craniopharyngiomas. J. Endocrinol. Invest. 37 (3), 219–228.

Kassam, A., Snyderman, C.H., Mintz, A., Gardner, P., Carrau, R.L., 2005a. Expanded endonasal approach: the rostrocaudal axis. Part I. Crista galli to the sella turcica. Neurosurg. Focus 19, E3.

Kassam, A., Snyderman, C.H., Mintz, A., Gardner, P., Carrau, R.L., 2005b. Expanded endonasal approach: the rostrocaudal axis. Part II. Posterior clinoids to the foramen magnum. Neurosurg. Focus 19, E4.

Kassam, A.B., Gardner, P.A., Snyderman, C.H., Carrau, R.L., Mintz, A.H., Prevedello, D.M., 2008a. Expanded endonasal approach, a fully endoscopic transnasal approach for the resection of midline suprasellar craniopharyngiomas: a new classification based on the infundibulum. J. Neurosurg. 108, 715–728.

Kassam, A.B., Prevedello, D.M., Thomas, A., Gardner, P., Mintz, A., Snyderman, C., Carrau, R., 2008b. Endoscopic endonasal pituitary transposition for a transdorsum sellae approach to the interpeduncular cistern. Neurosurgery 62, 57–72 discussion 72–74.

Kassam, A.B., Thomas, A., Carrau, R.L., Snyderman, C.H., Vescan, A., Prevedello, D., Mintz, A., Gardner, P., 2008c. Endoscopic reconstruction of the cranial base using a pedicled nasoseptal flap. Neurosurgery 63, ONS44–ONS52 discussion ONS52-ONS53.

Kassam, A.B., Prevedello, D.M., Carrau, R.L., Snyderman, C.H., Thomas, A., Gardner, P., Zanation, A., Duz, B., Stefko, S.T., Byers, K., Horowitz, M.B., 2011. Endoscopic endonasal skull base surgery: analysis of complications in the authors' initial 800 patients. J. Neurosurg. 114, 1544–1568.

Kelly, D.F., Oskouian, R.J., Fineman, I., 2001. Collagen sponge repair of small cerebrospinal fluid leaks obviates tissue grafts and cerebrospinal fluid diversion after pituitary surgery. Neurosurgery 49, 885–889 discussion 889–890.

Kitano, M., Taneda, M., 2008. Extended transsphenoidal surgery for suprasellar craniopharyngiomas: infrachiasmatic radical resection combined with or without a suprachiasmatic trans-lamina terminalis approach. Surg. Neurol. 290–298, discussion 298.

Komotar, R.J., Starke, R.M., Raper, D.M., Anand, V.K., Schwartz, T.H., 2012. Endoscopic endonasal compared with microscopic transsphenoidal and open transcranial resection of craniopharyngiomas. World Neurosurg. 77, 329–341.

Koutourousiou, M., Gardner, P.A., Fernandez-Miranda, J.C., Tyler-Kabara, E.C., Wang, E.W., Snyderman, C.H., 2013. Endoscopic endonasal surgery for craniopharyngiomas: surgical outcome in 64 patients. J. Neurosurg. 119, 1194–1207.

Kunihiro, N., Goto, T., Ishibashi, K., Ohata, K., 2014. Surgical outcomes of the minimum anterior and posterior combined transpetrosal approach for resection of retrochiasmatic craniopharyngiomas with complicated conditions. J. Neurosurg. 120, 1–11.

Kurosaki, M., Saeger, W., Ludecke, D.K., 2001. Immunohistochemical localisation of cytokeratins in craniopharyngioma. Acta. Neurochir. (Wien) 143, 147–151.

Larkin, S.J., Ansorge, O., 2013. Pathology and pathogenesis of craniopharyngiomas. Pituitary 16, 9–17.

Laws Jr, E.R., 1980. Transsphenoidal microsurgery in the management of craniopharyngioma. J. Neurosurg. 52, 661–666.

Lena, G., Paz Paredes, A., Scavarda, D., Giusiano, B., 2005. Craniopharyngioma in children: Marseille experience. Childs Nerv. Syst. 21, 778–784.

Leng, L.Z., Brown, S., Anand, V.K., Schwartz, T.H., 2008. "Gasket-seal" watertight closure in minimal-access endoscopic cranial base surgery. Neurosurgery 62, ONSE342–ONSE343 discussion ONSE343.

Leng, L.Z., Greenfield, J.P., Souweidane, M.M., Anand, V.K., Schwartz, T.H., 2012. Endoscopic, endonasal resection of craniopharyngiomas: analysis of outcome including extent of resection, cerebrospinal fluid leak, return to preoperative productivity, and body mass index. Neurosurgery 70, 110–123 discussion 123–124.

Lewis, D., 1910. A contribution to the subject of tumors of the hypophysis. JAMA 55, 1002–1008.

Lin, L.L., El Naqa, I., Leonard, J.R., Park, T.S., Hollander, A.S., Michalski, J.M., Mansur, D.B., 2008. Long-term outcome in children treated for craniopharyngioma with and without radiotherapy. J. Neurosurg. Pediatr. 1, 126–130.
Liu, J.K., Christiano, L.D., Gupta, G., Carmel, P.W., 2010. Surgical nuances for removal of retrochiasmatic craniopharyngiomas via the transbasal subfrontal translamina terminalis approach. Neurosurg. Focus 28, E6.
Liu, W., Fang, Y., Cai, B., Xu, J., You, C., Zhang, H., 2012. Intracystic bleomycin for cystic craniopharyngiomas in children (abridged republication of cochrane systematic review). Neurosurgery 71, 909–915.
Maira, G., Anile, C., Albanese, A., Cabezas, D., Pardi, F., Vignati, A., 2004. The role of transsphenoidal surgery in the treatment of craniopharyngiomas. J. Neurosurg. 100, 445–451.
Malik, M.U., Aberle, J.C., Flitsch, J., 2012. CSF fistulas after transsphenoidal pituitary surgery – a solved problem? J. Neurol. Surg. A. Cent. Eur. Neurosurg. 73, 275–280.
Mark, R.J., Lutge, W.R., Shimizu, K.T., Tran, L.M., Selch, M.T., Parker, R.G., 1995. Craniopharyngioma: treatment in the CT and MR imaging era. Radiology 197, 195–198.
Minamida, Y., Mikami, T., Hashi, K., Houkin, K., 2005. Surgical management of the recurrence and regrowth of craniopharyngiomas. J. Neurosurg. 103, 224–232.
Minniti, G., Saran, F., Traish, D., Soomal, R., Sardell, S., Gonsalves, A., Ashley, S., Warrington, J., Burke, K., Mosleh-Shirazi, A., Brada, M., 2007. Fractionated stereotactic conformal radiotherapy following conservative surgery in the control of craniopharyngiomas. Radiother. Oncol. 82, 90–95.
Minniti, G., Esposito, V., Amichetti, M., Enrici, R.M., 2009. The role of fractionated radiotherapy and radiosurgery in the management of patients with craniopharyngioma. Neurosurg. Rev. 32, 125–132 discussion 132.
Mortini, P., Gagliardi, F., Boari, N., Losa, M., 2013. Surgical strategies and modern therapeutic options in the treatment of craniopharyngiomas. Crit. Rev. Oncol. Hematol. 514–519.
Mott, F.W., Barret, J.O., 1899. Three cases of tumor of the third ventricle. Arch. Neurol. 1, 417–440.
Mottolese, C., Szathmari, A., Berlier, P., Hermier, M., 2005. Craniopharyngiomas: our experience in Lyon. Childs Nerv. Syst. 21, 790–798.
Pascual, J.M., Prieto, R., Carrasco, R., 2011. Infundibulo-tuberal or not strictly intraventricular craniopharyngioma: evidence for a major topographical category. Acta. Neurochir. (Wien) 153, 2403–2425 discussion 2426.
Paulus, W., Stockel, C., Krauss, J., Sorensen, N., Roggendorf, W., 1997. Odontogenic classification of craniopharyngiomas: a clinicopathological study of 54 cases. Histopathology 30, 172–176.
Reisch, R., Perneczky, A., 2005. Ten-year experience with the supraorbital subfrontal approach through an eyebrow skin incision. Neurosurgery 57, 242–255.
Sainte-Rose, C., Puget, S., Wray, A., Zerah, M., Grill, J., Brauner, R., Boddaert, N., Pierre-Kahn, A., 2005. Craniopharyngioma: the pendulum of surgical management. Childs Nerv. Syst. 21, 691–695.
Samii, M., Samii, A., 2000. Surgical management of craniopharyngiomas. In: Schmidek, H.H. (Ed.), Schmidek and Sweet Operative neurosurgical techniques. Indications, methods, and results. W. B. Saunders, Philadelphia.
Samii, M., Tatagiba, M., 1997. Surgical management of craniopharyngiomas: a review. Neurol. Med. Chir. (Tokyo) 37, 141–149.
Schloffer, H., 1907. Erforgleiche operationen eines hypophysentumors auf nasalem wege. Wien. Klin. Wochenschr. 20, 621–624.
Schulz-Ertner, D., Frank, C., Herfarth, K.K., Rhein, B., Wannenmacher, M., Debus, J., 2002. Fractionated stereotactic radiotherapy for craniopharyngiomas. Int. J. Radiat. Oncol. Biol. Phys. 54, 1114–1120.
Sekine, S., Shibata, T., Kokubu, A., Morishita, Y., Noguchi, M., Nakanishi, Y., Sakamoto, M., Hirohashi, S., 2002. Craniopharyngiomas of adamantinomatous type harbor beta-catenin gene mutations. Am. J. Pathol. 161, 1997–2001.
Shi, X.E., Wu, B., Zhou, Z.Q., Fan, T., Zhang, Y.L., 2006. Microsurgical treatment of craniopharyngiomas: report of 284 patients. Chin. Med. J. (Engl) 119, 1653–1663.
Spaziante, R., De Divitiis, E., 1997. Drainage techniques for cystic craniopharyngiomas. Neurosurg. Quart. 7, 183–208.
Spaziante, R., De Divitiis, E., Irace, C., Cappabianca, P., Caputi, F., 1989. Management of primary or recurring grossly cystic craniopharyngiomas by means of draining systems. Topic review and six case reports. Acta. Neurochir. (Wien) 97, 95–106.
Steno, J., Malacek, M., Bizik, I., 2004. Tumor-third ventricular relationships in supradiaphragmatic craniopharyngiomas: correlation of morphological, magnetic resonance imaging, and operative findings. Neurosurgery 54, 1051–1058 discussion 1058–60.

Symon, L., Pell, M.F., Habib, A.H., 1991. Radical excision of craniopharyngioma by the temporal route: a review of 50 patients. Br. J. Neurosurg. 5, 539–549.

Tateyama, H., Tada, T., Okabe, M., Takahashi, E., Eimoto, T., 2001. Different keratin profiles in craniopharyngioma subtypes and ameloblastomas. Pathol. Res. Pract. 197, 735–742.

Van Effenterre, R., Boch, A.L., 2002. Craniopharyngioma in adults and children: a study of 122 surgical cases. J. Neurosurg. 97, 3–11.

Varlotto, J.M., Flickinger, J.C., Kondziolka, D., Lunsford, L.D., Deutsch, M., 2002. External beam irradiation of craniopharyngiomas: long-term analysis of tumor control and morbidity. Int. J. Radiat. Oncol. Biol. Phys. 54, 492–499.

Weiss, M.H., 1987. The transnasal transsphenoidal approach. In: Apuzzo, M.L.J. (Ed.), Surgery of the third ventricle. Williams and Wilkins, Baltimore.

Xin, W., Rubin, M.A., Mckeever, P.E., 2002. Differential expression of cytokeratins 8 and 20 distinguishes craniopharyngioma from Rathke cleft cyst. Arch. Pathol. Lab. Med. 126, 1174–1178.

Yaşargil, M. G, 1984. Microneurosurgery. George Thieme Verlag, Stuttgart.

Yasargil, M.G., Curcic, M., Kis, M., Siegenthaler, G., Teddy, P.J., Roth, P., 1990. Total removal of craniopharyngiomas. Approaches and long-term results in 144 patients. J. Neurosurg. 73, 3–11.

Zenker, F.A., 1857. Enorme Cystenbildung im Gehirn, vom Hirnanhang ausgehend. Arch. Pathol. Anat. Physiol. Klin. Med. 12, 454–466.

Zhang, Y.Q., Ma, Z.Y., Wu, Z.B., Luo, S.Q., Wang, Z.C., 2008. Radical resection of 202 pediatric craniopharyngiomas with special reference to the surgical approaches and hypothalamic protection. Pediatr. Neurosurg. 44, 435–443.

CHAPTER

8

Endoscopic Resection of Craniopharyngiomas

Tyler J. Kenning, James J. Evans*[†]

*Department of Neurosurgery, Albany Medical Center, Albany, NY, USA; [†]Department of Neurological Surgery, Thomas Jefferson University Hospital, Philadelphia, PA, USA

"The nasal route is impractical and can never be otherwise." **Walter Dandy, 1945**

INTRODUCTION

Craniopharyngiomas remain one of the most challenging central nervous system tumors to treat effectively. Involvement of the pituitary stalk and hypothalamus, as well as adherence to cerebral blood vessels often make complete resection unattainable. Surrounding critical neurovascular structures, diminutive intraoperative visualization, distorted anatomical relationships, and limited sharp dissection often hinder complete resection, regardless of the approach taken (Stamm, 2008). Traditionally, these tumors have been removed surgically via a microscopic transcranial approach, whereas the transsphenoidal approach, either microsurgical or endoscopic, has been used more recently to access intrasellar or subdiaphragmatic tumors (Laws, 1980; Honegger, 1992). With the increasing use of endoscopic techniques and the improved illumination and expansive view they provide, endonasal approaches have been shown to be effective and safe for treating certain midline lesions of the cranial base beyond the sellar region (Jho, 1997; Esposito, 2004; Dehdashti, 2009). These approaches provide more direct access to pathology, reduce brain retraction and manipulation of the optic chiasm, and may decrease hospital stay and morbidity (Batra, 2005; Casler, 2005).

ENDOSCOPIC OPERATIVE TECHNIQUE

Patient Positioning

The patient is positioned supine with a neuronavigation mask in place. The head is not placed in fixation. A lateral thigh incision is prepared for fascia lata harvest on the side

Craniopharyngiomas
http://dx.doi.org/10.1016/B978-0-12-416706-3.00008-8

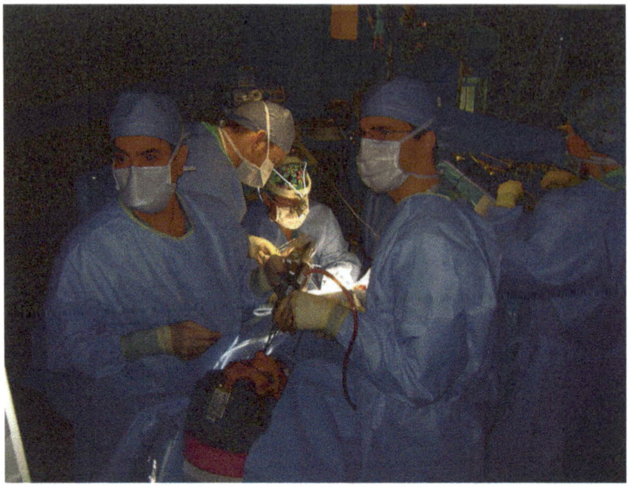

FIGURE 8.1 The neurosurgeon and the otolaryngologist stand on opposite sides of the patient's head so that they may work simultaneously.

contralateral to the scrub nurse setup. The neurosurgeon and the otolaryngologist stand on opposite sides of the patient's head so that they may work simultaneously in an ergonomic fashion (Figure 8.1).

Nasoseptal Flap Preparation

The nasal mucosa is prepared with pledgets soaked in 4% cocaine prior to surgical draping. Before introduction of the endoscope, the pledgets are removed and the base of the middle turbinates, the inferior turbinates, and the nasal septum are injected with 1% lidocaine with epinephrine (1:100,000). Bilaterally, the inferior and middle turbinates are then outfractured and lateralized. The next step is to mobilize a pedicled, vascularized nasoseptal mucoperiosteal flap (Figure 8.2). The mucosal surface of the nasoseptal flap is colored with a surgical marker to aid with proper orientation during cranial base repair at the end of the procedure. A monopolar electrocautery with a right-angled, needle tip is utilized to make the mucosal incisions. The first incision is made along the choana from the inferior nasal septum and along the nasoseptal floor below the level of the inferior turbinate. This incision is carried anteriorly to the level of the mucosa–epithelium junction. The septal incision is made from the superior aspect of the sphenoid os and extends up the nasal septum vertically. It is then carried anteriorly, staying approximately 1 cm below the most superior aspect of the septum in order to preserve the olfactory endothelium. At the anterior aspect of the middle turbinate, the incision is extended upwards to the superior aspect of the septum and again carried forward to the mucosa–epithelium junction. The third and final incision is made vertically behind the columella and connects the superior and inferior nasoseptal cuts. A Gorney suction elevator is then used to mobilize the flap from the nasal septum. One of the more difficult areas to separate is along the inferior aspect where the septum turns

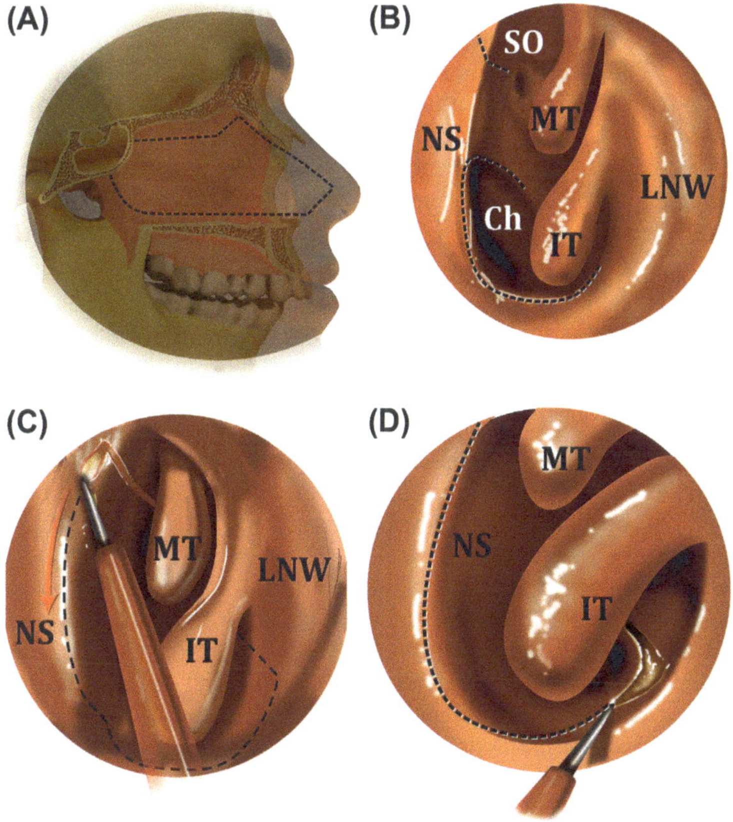

FIGURE 8.2 Design of the nasoseptal flap (NSF) for cranial base repair. **A,** A sagittal image detailing the series of cuts (dotted lines) necessary. **B,** The septal and inferior incisions are based on the vascular pedicle supplied by the sphenopalatine artery, which emerges between the sphenoid os and the choana. **C,** The vertical incision is made behind the columella and connects the superior and inferior nasoseptal cuts. **D,** The inferior incision is carried out inferiorly and laterally to the inferior turbinate to create a wider NSF for repair. *Ch: choana, IT: inferior turbinate, LNW: lateral nasal wall, MT: middle turbinate, NS: nasal septum, SO: sphenoid os.*

to the nasal floor. There are decussating fibers in this region and particular care must be taken to avoid tearing the flap. Once fully mobilized, the flap is then reflected down into the nasopharynx for storage during the tumor resection and until it is to be used for reconstruction.

Anterior Cranial Base Exposure and Osteotomy

Next, the sphenoid os is identified and opened using a straight thru-cut instrument. This is performed bilaterally and a small posterior septectomy is performed to allow binarial access to the sphenoid sinus. The sphenoid rostrum is removed with a Jansen-Middleton rongeur, a Kerrison punch, drill, or ultrasonic bone aspirator depending on the surgeon's preference. After widening the sphenoidotomy, a drill with a diamond burr is used to remove thick sphenoid septations, the vomer, and to begin opening the anterior cranial base. Ultimately, the sella, tuberculum sella, and the planum sphenoidale will be removed to allow adequate access to the sella, parasellar, and suprasellar areas. A Kerrison punch is used to remove thin remaining shells of bone. The anterior cranial base osteotomy is carried to the width of the internal carotid arteries bilaterally. In addition, the medial aspects of the optic canals are unroofed and decompressed. Large tumors may require removal of the entire planum sphenoidale as well as a posterior ethmoidectomy to allow access to the anterior aspect of the craniopharyngioma.

Dural Opening and Tumor Resection (Figure 8.3)

The dura is opened in the midline along the posterior aspect of the planum sphenoidale and tuberculum sellae, and carried down towards the superior aspect of the pituitary gland, allowing exposure of the suprasellar cistern and just below the diaphragma sella. The superior intercavernous sinus will need to be coagulated with bipolar electrocautery prior to its division. The arachnoid is then opened with a combination of sharp and blunt endoscopic microdissection. The anterior aspect of the tumor capsule will then often be seen below the level of the optic chiasm and above the pituitary gland. Small perforating vessels in this area will then have to be carefully inspected. Vasculature to the optic chiasm and the pituitary gland, including the superior hypophyseal arteries and their branches, must be preserved. Vessels supplying the tumor capsule may be carefully cauterized and divided.

The anterior tumor capsule is then cauterized with the bipolar electrocautery and opened by sharp and blunt endoscopic microdissection. Craniopharyngiomas are often both solid and cystic and have variable areas of calcification. First, internal debulking of the tumor is performed and a biopsy sample is obtained for pathological diagnosis. The cystic contents of the tumor are evacuated and the more solid and calcified portions are debulked. The latter can be performed with ring curettes and/or an ultrasonic aspirator. Sequential internal debulking is followed by extra-capsular sharp microdissection. With large, solid, and cystic craniopharyngiomas, extensive internal debulking is required in order to permit extracapsular mobilization of the tumor. The tumor walls can be densely adherent to surrounding neurovascular structures, including the optic chiasm, hypothalamus, ventricular walls, and cerebral vasculature. If present, the gliotic plane is utilized in order to fully mobilize the tumor capsule from the adjacent hypothalamus. In areas where this plane cannot be adequately developed, it is likely best to leave residual tumor capsule that can be treated with postoperative radiotherapy, rather than cause neurologic injury. However, whenever possible a gross total tumor resection is desired. Angled endoscopes (30, 45, and 70 degrees) can be used to examine and dissect tumor in the far reaches of the parasellar, suprasellar, and retrosellar regions. An area of particular controversy is management of the pituitary stalk. It remains unclear whether gross total resection of a craniopharyngioma can be reliably achieved with functional preservation of the pituitary stalk. This controversy is addressed elsewhere in this book.

Fascia Lata Harvest and Cranial Base Repair

A linear lateral thigh incision is used to harvest fascia lata (Figure 8.4). Prior to harvesting the fascia lata, a pituitary rongeur is used to measure the extent of the dural defect.

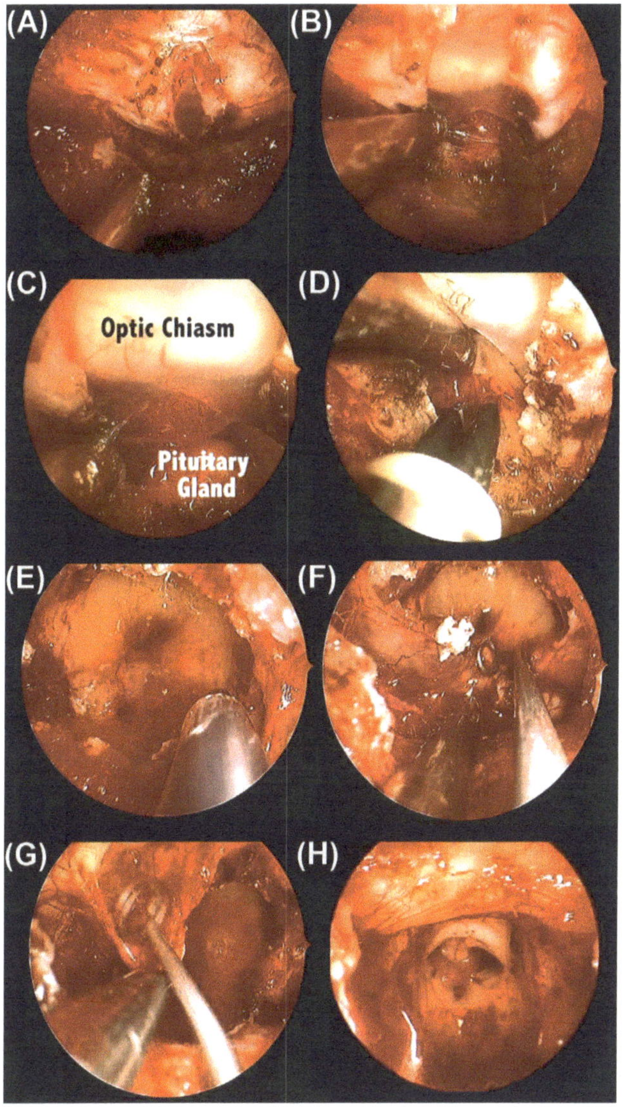

FIGURE 8.3 **A,** The dura is opened in the midline along the planum sphenoidale, tuberculum sellae, and the face of the sella turcica. **B,** The arachnoid is opened. **C,** The anterior aspect of the tumor capsule is visualized below the optic chiasm and above the pituitary gland. **D,** Vessels involved with the tumor capsule are cauterized and divided, sparing the vasculature supplying the optic chiasm and pituitary gland. **E,** Internal debulking of the tumor is performed with an ultrasonic aspirator. **F,** Ringed curettes and sharp microdissection allow for extra-capsular mobilization of the tumor. **G,** The gliotic plane is utilized in order to fully mobilize the tumor capsule from the adjacent hypothalamus. **H,** A 30-degree angled endoscope is used to inspect the resection cavity and the roof of the third ventricle.

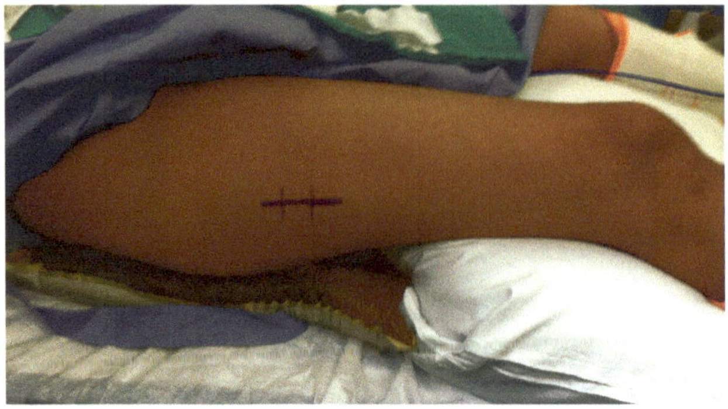

FIGURE 8.4 A linear lateral thigh incision is used to harvest fascia lata for primary dural repair.

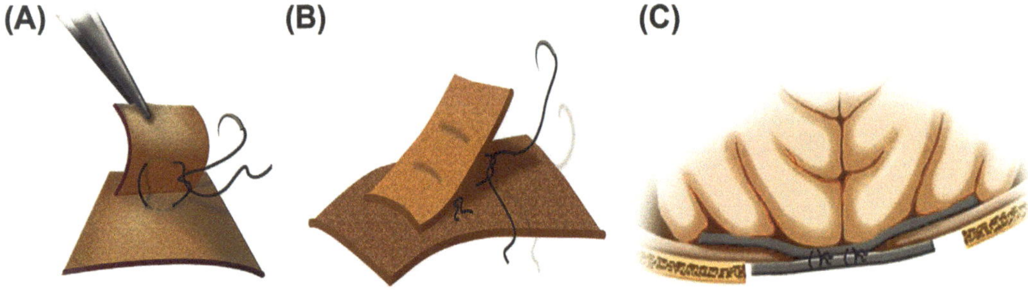

FIGURE 8.5 **A,** and **B,** The "button graft." Using two to four sutures, the two layers of fascia are sutured together, leaving room so the two layers can overlap the edge of the dural defect. **C,** There is no fat or other material placed within the intradural space.

Depending on patient size and the size of the graft needed, a 6–8 cm incision is made over the lateral thigh along the upper third of a line between the greater trochanter and the knee in a caudal/rostral orientation, followed by blunt dissection to expose the fascia lata. A piece of fascia lata is harvested that is large enough to allow for creation of a bilayer "button" graft (Luginbuhl, 2010).

The button is assembled on the back table from two layers of fascia lata (Figure 8.5). The inlay, which will eventually sit on the inside of the dural defect, is made 30% larger than the defect. The onlay graft is made to be only 5–10% larger than the opening. Using two to four 4–0 Neurolon sutures (Ethicon, Bridgewater, NJ), the two layers of fascia are sutured together, leaving enough room for the two layers to overlap the edge of the dural defect. No fat or other material is placed within the intradural space.

The mucoperichondrial septal flap is then reflected to cover the primary dural repair. No fat, balloon, or packing is necessary to ensure graft stability. Finally, a small amount of biological glue (DuraSeal, Covidien, Waltham, MA, USA) is applied over the edges of the flap, and an absorbable collagen sponge (NasoPore, Polyganics, Groningen, The Netherlands) supports the repair centrally. The middle turbinates are then returned medially to their natural anatomical position. Rolls of absorbable gelatin film (Gelfilm, Pfizer, New York, NY) are placed in the middle meatus bilaterally to prevent synechiae formation and to promote normal drainage from the sinuses. A single flat sheet of the absorbable gelatin film is then placed between the nasal septum and the inferior turbinate to prevent synechiae formation and nasal obstruction.

OUTCOMES

A review of studies examining the results of endoscopic endonasal resection of craniopharyngiomas is shown in Table 8.1. With nearly 80% of reported lesions measuring > 2 cm, these results demonstrate that larger tumors are amenable to endoscopic resection with acceptable morbidity and resection rates. These compare favorably with those published using traditional transcranial approaches (Maira, 1995; Fahlbusch, 1999; Honegger, 1999; Jung, 2009). Furthermore, endoscopic resection seems to provide a better chance of vision preservation (Komotar, 2012). The cerebrospinal fluid leak rates reported in the endoscopic literature are certainly higher than with open resections, but are likely a reflection of the early, limited experiences with endonasal techniques. As experience has evolved along with technology

TABLE 8.1 Summary of Studies Examining the Results of Endoscopic Endonasal Resection of Craniopharyngiomas

			Postop Endocrinology	Postop Ophthalmology			
Authors & Year	**No. of Patients**	**Tumor Size > 2 cm (%)**	**DI(%)/HP(%)**	**No Deficit (%)**	**Improved (%)**	**GTR (%)**	**CSF Leak (%)**
Cappabianca et al., 2002	4	NR	NR	NR	NR	100	NR
Frank et al., 2006	10	80	60/100	40	70	70	30
Laufer et al., 2007	4	75	100/100	NR	NR	100	0
de Divitiis et al., 2007	10	NR	60/60	30	50	70	20
Stamm et al., 2008	7	NR	85.7/NR	57.1	67	57	29
Gardner et al., 2008	16	81.3	56.3/88.3	50	75	50	58
Cavallo et al., 2009	22	91	72.7/91.0	36.4	68.1	40.9	13.6
Dehdashti et al., 2009	6	NR	50/NR	16.7	80	16.7	33.3
Campbell et al., 2010	14	85.7	64.3/57.1	42.9	85.7	28.6	35.7
Leng et al., 2011	24	62.5	42/38	NR	77	69	3.8
Cavallo et al., 2014	103	NR	48.1/46.8	NR	74.7	68.9	14.6

NR: not reported; DI: diabetes inspidus; HP: hypopituitarism; GTR: gross total resection; CSF: cerebrospinal fluid leak and improved repair materials, the rate of persistent CSF leaks has declined dramatically, approaching those in the transcranial literature, and this no longer seems to be a major drawback of the endonasal approach (Gardner, 2008; Cavallo, 2009; Campbell, 2010).

CONCLUSION

The extent of resection, along with the choice of surgical approach, has a significant effect on the rate of ophthalmological and endocrinological dysfunction after craniopharyngioma resection. Although not all tumors are amenable to an endonasal endoscopic approach, when applicable, its use can provide a high rate of endocrine function preservation and visual recovery, while simultaneously attaining substantial resections. A purely endoscopic technique, in appropriately selected patients, can substitute for classical transcranial approaches and allow safe and effective management of craniopharyngiomas with comparable, and likely favorable, outcomes.

References

Batra, P.S., Citardi, M.J., Lanza, D.C., 2005. Isolated sphenoid sinusitis after transsphenoidal hypophysectomy. Am. J. Rhinol. 19, 185–189.

Campbell, P.G., McGettigan, B., Luginbuhl, A., Yadla, S., Rosen, M.R., Evans, J.J., 2010. Endocrinological and ophthalmological consequences of an initial endonasal endoscopic approach for resection of craniopharyngiomas. Neurosurg. Focus. 28, E8.

Casler, J.D., Doolittle, A.M., Mair, E.A., 2005. Endoscopic surgery of the anterior skull base. Laryngoscope 115, 16–24.

Cavallo, L.M., Prevedello, D.M., Solari, D., Gardner, P.A., Esposito, F., Snyderman, C.H., Carrau, R.L., Kassam, A.B., Cappabianca, P., 2009. Extended endoscopic endonasal transsphenoidal approach for residual or recurrent craniopharyngiomas. J. Neurosurg. 111, 578–589.

Dandy, Walter E., 1945. Surgery of the Brain. W. F. Prior Company, Inc, Hagerstown. Print, p. 557.

de Divitiis, E., Cappabaianca, P., Cavallo, L.M., Esposito, F., de Divitiis, O., Messina, A., 2007. Extended endoscopic transsphenoidal approach for extrasellar craniopharyngiomas. Neurosurg. 61, 219–227.

Dehdashti, A.R., Ganna, A., Witterick, I., Gentili, F., 2009. Expanded endoscopicendonasal approach for anterior cranial base and suprasellar lesions: indications and limitations. Neurosurgery 64, 677–689.

Esposito, F., Cappabianca, P., Del Basso De Caro, M., Cavallo, L.M., Rinaldi, C., De Divitiis, E., 2004. Endoscopic endonasal transsphenoidal removal of an intra-suprasellar schwannoma mimicking a pituitary adenoma. Minim. Invasive Neurosurg. 47, 230–234.

Fahlbusch, R., Honegger, J., Paulus, W., Huk, W., Buchfelder, M., 1999. Surgical treatment of craniopharyngiomas: experience with 168 patients. J. Neurosurg. 90, 237–250.

Frank, G., Pasquini, E., Doglietto, F., Mazzatenta, D., Sciarretta, V., Farneti, G., Calbucci, A., 2006. The endoscopic extended transsphenoidal approach for craniopharyngiomas. Neurosurgery 59, ONS75–83.

Gardner, P.A., Kassam, A.B., Snyderman, C.H., Carrau, R.L., Mintz, A.H., Grahovac, S., et al., 2008. Outcomes following endoscopic, expanded endonasal resection of suprasellar craniopharyngiomas: a case series. J. Neurosurg. 109, 6–16.

Honegger, J., Buchfelder, M., Fahlbusch, R., Däubler, B., Dörr, H.G., 1992. Transsphenoidal microsurgery for craniopharyngioma. Surg. Neurol. 37, 189–196.

Jho, H.D., Carrau, R.L., 1997. Endoscopic endonasal transsphenoidal surgery: experience with 50 patients. J. Neurosurg. 87, 44–51.

Jung, T.Y., Jung, S., Choi, J.E., Moon, K.S., Kim, I.Y., Kang, S.S., 2009. Adult craniopharyngiomas: surgical results with a special focus on endocrinological outcomes and recurrence according to pituitary stalk preservation. J. Neurosurg. 111, 572–577.

Komotar, R.J., Starke, R.M., Raper, D.M., Anand, V.L., Schwartz, T.H., 2012. Endoscopic endonasal compared with microscopic transsphenoidal and open transcranial resection of craniopharyngiomas. World Neurosurg. 77, 329–341.

Laufer, I., Anand, V.K., Schwartz, T.H., 2007. Endoscopic, endonasal extended transsphenoidal, transplanum transtuberculum approach for resection of suprasellar lesions. J. Neurosurg. 106, 400–406.

Laws Jr., E.R., 1980. Transsphenoidal microsurgery in the management of craniopharyngioma. J. Neurosurg. 52, 661–666.

Leng, L.Z., Anand, V.K., Schwartz, T.H., 2011. Endoscopic, endonasal resection of craniopharyngiomas: analysis of outcome including extent of resection, cerebrospinal fluid leak, return to preoperative productivity, and body mass index. Neurosurgery 70, 110–123.

Luginbuhl, A.J., Campbell, P.G., Evans, J., Rosen, M., 2010. Endoscopic repair of high-flow cranial base defects using a bilayer button. Laryngoscope 120, 876–880.

Maira, G., Anile, C., Rossi, G.F., Colosimo, C., 1995. Surgical treatment of craniopharyngiomas: an evaluation of the transsphenoidal and pterional approaches. Neurosurgery 36, 715–724.

Stamm, A.C., Vellutini, E., Harvey, R.J., Nogeira Jr., J.F., Herman, D.R., 2008. Endoscopic transnasal craniotomy and the resection of craniopharyngioma. Laryngoscope 118, 1142–1148.

CHAPTER

9

The Microscopic Transsphenoidal Approach for Craniopharyngiomas

Wenya Linda Bi, Edward R. Laws, Jr, Ian F. Dunn

Department of Neurosurgery, Brigham and Women's Hospital and Harvard Medical School, Boston, MA, USA

"The neurosurgeon, trying his utmost to effect complete removal of a craniopharyngioma by employing meticulous microtechniques to separate normal from pathological structures, often reaches a point in dissection where to proceed further or to retreat, could, in the long term, be equally damaging to the patient." ***MG Yasargil, et al., 1990***

INTRODUCTION

First described over 150 years ago, craniopharyngiomas are thought to arise from squamous cell rests resulting from partial involution of the embryonic vestigial hypophyseal-pharyngeal duct, also known as the craniopharyngeal duct (Prabhu and Brown, 2005; Zada et al., 2010). They may represent one end of a spectrum of diseases spanning Rathke cleft cysts, arachnoid cysts, colloid cysts, cystic pituitary adenomas, epidermoid, and dermoid cysts (Zada et al., 2010). Two major pathologic subtypes of craniopharyngiomas, adamantinomatous, and squamous papillary, confer unique clinical, imaging, and histologic characteristics (Adamson et al., 1990; Weiner et al., 1994). Squamous papillary craniopharyngiomas are almost exclusively found in adults, are typically solid, rarely associated with calcifications, and tend not to recur if fully resected. The adamantinomatous subtype is represented in the pediatric subset as well as in two-thirds of the adult craniopharyngiomas.

The incidence of craniopharyngioma in the United States is estimated at 0.13 per 100,000 cases, with most studies reporting bimodal peaks at ages 5–14 and then 65–74 (Bunin et al., 1998). Two hypotheses regarding the oncogenesis of craniopharyngiomas seek to reconcile the bimodal distribution of diagnosis (Prabhu and Brown, 2005; Oskouian et al., 2006b; Zada et al., 2010). In the first, ectopic craniopharyngeal duct cells during pituitary development underlie the formation of the tumors, accounting for the high prevalence of adamantinomatous tumors among the pediatric population. The second hypothesis evokes metaplasia

Craniopharyngiomas
http://dx.doi.org/10.1016/B978-0-12-416706-3.00009-X

of residual squamous cell rests, accounting for adult tumors, especially of the papillary subtype (Oskouian et al., 2006b; Zada et al., 2010).

Although craniopharyngiomas are most commonly intimately associated with the infundibulum, they can be found anywhere along the path from the nasopharynx to the third ventricle, diversifying the array of potential surgical approaches needed to attack these tumors (Figure 9.1). They have long presented a management quandary and surgical challenge; Harvey Cushing declared them "the most formidable of intracranial tumors" (Cushing, 1932; Barkhoudarian and Laws, 2013). Surgery continues to be at the heart of therapeutic strategies to manage these tumors, though controversy remains regarding the precise goal of surgery for craniopharyngiomas (Al-Mefty, 2010; Yang et al., 2010). Complete surgical removal improves outcome, overall survival, and decreases recurrence risk, across both pediatric and adult populations (Matson and Crigler, 1969; Yasargil et al., 1990; Fahlbusch et al., 1999; Duff et al., 2000). However, the endocrinologic sequelae and concomitant operative risk for these large complex tumors that span the sellar, suprasellar, parasellar, and often intraventricular regions, has swayed some to pursue subtotal resection with adjuvant radiation therapy as the treatment goal, with increasingly comparable survival rates (Scott et al., 1994; Yang et al., 2010). It is important to recognize that each patient and each craniopharyngioma is unique, and that generalizations with regard to optimal treatment are dangerous. The mode of presentation often guides the aggressiveness and timing of surgery, and there is no "one size fits all" solution for this tumor.

RATIONALE FOR CHOICE OF SURGICAL APPROACH

A number of critical factors help determine whether the transcranial or the transsphenoidal approach is most suitable for sellar and parasellar lesions (de Divitiis and Laws, 2013). These include the pathology of the lesion, if known; the origin, epicenter, and extension of the lesion; its presumed consistency; the nature of visual loss; the involvement of the optic apparatus, circle of Willis, pituitary gland, infundibulum, and hypothalamus; and whether or not there is hydrocephalus or elevated intracranial pressure. Should there be equipoise regarding the appropriate strategy, the surgeon's fundamental comfort level with the approaches is decisive. However, the origin and epicenter of craniopharyngiomas are often related to the pituitary stalk, and many lesions in the suprasellar space extend posterior to the optic chiasm. Even if they extend up to the third ventricle, they are excellent candidates for the transsphenoidal approach, because the axis of the tumor lies along the axis of the plane of visualization (Laws, 2010).

TRANSSPHENOIDAL APPROACH

The first successful resection of a craniopharyngioma was performed through an oro-nasal approach by A. E. Halstead of Chicago in 1910, shortly after the inception of the transsphenoidal approach for pituitary lesions (Schloffer, 1907; Halstead, 1910). The patient, an express coach driver, presented with frontal headache and loss of vision, and was initially diagnosed with cerebral syphilis because of physical findings of a perforated nasal septum and aortic regurgitation (Roderick et al., 2008). Subsequent development of impotence and bitemporal

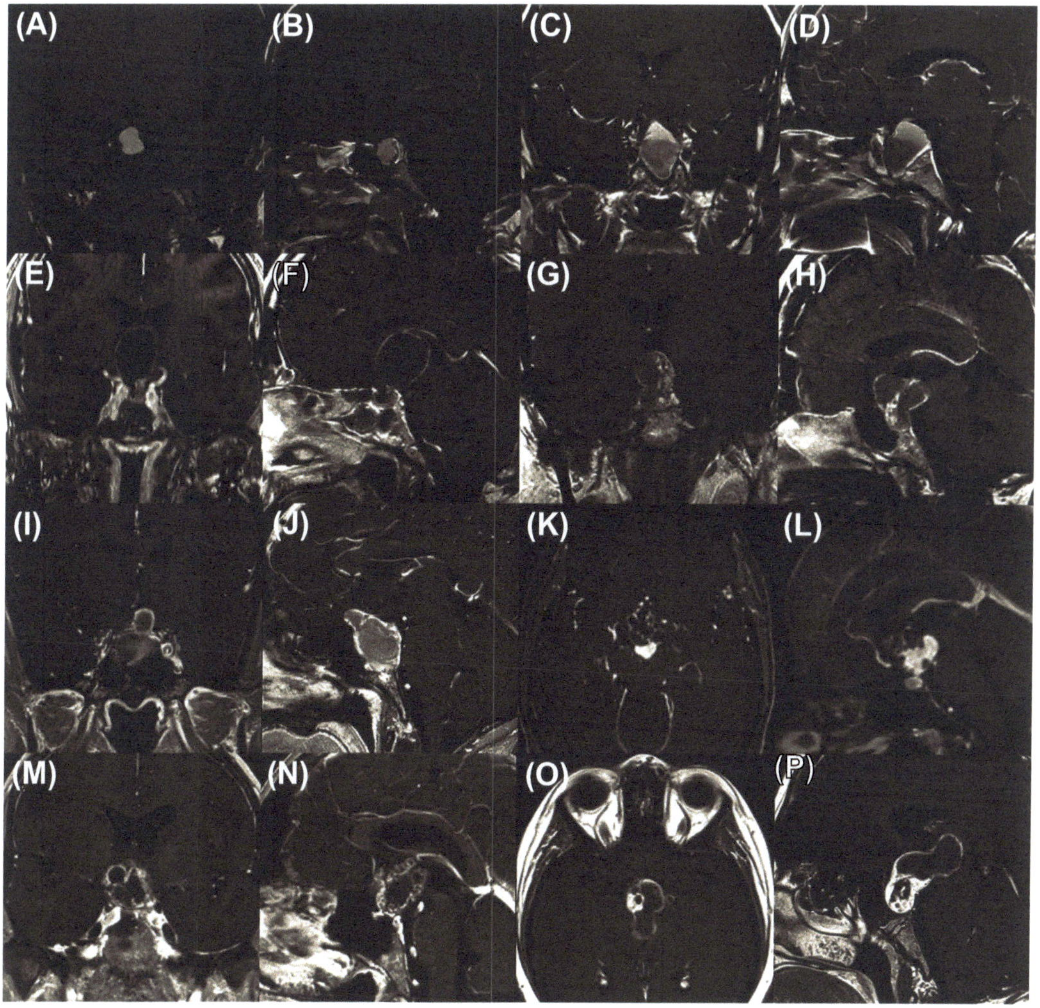

FIGURE 9.1 Craniopharyngiomas can localize to the sellar, suprasellar, parasellar, and intraventricular compartments, with a heterogeneous array of consistencies. Here we present a selection of gadolinium-enhanced MRI images for craniopharyngioma patients. **A, B**, A solid intrasellar craniopharyngioma, without significant sellar expansion, diagnosed in a child after a fainting spell. **C, D**, A recurrent intrasellar craniopharyngioma of mixed consistencies, with sellar expansion, in a patient with amenorrhea and visual loss. **E, F**, A suprasellar retrochiasmatic cystic craniopharyngioma with normal sella in a patient presenting with visual loss. **G, H**, A recurrent sellar and suprasellar multi-compartmental tumor in a patient with visual loss and hypothalamic weight gain. **I, J**, A cystic craniopharyngioma with suprasellar and subfrontal extension, as well as sellar expansion, in a patient with headache and panhypopituitarism. **K, L**, A suprasellar, mixed solid and multi-cystic tumor, extending to the interpeduncular cistern in a patient presenting with headache, polydipsia, and polyuria. **M, N**, A primarily suprasellar retrochiasmatic tumor associated with early hydrocephalus in a patient presenting with visual loss. **O, P**, A large craniopharyngioma extending from the intrasellar compartment to the third ventricle in a child presenting with headache, visual loss, and weight gain.

hemianopia raised suspicion of a pituitary tumor, resulting in surgical intervention and post-operative recovery of vision.

What followed is a fascinating chronicle of the development of cranial and endonasal techniques, multiple variations of which have in turn been used to approach craniopharyngiomas. Fedor Krause, Sir Victor Horsley, Harvey Cushing, and Walter Dandy pioneered early frontal and subtemporal approaches to the sella (Kanter et al., 2005). At the same time, endonasal and sublabial approaches without a disfiguring external rhinotomy incision were introduced by Hirsch (Lanzino and Laws, 2003) and Halstead (Halstead, 1910), respectively, leading to the sublabial submucosal transseptal approach innovated by Cushing and used for many decades thereafter (Cushing, 1914) (Figure 9.2). Presumably because of poor visualization, incomplete resections and early recurrences and suboptimal results with regard to visual improvement, Cushing abandoned the transsphenoidal approach in 1927, late in his surgical career. Another factor may have been his increasing confidence in transcranial methods after the introduction of electrocautery by Bovie in 1926. Through the untiring efforts of Norman Dott, Oskar Hirsch, Dott's trainee Gerard Guiot, who introduced fluoroscopy for image guidance (Guiot and Thibaut, 1959), and Jules Hardy, who introduced the operating microscope (Hardy and Wigser, 1965), transsphenoidal approaches resumed popularity for sellar lesions, including complex craniopharyngiomas that push the "edge of the envelope" (Lanzino and Laws, 2003; Zada et al., 2011).

Early transsphenoidal microsurgery experience with craniopharyngioma resection pertained primarily to subdiaphragmatic tumors, preferably with an enlarged sella, cystic character, and patients with pre-operative hypopituitarism (Laws, 1980, Laws, 1994). Hardy had emphasized the fact that craniopharyngioma patients with enlargement of the sella almost always had tumors

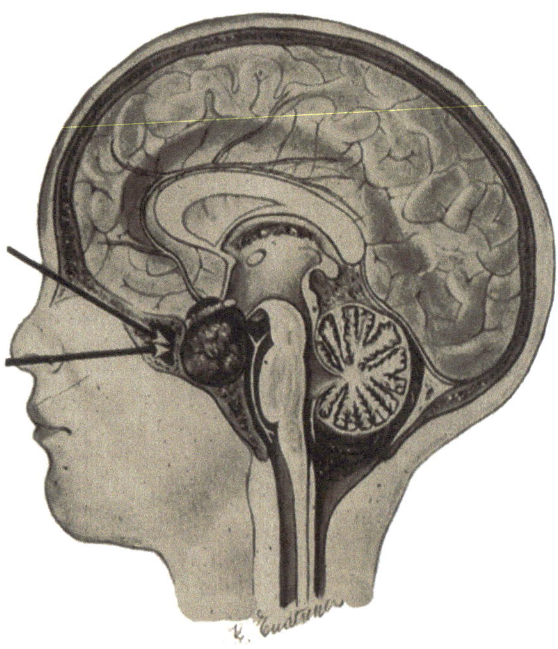

FIGURE 9.2 Transethmoid and transnasal approaches to the sella in the early evolution of transsphenoidal surgery. *(Figure adapted by Koos W., from the author's collection)*

that began below the diaphragm, and were well suited to the transsphenoidal approach, as the expanded diaphragm was a barrier against tumor invasion of the chiasm and the hypothalamus. Since then, suprasellar craniopharyngiomas, without sellar expansion, and with posterior extension, have been tackled by many using a transsphenoidal microsurgical approach (Weiss, 1987; Kaptain et al., 2001; Couldwell et al., 2004; Kim et al., 2011; Ikeda et al., 2012).

The cystic, multi-compartmental nature of craniopharyngiomas as well as their frequent adherence to the infundibulum, optic apparatus, and other nearby structures, are challenges for safe and effective resection. Thorough dissection of the craniopharyngioma capsule and preservation of the vascular supply to the hypophyseal, hypothalamic, and optic chiasm regions is abetted by microscopic inspection. Although the endoscope provides a broad scope of view, microscope-guided transsphenoidal approaches can afford higher resolution stereoscopic visualization and more facile surgical maneuverability with tactile feedback when dissecting tumor capsule, delicate adherent vessels, or reconstructing the sellar floor (Kim et al., 2011; Ikeda et al., 2012).

Transsphenoidal approaches for craniopharyngiomas have been associated with increased gross total resection, decreased recurrence, and a lower incidence of permanent diabetes insipidus when compared to transcranial approaches in recent meta-analysis, although reported rates vary widely (Komotar et al., 2012), and we emphasize the need to evaluate the merits of each case individually. Endonasal methods may also lead to comparable or improved visual outcome compared to open transcranial approaches (Fahlbusch et al., 1999; Komotar et al., 2012). Selection bias should also be taken into account when comparing the two approaches.

Pre-operative Evaluation

Magnetic resonance imaging (MRI), with gadolinium enhancement, is best suited to delineate tumor architecture and adjacent structures. Computed tomography (CT) discloses the presence and amount of calcification in the tumor, and optimizes visualization of bony landmarks, including nasal septal deviation, and alterations in sphenoid sinus or carotid canal anatomy. High-resolution MRI or CT can be used for image guidance, which may be especially beneficial for large lesions with significant parasellar or caudal extent.

A full endocrinological work-up is pursued before surgery, including laboratory measurement of prolactin, the thyroid panel, growth hormone, IGF-1, fasting cortisol, and ACTH. Hypocortisolemia should be treated with stress dose steroids prior to induction of anesthesia. The introduction of peri-operative steroids by Ingraham, Matson, and colleagues transformed craniopharyngioma peri-operative morbidity from formidable to acceptable (Ingraham et al., 1952; Matson and Crigler, 1969). The presence of diabetes insipidus prior to surgery may allow more latitude in transecting the infundibulum during surgery, resulting in a wider aperture for manipulation of the tumor.

Operative and Pathologic Anatomy

Nasal, sphenoid, and sellar anatomy are all pertinent to the surgical approach. Septal spurs, pneumatization of the sphenoid sinus, which is often age-dependent, expansion of the sella, and erosion of any local bony structures are noted. We attempt to identify the position of the normal pituitary on pre-operative MRI and note any deviation of the stalk, though this may be difficult to locate. The location of the optic chiasm with respect to infundibulum and the tumor dictates the operative window for craniopharyngiomas with superior extension; while tumors centered on the stalk may extend behind the chiasm high into the third ventricle, this extension along the nasal axis may render these tumors ideal for transsphenoidal surgery. The distance between the carotid arteries and the optic canals may constrain the coronal plane working distance. Tumor epicenter, morphology, the presence of cystic and calcific features, and degree of mass effect exerted on the hypothalamus, including any signs of hydrocephalus, also influence the working angles and the aperture needed for resection. Lastly, surgery on recurrent, residual, or previously radiated tumors carries a significantly higher risk of complications (Laws, 1980; Yasargil et al., 1990; Fahlbusch et al., 1999).

SURGICAL TECHNIQUE

Operative Set-up

Patient positioning aims to maximize exposure of the nasal passage and sphenoid while maintaining surgeon comfort and spatial orientation. The room is set up to allow the surgeon to stand on the patient's right side, looking at the face, with the scrub nurse on the patient's left side and anesthesia at the feet. The operating table is turned approximately 170 degrees from anesthesia and the patient's vertex is turned to the left, to align the dorsum of the nose with the walls of the room. The patient is adjusted to a semi-recumbent position, with the torso elevated 20–30 degrees and the knees gently flexed, to minimize venous congestion and to promote drainage of blood from the sellar region during the operation. The table is tilted slightly to the right, minimizing the need to lean over the torso to maintain the midline approach. Tilting especially improves surgeon's comfort when operating on larger-built patients and those with limited neck flexion (Jane et al., 2002).

The head is further adjusted to ensure parallel orientation of the nasal dorsum with the floor, which allows a straight-on view into the nose. One may extend the head slightly should the tumor extend toward the planum sphenoidale. The patient's right arm is tucked while the left arm is made available for anesthesia access during the operation. The assistant and operating microscope are positioned to the surgeon's left.

We routinely employ neuro-navigation (Asthagiri et al., 2006). For particularly complex and large tumors, intra-operative MRI may also improve ability to maximize resection. A rigid fixation system, such as the Mayfield head holder with pins, is commonly used in conjunction with the stereotaxic image guidance systems. In contrast, a horseshoe headrest allows delicate manipulation of the operative view when working with a narrow corridor, and some image guidance systems that use facemask registration technology are compatible with this strategy.

Patient Preparation

Administration of intranasal oxymetazoline (0.05% solution, Afrin™) spray to promote vasoconstriction and minimize nasal mucosa bleeding begins in the pre-operative area, with two sprays into each nostril every 10 minutes. Immediately before induction, long cotton pledgets saturated with oxymetazoline are placed into both nostrils for 5 to 10 minutes, followed by pledgets soaked in 1% lidocaine with 1:200,000 epinephrine for another 5–10 minutes. The eyes are covered with protective dressings and the mid-face is scrubbed with an aqueous surgical prep solution.

The orotracheal tube is taped to the left side of the mouth. An orogastric tube is placed on induction, to allow suctioning of dependent and swallowed blood at the end of surgery. An abdominal site (lower quadrant or sub-umbilical) is prepared on all patients to allow for potential fat and/or rectus fascia graft harvest should cerebrospinal fluid (CSF) leak be encountered. A lumbar drain is placed pre-operatively, on rare occasion, to facilitate delivery of suprasellar tumor components, especially in the setting of a small sella or a narrow diaphragmatic aperture.

Broad-spectrum antibiotic is given at the beginning of surgery and through the first 24 hours, or while nasal packing is in place. One hundred mg of hydrocortisone (Solu-Cortef) is given prior to induction if pre-operative adrenal axis testing suggests insufficiency.

Operative Phases

The transsphenoidal approach progresses in several discrete stages (Dunn and Laws, 2010). First, either the sublabial region or the nasal orifices are manipulated to gain entry into the sphenoid sinus. Next, the sphenoid sinus is traversed to reach the sellar floor. The sellar floor is widely removed and the sellar dura is opened, exposing the edges of the cavernous sinus laterally and exposing both the superior and inferior intercavernous sinuses. The superior intercavernous sinus may need to be cauterized and divided to reach the intracranial portion of the tumor and to separate its capsule safely from the optic chiasm. The pituitary fossa and adjacent spaces are then exposed for tumor removal. Craniopharyngiomas are subarachnoid lesions and the arachnoid needs to be dissected away from the tumor capsule. Lastly, and at times the most challenging, CSF leaks are repaired and the sella floor is reconstructed.

Nasal Phase

Entry into the nasal portal can be gained through a sublabial or a transnasal approach. One percent lidocaine with 1:200,000 epinephrine may be injected into the submucosal plane along the two sides of the nasal septum to promote hemostasis for subsequent dissection. Some omit this step and rely on only topical application of local anesthetics to minimize the risk of subsequent devascularization and septal perforation.

The sublabial approach used by Cushing, Guiot, and Hardy has subsided in popularity compared to modern endonasal approaches. The wide exposure afforded by this approach remains useful for patients with small nostrils, especially children, and when additional lateral reach is desired. The sublabial submucosal transseptal approach begins with a transverse gingival incision along the face of the maxilla, extending between the two incisor teeth, taking care to avoid excessive cautery and devitalization of the upper teeth. The mucosa is dissected away from the superior surface of the hard palate to reveal the piriform aperture and the anterior nasal septum. A unilateral hemi-transfixion incision allows the creation of a submucosal tunnel along the nasal septum. The cartilaginous portion is dislocated at its junction with the bony septum and reflected to the contralateral side, producing an opening to create a contralateral posterior submucosal tunnel next to the perpendicular plate of the ethmoid and vomer. The sublabial incision can also be combined with a transnasal submucosal transseptal approach to provide a wider aperture.

For transnasal and endonasal approaches, the initial opening varies from a superficial transcolumellar incision (Kim et al., 2001), a hemi-transfixion incision immediately posterior to the columella (Kern et al., 1979), an incision at the junction of the bony and cartilaginous septum (Wilson et al., 1990), or at the junction of the bony nasal septum with the sphenoid rostrum (Griffith and Veerapen, 1987).

The transnasal submucosal transseptal approach starts with a vertical hemi-transfixion incision, with the columella retracted to the contralateral side (Kern et al., 1979). The cartilaginous septum is exposed through submucosal perichondral dissection, creating the anterior tunnel, to reach the junction of the bony septum. Another vertical incision is made at this junction to allow further separation of the mucosa from both sides of the bony septum, or the perpendicular plate of the ethmoid, and to create bilateral posterior tunnels (Figure 9.3). This potential space is expanded along the nasal floor after freeing the cartilaginous septum from the maxilla, to create inferior tunnels, and allow displacement of the anterior septum without causing mucosal tears. A relaxing incision extending from the base of the hemi-transfixion incision or the right ala may be used in the setting of a small nostril with limited space. A nasal speculum is then introduced on the two sides of the perpendicular plate to expose the anterior surface of the sphenoid sinus. At the end of surgery, nasal packing is traditionally used to prevent submucosal hematoma. Modifications of the closure have been described to accelerate recovery and obviate the need for packing (Liu et al., 2004).

The septal displacement technique is probably the most common of the microscopic approaches used today, as it avoids the extensive anterior submucosal perichondral dissection, and the consequent risks of septal perforation. It was initially described in patients undergoing repeat transsphenoidal surgery with prior injury to the septum (Wilson and Laws, 1992). In contrast to the original hemi-transfixion incision described, the incision is made at the junction of the bony and cartilaginous septum, with subsequent submucosal dissection along the perpendicular plate to create posterior tunnels. The anterior septum, covered by both layers of mucosa, is displaced towards one side. The posterior bony septum is removed. In this fashion, the sphenoid face is rapidly exposed within minutes, allowing for placement of the nasal speculum.

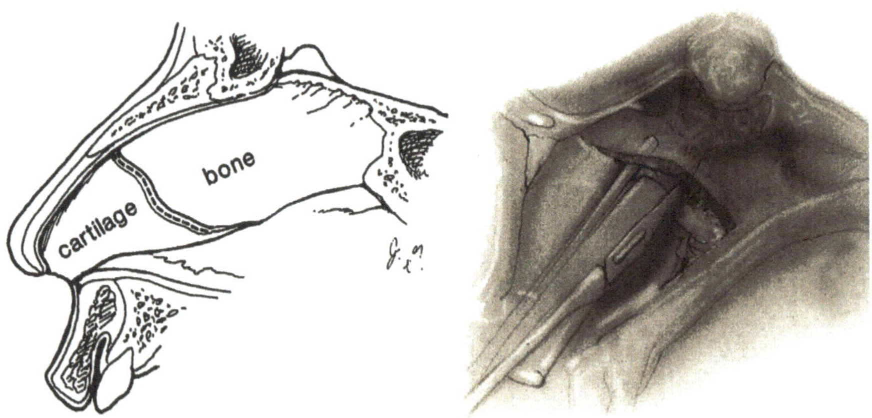

FIGURE 9.3 Schematic representation of the septal displacement approach with an incision made at the junction of the cartilaginous and bony nasal septum. *(Figures adapted from Wilson and Laws, 1990 and Jane, Thapar, et al., 2002).*

Direct anterior sphenoidotomy offers an even more posterior initial entry, directly at the junction of the bony nasal septum with the sphenoid rostrum (Griffith and Veerapen, 1987). Early introduction of a nasal speculum under direct microscopic visualization forces the ipsilateral middle turbinate laterally and is then used to fracture the posterior septum to the other side (Zada et al., 2003). A longer speculum is replaced to allow visualization of the sphenoid rostrum. Because of the posterior extent of this approach, the resultant exposure is significantly narrower than other transnasal approaches. Furthermore, the oblique unilateral trajectory may challenge correct orientation during the subsequent phases of tumor resection.

A bivalve nasal speculum retracts open the nasal corridor during microscopic transsphenoidal surgery, which is also evolving in design to match developing technical needs (Chole et al., 2011). Caution should be exerted in spreading the speculum to avoid fractures extending into the optic foramen or adjacent maxillary structures, which may lead to facial numbness and lacrimal dysfunction (Kern et al., 1979).

Sphenoidal Phase

The anterior face of the sphenoid sinus is demarcated by the keel of the vomer in the midline and the sphenoid ostia in the inferolateral quadrants. A pneumatized sphenoid sinus can be entered by fracturing the vomer or using a chisel or drill. The sphenoidectomy is carried out superiorly to the planum sphenoidale, inferiorly to the floor of the sinus, and laterally just prior to reaching the sphenopalatine foramen. Care is taken to avoid injuring the sphenopalatine artery near the inferolateral border of the sphenoid ostium (at the 7 o'clock position for the right side and the 5 o'clock position for the left side). A fragment of the vomer is preserved to mark the midline. Mucosa within the sphenoid sinus is stripped with a cup forcep to reduce risk of post-operative mucocele. Septae within the sphenoid sinus are removed, after noting their relation to the cavernous carotid canals on pre-operative image. Inspection at this point, prior to entering the sella, should reveal the carotid canals, the planum, the opticocarotid recesses, and the clivus.

Next, the sellar floor is widely exposed after verification of the midline and adjacent structures. A chisel or blunt nerve hook or drill is used to penetrate the floor. A 1 or 2 mm Kerrison punch extends bony removal to reach the inferior border of the superior intercavernous sinus, the optic canals superolaterally, and the bilateral cavernous sinuses laterally in traditional transsphenoidal approaches. Removal of the posterior planum sphenoidale and tuberculum sellae, with adjustments in the speculum orientation, tailors the operative approach to address tumors with suprasellar, pre-chiasmatic, parasellar, or third ventricular extension (Weiss, 1987; Kaptain et al., 2001; Couldwell et al., 2004).

Sellar Phase

A microvascular Doppler probe is used routinely to verify the position of the cavernous carotid arteries and to define the lateral limits of dural opening (Oskouian et al., 2006a). Pulsatile flow may occasionally be transmitted in the midline position through a cystic mass from the basilar artery. This should be distinguished from vascular pathologies, such as an aneurysm, which may pose as a rare mimic for a sellar mass (Hanak et al., 2012).

After determining the safe entry zone, the dura is coagulated and opened in a cruciate manner or excised in a rectangular fashion (Figure 9.4). Considerable bleeding can be encountered during opening from the bisecting intercavernous sinus or even from between the dural leaves. Hemostasis is achieved through cauterization, application of gelatin hemostasis matrix mixed with thrombin, such as SurgiFlo™ (Ethicon, Inc, NJ) or Gelfoam® (Pharmacia and Upjohn Company, Kalamazoo, MI), with subsequent cottonoid tamponade, or fibrin sealant, such as Evicel® (Ethicon, Inc, NJ) administered through a long malleable nozzle.

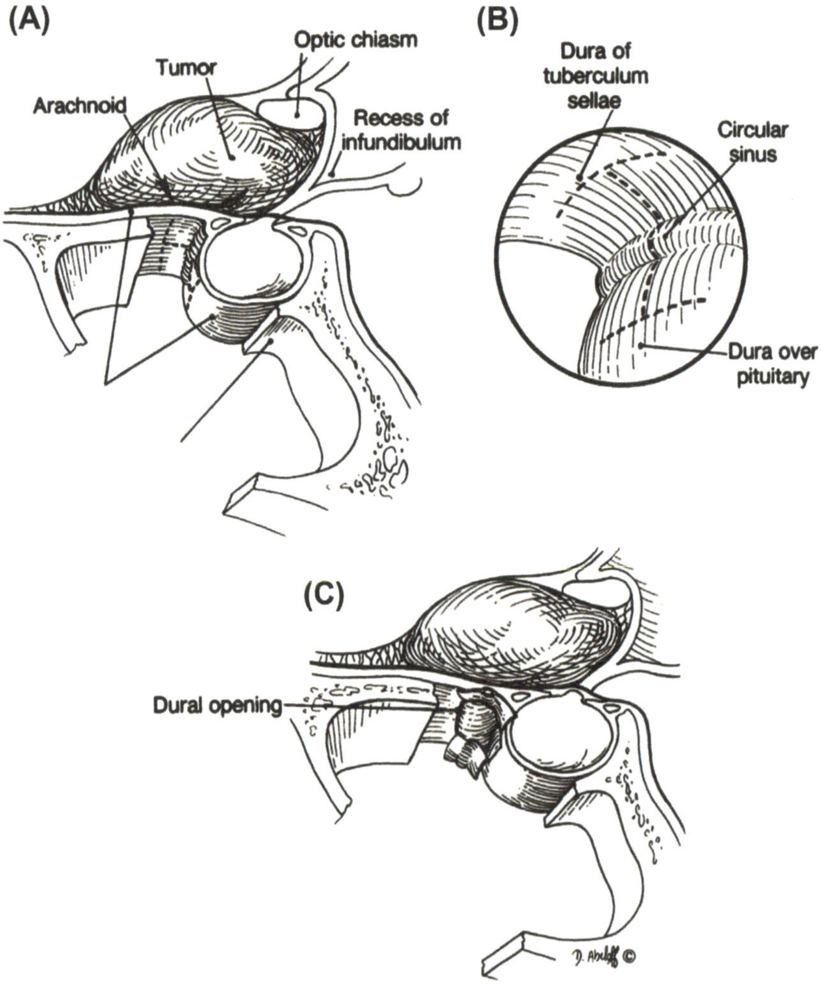

FIGURE 9.4 Essential steps in the extended transsphenoidal exposure adapted from Weiss (1987). **A**, Exposure of the sella and posterior planum sphenoidale. **B**, Dural incision incorporating the superior intercavernous sinus. **C**, Dural exposure. *(Figure courtesy of Lippincott Williams and Wilkins.)*

After the dura is opened, the pituitary gland can be mobilized laterally or inferiorly to increase exposure; the dural opening more anteriorly after intercavernous sinus coagulation and division may allow an enhanced view of the anterior border of the tumor with the optic chiasm. A right angle dissector or blunt hook is used to define the subdural plane before distortion from tumor resection. For intrasellar and paradiaphragmatic craniopharyngiomas, tumor resection begins in the inferior and lateral portions to allow the superior extent to descend into the field. Exploration of the lateral sella with a blunt ring curette should be pursued gently to avoid injury to the cavernous sinus and adjacent cranial nerves.

For suprasellar lesions, the diaphragm can be sharply dissected from the roof of the sella detaching it from just behind the tuberculum. The tumor capsule is defined behind the arachnoid, capsular feeder vessels are cauterized, cystic components are evacuated first, and solid and calcified fragments resected next. Adhesions to the optic nerve, chiasm, and pituitary stalk are sharply dissected, and extreme care is taken in separating the tumor from the hypothalamus. In subdiaphragmatic craniopharyngiomas, before a CSF leak occurs, delivery of suprasellar components may be facilitated by jugular vein compression, Valsalva, or injection of air or saline via a lumbar drain (Zada et al., 2011). Staged or simultaneous transcranial and endonasal approaches may also be indicated for certain tumors.

Closure

The dural opening in craniopharyngioma surgery often results in an immediate significant cerebrospinal fluid (CSF) leak. More occult leaks may appear as dark streaks against a background of venous bleeding. Presence or suspicion of CSF leak during surgery, or with provocative maneuvers, such as on Valsalva, is managed with placement of a fat graft. Abdominal fat is harvested from a curvilinear subumbilical incision for cosmesis using a dedicated clean set of instruments and after exchange of gloves. The fat is dissected into small portions, soaked in a 10% chloramphenicol solution, blotted dry, lightly dusted with wisps of cotton to provoke an inflammatory response which improves the sealant effect, and finally coated in Avitene™ (Davol Inc, Cranston, RI) collagen powder to promote hemostasis (Jane et al., 2002). Care is taken to avoid over-packing of fat into the sella, which may be associated with post-operative visual loss due to compression of the optic chiasm. The sellar floor is reconstructed with autologous bone from the initial opening or with a biosynthetic substitute such as the MedPor® polyethylene plate (Stryker, Kalamazoo, MI).

When the extended transsphenoidal methods are utilized in the setting of complex suprasellar craniopharyngiomas, especially those with significant parasellar or intraventricular components, additional steps are taken during closure. An in-lay autologous or cadaveric fascial graft may be placed subdurally, and, although not traditionally employed with straight microscopic transsphenoidal cases, a pedicled nasoseptal flap based on the sphenopalatine artery confers a highly effective biological barrier against persistent CSF leak (Hadad et al., 2006; Kassam et al., 2008b; Rivera-Serrano et al., 2011; Otto et al., 2013).

We do not routinely use lumbar drainage for management of CSF leak from transsphenoidal operations. When a post-operative leak is noted, the patient is taken back for exploration and repacking of the sella.

POST-OPERATIVE CONSIDERATIONS AND OUTCOMES

From early experiences with transsphenoidal microscopic techniques for resection of craniopharyngiomas to the modern era endoscopic-assisted microscopic approaches, neurological and endocrinological outcomes continue to vary significantly (Laws, 1980; Adamson et al., 1990; Yasargil et al., 1990; Laws, 1994; Maira et al., 1995; Villani et al., 1997; Fahlbusch et al., 1999; Honegger et al., 1999; Van Effenterre and Boch, 2002; Couldwell et al., 2004; Chakrabarti et al., 2005; Dusick et al., 2005; Gardner et al., 2008; Jane et al., 2010a, 2010b; Yamada et al., 2010; Kim et al., 2011; Mortini et al., 2011; Hofmann et al., 2012; Ikeda et al., 2012; Lopez-Serna et al., 2012). Several trends hold throughout reported studies: gross total resection ranges from 50–90% when the surgical intent is for full resection; subtotal resections lead to earlier and more frequent recurrences; recurrent craniopharyngiomas present with higher rates of visual loss, hypopituitarism, and diabetes insipidus, and also incur higher risks of new-onset deficits after transsphenoidal resection; adamantinous craniopharyngiomas are more apt to recur than papillary ones; and pediatric craniopharyngiomas may be associated with greater symptomology on presentation as well as post-operatively when compared to adult craniopharyngiomas.

Resection Rates

In one of the earliest series on using a dedicated transsphenoidal microscopic approach for resecting craniopharyngiomas, Laws reported 64% gross total resection among patients undergoing initial treatment, but only 17% gross total resection among those with prior craniotomy for craniopharyngioma and recurrent or residual tumor (Laws, 1980). This is comparable with the transsphenoidal resection results of 50–90% within later single-institution series of mixed transcranial and transsphenoidal approaches, as well as solely transsphenoidal microscopic approaches (Maira et al., 1995; Fahlbusch et al., 1999; Chakrabarti et al., 2005; Jane et al., 2010b; Hofmann et al., 2012). More recent experiences with extended transsphenoidal microscopic approaches, with or without endoscopic assistance, which focus on craniopharyngiomas with previously contraindicated surgical characteristics, suggest improving resection rates with all new methodologies (Dusick et al., 2005; Kim et al., 2011; Ikeda et al., 2012). Namely, Dusick et al. reported 12.5% gross total resection and 50% near-gross total resection in eight craniopharyngiomas analyzed in their extended direct endonasal transsphenoidal series, with tumor size ranging from 3 to 6 cm (Dusick et al., 2005). Kim et al. report total resection in all suprasellar craniopharyngiomas in their series (Kim et al., 2011), while Ikeda et al. achieved 60% gross total resection among their suprasellar craniopharyngiomas (Ikeda et al., 2012). Factors predisposing to subtotal resection included suprasellar and retrosellar extension, far lateral extension, firm consistency including calcification, hypothalamic invasion, encasement of optic apparatus, displacement of circle of Willis vessels and perforating arteries, severe bradycardia during dissection, advanced age of patient, and false intra-operative impression (Fahlbusch et al., 1999; Zada et al., 2011). Prior surgery and radiation treatment also contribute to subtotal resection on repeat surgery, likely due to enhancement of the above-mentioned factors.

Recurrence and Survival

Craniopharyngioma recurrence directly correlates to the degree of resection from all operative modalities, transcranial or transsphenoidal. Villani et al. reported 17.6% recurrence after radical resection of pediatric craniopharyngiomas compared to 42.8% after subtotal resection with adjuvant radiotherapy (Villani et al., 1997). Similarly, Jane et al. found an 18% recurrence rate in their series of pediatric craniopharyngiomas, with 13% following gross total resection and 28.5% after all other degrees of resection or 30% with prior treatment (Jane et al., 2010b). Among adult craniopharyngiomas treated through a transsphenoidal approach, recurrence rates are often lower, with 5.9% reported in a series of 18 patients (Kim et al., 2011), possibly due to the virtually exclusive presence of the papillary subtype among adults, which is associated with a more benign profile. In their large series of 168 craniopharyngiomas with long follow-up, Fahlbusch et al. noted an overall recurrence rate of 11% after gross total resection, but that no recurrences occurred after complete tumor removal by a transsphenoidal approach (Fahlbusch et al., 1999).

Although craniopharyngiomas are considered benign tumors by histopathological criteria, their intimate relationship with and frequent invasion of critical neurovascular structures contributes to peri-operative mortality. In case series of craniopharyngiomas, those undergoing transsphenoidal resection are sometimes reported as having lower mortality than those following transcranial resection; however, this may reflect the inherent selection bias in choosing the transsphenoidal cohort at institutions offering both modalities (Fahlbusch et al., 1999). After gross total resection, patients achieve approximately 90% survival at 5 years and 80–85% at 10 years after surgery (Fahlbusch et al., 1999; Van Effenterre and Boch, 2002).

Large, parasellar tumors with significant lateral extension may still be more safely approached through transcranial methods, especially on recurrence after an initial transsphenoidal approach. Focal radiation therapy or stereotactic radiosurgery are commonly applied after subtotal resection of craniopharyngiomas, with some promising results (Yang et al., 2010).

Neurological Outcome

Visual impairment is one of the most frequent presenting symptoms among adult and pediatric craniopharyngiomas, occurring in half to three-quarter of patients (Laws, 1980; Yasargil et al., 1990). At the same time, visual acuity and visual field deficits demonstrate dramatic improvement following resection of craniopharyngiomas in all series, with a propensity for even more significant results with the transsphenoidal approach as compared to transcranial approaches (Laws, 1980; Chakrabarti et al., 2005; Yamada et al., 2010; Kim et al., 2011).

The incidence of CSF leak following microscopic transsphenoidal surgery for craniopharyngiomas ranges from 1.5% to 17% among reported case series (Laws, 1994; Maira et al., 1995; Fahlbusch et al., 1999; Maira et al., 2004; Chakrabarti et al., 2005; Dusick et al., 2005; Kim et al., 2011). Meningitis, when reported, was an infrequent occurrence across all large modern transsphenoidal series.

Endocrinological Status

Hypopituitarism in the form of growth or sexual maturation delay or amenorrhea is a frequent presenting symptom among craniopharyngioma patients. Following surgery, some form of transient or permanent hypopituitarism would seem inevitable, given the route of access for tumor resection, following the trajectory of the infundibulum. However, although pre-existing hypopituitarism ordinarily does not improve after surgery, new-onset panhypopituitarism following transsphenoidal microscopic resection of craniopharyngiomas ranges from 12.8% (Dusick et al., 2005) to 67% (Jane et al., 2010b).

Diabetes insipidus ensues in up to half of patients following surgical resection of craniopharyngioma, although some improvement is noted on long-term follow-up. Laws reported an incidence of 14% among craniopharyngiomas following initial transsphenoidal resection (Laws, 1980). In two pediatric craniopharyngioma series resected by the transsphenoidal approach, a 50–56% incidence of new-onset diabetes insipidus was noted post-operatively (Villani et al., 1997; Jane et al., 2010b). Similarly, extended transsphenoidal microscopic series for craniopharyngioma resection in adults reported permanent diabetes insipidus in 37.5–41% of patients (Dusick et al., 2005; Kim et al., 2011), while series of mixed adult and pediatric populations also note 52% new incidence (Yamada et al., 2010). In cases where the infundibulum must be transected to improve surgical exposure, sharp sectioning of the stalk to minimize injury to the upstream neuronal cell bodies may reduce the risk of permanent diabetes insipidus.

Morbid obesity, ensuing from distortion of hypothalamic regulation, memory problems, and psychological derangement are other major challenges in peri-operative management.

Limitations

The frequently suprasellar nature of craniopharyngiomas, often with hypothalamic or intraventricular involvement, may challenge the working distance and visualization afforded by the operative microscope via a ventral approach. A purely microscopic approach via a transsphenoidal exposure naturally limits the angles from which vital structures can be visualized. The utilization of an endoscope to inspect hidden corners complements the microscopic approach (Ikeda et al., 2012). Furthermore, the heterogeneity and challenges of craniopharyngioma surgery have prompted significant development of endoscopic-assisted techniques, especially extended endoscopic endonasal transsphenoidal approaches (Couldwell et al., 2004; Gardner et al., 2008; Kassam et al., 2008a; Cavallo et al., 2009; Komotar et al., 2012).

PROSPECTS

Craniopharyngiomas epitomize the challenges and intrigue inherent in skull base lesions. The early adoption of the transsphenoidal approach by Halstead and Cushing, to its loss of popularity in the face of poor visualization and disheartening outcomes, and subsequent revival by Guiot and Hardy reflects not only a technological but also a conceptual evolution within skull base surgery. The goals of optimal visualization, maximal exposure through removal of obstructing bone, minimization of working distance, preservation of intrinsic neurovascular structures, avoidance of brain retraction, and functional and cosmetic reconstruction drove the progression from sublabial to transethmoidal and endonasal approaches. Microsurgical techniques revolutionized the ability to bimanually manipulate delicate neurovascular structures under proper illumination to abet tumor resection. Likewise, endoscopic tools and extended endoscopic endonasal techniques may represent the next frontier for the appropriate craniopharyngioma patient. Early experience with the endoscope was constrained by relative handicaps of surgical maneuverability and stereoscopic visualization. With an assistant holding the endoscope and providing visualization, and growing experience, the surgeon is still afforded bimanual microsurgical control and dexterity with endoscopic techniques. Lastly, proficiency in both the microscopic and endoscopic techniques may offer the broadest and safest spectrum of management options for a major part of the diverse spectrum of craniopharyngiomas.

References

Adamson, T.E., Wiestler, O.D., Kleihues, P., Yasargil, M.G., 1990. Correlation of clinical and pathological features in surgically treated craniopharyngiomas. J. Neurosurg. 73, 12–17.

Al-Mefty, O., 2010. Less is less. J. Neurosurg. Pediatr. 6, 401–402 discussion 402.

Asthagiri, A.R., Laws Jr., E.R., Jane Jr, J.A., 2006. Image guidance in pituitary surgery. Front. Horm. Res. 34, 46–63.

Barkhoudarian, G., Laws, E.R., 2013. Craniopharyngioma: history. Pituitary 16, 1–8.

Bunin, G.R., Surawicz, T.S., Witman, P.A., Preston-Martin, S., Davis, F., Bruner, J.M., 1998. The descriptive epidemiology of craniopharyngioma. J. Neurosurg. 89, 547–551.

Cavallo, L.M., Prevedello, D.M., Solari, D., Gardner, P.A., Esposito, F., Snyderman, C.H., Carrau, R.L., Kassam, A.B., Cappabianca, P., 2009. Extended endoscopic endonasal transsphenoidal approach for residual or recurrent craniopharyngiomas. J. Neurosurg. 111, 578–589.

Chakrabarti, I., Amar, A.P., Couldwell, W., Weiss, M.H., 2005. Long-term neurological, visual, and endocrine outcomes following transnasal resection of craniopharyngioma. J. Neurosurg. 102, 650–657.

Chole, R.A., Lim, C., Dunham, B., Chicoine, M.R., Dacey Jr, R.G., 2011. A novel transnasal transsphenoidal speculum: a design for both microscopic and endoscopic transsphenoidal pituitary surgery. J. Neurosurg. 114, 1380–1385.

Couldwell, W.T., Weiss, M.H., Rabb, C., Liu, J.K., Apfelbaum, R.I., Fukushima, T., 2004. Variations on the standard transsphenoidal approach to the sellar region, with emphasis on the extended approaches and parasellar approaches: surgical experience in 105 cases. Neurosurgery 55, 539–547 discussion 547–550.

Cushing, H., 1914. The Weir Mitchell Lecture. Surgical experiences with pituitary adenoma. JAMA 63, 1515–1525.

Cushing, H., 1932. Intracranial tumors: notes upon a series of two thousand cases with surgical mortality percentages pertaining thereto. Thomas, Springfield, IL.

De Divitiis, E., Laws Jr, E.R., 2013. The transnasal versus transcranial approach to lesions of the anterior skull base. World Neurosurg. 728–729.

Duff, J., Meyer, F.B., Ilstrup, D.M., Laws Jr., E.R., Schleck, C.D., Scheithauer, B.W., 2000. Long-term outcomes for surgically resected craniopharyngiomas. Neurosurgery 46, 291–302 discussion 302–305.

Dunn, I.F., Laws, E.R., 2010. Microsurgical approaches for transsphenoidal surgery. In: Laws, E.R., Lanzino, G. (Eds.), Transsphenoidal Surgery, First ed. Elsevier, Philadelphia, PA: Saunders.

Dusick, J.R., Esposito, F., Kelly, D.F., Cohan, P., Desalles, A., Becker, D.P., Martin, N.A., 2005. The extended direct endonasal transsphenoidal approach for nonadenomatous suprasellar tumors. J. Neurosurg. 102, 832–841.

Fahlbusch, R., Honegger, J., Paulus, W., Huk, W., Buchfelder, M., 1999. Surgical treatment of craniopharyngiomas: experience with 168 patients. J. Neurosurg. 90, 237–250.

Gardner, P.A., Prevedello, D.M., Kassam, A.B., Snyderman, C.H., Carrau, R.L., Mintz, A.H., 2008. The evolution of the endonasal approach for craniopharyngiomas. J. Neurosurg. 108, 1043–1047.

Griffith, H.B., Veerapen, R., 1987. A direct transnasal approach to the sphenoid sinus. Technical note. J. Neurosurg. 66, 140–142.

Guiot, G., Thibaut, B., 1959. [Excision of pituitary adenomas by trans-sphenoidal route]. Neurochirurgia (Stuttg) 1, 133–150.

Hadad, G., Bassagasteguy, L., Carrau, R.L., Mataza, J.C., Kassam, A., Snyderman, C.H., Mintz, A., 2006. A novel reconstructive technique after endoscopic expanded endonasal approaches: vascular pedicle nasoseptal flap. Laryngoscope 116, 1882–1886.

Halstead, A.E., 1910. Remarks on the operative treatment of tumors of the hypophysis with the report of two cases operated on by an oro-nasal method. Surg. Gynecol. Obstet., 494–502.

Hanak, B.W., Zada, G., Nayar, V.V., Thiex, R., Du, R., Day, A.L., Laws, E.R., 2012. Cerebral aneurysms with intrasellar extension: a systematic review of clinical, anatomical, and treatment characteristics. J. Neurosurg. 116, 164–178.

Hardy, J., Wigser, S.M., 1965. Trans-sphenoidal surgery of pituitary fossa tumors with televised radiofluoroscopic control. J. Neurosurg. 23, 612–619.

Hofmann, B.M., Hollig, A., Strauss, C., Buslei, R., Buchfelder, M., Fahlbusch, R., 2012. Results after treatment of craniopharyngiomas: further experiences with 73 patients since 1997. J. Neurosurg. 116, 373–384.

Honegger, J., Buchfelder, M., Fahlbusch, R., 1999. Surgical treatment of craniopharyngiomas: endocrinological results. J. Neurosurg. 90, 251–257.

Ikeda, H., Gotoh, H., Watanabe, K., 2012. Outcome of endoscopy-assisted microscopic extended transsphenoidal surgery for suprasellar adult craniopharyngiomas. Front. Endocrinol. (Lausanne) 3, 25.

Ingraham, F.D., Matson, D.D., Mc, L.R., 1952. Cortisone and ACTH as an adjunct to the surgery of craniopharyngiomas. N. Engl. J. Med. 246, 568–571.

Jane Jr., J.A., Kiehna, E., Payne, S.C., Early, S.V., Laws Jr, E.R., 2010a. Early outcomes of endoscopic transsphenoidal surgery for adult craniopharyngiomas. Neurosurg. Focus, 28, E9.

Jane Jr., J.A., Prevedello, D.M., Alden, T.D., Laws Jr, E.R., 2010b. The transsphenoidal resection of pediatric craniopharyngiomas: a case series. J. Neurosurg. Pediatr. 5, 49–60.

Jane Jr., J.A., Thapar, K., Kaptain, G.J., Maartens, N., Laws Jr, E.R., 2002. Pituitary surgery: transsphenoidal approach. Neurosurgery 51, 435–442 discussion 442–444.

Kanter, A.S., Dumont, A.S., Asthagiri, A.R., Oskouian, R.J., Jane Jr., J.A., Laws Jr, E.R., 2005. The transsphenoidal approach. A historical perspective. Neurosurg. Focus, 18, e6.

Kaptain, G.J., Vincent, D.A., Sheehan, J.P., Laws Jr, E.R., 2001. Transsphenoidal approaches for the extracapsular resection of midline suprasellar and anterior cranial base lesions. Neurosurgery 49, 94–100 discussion 100–101.

Kassam, A.B., Gardner, P.A., Snyderman, C.H., Carrau, R.L., Mintz, A.H., Prevedello, D.M., 2008a. Expanded endonasal approach, a fully endoscopic transnasal approach for the resection of midline suprasellar craniopharyngiomas: a new classification based on the infundibulum. J. Neurosurg. 108, 715–728.

Kassam, A.B., Thomas, A., Carrau, R.L., Snyderman, C.H., Vescan, A., Prevedello, D., Mintz, A., Gardner, P., 2008b. Endoscopic reconstruction of the cranial base using a pedicled nasoseptal flap. Neurosurgery 63, ONS44–ONS52 discussion ONS52–ONS53.

Kern, E.B., Pearson, B.W., Mcdonald, T.J., Laws Jr, E.R., 1979. The transseptal approach to lesions of the pituitary and parasellar regions. Laryngoscope 89, 1–34.

Kim, E.H., Ahn, J.Y., Kim, S.H., 2011. Technique and outcome of endoscopy-assisted microscopic extended transsphenoidal surgery for suprasellar craniopharyngiomas. J. Neurosurg. 114, 1338–1349.

Kim, S.H., Yoon, J.H., Choi, J.U., Chung, S.S., Lee, K.C., 2001. Transcolumellar approach in transsphenoidal pituitary surgery for patients with small nostril. Otolaryngol. Head Neck. Surg. 125, 609–612.

Komotar, R.J., Starke, R.M., Raper, D.M., Anand, V.K., Schwartz, T.H., 2012. Endoscopic endonasal compared with microscopic transsphenoidal and open transcranial resection of craniopharyngiomas. World Neurosurg. 77, 329–341.

Lanzino, G., Laws Jr, E.R., 2003. Key personalities in the development and popularization of the transsphenoidal approach to pituitary tumors: an historical overview. Neurosurg. Clin. N. Am. 14, 1–10.

Laws Jr, E.R., 1980. Transsphenoidal microsurgery in the management of craniopharyngioma. J. Neurosurg. 52, 661–666.

Laws Jr, E.R., 1994. Transsphenoidal removal of craniopharyngioma. Pediatr. Neurosurg. 21 (Suppl. 1), 57–63.

Laws Jr, E.R., 2010. Surgical outcome in 90 patients with craniopharyngiomas: an evaluation of the transsphenoidal approach. World. Neurosurg. 74, 254–255.

Liu, J.K., Orlandi, R.R., Apfelbaum, R.I., Couldwell, W.T., 2004. Novel closure technique for the endonasal transsphenoidal approach. Technical note. J. Neurosurg. 100, 161–164.

Lopez-Serna, R., Gomez-Amador, J.L., Barges-Coll, J., Nathal-Vera, E., Revuelta-Gutierrez, R., Alonso-Vanegas, M., Ramos-Peek, M., Portocarrero-Ortiz, L., 2012. Treatment of craniopharyngioma in adults: systematic analysis of a 25-year experience. Arch. Med. Res. 43, 347–355.

Maira, G., Anile, C., Albanese, A., Cabezas, D., Pardi, F., Vignati, A., 2004. The role of transsphenoidal surgery in the treatment of craniopharyngiomas. J. Neurosurg. 100, 445–451.

Maira, G., Anile, C., Rossi, G.F., Colosimo, C., 1995. Surgical treatment of craniopharyngiomas: an evaluation of the transsphenoidal and pterional approaches. Neurosurgery 36, 715–724.

Matson, D.D., Crigler Jr, J.F., 1969. Management of craniopharyngioma in childhood. J. Neurosurg. 30, 377–390.

Mortini, P., Losa, M., Pozzobon, G., Barzaghi, R., Riva, M., Acerno, S., Angius, D., Weber, G., Chiumello, G., Giovanelli, M., 2011. Neurosurgical treatment of craniopharyngioma in adults and children: early and long-term results in a large case series. J. Neurosurg. 114, 1350–1359.

Oskouian, R.J., Kelly, D.F., Laws Jr, E.R., 2006a. Vascular injury and transsphenoidal surgery. Front. Horm. Res. 34, 256–278.

Oskouian, R.J., Samii, A., Laws Jr, E.R., 2006b. The craniopharyngioma. Front. Horm. Res. 34, 105–126.

Otto, B.A., Bowe, S.N., Carrau, R.L., Prevedello, D.M., Ditzel Filho, L.F., De Lara, D., 2013. Transsphenoidal approach with nasoseptal flap pedicle transposition: Modified rescue flap technique. Laryngoscope.

Prabhu, V.C., Brown, H.G., 2005. The pathogenesis of craniopharyngiomas. Childs. Nerv. Syst. 21, 622–627.

Rivera-Serrano, C.M., Snyderman, C.H., Gardner, P., Prevedello, D., Wheless, S., Kassam, A.B., Carrau, R.L., Germanwala, A., Zanation, A., 2011. Nasoseptal "rescue" flap: a novel modification of the nasoseptal flap technique for pituitary surgery. Laryngoscope 121, 990–993.

Roderick, E., Karavitaki, N., Wass, J.A., 2008. Craniopharyngiomas. Historical aspects of their management. Hormones (Athens) 7, 271–274.

Schloffer, H., 1907. Erfolgreiche Operationen eines Hypophysentumors auf Nasalem Wege. Wien. Klin. Wochenschr. 20, 621–624.

Scott, R.M., Hetelekidis, S., Barnes, P.D., Goumnerova, L., Tarbell, N.J., 1994. Surgery, radiation, and combination therapy in the treatment of childhood craniopharyngioma – a 20 year experience. Pediatr. Neurosurg. 21 (Suppl. 1), 75–81.

Van Effenterre, R., Boch, A.L., 2002. Craniopharyngioma in adults and children: a study of 122 surgical cases. J. Neurosurg. 97, 3–11.

Villani, R.M., Tomei, G., Bello, L., Sganzerla, E., Ambrosi, B., Re, T., Giovanelli Barilari, M., 1997. Long-term results of treatment for craniopharyngioma in children. Childs. Nerv. Syst. 13, 397–405.

Weiner, H.L., Wisoff, J.H., Rosenberg, M.E., Kupersmith, M.J., Cohen, H., Zagzag, D., Shiminski-Maher, T., Flamm, E.S., Epstein, F.J., Miller, D.C., 1994. Craniopharyngiomas: a clinicopathological analysis of factors predictive of recurrence and functional outcome. Neurosurgery 35, 1001–1010 discussion 1010–1011.

Weiss, M.H., 1987. Transnasal transsphenoidal approach. In: Apuzzo, M.L. (Ed.), Surgery of the Third Ventricle. Williams and Wilkins, Baltimore.

Wilson, W.R., Khan, A., Laws Jr, E.R., 1990. Transseptal approaches for pituitary surgery. Laryngoscope 100, 817–819.

Wilson, W.R., Laws Jr, E.R., 1992. Transnasal septal displacement approach for secondary transsphenoidal pituitary surgery. Laryngoscope 102, 951–953.

Yamada, S., Fukuhara, N., Oyama, K., Takeshita, A., Takeuchi, Y., Ito, J., Inoshita, N., 2010. Surgical outcome in 90 patients with craniopharyngioma: an evaluation of transsphenoidal surgery. World. Neurosurg. 74, 320–330.

Yang, I., Sughrue, M.E., Rutkowski, M.J., Kaur, R., Ivan, M.E., Aranda, D., Barani, I.J., Parsa, A.T., 2010. Craniopharyngioma: a comparison of tumor control with various treatment strategies. Neurosurg. Focus 28, E5.

Yasargil, M.G., Curcic, M., Kis, M., Siegenthaler, G., Teddy, P.J., Roth, P., 1990. Total removal of craniopharyngiomas. Approaches and long-term results in 144 patients. J. Neurosurg. 73, 3–11.

Zada, G., Du, R., Laws Jr, E.R., 2011. Defining the "edge of the envelope": patient selection in treating complex sellar-based neoplasms via transsphenoidal versus open craniotomy. J. Neurosurg. 114, 286–300.

Zada, G., Kelly, D.F., Cohan, P., Wang, C., Swerdloff, R., 2003. Endonasal transsphenoidal approach for pituitary adenomas and other sellar lesions: an assessment of efficacy, safety, and patient impressions. J. Neurosurg. 98, 350–358.

Zada, G., Lin, N., Ojerholm, E., Ramkissoon, S., Laws, E.R., 2010. Craniopharyngioma and other cystic epithelial lesions of the sellar region: a review of clinical, imaging, and histopathological relationships. Neurosurg. Focus 28, E4.

CHAPTER

10

Pterional Approach for the Resection of Craniopharyngioma

Ravi H. Gandhi, Troy D. Payner

Goodman Campbell Brain and Spine, Indiana University School on Medicine, IN, USA

"Disheartening from an operative standpoint, for they represent one of the most baffling of surgical problems." **Harvey Cushing, 1932**

INTRODUCTION

It is well known that resections of craniopharyngiomas are surgically challenging. The vital structures surrounding these lesions, including the optic and oculomotor nerves, the hypothalamus, the third ventricle, the arteries and perforators of the circle of Willis, and the pituitary stalk make the risk of surgical morbidity and mortality significant. The soft and cystic nature of craniopharyngiomas allows them to grow around and between critical structures, but can also lead to distorted anatomy. This complexity has forced skull-based neurosurgeons to select surgical approaches to maximize exposure, improve visualization from different vantage points, and use microsurgical techniques that help mitigate the risks.

The location of craniopharyngiomas can be divided into four categories on the basis of pre-operative imaging: suprasellar-prechiasmatic, suprasellar-retrochiasmatic, third ventricular, and sellar. The locations help dictate the surgical approach, which falls into three broad categories: anterior midline, frontotemporal or pterional, and transphenoidal. This chapter presents the pterional approach. (Transphenoidal and subfrontal approaches are discussed elsewhere in this book.)

Craniopharyngiomas arise from the pituitary stalk and grow subarachnoid extrapial (Wang et al., 2005). Tumor growth leads to compression of the normal arachnoid planes in the early phases, allowing extracapsular dissection of the tumor. Giant tumors may extend beyond the normal arachnoid planes and lead to pial adhesions, making dissection more difficult. Recurrent tumors, those that have been irradiated, or tumors that are purely intraventricular certainly add to the complexity of subarachnoid dissection.

Selection of the appropriate surgical approach or combination of approaches requires careful evaluation of the pre-operative images in regard to the neural and vascular structures

Craniopharyngiomas
http://dx.doi.org/10.1016/B978-0-12-416706-3.00010-6

that are involved, along with careful consideration of the patient's pre-operative status and goals of surgery. In general, the goal of surgery should be to maximize resection and minimize the risk of post-operative morbidity. However, this must be based on anatomical and tumor-specific characteristics, and patient-specific circumstances.

PTERIONAL CRANIOTOMY

The pterional approach is the workhorse of the transcranial approaches for many pathologies, including craniopharyngiomas (Yasargil et al., 1990). It offers the shortest working distance to the suprasellar space, and with little modification, it can be used to treat craniopharyngiomas in nearly all tumor extensions. It can be used to treat tumors that extend into the prechiasmatic, retrochiasmatic, suprasellar, intrasellar, and lateral parasellar spaces. By opening the lamina terminalis, tumors extending into the third ventricle can also be removed (Maira et al., 2000). It must be understood that not all pterional craniotomies are the same. The exposure necessary for removal of a large craniopharyngioma requires the surgeon to push the limits of the standard pterional craniotomy, usually without the need for a skull base adjunct such as an orbitozygomatic oseotomy. In this chapter, the details of maximizing the pterional approach, the "pturbo pterional," are presented as they apply to craniopharyngiomas.

PTURBO PTERIONAL

Patient Positioning

The pterional craniotomy for craniopharyngiomas is most commonly performed on the right side unless the patient has worse vision on the left, or the tumor is significantly eccentric to the left. The patient is placed in a supine position with the head in the Mayfield three-point fixation device. Two pins are placed on the occiput and the third pin in the forehead as far lateral as possible without involving the temporalis muscle. This position of the Mayfield optimizes the subsequent position of the Doro Halo (Pro Med Instruments; Freiburg, Germany) brain protection system. There are four planes of movement for the head starting from the neutral position. First, the head is lifted straight up about by 2 inches (5 cm) with the patient facing the ceiling. Second, the head is rotated by no more than 15 degrees to the opposite side of the approach. Third, the head is extended to allow the frontal lobe to fall away from the skull base. The fourth plane of movement is a tilt of the head to the opposite side, opening up the angle between the patient's ear and shoulder on the side of the approach. This last maneuver gives more working space to the surgeon and his assistant, while allowing the scrub nurse access to pass instruments freely. It also expands the space for the microscope, which is always brought in from the patient's left side.

Skin Incision and Extracranial Exposure

A curvilinear incision (Figure 10.1) is made 5 mm anterior to the tragus, starting just above the root of the zygoma and extending to the midline just behind the hairline. A cutaneous flap is then reflected anteriorly. Deep sharp dissection to the superficial fat pad is performed to

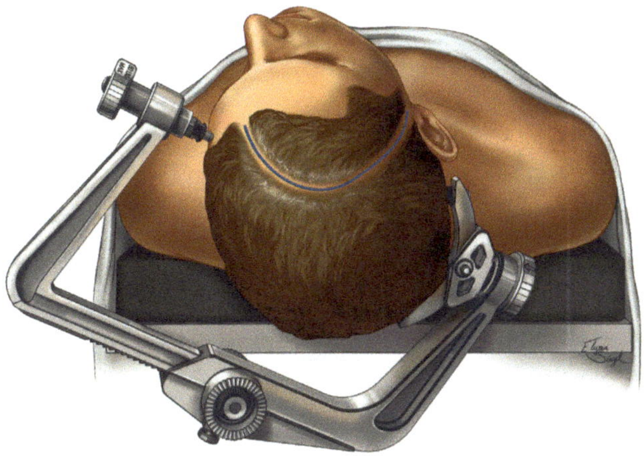

FIGURE 10.1 An illustration of the senior author's incision for a pterional craniotomy. A strip of hair is left anterior to the incision.

reflect the fat pad anteriorly and protect the frontalis branch of the facial nerve. The temporalis muscle is incised along the superior temporal line, leaving a cuff of muscle for reattaching it when closing. This flap is then reflected antero-inferiorly and secured with fish hooks. It is not enough to simply hold back the flap with fish hooks. The flap must be held low enough to keep it from obstructing the surgeon's view along the skull base. This can be accomplished by securing a Kerlix gauze to the foot of the table and attaching the fish hooks to the sterile Kerlix with a clamp. Because the gauze is fixed to the table, it will not give way during the operation and the flap will remain securely retracted. The surgeon makes a single burr hole at the keyhole area and creates a craniotomy, carefully staying low along the anterior skull base over the orbital rim and extending medially. The frontal sinus can be avoided in most patients unless it is quite large. The craniotomy should also include temporal lobe exposure.

Once the craniotomy is completed, attention is given to removing the sphenoid wing. The first step in doing this is to free the dura from the frontal floor and the anterior temporal fossa on each side of the pterion past the superior orbital fissure on each side. The second is to remove the bone overlying the anterior temporal tip. This can be done with a rongeur. Next, the lesser wing of the sphenoid is drilled flat, leaving a thin cortical bone on the orbital roof and lateral wall. An important modification of the traditional pterional craniotomy devised by the senior author (TDP) is removal of bone 270 degrees around the superior orbital fissure to enhance visualization via improved dural retraction (Figure 10.2). The periorbita is exposed around the superior orbital fissure. The sphenoid wing is curved from its lateral extent to its medial extent at the anterior clinoid process; however, the wing is essentially straight from the superior orbital fissure to the anterior clinoid. By drilling the wing down to the superior orbital fissure, a completely flat surface is created. A subfrontal approach can be taken all the way to the optic nerve with virtually no brain retraction. This is similar to an orbitozygomatic osteotomy, but without removal of the orbital rim.

Dural Opening

The dura is opened in a C-shaped fashion, with the base at the sphenoid wing and sutured to the cutaneous flap. Some temporal lobe exposure is beneficial, so the dural opening should

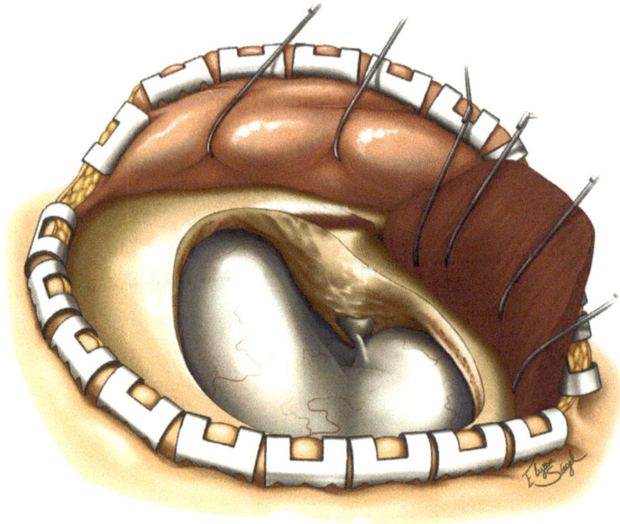

FIGURE 10.2 An illustration of removal of bone around the meningo-orbital band (MOB). This addition to the traditional pterional improves the retraction of dura.

cross the Sylvian fissure. In addition to suturing the dural flap, a single suture can be placed to tack back the edge of the temporal dura to provide more temporal lobe exposure and create a "ledge" to delay any extradural ooze of blood from dripping into the intradural compartment. There should be no dural folds in the flap that could obstruct the surgeon's view across the skull base.

Microscopic Exposure

A brain protector is placed subfrontally along the skull base straight to the optic nerve. The protector blade should remain flat along the dura of the skull base to avoid brain injury. Once the nerve is identified, the optico-carotid cistern is opened to allow the cerebrospinal fluid egress to facilitate brain relaxation. At this point, the arachnoid is sharply dissected over the optic nerve and the carotid. Once the carotid is identified, the proximal portion of the Sylvian fissure is opened to expose the A1 segment of the anterior cerebral artery and enlarge the working corridor (Figure 10.3).

The tumor will usually be seen first in the prechiasmatic space, and the arachnoid should be opened over it to further relax the frontal lobe. The falciform ligament should always be opened early in the surgery to allow greater mobility of the optic nerve. The bone overlying the optic canal is often thinned by the tumor and can be removed with a sickle knife. After the surgeon identifies the optic nerve, it is followed back to the optic chiasm and ultimately to the contralateral optic nerve. The tumor is then dissected through various corridors, including the prechiasmatic space, the optico-carotid triangle, the carotid-oculomotor triangle, and, for extension into the third ventricle, through the lamina terminalis.

Depending on the tumor's size, initial dissection of the tumor capsule may be left intact because the tumor's turgor can help with microdissection. Usually the tumor capsule is opened in the prechiasmatic cistern first to drain any cystic portion. The surgeon attempts to suction the cystic contents to reduce the risk of chemical meningitis and cerebrospinal fluid

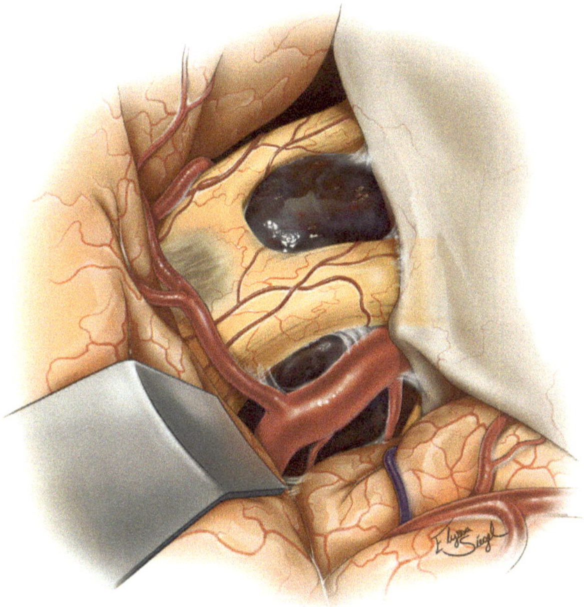

FIGURE 10.3 An illustration demonstrating the various corridors for tumor resection.

seeding. Once the cyst is drained, the tumor can be removed piecemeal by debulking it internally and then removing portions of the capsule.

When using the pterional approach, it is best to first remove the tumor from the medial side of the contralateral optic nerve and the carotid artery. The capsule will generally "peel" away with blunt and sharp dissection. Further dissection can proceed by following the contralateral optic nerve back to the optic chiasm. The contralateral A1 can also be seen at this point. The bulk of the remaining tumor will be behind the ipsilateral optic nerve and possibly in the third ventricle if the tumor is large enough. There may also be tumor protruding back to the membrane of Lillequist. By working in the plane between the optic nerve and the carotid, the capsule can be dissected off the posterior communicating artery and its perforators, as well as the anterior choroidal artery. Typically these vessels can be visualized through the window between the carotid and the oculomotor nerve, but dissection between these vessels in this window is not advised. Once the vessels are identified, the tumor capsule should be dissected from the medial side of the carotid teasing the capsule into the space created by debulking the tumor. This affords the best chance of preserving these vessels and their perforators without injury.

There are three areas of greatest challenge when removing a craniopharyngioma via a pterional approach. These include removing:

1) The portion behind the ipsilateral optic nerve,
2) The portion in the third ventricle, and
3) The portion involving the infundibulum.

The portion behind the ipsilateral optic nerve should be removed only after the tumor has been debulked and the falciform ligament opened as described above. At this point, the surgeon should use sharp dissection to open the arachnoid along the medial border of the nerve from proximal to distal. It is then usually possible to use blunt dissection to "peel" the tumor away from the nerve on the medial and lateral sides as the surgeon tries to bring the tumor into the center which has already been removed. It is easiest to find this plane near the skull base between the optic nerve and carotid artery.

The ophthalmic artery should be identified early to avoid injuring it. Once the plane of the capsule of the tumor is mobilized proximally along the nerve, it can be debulked while it is dissected free of the underside of the nerve distally and then followed out to the ipsilateral chiasm, ultimately meeting the dissection plane from the contralateral side of the chiasm dissected earlier. It is vital to preserve the vasculature of the optic nerve and avoid excessive manipulation. If any tumor is to be left behind, the underside of the ipsilateral optic nerve is the likely place.

Tumor in the third ventricle can be removed through the lamina terminalis. By exposing the lamina terminalis behind the chiasm and below the anterior communicating artery, an opening can be made. The opening should start just behind the chiasm and be extended posteriorly. Usually the lamina terminalis is discolored, expanded, and quite obvious. If the tumor is large enough to extend into the third ventricle, the surgeon can create a large enough space in the lamina terminalis and resect the tumor through this opening. First the tumor is debulked. The capsule can be identified along the contralateral wall of the third ventricle. As the tumor is debulked, it will "deliver" itself from a position higher in the third ventricle with gentle traction. Often there will be a cystic portion of the tumor in the third ventricle, and this can make it easier to debulk so that the capsule can be identified. It is also possible to deliver this portion of the tumor downward behind the chiasm and remove it through the prechiasmatic space, rather than by pulling it out through the lamina terminalis. Typically, as the superior pole of the tumor is delivered from the superior third ventricle there will be a gush of cerebrospinal fluid (CSF), indicating that the top of the tumor has been reached. At this point a movable Yasargil mirror (Braun, Melsungen, Germany) or even a small endoscope can be used to look up into the third ventricle and ensure that the tumor has been removed.

The infundibulum can often be spared with microdissection. The challenge is to identify it before injuring it, because it may blend into the capsule of the tumor. The infundibulum courses along the back of the tumor, usually eccentric to one side. As more and more tumor is debulked and the anterior portion of the tumor is removed, it becomes easier to develop the plane behind the capsule of the tumor in front of the membrane of Lillequist. It is here that the infundibulum can be identified. Typically the infundibulum will be seen coming out of the sella and "merging" with the tumor. It can even be splayed out over the tumor capsule. Again, sharp dissection is best to identify its margins and cut along them on each side.

A plane can usually be developed to peel the tumor capsule away from the infundibulum, but sometimes the tumor blends into it and small remnants of tumor must be left behind. As the infundibulum courses toward the hypothalamus behind the chiasm, it can be difficult to follow, but the tumor capsule removed from the third ventricle will spare the infundibulum superiorly.

Tips for Success

It is much easier to remove tumor from the contralateral nerve and carotid when using the pterional approach, and this should be done early in the operation. Tumor should be removed from behind the ipsilateral nerve before working along the infundibulum or on the portion in the third ventricle. To protect the ipsilateral nerve, widely open the falciform ligament and the optic foramen. This allows increased mobilization of the nerve with less risk of injury. Sharp dissection should be used along the medial border of the ipsilateral nerve, and then blunt dissection to further mobilize the tumor away from it. Electrocauterization should be avoided near the optic nerve. A Yasargil movable mirror can be used to inspect the inferior surface of the optic chiasm for residual tumor. It can also be used to see into the third ventricle and identify any remaining tumor. The most likely places for residual tumor are on the underside of the ipsilateral optic nerve and chiasm and adherent to the infundibulum.

Overall, adherence to the principles presented here will lead to very successful resection of craniopharyngiomas with low morbidity. This approach affords many advantages, including the familiarity of the normal anatomy to most neurosurgeons. It also affords a wide view of both optic nerves, the chiasm, and the carotid arteries, and it allows access to the third ventricle via the lamina terminalis. The limitation of this approach may be if the tumor has a very cephalad or posterior extension into the third ventricle. In rare circumstances, this may require the addition of an orbitozygomatic modification to the craniotomy to maximize superior visualization and access.

ILLUSTRATIVE CASE

A 23-year-old man presented with severe headaches and rapid progression of vision loss. Magnetic resonance imaging (MRI) demonstrated a large cystic suprasellar mass with compression of the optic chiasm and extension into the third ventricle and interpeduncular cistern (Figure 10.4). The senior author (TDP) performed a pterional approach to the tumor. A small remnant of tumor was left on the inferior aspect of the optic chiasm and the right internal carotid artery (Figure 10.5). The pituitary stalk was preserved. After surgery, the patient had transient diabetes insipidus and near complete resolution of his bitemporal hemianopsia.

EXPERIENCE

We retrospectively reviewed 28 pterional craniotomies in 26 patients performed by the senior author (TDP) from 1996 through 2013. This is compared with the literature in regard to extent of resection, recurrence, and outcome.

All patients had a resection performed by the senior author via a "Pturbo" pterional approach with an attempt at gross total resection without compromising neurologic function and preservation of the pituitary stalk when possible. All patients had a post-operative MRI with contrast within 3 months of surgery, and follow-up imaging on an annual basis after that unless there was evidence of growth.

The patients' ages ranged from seven to 86 years (mean 49). Ten patients were female and 16 were male. The primary complaint was vision loss in 23 patients (88.5%) and endocrine symptoms in three patients (11.5%). Other symptoms included headache, memory loss,

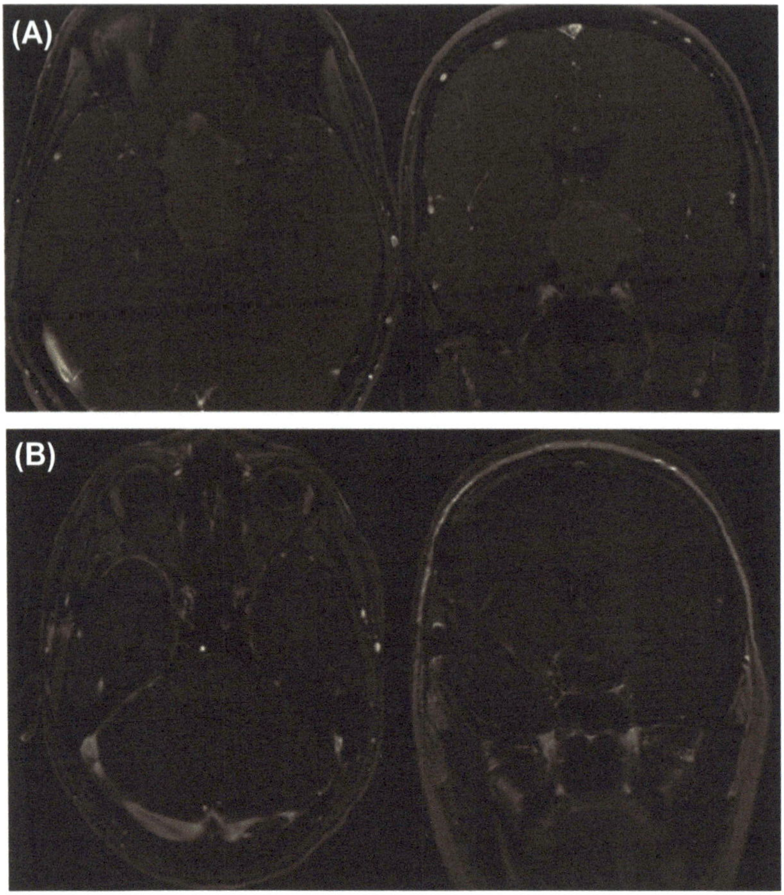

FIGURE 10.4 **A,** A pre-operative gadolinium-enhanced MRI (axial and coronal) demonstrating a large suprasellar craniopharyngioma with extension into the third ventricle. **B,** A post-operative gadolinium-enhanced MRI (axial and coronal) after resection. This demonstrates a small remnant of tumor inferior to the chiasm.

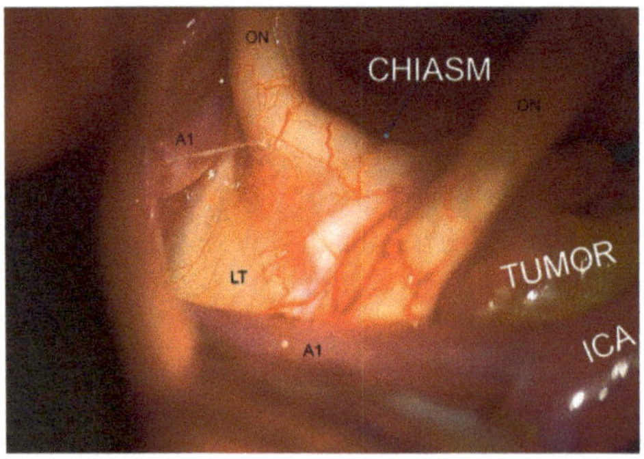

FIGURE 10.5 Intra-operative photograph of the pterional approach to a suprasellar craniopharyngioma after partial resection of the tumor. (ICA: internal carotid artery; ON: optic nerve; A1: First division of the ACA.)

and confusion. Two patients had had previous surgery for craniopharyngioma before presenting to the senior author. One of these had undergone resection via a pterional craniotomy and the other had undergone a previous transphenoidal resection. Both of these patients experienced worsening of their visual symptoms, and this prompted resection of the recurrence.

The tumors ranged in size from 1 to 5.5 cm (mean 2.4 cm), and ten extended into the third ventricle. Based on the operative reports, 20 of 26 (77%) had a gross total resection. In the six cases of residual tumor, the reason for leaving tumor was adherence to the inferior surface of the chiasm or incorporation into the pituitary stalk. Six patients had post-operative tumor growth evident on follow-up imaging. Only three of these patients had residual tumor at the time of the initial surgery; the other three patients did not have any residual tumor evident on an MRI immediately after surgery.

Two patients were returned to the operating room for resection of the recurrence because of progressive vision loss. Patients with a subtotal resection or recurrence were referred for radiation therapy. There were two post-operative deaths. Both of these patients had significant medical co-morbidities, and they were the two oldest patients in this series. One of these patients had a subarachnoid hemorrhage evident on the immediate post-operative CT and the other experienced a delayed intraparenchymal hemorrhage.

Of the 23 patients with visual deficit, 13 had resolution of their visual symptoms, three had some improvement, three patients' vision remained stable, two were not assessed because they died, and two had worsening visual symptoms. The two that worsened had decreased vision in the side that was worse before surgery, but improved visual fields in the contralateral eye.

Other authors have reported gross resection rates between 73 and 93%; similar to our series (Yasargil et al., 1990; Dehdashti and de Tribolet, 2008; Jung et al., 2009; Elliott and Wisoff, 2010; Gerganov et al., 2014; Kunihiro et al., 2014). Although six patients (23%) had recurrence, only two patients became symptomatic and required subsequent surgery. Large operative series of craniopharyngioma have reported mortality rates of 1.1–13.5% (Yasargil et al., 1990; Fahlbusch and Hofmann, 2008; Mortini et al., 2011), and the rate is our series was 8.7% (two of 23), so it is within the range reported by other studies. A total of 16 of 23 patients (69.6%) had improvement in their visual fields. This series demonstrates that the "Pturbo" pterional approach is a safe and efficacious approach to the resection of craniopharyngioma.

References

Cushing, H., 1932. Papers relating to the pituitary body, hypothalamus and parasympathetic nervous system. Charles C. Thomas, Springfield, p 51.

Dehdashti, A.R., de Tribolet, N., 2008. Frontobasal interhemispheric trans-lamina terminalis approach for suprasellar lesions. Neurosurgery 62 (6 Suppl. 3), 1233–1239.

Elliott, R.E., Wisoff, J.H., 2010. Surgical management of giant pediatric craniopharyngiomas. J. Neurosurg. Pediatr. 6 (5), 403–416.

Fahlbusch, R., Hofmann, B.M., 2008. Surgical management of giant craniopharyngiomas. Acta. Neurochir. 150 (12), 1213–1226.

Gerganov, V., Metwali, H., Samii, A., Fahlbusch, R., Samii, M., 2014. Microsurgical resection of extensive craniopharyngiomas using a frontolateral approach: operative technique and outcome. J. Neurosurg. 120 (2), 559–570.

Jung, T.Y., Jung, S., Choi, J.E., Moon, K.S., Kim, I.Y., Kang, S.S., 2009. Adult craniopharyngiomas: surgical results with a special focus on endocrinological outcomes and recurrence according to pituitary stalk preservation. J. Neurosurg. 111 (3), 572–577.

Kunihiro, N., Goto, T., Ishibashi, K., Ohata, K., 2014. Surgical outcomes of the minimum anterior and posterior combined transpetrosal approach for resection of retrochiasmatic craniopharyngiomas with complicated conditions. J. Neurosurg. 120 (1), 1–11.

Maira, G., Anile, C., Colosimo, C., Cabezas, D., 2000. Craniopharyngiomas of the third ventricle: trans-lamina terminalis approach. Neurosurgery 47 (4), 857–863 discussion 863–855.

Mortini, P., Losa, M., Pozzobon, G., et al., 2011. Neurosurgical treatment of craniopharyngioma in adults and children: early and long-term results in a large case series. J. Neurosurg. 114 (5), 1350–1359.

Wang, K.C., Hong, S.H., Kim, S.K., Cho, B.K., 2005. Origin of craniopharyngiomas: implication on the growth pattern. Childs. Nerv. Sys. 21 (8-9), 628–634.

Yasargıl, M.G., Curcic, M., Kis, M., Siegenthaler, G., Teddy, P.J., Roth, P., 1990. Total removal of craniopharyngiomas. Approaches and long-term results in 144 patients. J. Neurosurg. 73 (1), 3–11.

CHAPTER

11

The Frontolateral Approach to Adult Craniopharyngiomas

Alessandra Mantovani, Manuel Ferreira, Jr., Laligam N. Sekhar

Department of Neurological Surgery, University of Washington, Harborview Medical Center, Seattle, WA, USA

"Meticulous attention to details in the preoperative and postoperative care of patients, through innumerable small maneuvers before, but especially during and after operation, may avert disaster or shorten convalescence; if neglected, they may cost a patient's life." ***Ernest Sachs, 1949***

Craniopharyngiomas are histologically benign, extra-axial, epithelial tumors. Although classified as low-grade neoplasms, the natural history of these tumors is unpredictable and they often present with locally invasive growth patterns and an aggressive clinical course, resulting in significant morbidity. Craniopharyngiomas represent 1–4.6% of all intracranial tumors and 13% of sellar and suprasellar tumors. The incidence of these tumors is estimated as 0.5–2.5 new cases per 1 million population per year. From a histopathological perspective, craniopharyngiomas are broadly classified into adamantinomatous and papillary types. The papillary craniopharyngiomas present almost exclusively in adults, at a mean age of 40–55 years, while adamantinomatous craniopharyngiomas have a bimodal distribution: they occurr either in children aged 5–15 years and in adults aged 40–55 years (Rushing et al., 2007). This chapter mainly discusses the lesions in adults, although it is broadly applicable to children also.

SURGICAL ANATOMY

Craniopharyngiomas are solid tumors with a variable cystic component. The adamantinomatous type may be multicystic, containing a cholesterol-rich fluid, while the papillary type usually lacks the cystic component. Calcifications are often present and they may be abundant.

These epithelial tumors take origin from the remnants of the craniopharyngeal duct or Rathke's pouch. Cell rests of this embryonic structure can be found from the infundibulum to

Craniopharyngiomas
http://dx.doi.org/10.1016/B978-0-12-416706-3.00011-8

the pituitary gland. The site of origin of these lesions can predict their growth pattern, as can the appearance of the optic chiasm and the relationship with the surrounding structures. The normal location of the optic chiasm is over the sellar diaphragm and pituitary gland, but it may manifest variations on the horizontal plane. The chiasm is referred to as prefixed when it is positioned superior to the tuberculum sellae, and postfixed when it is superior to the dorsum sellae (Gulsen et al., 2010). According to the position of the optic chiasm, the tumor can grow anteriorly in the case of postfixed chiasm, or posteriorly in the case of prefixed chiasm. Knowledge of the relationship of the tumor with the surrounding structures, especially the location of the optic chiasm and the pituitary gland, is essential when planning the best approach to the lesion.

Craniopharyngiomas can grow either below or above the sellar diaphragm. In the first case, the lesion grows intrasellar and suprasellar under the chiasm, which is gradually displaced upward and compressed, as is the floor of the third ventricle. Supradiaphragmatic craniopharyngiomas may have their origin in the pituitary stalk into the chiasmatic cistern or inside the infundibulum. Lesions taking origin from the pituitary stalk can extend inside the subarachnoid space under the chiasm and the floor of the third ventricle. They can be either prechiasmatic or retrochiasmatic, but this second extension is less common and can be due to a prefixed chiasm. Tumors starting from the infundibulum grow behind the chiasm, and they may invade the floor of the third ventricle, extending up to the lateral ventricles. Rarely, the tumor may be confined within the third ventricle, and extend into the lateral ventricles.

Giant craniopharyngiomas can grow in various directions and can extend into the posterior fossa. In the case of a lateral growth, the tumor may encase the internal carotid arteries (ICAs) or can be firmly attached to the wall of the cavernous sinus.

PRE-OPERATIVE STUDIES

Radiology

Magnetic resonance imaging (MRI) provides information about the heterogeneous nature of craniopharyngiomas, their topography, and relation with the other structures. Solid components of the tumor are usually isointense in T1-weighted images and, along with the wall of any cystic components, demonstrate contrast enhancement. On the T2-weighted images, it is sometimes possible to note an arachnoidal plane between the tumor and the neural structures. Fine cut post-gadolinium images are used for identifying the pituitary stalk. Calcifications are often present, and are better visualized by computed tomography (CT). A CT scan can demonstrate the bony anatomy of the skull base as well as the extent of calcification in the tumor. MR angiography or four-vessel angiography is sometimes necessary to show the relationship with the major vessels and their displacement. A catheter intra-arterial angiogram is performed when the ICA or other arteries are encased. Simultaneously, the surgeon may wish to evaluate the collateral circulation by a carotid occlusion test or a cross compression (common carotid compression angiogram).

Endocrinological Evaluation

Hypopituitarism or diabetes insipidus (DI) are common manifestations of craniopharyngiomas at diagnosis. However, they are rarely the reason for referral. Since the patient is likely to have post-operative panhypopituitarism, a complete endocrinological evaluation is performed before any treatment of craniopharyngiomas. The pre-operative endocrinological status is important for adequate pre-operative hormone replacement (particularly corticosteroids and thyroid medications), in order to reduce morbidity.

Neuro-Ophthalmological Evaluation

The pre-operative neuro-ophthalmic status should be carefully evaluated in patients. Damage to the visual pathway can be manifested as defects of the visual fields or visual acuity. Among the various visual fields defects, asymmetrical bitemporal hemianopia is the most common and is caused by compression of the optic chiasm. The patient's visual status is essential for estimating the damage caused by the tumor itself and comparing that to the visual status at follow-up.

Neurobehavioral Evaluation

Personality changes and cognitive and memory impairment may be present in adults and should be tested before surgery, for assessing the neurobehavioral status. This will impact the patient's discharge planning. Memory disorders are caused by a lesion of the mammillary bodies or by any disconnections along the limbic system. Hypothalamic hyperphagia syndrome is seen in patients with lesions located in the hypothalamic region. It is characterized by fatigue, decreased physical activity, uncontrolled appetite, and morbid obesity, and it may be associated with insulin and leptin resistance (Roth, 2011). Patients with large tumors may exhibit behavioral disorders post-operatively on a temporary basis, and the family of the patient should be prepared for this.

GOALS OF SURGERY

Surgical resection is the main treatment for craniopharyngiomas. Modern radiosurgery may be used as an option for residual or recurrent lesions (Niranjan et al., 2010; Khamlichi et al., 2013). Complete tumor removal is preferred; if a small remnant is left in order to preserve any structures, then radiation or radiosurgery may be performed. The goals of surgery are control of tumor growth, preservation, or improvement of the patient's vision, and pituitary/hypothalamic preservation. Other factors influencing the decision about the treatment include the patient's age and gender, informed consent, and the patient's goals.

CHOICE OF OPERATIVE APPROACH

Different transcranial approaches with variable modifications have been proposed, depending on the preferences and experience of the surgeon and on the position and characteristics of the tumor. The senior authors' choices have evolved over the years, according to their experience with different approaches; the authors' currently preferred approaches are summarized in Table 11.1. Retrochiasmatic tumors extending superiorly up to the third

TABLE 11.1 Authors' Preferred Approaches for Craniopharyngiomas and Patients Series

Approaches	Characteristic of Tumors	Number of Patients (%) in Our Series
Frontolateral/Transorbital	Most tumors	14 (56%)
Petrosal	Very high extending retrochiasmatic tumors (up to third and lateral ventricles)	4 (16%)
Bifrontal interhemispheric	Very high extending retrochiasmatic tumors, mainly growing inside the third ventricle	3 (12%)
Transsphenoidal endoscopic	Tumor in the midline, patients with intact pituitary function	3 (12%)
Transcallosal	Tumors extending into the lateral ventricle or frontal lobe	1 (4%)

and lateral ventricles can be reached through a *transpetrosal approach*, as well as prepeduncular or prepontine lesions. The *transcallosal approach* is reserved for tumors extending into the lateral ventricle or frontal lobe. A *bifrontal, interhemispheric approach* is sometimes used for tumors mainly growing inside the third ventricle. An *endonasal endoscopic transsphenoidal approach* minimizes the risk of damage of the pituitary stalk and gland, hypothalamus, and optic apparatus. It is mainly preferred for midline tumors, especially when the pituitary function is intact, and no vascular encasement is present. The *frontolateral approach*, utilized for most tumors, offers a short distance to the suprasellar region as well as an optimal visualization of the anatomical structures. The basal cisterns can be easily opened, resulting in early cerebrospinal fluid (CSF) drainage and subsequent decompression. The orbital osteotomy permits a lower, basal approach than the classic pterional approach. Compared to the bifrontal approach, the frontolateral approach avoids olfactory nerve injuries and bifrontal lobe retractions (Shirane et al., 2002; Chi et al., 2006; Gerganov et al., 2013).

FRONTOLATERAL APPROACH

Position and Initial Exposure

The patient is placed in the supine position and the head is fixed in extension, rotated 30° to the opposite side of the craniotomy using a Mayfield head holder. A bicoronal skin incision is made. The flap is then reflected forward, along with pericranium. The pericranial flap should be preserved for the reconstruction of skull base defects. After elevating the temporalis muscle and separating the dura mater in the frontal region, a frontal craniotomy and a small temporal craniotomy are performed. Regardless of the side with worse vision, a right-sided approach is usually preferred, unless the lateral extension of the tumor is mainly on the left side. The orbital osteotomy is then performed on the side of the craniotomy.

The frontal and temporal dura mater are carefully separated from the roof and lateral walls of the orbit. The periorbita is separated as well, and the supraorbital nerve is preserved. An osteotomy of the roof and lateral wall of the orbit is performed. Under the surgical microscope, the superior orbital fissure is first unroofed, with the removal of the greater and lesser wings of the sphenoid bone. The anterior clinoid process is extradurally removed, completely if possible, and the ipsilateral optic nerve is unroofed extradurally.

The frontotemporal dura is opened in a C-shaped fashion, in order to visualize the Sylvian anatomy. The optic nerve and carotid cisterns, as well as the medial part of the Sylvian fissure, are opened. The ipsilateral optic nerve, which is often stretched over the tumor, is relaxed by opening the dural sheath of the optic canal completely. The rest of the anterior clinoid process is removed intradurally, if necessary.

Exposure of the Tumor and Resection

At this point the tumor can be well seen, and the operative approach depends upon the extensions of the tumor and the position of the chiasm: normal position, prefixed, or postfixed chiasm.

In the case of postfixed chiasm, and when the tumor extends laterally, an approach through the interoptic, optico-carotid, and carotid-tentorial space is preferred (Figure 11.1): the tumor is debulked through the subchiasmatic space, and working through the three avenues, gradually separated from important neurovascular structures and removed. Special attention is paid to the superior hypophyseal arteries, which have to be carefully preserved.

For a prefixed chiasm, a translamina terminalis avenue is added to the other routes: the lamina terminalis is opened in the midline behind the crossing of the macular fibers of the optic chiasm, and the craniopharyngioma is dissected from the hypothalamic area and the posterior part of the circle of Willis. More dissection is also performed through the carotid-tentorial, and optico-carotid spaces. The planum sphenoidale is removed after opening a dural flap, and the tumor can be accessed inside an enlarged sella if needed (Figure 11.2A, B).

In the case of a cystic lesion, the tumor is drained first, and then the capsule is grasped and gently pulled, while dissection is performed in the arachnoid plane with Rhoton 3, 6, or

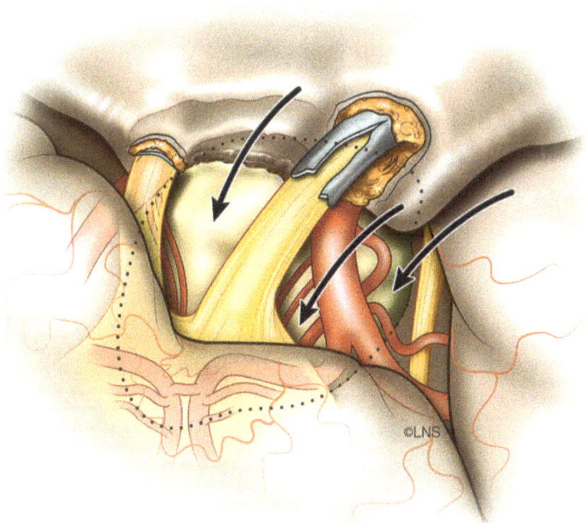

FIGURE 11.1 Optico-carotid, carotid-tentorial space approach for removal of the tumor in the case of a postfixed chiasm. The tumor extends to the lateral side and it is removed through the interoptic, carotid-oculomotor and carotid-tentorial spaces, carefully preserving the superior hypophyseal arteries.

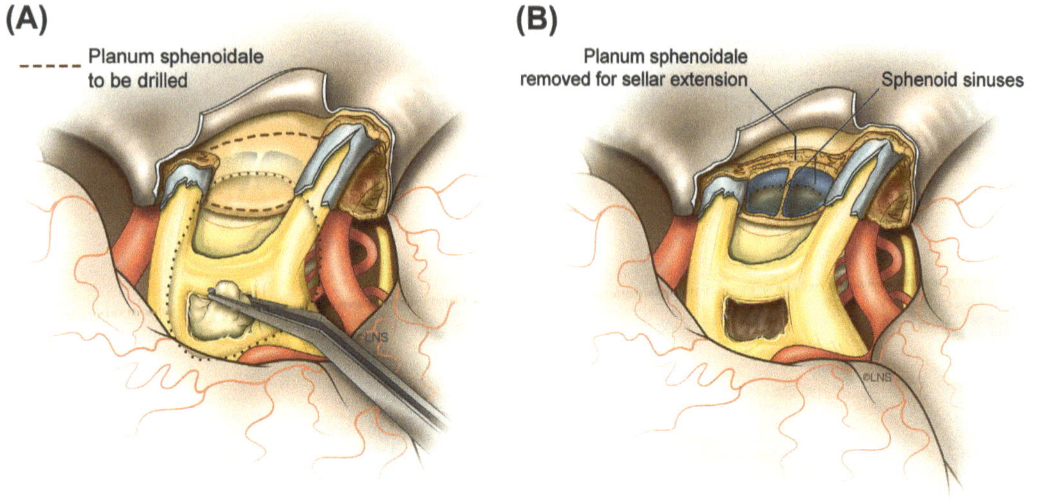

FIGURE 11.2 Approach for prefixed chiasm. **A**, A translamina terminalis approach is added to the frontolateral approach for the removal of the tumor. **B**, The planum sphenoidale is drilled and removed after opening a dural flap, to aid in the removal of the sellar and intrachiasmatic tumor.

9 instruments or microscissors. The assistant provides suction (the three hands method). Then the tumor is sharply dissected from the surrounding structures using scissors or fine microinstruments. The main attachments are expected to be to the pituitary stalk or hypothalamic area. The tumor may be quite adherent to arteries as well, even more densely than to nervous structures. In some cases a tiny remnant may be left, in order to preserve the nervous or vascular structure, especially chiasm, ICA, superior hypophyseal arteries, or hypothalamus.

Once the tumor has been partially dissected, the pituitary stalk may be identified as a longitudinally striated vascularized structure, which can be seen on any part of the capsule, but most frequently it is found on its fixed entrance through the diaphragm sellae. If the pituitary stalk is not infiltrated by the tumor, then it can be gently dissected by pulling the capsule from the lower part of the pituitary stalk. Otherwise, in order to prevent a recurrence, the stalk may be sacrificed and cut as low as possible (when pituitary functional preservation is not a goal of the surgery).

In the case of solid, fleshy, or calcified lesions, the tumor is resected piecemeal with the aid of a pituitary forceps, microscissors, ultrasonic aspirators, or the hand-held CO_2 laser (OmniGuide, Boston, Massachusetts). Sometimes the lesion is very firm and needs to be broken into smaller pieces. The tumor should be delivered into the field by a three hands technique. Sometimes, another approach (for example the transpetrosal approach or a subtemporal approach) may be needed for reaching a remaining part of the lesion.

Inspection of the tumor bed should be performed under the miscroscope. Also, an angled endoscope can be used to best visualize the surface of the nervous and vascular structures, for ensuring complete resection.

CLOSURE

If the sphenoid sinus was opened, the skull base defect has to be repaired. Abdominal fat is harvested and packed into the upper portion of the sinus. A free and large piece of pericranium is sutured circumferentially to the dural defect, and secured with fibrin glue. If the frontal sinus was opened, the mucosa is stripped off the bone first, then the frontonasal duct is packed with oxidized cellulose and a small abdominal fat graft. The sinus is then completely sealed with bone cement, and covered with a vascularized flap of pericranium, which is sutured to the basal dura. The bone flap and the orbital piece are repositioned and fixed by miniplates. Any bone defect should also be reconstructed with absorbable mesh and bone cement. In young patients, and patients with thin skin, we prefer to use the absorbable plates, in order to obtain the best aesthetic and functional result. The temporal muscle, fascia temporalis and skin layers are sutured in the usual manner.

COMPLICATIONS

Diabetes Insipidus

Transient diabetes insipidus (DI) is almost always present after surgery and it is due to surgical manipulation of the pituitary stalk. A triphasic response is expected over the first week with DI giving way to hyponatremia, followed by mild DI, or no DI at all. In the post-operative period daily fluid and electrolyte control and balance are essential and serum sodium should be monitored once every 6 hours until stable. If the pituitary stalk was damaged or cut during the operation, patients may present with permanent DI. In this case they may need a long-term vasopressin replacement. A permanent DI can sometimes be present with an intact pituitary stalk: in this case, it may be due to hypothalamic dysfunction.

Hypopituitarism

Hypopituitarism is common after the operation. It is usually caused by the compression applied by the tumor to the anterior pituitary gland, but it sometimes can be iatrogenic, caused by a direct injury during surgery. For patients with apparently intact pituitary function it is recommended to check the morning fasting cortisol level and to undergo a delayed cosyntropin stimulation test to assess the function of the pituitary–adrenal gland axis. Hypoadrenalism is very common and should always be suspected: for this reason, high doses of corticosteroids are provided before the operation and in the first 2 weeks after surgery. They may then be tapered. Further endocrinological disorders may be experienced and they are treated according to the hormone levels and physiological requirements. The patient should be managed post-operatively by an endocrinologist.

Injury to the ICA

The arachnoid plane between the tumor capsule and the ICA usually allows a sharp dissection of the lesion. The tumor capsule may sometimes be firmly adherent to the ICA, however. Special attention should be paid to patients who have undergone previous operations or radiosurgery for the tumor. If damage to the ICA occurs, the best option for repairing is by direct suture under temporary occlusion. Rarely, some patients may need a bypass when a direct repair is not feasible.

Injury of the Optic Nerve and Chiasm

Injuries of the optic nerve and chiasm are quite rare. They may occur due to excessive retraction and decompression of these structures. The chiasm and optic nerve are very sensitive to vascular damage as well. The superior hypophyseal arteries may be stretched or damaged during their tortuous course to the optic nerve (van Overbeeke and Sekhar, 2003).

Vasospasm

Vasospasm can occur up to 4 weeks after surgery, and can be the cause of delayed neurological deficits. Special vigilance is needed, especially in patients with tumors encasing the arteries. When this complication is recognized, prompt treatment is started, consisting of hydration, induced arterial hypertension, and endovascular angioplasty when needed.

OUR SERIES

From September 2005 to November 2013, 25 patients with craniopharyngiomas underwent surgical resection at Haborview Medical Center in Seattle, Washington, by the two senior authors (LNS and MFJ). Thirteen patients were men and 12 were women, with ages ranging from 14 to 81 years (mean ± standard deviation 42.6 ± 19 years). All patients were subjected to pre-operative MRI, endocrinological, and neuro-ophthalmological evaluations. Nine craniopharyngiomas (36%) were positioned in the sellar/suprasellar region, 14 (56%) were suprasellar retrochiasmatic lesions, seven of them extending to the third ventricle and one also extending to the posterior fossa. One lesion (4%) was positioned predominantly in the third ventricle, the last one (4%) was a sellar lesion extending to the right side. The mean pre-operative modified Rankin Scale (mRS) score was 1.16, ranging from 0 to 3. A total of 15/25 patients (60%) presented with visual loss, 10/25 patients (40%) with endocrinological dysfunctions, mainly due to anterior hypopituitarism. Eight patients (32%) had previous operations and presented with a remnant or a recurrent lesion.

Table 11.1 shows the operative approaches utilized in this series according to the characteristics of the tumors. Seventeen patients (68%) had a gross total resection of the tumor, while a tiny remnant was left in the other eight patients (32%), in order to preserve nervous or vascular structures. One patient, who presented in a poor condition, died during hospitalization due to multiple medical complications. The length of the follow-up for this series is 29.37 ± 23.74 months (mean ± standard deviation) and the mean mRS score at the last follow-up was 1.3. Table 11.2 shows the patients' visual and endocrine status at presentation and at follow-up. A total of 7/15 (46.7%) patients presenting with visual loss improved postoperatively. The improvement was not as positive for patients with endocrine deficiency: only 1/10 patient improved after surgery, while 10/15 (66.7%) patients presenting with intact pituitary function manifested hypopituitarism or DI at the follow-up.

TABLE 11.2 Visual and Endocrine Patients' Status at Presentation and at Follow-up

	Pre-operative status	Follow-up
Visual status	Normal: 10 (40%)	Normal: 9 (90%)
		Visual deficit: 1 (10%)
	Visual loss: 15 (60%)	Stable: 8 (53.3%)
		Improved: 7 (46.7%)
Endocrine status	Normal: 15 (60%)	Normal: 5 (33.3%)
		Endocrine deficiency/DI: 10 (66.7%)
	Endocrine deficiency: 10 (40%)	Stable: 9 (90%)
		Improved: 1 (10%)

Illustrative Case 1

This is a 65-year-old man who presented with increasing mental confusion. The MRI showed a suprasellar, retrochiasmatic lesion, measuring 25 x 25 x 31 mm (Figure 11.3A, B, C). He underwent a frontolateral approach with a total tumor resection. After the operation he manifested hypopituitarism, which necessitated hormonal replacement. At the last follow-up, 4 years after surgery, the patient exhibited chronic hypopituitarism, and no other symptoms. His MRI showed no evidence of tumor recurrence (Figure 11.4A, B, C).

Illustrative Case 2

This 17-year-old boy presented with 2 months of severe headaches, fatigue, and defects of the visual fields. His MRI showed the presence of a retrosellar lesion extending to the posterior fossa, with severe compression of the hypothalamus, the third ventricle, and the

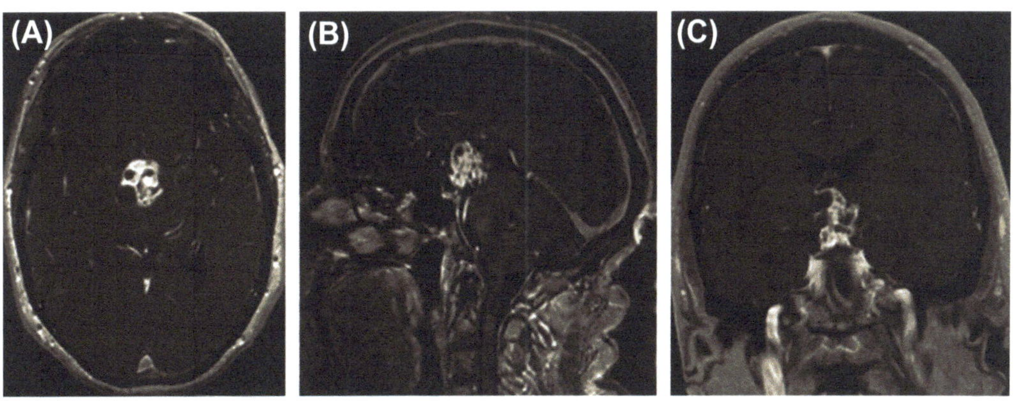

FIGURE 11.3 **A, B, C**: Pre-operative MRI for illustrative case 1. Suprasellar, retrochiasmatic lesion, removed via frontolateral approach.

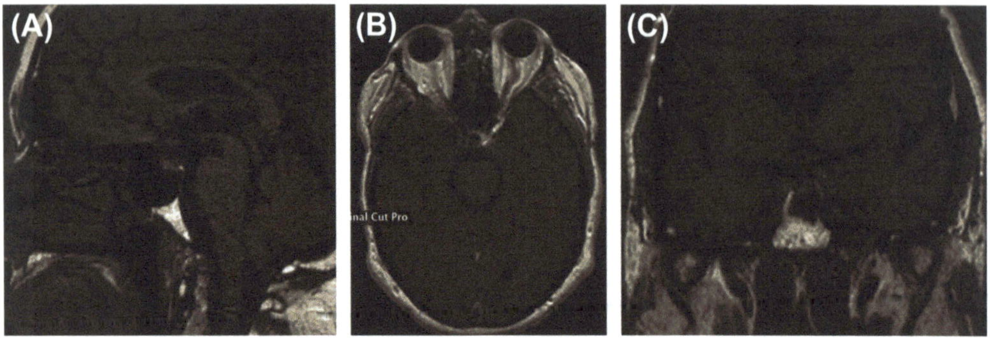

FIGURE 11.4 **A, B, C**: Post-operative MRI for illustrative case 1, showing a complete removal of the tumor.

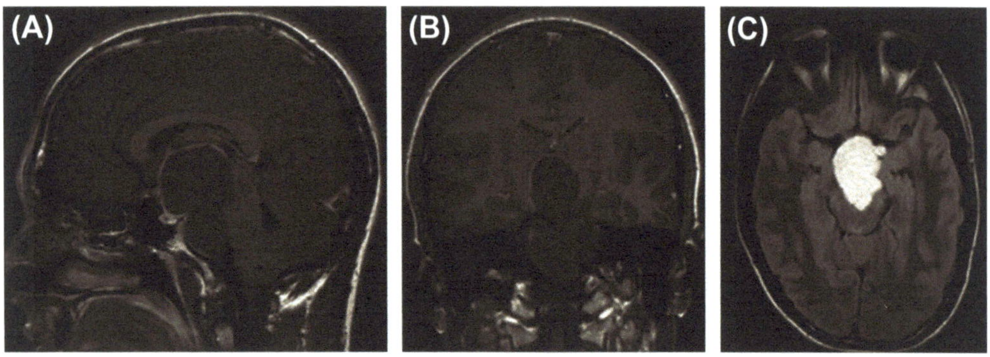

FIGURE 11.5 **A, B, C**: Pre-operative MRI for illustrative case 2. Retrosellar lesion extending to the posterior fossa, with severe compression of the hypothalamus, the third ventricle, and the brainstem, removed via the transpetrosal approach.

brainstem (Figure 11.5A, B, C). The pre-operative endocrinological evaluation also revealed low levels of cortisol and testosterone. He underwent a complete removal of the lesion through a presigmoidal transpetrosal approach. During the post-operative period the patient experienced transient DI, and transient cranial nerves III and VI palsy, which recovered completely within 3 months. At the last follow-up, 3 years after surgery, the patient was doing well, and was attending college. He had no endocrine or visual deficits and his MRI did not show any recurrence (Figure 11.6A, B).

Illustrative Case 3

This 20-year-old man had undergone removal of a craniopharyngioma at the age of 6 and had been followed by his endocrinologist for hypopituitarism. He presented to the emergency room complaining of near complete loss of vision in the left eye for about 4 days. His MRI showed a recurrent complex suprasellar retrochiasmatic lesion, measuring 17 x 18 x 18 mm, with encasement of the basilar artery (Figure 11.7A, B, C). Because of the

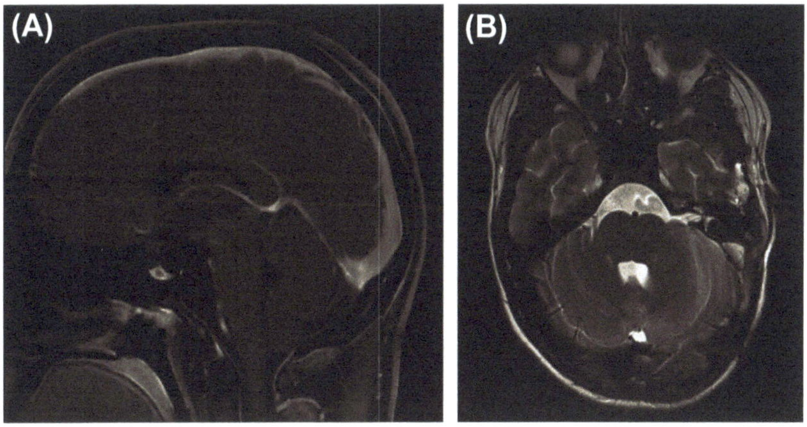

FIGURE 11.6 **A, B**: Post-operative MRI for illustrative case 2. The tumor was completely removed, no endocrine deficiency.

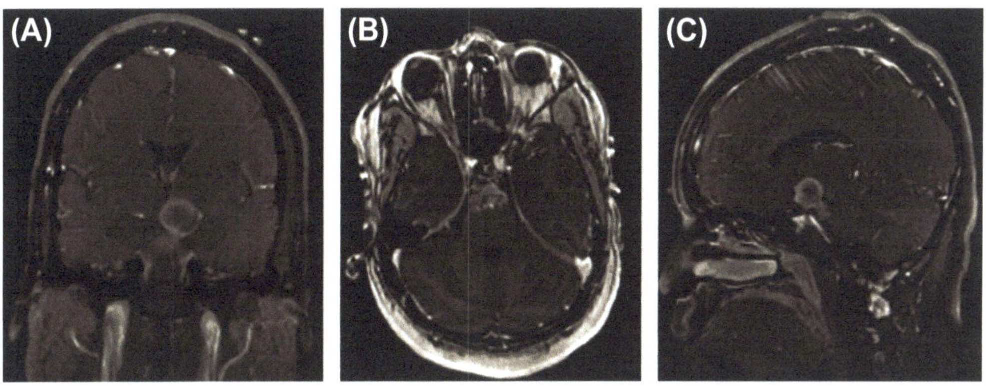

FIGURE 11.7 **A, B, C**: Pre-operative MRI for illustrative case 3. Recurrent complex suprasellar retrochiasmatic lesion, with encasement of the basilar artery. A two-stage surgery was planned, and the tumor was removed via the frontolateral approach first and the tranpetrosal approach in the second stage.

complexity and the extension of the lesion, an operation in two stages was planned. He underwent a frontolateral approach with a partial removal of the lesion first, followed by a transpetrosal approach for removing the residual posterior part of the craniopharyngioma located anterior to the brain stem with encasement of the basilar artery. Post-operatively he manifested hydrocephalus and a lumboperitoneal shunt was placed. At the last follow-up, 5 years after the operation, the patient was doing well, and functioning normally. He had completed high school, and was seeking employment. He had chronic hypopituitarism and visual deficit in the left eye: he had light perception, but was unable to discern objects with it. His MRI showed a stable small amount of enhancement in the left parasellar region (Figure 11.8A, B).

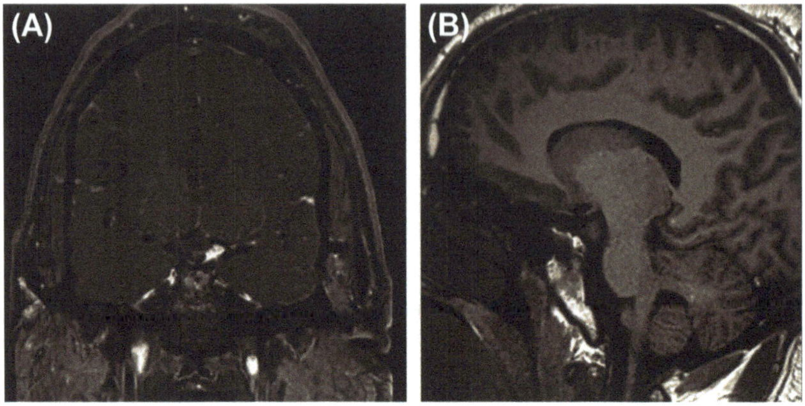

FIGURE 11.8 **A, B**: Post-operative MRI for illustrative case 3, showing a near-complete tumor removal, with a stable small amount of enhancement in the left parasellar region.

Illustrative Case 4

This is a 29-year-old woman presenting with progressive vision loss that was greater in the left eye than in the right, and bilateral visual fields cuts. Her MRI showed a suprasellar retrochiasmatic lesion, extending up to the third ventricle (Figure 11.9A, B, C). She underwent an endonasal transsphenoidal approach, with a complete removal of the tumor. Her post-operative course was complicated by a CSF leak requiring a re-exploration, and the placement of a nasal septal flap. At her last follow-up, 16 months after surgery, she was doing very well, not presenting any symptoms. Her visual deficits had completely recovered, she had intact pituitary function, no signs of DI, and she was pregnant. Her MRI did not show any recurrence (Figure 11.10A, B).

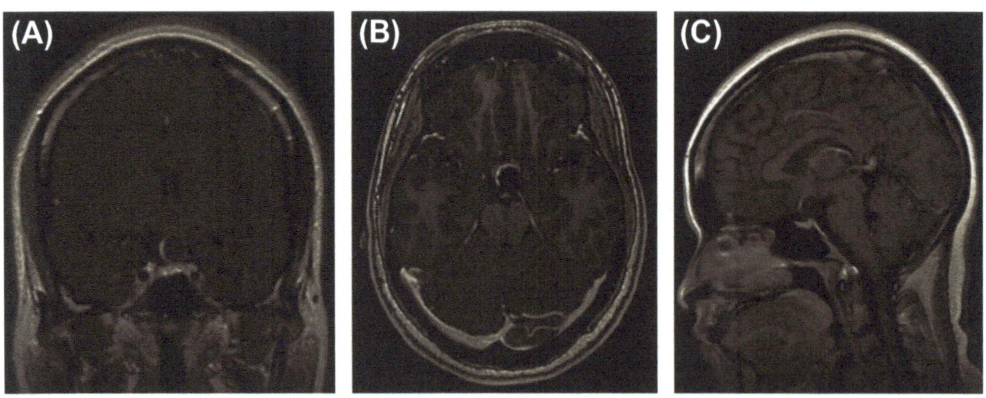

FIGURE 11.9 **A, B, C**: Pre-operative MRI for illustrative case 4. Suprasellar retrochiasmatic lesion, extending up to the third ventricle, removed via transsphenoidal approach.

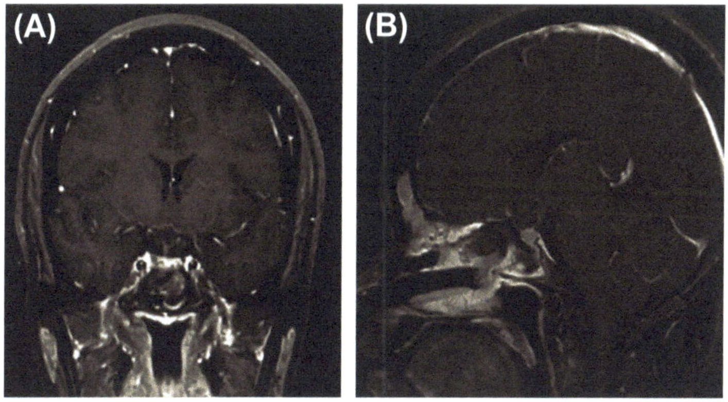

FIGURE 11.10 **A, B**: Post-operative MRI for illustrative case 4. The tumor was completely removed and the pituitary stalk was intact.

CONCLUSIONS

Craniopharyngiomas in adults are complex lesions. The majority of tumors can be removed completely, or nearly completely, with the preservation or the improvement of patients' vision. The frontolateral, transpetrosal, and endoscopic transsphenoidal are the currently preferred operative approaches. A careful endocrine management is required in both the pre-operative and post-operative phases.

Acknowledgments

The illustrations were prepared by Jennifer Pryll, medical illustrator.
Doctor Laligam N. Sekhar retains the copyright for the illustrations.

References

Chi, J.H., Parsa, A.T., Berger, M.S., Kunwar, S., McDermott, M.W., Oct 2006. Extended bifrontal craniotomy for midline anterior fossa meningiomas: minimization of retraction-related edema and surgical outcomes. Neurosurgery 59 (4 Suppl. 2). ONS426–433; discussion ONS433–424.

Gerganov, V., Metwali, H., Samii, A., Fahlbusch, R., Samii, M., Nov 22 2013. Microsurgical resection of extensive craniopharyngiomas using a frontolateral approach: operative technique and outcome. J. Neurosurg..

Gulsen, S., Dinc, A.H., Unal, M., Canturk, N., Altinors, N., Mar 2010. Characterization of the anatomic location of the pituitary stalk and its relationship to the dorsum sellae, tuberculum sellae and chiasmatic cistern. J. Korean. Neurosurg. Soc. 47 (3), 169–173.

Khamlichi, A.E., Melhaoui, A., Arkha, Y., Jiddane, M., Gueddari, B.K., 2013. Role of gamma knife radiosurgery in the management of pituitary adenomas and craniopharyngiomas. Acta. Neurochir. Suppl. 116, 49–54.

Niranjan, A., Kano, H., Mathieu, D., Kondziolka, D., Flickinger, J.C., Lunsford, L.D., Sep 1 2010. Radiosurgery for craniopharyngioma. Int. J. Radiat. Oncol. Biol. Phys. 78 (1), 64–71.

Roth, C.L., 2011. Hypothalamic obesity in patients with craniopharyngioma: profound changes of several weight regulatory circuits. Front. endocrinol. 2, 49.

Rushing, E.J.G.F., Paulus, W., Burger, P.C., 2007. Craniopharyngioma. In: Louis, D.N.O.H., Wiestler, O.D., Cavenee, W.K. (Eds.), WHO Classification of Tumours of the Central Nervous System, fourth ed. IARC Press, Lyon, pp. 238–240.

Sachs, E., 1949. Diagnosis and treatment of brain tumors and care of the neurosurgical patient. C.V. Mosby Company, St. Louis, p 13.

Shirane, R., Ching-Chan, S., Kusaka, Y., Jokura, H., Yoshimoto, T., Apr 2002. Surgical outcomes in 31 patients with craniopharyngiomas extending outside the suprasellar cistern: an evaluation of the frontobasal interhemispheric approach. J. Neurosurg. 96 (4), 704–712.

van Overbeeke, J., Sekhar, L., Jun 2003. Microanatomy of the blood supply to the optic nerve. Orbit 22 (2), 81–88.

CHAPTER

12

Supraorbital Eyebrow Approach for Craniopharyngiomas

Brian J. Dlouhy,†, Charles Teo†*

*Department of Neurosurgery, University of Iowa Hospitals and Clinics, Iowa City, IA, USA;
†Centre for Minimally Invasive Neurosurgery, Prince of Wales Hospital, Sydney, New South Wales, Australia

"These cases offer the baffling problem which confronts the neurosurgeon; and the fact that the mortality which accompanies radical attempts to extirpate a large solidified tumor must approximate 100% probably accounts for the few reports of these lesions other than by pathologists." **Harvey Cushing, 1932**

INTRODUCTION

The supraorbital eyebrow approach is a keyhole technique in which a small anterolateral supraorbital craniotomy is used to reach a wide range of anterior and midline skull base pathologies (van Lindert et al., 1998; Reisch et al., 2003, 2009; Reisch and Perneczky, 2005; Teo, 2005; Little et al., 2010; Wilson et al., 2013). Relying on keyhole principles (Fries and Perneczky, 1998; Perneczky and Fries, 1998) a small incision in the eyebrow is used for an appropriately placed craniotomy, which limits tissue damage, but allows for a wide surgical exposure, making it minimally invasive yet maximally effective.

This approach provides effective surgical access to the anterior cranial fossa floor, the basal frontal lobe, frontal pole, the suprasellar and parasellar regions, the circle of Willis, the ventral brainstem, the proximal Sylvian fissure, and the medial temporal lobe. The endoscope can expand the reach of this microscopic approach and provide or enhance access to adjacent areas. These include the sella/pituitary fossa, region under the ipsilateral optic nerve/carotid artery, contralateral segments of the circle of Willis, anterior third ventricle, anterior interhemispheric fissure, upper third of the clivus, interpeduncular cistern, medial aspect of the ipsilateral middle cranial fossa and temporal lobe, and anterior olfactory groove.

The efficiency and practicality of the endoscopic-assisted, supraorbital keyhole approach makes it a frequently used approach for providing access to lesions in the sella and suprasellar and parasellar regions, and therefore, ideal for resection of craniopharyngiomas (Teo, 2005). When practiced correctly, it offers great exposure with a small cosmetic incision and minimal bony drilling (Teo, 2005).

Craniopharyngiomas
http://dx.doi.org/10.1016/B978-0-12-416706-3.00012-X

CLINICAL HISTORY

One must obtain a clinical history from the patient or the patient's family regarding previous surgery or radiation (Teo, 2005). Recurrent or previously radiated craniopharyngiomas have poorly defined planes and may require more extensive cranial access. This will also help guide preoperative counseling in terms of expected functional outcomes, including neurological and hypothalamic/endocrinological outcomes (Teo, 2005).

PHYSICAL EXAMINATION

The presence of frontal protuberances occasionally offers assistance in locating the whereabouts of the underlying frontal sinuses. Also, in the elderly, the skin creases in the forehead may be prominent enough to "hide" a scar. If so, the eyebrow incision may be replaced with a forehead skin crease incision. However, we prefer an eyebrow incision; as in almost all cases the cosmetic results have been excellent (Teo, 2005; Wilson et al., 2013).

INDICATIONS AND CONTRAINDICATIONS

Craniopharyngiomas can be accessed through a variety of different approaches (Liu et al., 2005; Komotar et al., 2009). The tumor location (Hoffman et al., 1992; Samii and Tatagiba, 1997). and extension with respect to the sella, chiasm, and third ventricle greatly influences the appropriate surgical approach (Fatemi et al., 2009). It is important to consider each case on an individual basis, as the characteristics of a given tumor and individual anatomical variation strongly influence whether a tumor is amenable to resection via a particular approach. Even then, the optimal approach is debatable and may rely on the surgeon's familiarity with it (Komotar et al., 2009).

The majority of craniopharyngiomas can be removed using the supraorbital eyebrow approach (Teo, 2005). Although a prefixed optic chiasm and retrochiasmal tumor may make the approach technically more complicated, in such cases the supraorbital approach and subfrontal corridor still allow access behind the chiasm and through the lamina terminalis to a tumor within the third ventricle (Liu et al., 2005). Retrochiasmal craniopharyngiomas may be approached via an extended endonasal route, as this provides direct access underneath and posterior to the optic chiasm and allows direct access up to the third ventricle (Fatemi et al., 2009).

When selecting a keyhole supraorbital approach, care must be taken in reviewing pertinent imaging and in assessing the anticipated surgical trajectory. Significant superior midline extension of the tumor challenges the access provided by the supraorbital approach, as the flat trajectory along the floor of the frontal fossa may not provide access to the superior extent of the tumor. However, supplementing this approach with neuroendoscopy augments the exposure to include the anterior third ventricle, which can assist in achieving a complete resection (Teo, 2005). Alternatively, extending the supraorbital craniotomy to include the orbital bar or performing a mini orbito-zygomatic craniotomy can allow for a more cephalad trajectory and therefore more superior access in such cases (Jho, 1997; Maus and Goldman, 1999; Dare et al., 2001; Shanno et al., 2001; Ramos-Zuniga et al., 2002; Kanaan, 2005; Warren and Grant, 2009; Cavalcanti et al., 2010). Additionally, the endonasal transsphenoidal approach may offer a more advantageous inferior-to-superior surgical trajectory (Fatemi et al., 2009).

Craniopharyngiomas with lateral extension beyond the supraclinoid carotid arteries or large anterior extensions are often best approached via the supraorbital or pterional route. The supraorbital eyebrow approach may also be used in young children with small nasal cavities and poorly pneumatized sinuses (Teo, 2005). Recurrent craniopharyngiomas, especially those with cystic progression into the suprachiasmatic space, are also accessible via the supraorbital route (Teo, 2005).

One important concern in planning a supraorbital craniotomy is the position and size of the frontal sinus. A large lateral extension of the frontal sinus may discourage one from using the supraorbital approach, but in general this is only an issue in a minority of cases. In children, this is usually not a concern, as the frontal sinus is small or non-existent. However, a large frontal sinus requires a more lateral craniotomy that may further limit the surgical working area and alter the achievable surgical trajectory. Image-based frameless stereotaxy is helpful in assessing the operative trajectory in each case.

In many cases, the supraorbital eyebrow approach is an effective, less-invasive alternative to the standard pterional or orbitozygomatic craniotomies for resection of craniopharyngiomas.

PREOPERATIVE PLANNING

Preoperative MR imaging is essential, both in assessing involvement of surrounding neurovascular structures and in determining the surgical accessibility of the craniopharyngioma. Close examination of axial sequences will demonstrate the lateral and posterior extent of the lesion in relation to the sella, the carotid arteries and the sphenoid ridge. Coronal sequences will also provide important details regarding the lateral extent of the lesion into the adjacent middle cranial fossa, involvement of the cavernous and supraclinoid carotid arteries, and the position of the optic nerves and chiasm. A careful examination of sagittal sequences will demonstrate potential intrasellar extension, the position of the infundibulum and optic apparatus, and the cephalad extent of the lesion. All sequences will be helpful in determining the presence of hydrocephalus and the site of cerebrospinal fluid (CSF) blockage (e.g., foramina of Monro, third ventricle, aqueduct). Additionally, MR imaging assists in determining the presence of a cystic component that may be amenable to drainage. A thoughtful assessment of the radiographic features of the lesion is crucial before one selects the supraorbital approach.

Before surgery, patients for whom a supraorbital approach is selected should be counseled regarding the risk of numbness of the forehead, frontalis palsy, and nasal CSF leak, although these rates are very low in experienced hands. In the senior author's series of over 450 cases, the CSF leak rate was negligible and only two patients experienced permanent frontalis palsy.

SURGICAL TECHNIQUE

After intubation and induction of general anesthesia, the patient's head is placed in a three-point rigid head-holder, gently translated anteriorly, extended, and rotated to the contralateral side approximately 15 degrees (Figure 12.1A). If the patient is a young child, the head may be

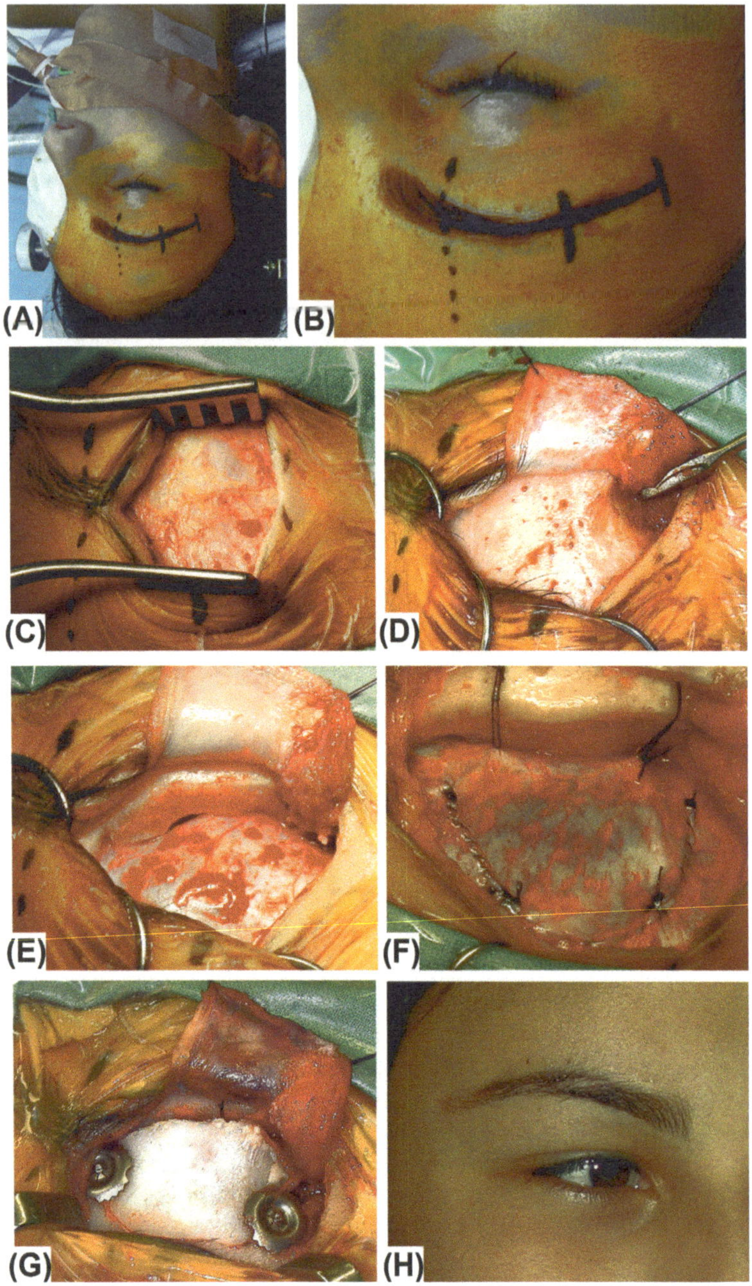

FIGURE 12.1 **A right supraorbital eyebrow approach in a 9-year-old girl for craniopharyngioma resection. A,** The head is placed in a three-pin head-holder and extended and rotated to the left approximately 15 degrees. **B,** The supraorbital notch is palpated and marked with a dashed line. The incision is marked in the superior aspect of the eyebrow (in the hairline, not completely superior to the brow) and extends from the supraorbital notch to the lateral

placed on a padded headrest and positioned in the same way as would be done in a three-point rigid head-holder as described above. The 15-degree rotation allows a perpendicular approach to the sella and parasellar region. Extension of the head facilitates the natural "retraction" of the frontal lobe by gravity and is essential for opening the subfrontal corridor through which microsurgery will proceed, so avoiding the use of retractors. The ipsilateral eye is lubricated and closed with a temporary nylon tarsorrhaphy suture (Figure 12.1B). This prevents surgical prep solution from contacting the cornea, and allows exposure of the nose and ipsilateral eye during draping, which provides external landmarks useful in opening and closing and allows visualization of the orbit at all times during the case. Use of image-based, frameless, stereotaxic guidance determines the position of the frontal sinus and ensures an optimal trajectory to the lesion of interest. It is prudent to avoid the frontal sinus. In children, the frontal sinus is often small and therefore is generally never encountered.

The lateral margin of the frontal sinus is marked and the supraorbital notch is palpated (Figure 12.1B). The supraorbital notch represents the medial limit of the skin incision. When the supraorbital notch is lateral to the frontal sinus, it also marks the medial limit of the craniotomy. In cases where a large frontal sinus extends lateral to the supraorbital notch, the lateral margin of the frontal sinus marks the medial limit of the craniotomy.

After prepping and draping, a skin incision is made within the superior aspect of the eyebrow, extending from the supraorbital notch medially (to avoid the supraorbital nerve) to the lateral aspect of the eyebrow (Figure 12.1B). We prefer to place the incision within the eyebrow, as it is more cosmetically pleasing hiding the scar within the brow hairline. We have not observed alopecia with proper tissue closure (Teo, 2005). The subgaleal layer is undermined superiorly, the skin is retracted superiorly with fish hooks, and a U-shaped pericranial flap is reflected inferiorly and held in place with stay sutures (Figure 12.1C, D). Laterally, the superior portion of the temporalis muscle is dissected to allow placement of a burr hole below the superior temporal line in the keyhole region (Figure 12.1D). A craniotomy is fashioned as low on the frontal bone and nearest to the orbital roof as possible. Using a Penfield dissector, the dura is dissected free from the orbital roof. This allows the protuberances of the orbital roof to be drilled flat, as well as the inner table of the inferior ledge of the craniotomy (Figure 12.1E). This assists in maximizing exposure and visualization and is essential. The craniotomy should be approximately 2–3 cm in width and 1.5–2 cm in height.

The dura is then opened in a U-shaped fashion. The subfrontal corridor is dissected under microscopic visualization. The ipsilateral optic nerve and carotid artery are identified. The arachnoid of the interchiasmatic, optic-carotid, and carotid-occulomotor cisterns, as well as the proximal Sylvian fissure, may be opened. With dissection of arachnoid adhesions and CSF egress, the frontal lobe falls away. The craniopharyngioma is identified and treated using the appropriate

aspect of the brow. The eyelid is suture closed. **C,** Tissue dissection proceeds down to the periosteum. **D,** The subgaleal layer is undermined superiorly above the periosteum, the skin retracted superiorly with fish hooks, and a U-shaped pericranial flap is reflected inferiorly. **E,** The craniotomy is made along the bony exposure and as close to the orbital rim as possible. The dura is opened in a U-shaped fashion and reflected inferiorly to exposure the subfrontal corridor. **F,** After resection of the craniopharyngioma, the dura is closed in a watertight fashion. **G,** A single epidural tack-up is placed and attached to the periosteum of the orbital rim. The bone flap is fixed with titanium plates ensuring the superior margin is flush with the skull. **H,** Six weeks post-operatively, the incision line is undetectable and there is no alopecia noted.

microsurgical techniques. One should anticipate and preserve the bilateral meningohypophyseal arteries arising from medial supraclinoid carotid arteries. Additionally, tumor cysts should be decompressed early if possible to reduce distortion of the optic apparatus. And lastly, tumor remnants densely adherent to the optic nerves and chiasm should be left to avoid new visual loss.

Neuroendoscopy with a 30-degree endoscope may augment visualization of the sella, interpeduncular cistern, interhemispheric cistern, contralateral circle of Willis, basal frontal lobe, and middle cranial fossa, if necessary. In all cases, the endoscope is utilized to either assist in treatment of the lesion or for final inspection to ensure complete resection.

After the craniopharyngioma has been surgically treated, hemostasis is achieved, and the dura is closed in a watertight fashion and sutured to the lower rim of the craniotomy or to periosteum on the orbital rim as an epidural tack-up (Figure 12.1F). The bone is replaced with low-profile titanium plates (Figure 12.1G). Care is taken to minimize the gap between the skull and bone flap at the more cosmetically noticeable superior margin. The pericranium, frontalis muscle and galea are closed in layers. The skin of the eyebrow is re-approximated with a subcuticular nylon suture with no knots. Prior to tying the suture, its free ends are flossed back and forth to ensure that it can be freely removed in 5–7 days. The free ends of this suture are tied so that the skin edges are re-approximated under gentle tension. Proper placement of this final skin suture is essential for obtaining a cosmetically acceptable result (Figure 12.1H). A non-absorbable dressing is placed under the tied ends of the extra-dermal portion of the suture to prevent it from burrowing into the incision. Immediately after the skin is closed, gentle continuous pressure is held over the incision until the patient is extubated and breathing comfortably. This maneuver prevents pseudomeningocele formation that could be promoted by coughing or straining as the patient emerges from anesthesia. The skin suture is removed 5–7 days post-operatively.

POST-OPERATIVE MANAGEMENT

In general, the supraorbital keyhole approach is associated with minimal discomfort and the hospital stay is generally limited by the endocrinological/neurological outcome. Some degree of periorbital edema is to be expected if the periorbita is violated during pericranial dissection or placement of the craniotomy. This generally resolves within 5 days.

COMPLICATIONS

Aside from general surgical complications, the following complications are specific to the supraorbital approach:

- Numbness of the forehead (caused by injury to the supraorbital nerve)
- Frontalis palsy (caused by injury to the frontalis branch of the facial nerve)
- Nasal CSF leak (caused by violation of the frontal sinus and inadequate repair)
- Poor cosmetic appearance. This may be the result of poor skin closure, partial- or full-thickness burns from the surgical microscope set at greater than 75% intensity for any length of time, infection, or persistent pseudomeningocele.

Overall, because the supraorbital approach requires only a small skin incision with minimal temporalis dissection, scalp pain, swelling, and difficulty with mastication are observed with less frequency than with standard pterional or orbitozygomatic approaches.

RESULTS

The senior author has used the supraorbital keyhole approach in over 450 cases in total, including tumors, aneurysms, and trauma. In more than 40 cases, the supraorbital approach has been used to resect all the different types of craniopharyngiomas (Figures 12.2–12.4) (Teo, 2005). In no case was conversion to a larger craniotomy required. The frequency with which we use this approach is a testament to its versatility. Our 0% incidence of conversion to a larger craniotomy demonstrates that, with proper selection and execution, the supraorbital keyhole does not compromise necessary anatomic access.

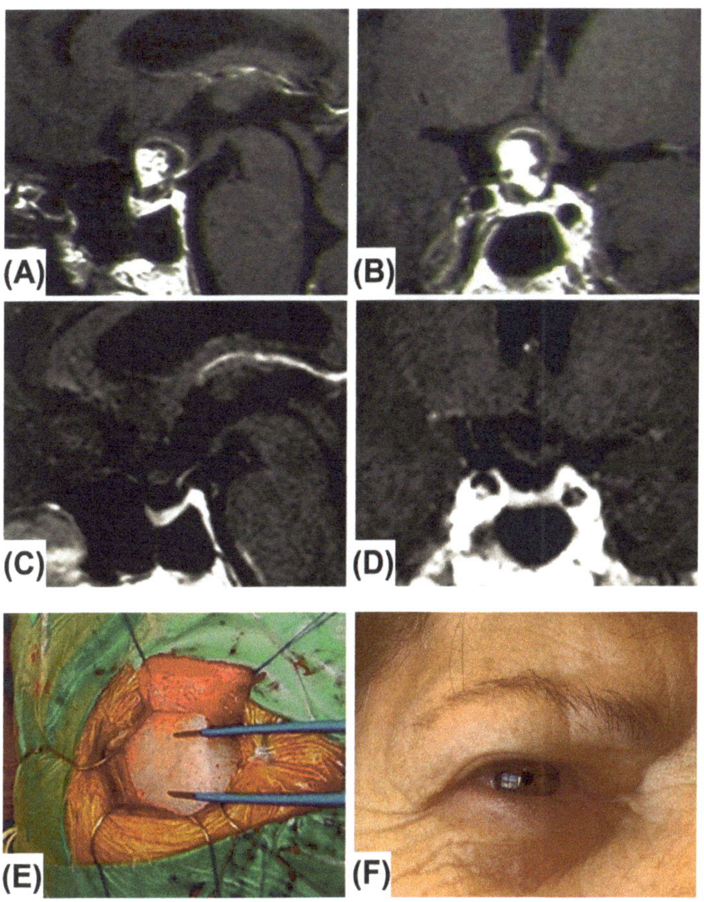

FIGURE 12.2 **A right supraorbital eyebrow approach in a 53-year-old woman for resection of a suprasellar craniopharyngioma. A,** Preoperative sagittal MRI and **B,** preoperative coronal MRI revealing a heterogeneously enhancing suprasellar craniopharyngioma with upward displacement of the optic chiasm. **C,** Post-operative sagittal MRI and **D,** post-operative coronal MRI demonstrating complete resection of the lesion after a right supraorbital eyebrow approach. **E,** Bony exposure prior to craniotomy. Only a craniotomy the size of an open bipolar instrument is needed for adequate working space. **F,** Six weeks post-operatively the incision line is undetectable and there is no alopecia noted.

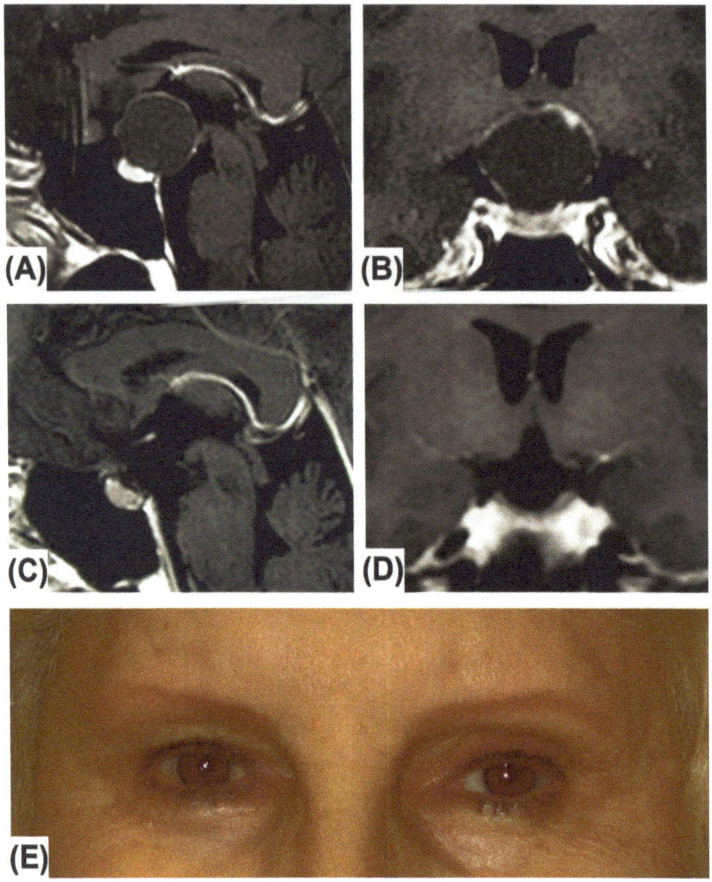

FIGURE 12.3 **A right supraorbital eyebrow approach in a 56-year-old woman for resection of a cystic craniopharyngioma. A,** Preoperative sagittal MRI and **B,** preoperative coronal MRI revealing a large cystic sellar and suprasellar craniopharyngioma with upward displacement of the optic chiasm. **C,** Post-operative sagittal MRI and **D,** post-operative coronal MRI demonstrating complete resection of the lesion after a right supraorbital eyebrow approach. **E,** Six weeks post-operatively and the incision line is undetectable and there is no alopecia noted.

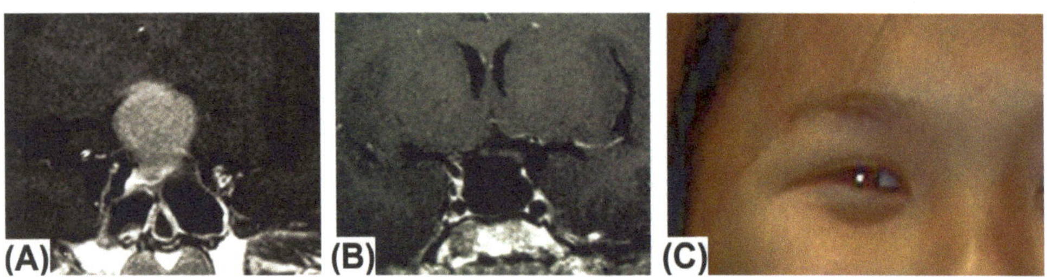

FIGURE 12.4 **A right supraorbital eyebrow approach in an 11-year-old girl for resection of a large craniopharyngioma with superior extension. A,** Preoperative coronal MRI revealing a large enhancing craniopharyngioma with considerable superior suprasellar extension. **B,** Post-operative coronal MRI demonstrating complete resection of the lesion after a right supraorbital eyebrow approach. **C,** Six weeks post-operatively and the incision line is undetectable and there is no alopecia noted.

SURGICAL PEARLS

The following surgical pearls will help ensure a satisfactory outcome with the supraorbital eyebrow approach to craniopharyngiomas

- *Preoperative imaging is essential.* Close inspection of the preoperative MRI is the most important step in properly selecting the supraorbital approach and ensuring that the craniopharyngioma can be accessed appropriately, and safely and completely resected.
- *Extend the head to allow the frontal lobe to fall away.* This simple positioning maneuver allows gravity to work in the surgeon's favor. Mild head extension allows the frontal lobe to fall away, naturally opening the subfrontal corridor and obviating the need for retractors (Figure 12.1A).
- *Avoid the frontal sinus.* The frontal sinus can be easily avoided with image-based frameless stereotaxis. Avoiding a sinus breach eliminates the risk of nasal CSF leak and decreases risk of infection and mucocele formation.
- *Position the craniotomy flush with the orbital roof.* Because the supraorbital craniotomy is a keyhole approach, each millimeter of bone left superficially above the orbital roof disproportionately limits the surgical trajectory to deeper targets. The goal is to achieve a low anterior-to-posterior working trajectory along the base of the frontal lobe, directly along the roof of the orbit.
- *Drill the roof of the orbit flat.* This step is critical in achieving a flat trajectory along the orbital roof.
- *Patiently allow CSF egress to relax the brain.* Patience is essential in allowing the frontal lobe to fall away. Aggressive retraction of a full frontal lobe risks cerebral contusions and potential aphasia when on the dominant side. Such retraction is dangerous and unnecessary. With proper dissection of the arachnoid, systematic opening of the subarachnoid cisterns and proximal Sylvian fissure, and patience, CSF egress will allow a full frontal lobe to eventually fall away and widen the field.
- *Supplement microsurgery with neuroendoscopy.* While the anatomical limits of the supraorbital approach must be respected, in experienced hands these limits can be pushed with the use of angled endoscopes. A 30-degree endoscope may provide access to the sella, the contralateral circle of Willis, the interhemispheric fissure, and a portion of the middle cranial fossa.
- *Utilize proper microsurgical techniques.* As with any transcranial approach, proper microsurgical technique will assist in achieving the desired outcome.
- *Achieve a watertight dural closure.* A watertight closure minimizes the risk of pseudomeningocele and offers additional protection against a nasal CSF leak if the sinus is breached.
- *Careful cosmetic closure.* Because the incision is made in the eyebrow, a cosmetic closure is of utmost importance. While cosmetic concerns are one reason that some neurosurgeons avoid the eyebrow incision, with proper technique excellent cosmesis can be achieved. The following steps are key in performing an optimal cosmetic closure:
  - Close with a subcuticular suture with no buried knots
  - Floss the skin stitch
  - Tie the loose ends under gentle tension
  - Place a non-absorbable dressing under the tied ends
  - Hold pressure until the patient is extubated.

PITFALLS

The following common pitfalls may complicate the supraorbital approach. Each, however, can usually be avoided with proper planning and technique.

- *Inadequate surgical access.* This is generally a result of inadequate review of the preoperative imaging or an incomplete understanding of the anatomical limits of the supraorbital approach. With proper patient selection, this pitfall can be avoided.
- *Breach of the frontal sinus.* Potential negative sequelae of breaching the frontal sinus include infection, pneumocranium, CSF fistula and formation of a mucocele in the long term (Figure 12.5). This can be avoided by identifying the lateral edge of the frontal sinus with image guidance prior to performing the craniotomy. In rare circumstances, a breach of the frontal sinus may be unavoidable. If the frontal sinus is inadvertently or deliberately entered, our current recommendation is to dissect the mucosa off the breach and push it towards the ostium. We then fill the sinus with Surgicel (Ethicon, Inc., USA) and seal the breach with bone wax. Our initial technique was to "cranialize" the sinus by drilling away the posterior wall but this was time-consuming and more destructive. After consultation with more senior colleagues, for the past 10 years we have done a more limited repair as described above, with not a single case of CSF fistula or mucocele formation.
- *Injury to the supraorbital nerve.* Generally, the supraorbital nerve may be preserved by palpating the supraorbital notch to identify the medial limit of the skin incision.
- *Injury to the frontalis branch of the facial nerve.* The risk of injury to the frontalis branch of the facial nerve is reduced by limiting the extent of the lateral incision and minimizing lateral dissection of the subcutaneous tissue.

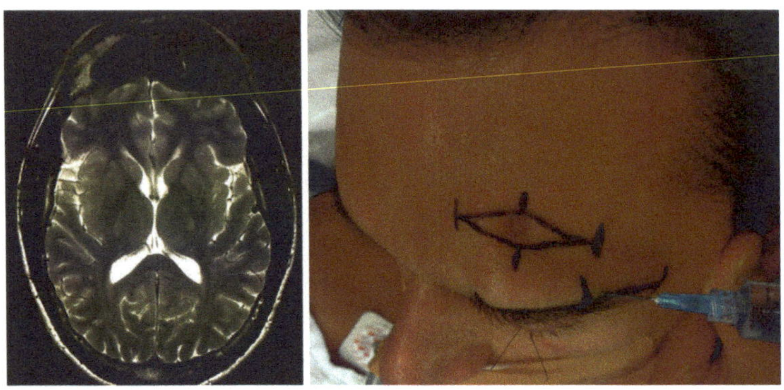

FIGURE 12.5 **Mucocele formation 10 years after breach of the left frontal sinus during a left supraorbital eyebrow craniotomy.** The case shown here was one of the first eyebrow incisions ever performed by the senior author in a man with an aggressive pituitary adenoma and acromegaly. The patient had an extremely large frontal sinus that was deliberately entered and "cranialized" at the end of the procedure. His immediate post-operative course was complicated by a wound infection that necessitated removal of the bone flap. Ten years later he presented with a discharging frontal sinus and was found to have an underlying mucocele. (Left) Preoperative axial MRI revealing the large frontal sinus and mucocele formation in the left frontal sinus. (Right) Draining sinus tract to the skin of the left forehead from underlying mucocele formation.

- *Pseudomeningocele.* May be avoided with a watertight dural closure and by holding pressure on the closed incision until after extubation.
- *Poor cosmesis.* An optimal cosmetic result is achievable by following the pearls outlined above.

References

Cavalcanti, D.D., Garcia-Gonzalez, U., Agrawal, A., Crawford, N.R., Tavares, P.L., Spetzler, R.F., Preul, M.C., 2010. Quantitative anatomic study of the transciliary supraorbital approach: benefits of additional orbital osteotomy? Neurosurgery 66 (6 Suppl. Operative), 205–210.

Cushing, H., 1932. Intracranial tumors. Notes upon a series of two thousand verified cases with surgical mortality percentages pertaining thereto. Thomas, Springfield, p 93–98.

Dare, A.O., Landi, M.K., Lopes, D.K., Grand, W., 2001. Eyebrow incision for combined orbital osteotomy and supraorbital minicraniotomy: application to aneurysms of the anterior circulation. Technical note. J. Neurosurg. 95 (4), 714–718.

Fatemi, N., Dusick, J.R., de Paiva Neto, M.A., Malkasian, D., Kelly, D.F., 2009. Endonasal versus supraorbital keyhole removal of craniopharyngiomas and tuberculum sellae meningiomas. Neurosurgery 64 (5 Suppl. 2), 269–284 discussion 284–266.

Fries, G., Perneczky, A., 1998. Endoscope-assisted brain surgery: part 2 – analysis of 380 procedures. Neurosurgery 42 (2), 226–231 discussion 231–222.

Hoffman, H.J., De Silva, M., Humphreys, R.P., Drake, J.M., Smith, M.L., Blaser, S.I., 1992. Aggressive surgical management of craniopharyngiomas in children. J. Neurosurg. 76 (1), 47–52.

Jho, H.D., 1997. Orbital roof craniotomy via an eyebrow incision: a simplified anterior skull base approach. Minim. Invasive Neurosurg. 40 (3), 91–97.

Kanaan, I.N., 2005. Trans-eyebrow mini-orbitozygomatic pterional approach for minimally invasive skull base surgery. Minim. Invasive Neurosurg. 48 (1), 34–38.

Komotar, R.J., Roguski, M., Bruce, J.N., 2009. Surgical management of craniopharyngiomas. J. Neuro. Oncol. 92 (3), 283–296.

Little, A.S.G.P., Darbar, A., Teo, C., 2010. Supraorbital eyebrow approach: less invasive corridor to lesions of the anterior cranial fossa, parasellar region, and ventral brainstem. In: Cappabianca (Ed.), Cranial, Cranio-Facial and Skull Base Surgery. Springer-Verlag, Italia.

Liu, J.K., Cole, C.D., Kestle, J.R., Brockmeyer, D.L., Walker, M.L., 2005. Cranial base strategies for resection of craniopharyngioma in children. Neurosurg. Focus 18 (6A), E9.

Maus, M., Goldman, H.W., 1999. Removal of orbital apex hemangioma using new transorbital craniotomy through suprabrow approach. Ophthal. Plast. Reconstr. Surg. 15 (3), 166–170.

Perneczky, A., Fries, G., 1998. Endoscope-assisted brain surgery: part 1 – evolution, basic concept, and current technique. Neurosurgery 42 (2), 219–224, discussion 224–215.

Ramos-Zuniga, R., Velazquez, H., Barajas, M.A., Lopez, R., Sanchez, E., Trejo, S., 2002. Trans-supraorbital approach to supratentorial aneurysms. Neurosurgery 51 (1), 125–130, discussion 130–121.

Reisch, R., Perneczky, A., 2005. Ten-year experience with the supraorbital subfrontal approach through an eyebrow skin incision. Neurosurgery 57 (Suppl. 4), 242–255, discussion 242–255.

Reisch, R., Stadie, A., Kockro, R., Gawish, I., Schwandt, E., Hopf, N., 2009. The minimally invasive supraorbital subfrontal key-hole approach for surgical treatment of temporomesial lesions of the dominant hemisphere. Minim. Invasive Neurosurg. 52 (4), 163–169.

Reisch, R., Perneczky, A., Filippi, R., 2003. Surgical technique of the supraorbital key-hole craniotomy. Surg. Neurol. 59 (3), 223–227.

Samii, M., Tatagiba, M., 1997. Surgical management of craniopharyngiomas: a review. Neurol. Med. chir. 37 (2), 141–149.

Shanno, G., Maus, M., Bilyk, J., Schwartz, S., Savino, P., Simeone, F., Goldman, H.W., 2001. Image-guided transorbital roof craniotomy via a suprabrow approach: a surgical series of 72 patients. Neurosurgery 48 (3), 559–567, discussion 567–558.

Teo, C., 2005. Application of endoscopy to the surgical management of craniopharyngiomas. Childs. Nerv. Syst. 21 (8–9), 696–700.

van Lindert, E., Perneczky, A., Fries, G., Pierangeli, E., 1998. The supraorbital keyhole approach to supratentorial aneurysms: concept and technique. Surg. Neurol. 49 (5), 481–489, discussion 489–490.

Warren, W.L., Grant, G.A., 2009. Transciliary orbitofrontozygomatic approach to lesions of the anterior cranial fossa. Neurosurgery 64 (5 Suppl. 2), 324–329 discussion 329–330.

Wilson, D.A., Duong, H., Teo, C., Kelly, D.F., 2013. The supraorbital endoscopic approach for tumors. World. Neurosurg.

CHAPTER

13

Surgical Approaches: Transcortical-Transventricular Removal of Craniopharyngioma

Walavan Sivakumar, Khaled M. Krisht, William T. Couldwell

Department of Neurosurgery, Clinical Neurosciences Center, University of Utah, Salt Lake City, UT, USA

*"Even from the mere standpoint of preservation of vision the problem is a highly complicated and difficult one." **Harvey Cushing, 1932***

INTRODUCTION

Although craniopharyngiomas are benign tumors, numerous factors have caused these lesions to remain a neurosurgical challenge for over a century. The relationship of these tumors to critical neurovascular structures (namely the circle of Willis, optic pathways, and the hypothalamus) results in potential significant morbidity and mortality associated with surgical access (Adamson et al., 1990; Yasargil et al., 1990). Additionally, even though 90% of tumors arise in the sellar and parasellar regions, they can originate anywhere along the obliterated craniopharyngeal duct, including the nasopharynx, sphenoid bone, third ventricle, pineal region, infrasellar region, and cerebellopontine angle (Falavigna and Kraemer, 2001; Ragel et al., 2007). As understanding of the anatomic variability of this tumor has grown through the use of advanced microsurgical, skull base, and endoscopic techniques, so too has the surgical armamentarium. An individualized, multi-disciplinary approach has become the standard of care for treatment, with either subtotal or gross total neurosurgical resection retaining a vital role. In this chapter, we describe the transcortical-transventricular approach to the resection of craniopharyngiomas and include a discussion of the transcallosal-transventricular approach and the authors' indications for these approaches.

Craniopharyngiomas
http://dx.doi.org/10.1016/B978-0-12-416706-3.00013-1

HISTORY

Jacob Erdheim first described the histopathological appearance of craniopharyngeal duct tumors in 1901 (Erdheim, 1904). The term "craniopharyngioma" was later coined by Charles Frazier in 1931 and further popularized by Harvey Cushing in his series in 1932 (Frazier and Alpers, 1931; Cushing, 1932). The first successful resection of a craniopharyngioma, or "Erdheim tumor," was reported by A. E. Halstead in 1910 using the sublabial gingival incision and transsphenoidal approach to resect the sellar mass (Halstead, 1910; Liu et al., 2001; Barkhoudarian and Laws, 2013).

Surgical approaches for the removal of craniopharyngiomas have evolved significantly over the last 100 years (Choux and Lena, 1998). The frontal craniotomy described by Cushing in 1932 was adopted as the preferred route for access to these tumors because of the trouble with visualization and difficulty of performing reoperations with the transsphenoidal route (Cushing, 1932; Barkhoudarian and Laws, 2013). From the 1950s until the 1970s, typical intervention involved subtotal surgical resection with aggressive adjuvant radiation therapy as there was concern over operative mortality. In 1950, Love and Marshall (Love and Marshall, 1950) reported their experience with 96 patients from the Mayo Clinic, citing a gross total resection rate of only 15% and an operative mortality of 40%. Beginning in the 1970s, there was a shift in surgeon preference towards attempting total resection of craniopharyngioma (Katz, 1975; Sweet, 1976; Hoffman et al., 1977; Rougerie, 1979). The transpetrosal-transtentorial approach was recommended for tumors that extended into the posterior fossa in the mid-1980s (Hakuba et al., 1985). Bifrontal interhemispheric approaches to this region were first described in the 1980s (Suzuki et al., 1984, 1986; Samii and Bini, 1991; Shibuya et al., 1996). For tumors primarily within the third ventricle, the most common technique historically has been the transcortical-transventricular, originally described by Dandy in 1922 (Dandy, 1922). The transcallosal-transventricular technique using an anterior callosotomy was first described by Milhorat in 1966 (Milhorat and Baldwin, 1966). Its use grew in the mid-1980s because of new reports that sectioning the anterior corpus callosum did not result in significant morbidity (Ehni, 1984). The concern regarding increased risk of post-operative seizures in the transcortical group during the pre-magnetic resonance imaging (MRI) era and the overall decreased morbidity with the transcallosal approach caused the transcortical approach to lose favor with many surgeons. Currently, there are advocates of both the transcortical-transventricular and the transcallosal-transventricular approach to tumors extending into the anterior third ventricle.

SURGICAL APPROACHES

When considering surgical resection for a suspected craniopharyngioma, great importance is placed on clarifying the localization and extension of the tumor in relation to the sella and third ventricle. Many have advocated for classification systems of these tumors by location, but there is currently no universally accepted system (Choux and Lena, 1998). We consider the transcortical-transventricular or transcallosal-transventricular approach mainly for tumors that invade or appear to be completely within the third ventricle.

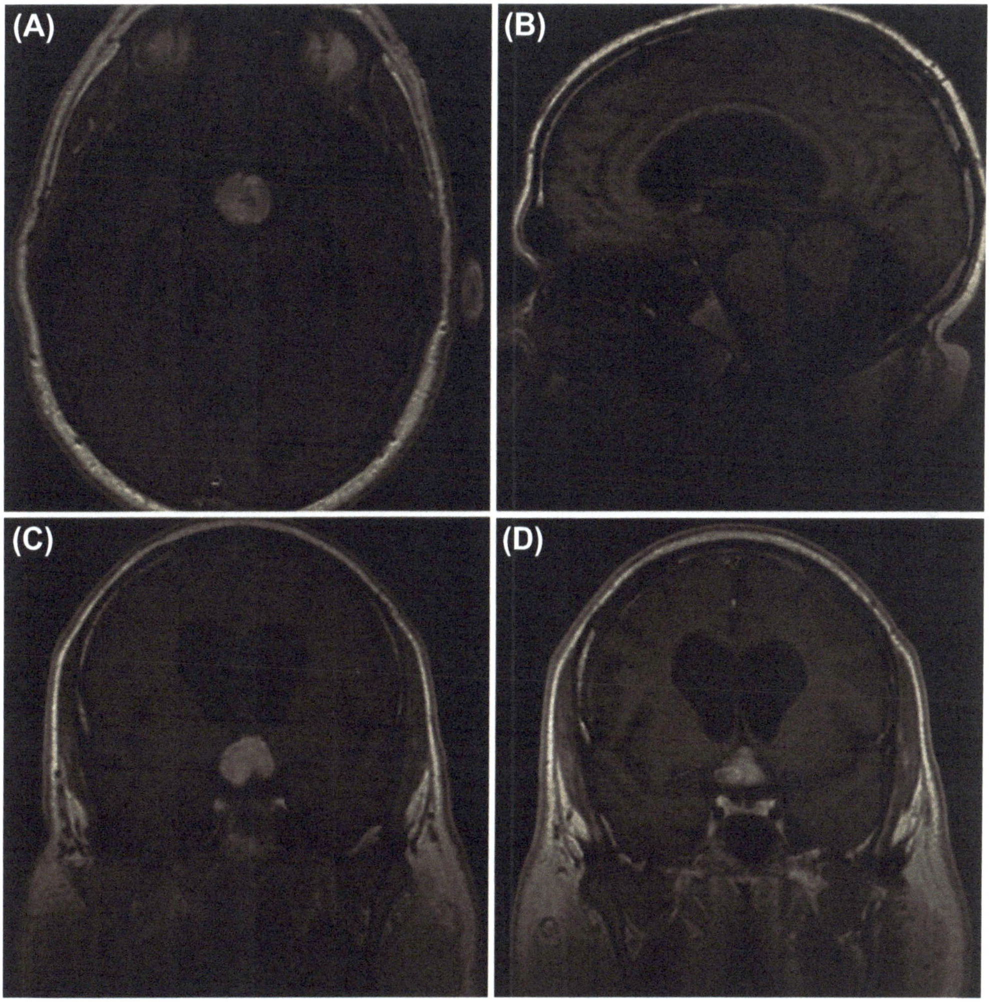

FIGURE 13.1 **A,** Axial T1-weighted MRI showing large contrast-enhancing lesion occupying the inferior part of the third ventricle. **B,** Sagittal T1-weighted MRI without contrast showing large lesion within the anterior portion of the third ventricle. **C,** Coronal T1-weighted MRI with contrast showing large contrast-enhancing lesion within the third ventricle. **D,** Coronal T1-weighted MRI with contrast showing large contrast-enhancing lesion within the third ventricle. The pituitary stalk is located in the midline and not displaced by the tumor.

When tumors lie primarily within the ventricle, the pituitary midline stalk tends to be midline on coronal MRI, a clue that the entire tumor is within the third ventricle (Figure 13.1) (Chamoun and Couldwell, 2013). Additionally, a recent study by Pascual et al. (2013) suggested that combining the patient's clinical history with an objective measure of mammillary body displacement on MRI can allow the surgeon to accurately predict whether a craniopharyngioma is suprasellar or intraventricular in 74–90% of lesions. For primarily intraventricular tumors, we prefer the transcortical-transventricular or transcallosal-transventricular approach, avoiding the need to violate the lamina terminalis or third ventricular floor and thereby potentially preserving pituitary function.

There are advocates for both the transcortical and the transcallosal approach to these ventricular tumors. Our decision regarding the approach with anterior third ventricular craniopharyngiomas is made on a case-by-case basis. The decision is made with consideration of the size of the lateral ventricles. If there is enlargement of the lateral ventricles, the senior author prefers a transcortical-transforaminal approach. In cases where the lateral ventricles are smaller, a transcallosal approach is chosen. Both approaches, with the utilization of neuronavigation techniques, have proven very accurate with regard to the trajectory into the ventricle, and each has associated risks.

Cerebrospinal Fluid Diversion

In patients who present with hydrocephalus as a result of the craniopharyngioma, the decision to initiate cerebrospinal fluid (CSF) diversion is made on the basis of the findings of a clinical examination. If the patient is mildly symptomatic from the hydrocephalus or has a long-standing history, we prefer to place an external ventricular drain in the operating room at the end of the surgical resection for post-operative control and wean the catheter if possible. If a patient is experiencing acute decline secondary to hydrocephalus, temporary CSF diversion is undertaken promptly and supportive care is given until the patient is considered stable enough to undergo surgery.

Neuronavigation

In almost all recent cases of anterior third ventricle surgery, we have utilized neuronavigation, both for placement of an external ventricular drain and for confirmation of our surgical trajectory. Either stereotactic computed tomography (CT) or MRI may be used, based on the available software on the neuronavigation system. Stereotactic CT scans serve the additional purpose of evaluating the extent of calcifications within this tumor, giving the surgeon additional information about what will be encountered in the operating room.

OPERATIVE TECHNIQUE

Transcortical-Transventricular Approach

The patient is placed under general anesthesia and positioned in the supine position with the head in a surgical head holder. The head is maintained in the midline and raised approximately 25 degrees to facilitate venous return (Figure 13.2). While the somatosensory evoked potential (SSEP) and motor evoked potential (MEP) electrodes are placed, the neuronavigation system is registered to the pre-operative imaging. A right-sided exposure is preferred in almost all cases unless the tumor extends primarily into the left lateral ventricle. The locations of the craniotomy and the anterior cortical incision are planned using the navigation software to gain optimal access through the lateral ventricle into the third ventricle through the foramen of Monro.

A curvilinear incision is made to encompass the small craniotomy, centered at the coronal suture about 3 cm from midline. The incision should allow the scalp flap to be reflected far

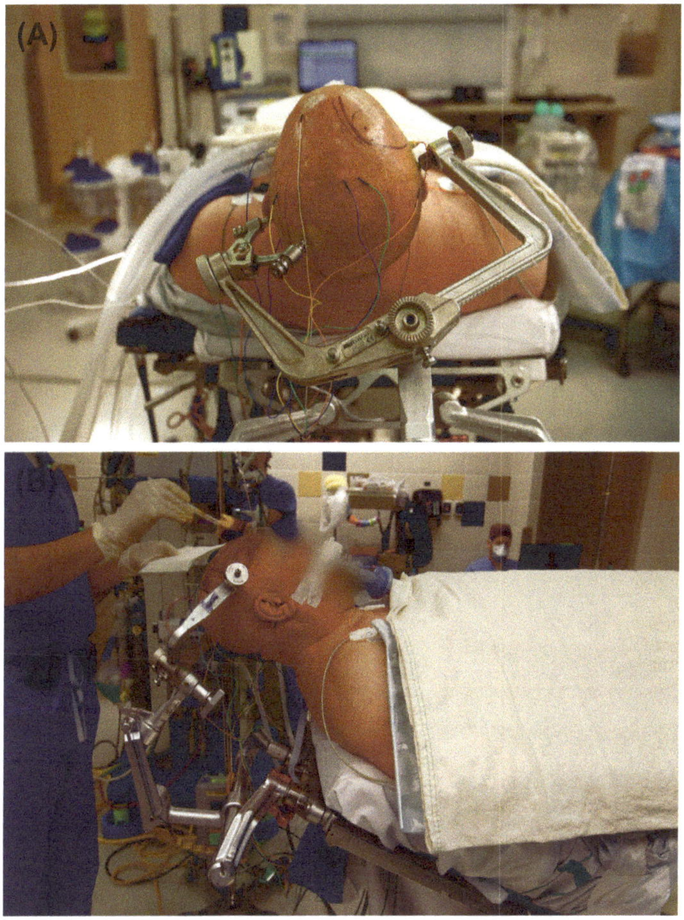

FIGURE 13.2 **A, B Intra-operative images of patient positioning.** The patient's head is maintained in the midline in the Mayfield head holder and angled to 25 degrees. SSEP and MEP wires are placed pre-operatively.

enough to expose the planned craniotomy and secured. A single burr hole is made using the high-speed drill, and a craniotomy, centered on the coronal suture, is turned. If the tumor is large and extends into the posterior third ventricle, the craniotomy may be extended slightly more posteriorly. The bony exposure posterior to the coronal suture is limited to approximately 2 cm in an attempt to avoid the motor strip. The dura is then opened in either a flap or a cruciate fashion.

The point of the cortical incision is reconfirmed with neuronavigation and the intra-operative microscope is brought into the field. Once a pathway of optimal access through the lateral ventricle and foramen of Monro to the third ventricle has been confirmed, a cortical incision is made. The pia mater surrounding the incision is cauterized, and small malleable self-retaining retractors are brought into the field. The size of the cortical incision is 1–2 cm. To reduce cerebral tissue retraction in patients with smaller ventricles, osmotic diuretics or hypertonic saline can be used in combination with the longer cortical incision. The trajectory towards the ipsilateral foramen of Monro can be confirmed using neuronavigation.

When the right lateral ventricle is penetrated, orientation can be confirmed by identifying the choroid plexus, septal vein, and thalamostriate vein. The septum pellucidum may be attenuated if significant, long-standing hydrocephalus is present. The foramen of Monro, which is usually dilated in patients with long-standing hydrocephalus, can be identified by tracing the choroid plexus and thalamostriate vein anteriorly and medially, respectively (Figure 13.3A). The direction of the choroid plexus as it courses lateral to the fornix and enters the foramen of Monro helps to differentiate between the right and left ventricles, and in rare cases, a cavum septum pellucidum. This is usually recognized by its presence on pre-operative imaging and the lack of the expected intraventricular structures.

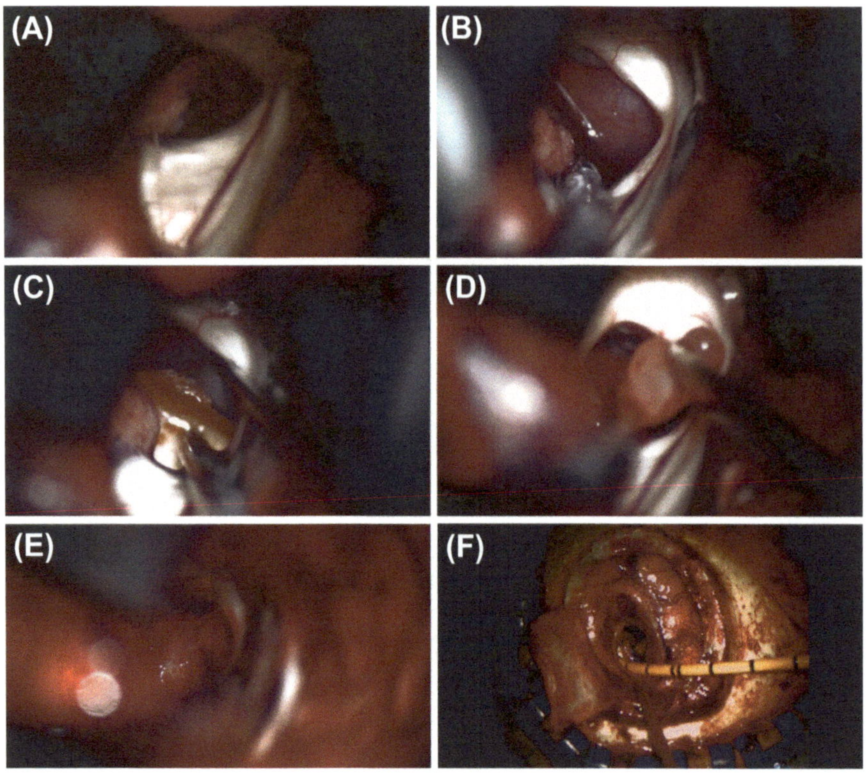

FIGURE 13.3 **A**, Intra-operative image showing third ventricle visualized through the dilated right foramen of Monro. The choroid plexus is noted medially. **B**, Intra-operative image showing the craniopharyngioma noted anteriorly by mildly displacing foramen of Monro posteriorly. The choroid plexus is displaced medially to better visualize tumor. **C**, Intra-operative image showing craniopharyngioma carefully displaced anteriorly to highlight the intact floor of the third ventricle. **D**, Intra-operative imaging showing craniopharyngioma being carefully morcellated and removed in a piecemeal fashion. **E**, Intra-operative image. Evaluation of the region post-resection shows no residual tumor, no significant bleeding, and no forniceal injury. **F**, Intra-operative image showing external ventricular drain being placed prior to closing.

If the intraventricular portion of the craniopharyngioma extends into the lateral ventricle, it should be easily visualized at this point, and careful exploration and dissection may begin. For tumors primarily within the third ventricle, dissection may begin after careful exploration of the ventricle (Figure 13.3B,C). The capsule is opened and the tumor is morcellated in a piecemeal fashion using microscissors and pituitary rongeurs. Using microdissectors and rhoton cup forceps, a careful, circumferential dissection around the extent of the tumor is undertaken. As it is released from the walls and floor of the third ventricle, it may continue to be morcellated (Figure 13.3D). There is significant variability in the vascularity of these lesions. Cottonoids may be used to prevent back-bleeding from the tumor into the aqueduct of Sylvius. Tremendous caution needs to be exercised when peeling the tumor off the walls and floor of the third ventricle. After the tumor is thought to be completely resected, the floor and walls of the third ventricle are explored for residual tumor (Figure 13.3E). There may be residual capsule identified during exploration. If it adheres firmly to surrounding critical brain structures, we choose to leave the capsule intact. Once adequate resection has been achieved, the region is irrigated and attention is turned to attaining meticulous hemostasis. An external ventricular drain is placed at this point, with plans to remove it on post-operative day two or three (Figure 13.3F). SSEPs and MEPs are once again reconfirmed to be stable (Chamoun and Couldwell, 2013). The dura is then reapproximated with 4–0 silk sutures and supplemented with a dural substitute for duraplasty. The ventricular drain is brought out through a burr hole. The bone flap is then replaced, and the skin is closed in the standard fashion. The patient is then extubated and transferred to the neurocritical care unit for close observation. Imaging is performed on post-operative day one or two to evaluate for peri-operative complications and repeated as follow-up to evaluate for extent of tumor resection (Figure 13.4).

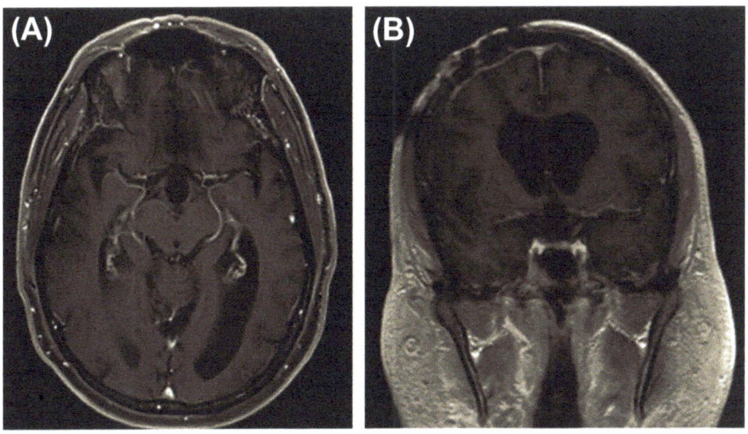

FIGURE 13.4 **A,** Post-operative axial T1-weighted MRI with contrast showing complete resection of tumor. **B,** Post-operative coronal T1-weighted MRI image with contrast showing complete resection of tumor. Right transcortical tract demonstrates no evidence of a porencephalic cyst.

Pre-Operative External Ventricular Drain Placement

If a patient presents with signs and symptoms consistent with worsening hydrocephalus, an external ventricular drain may be placed at admission or during surgery in the operating room. This latter method may be performed with stereotactic image guidance, which allows for more accurate placement of the drain into the right frontal horn of the lateral ventricle and subsequent easier blunt dissection as the drain can confirm the trajectory down to the ventricle.

Use of the Intra-Operative Endoscope

If the craniopharyngioma extends posteriorly in the third ventricle beyond the view of the microscope, an angled endoscope may be used to confirm complete resection of the tumor from the posterior walls or to assist in further resection.

TRANSCALLOSAL-TRANSVENTRICULAR APPROACH

The transcallosal-transventricular approach to craniopharyngioma resection is performed in much the same way as the transcortical-transventricular approach. The positioning of the patient and the planned incision are typically the same. The craniotomy is extended slightly more medially to expose the superior sagittal sinus. Great care must be taken when stripping the dura on the undersurface of the bone, especially medially, to prevent potential injury to the sinus or the large draining veins extending into the sinus. Additionally, the medial edge of the bony margin should be over the lateral edge of the sinus. This will allow the retractors to be placed directly inferior to the corpus callosum, with minimal inadvertent pressure on the sagittal sinus during tissue manipulation.

The dural opening is also extended slightly medially to expose the edge of the sagittal sinus, so that the falx cerebri can be easily visualized. Because the approach is typically reserved for ventricular extension of craniopharyngiomas with an absence of ventriculomegaly, osmotic diuretics or hypertonic saline are given to induce brain relaxation. This decreases the distance of blunt dissection as well as the amount of brain retraction needed. The bone flap should encompass the region of the coronal suture, and the trajectory is from this region, pending inspection of bridging veins. Under the intra-operative microscope, retractors are placed and a gentle surgical corridor is achieved. Fixed retraction should be minimized. The corpus callosum will be visualized at this point; however, the cingulate gyrus can sometimes be fused, creating a false impression of the corpus callosum. They can be differentiated by the glossy white appearance of the corpus callosum and the presence of overlying pericallosal arteries. Identifying the callosomarginal arteries and tracing them proximally to their origin near the anterior corpus callosum will also differentiate the structures.

Once the corpus callosum is clearly visualized, neuronavigation is used to plan the callosotomy. We aim for the callosotomy opening to be directly in line with the foramen of Monro. This allows for a very small callosotomy, ideally approximately 1 cm long. Occasionally, there may be small connecting branches between the pericallosal arteries overlying the planned callosotomy. If these vessels do not appear to penetrate the cingulum, they may be safely cauterized and transected. Opening the arachnoid membranes anterior and posterior to the planned callosotomy will increase the line of sight and further minimize the required hemispheric retraction. The callosotomy can then be completed using a Penfield 4 instrument to bluntly dissect the corpus callosum until the ependyma is visualized (Cohen-Gadol, 2013). After the orientation is confirmed, the surgical resection of the craniopharyngioma may be completed in a similar fashion to the transcortical-transventricular approach. The senior author prefers to work laterally around the columns of the fornix on one side to avoid risk of bilateral forniceal injury. The fornix is not divided.

Combined Approaches

While craniopharyngiomas can occur anywhere along the craniopharyngeal duct, 90% occur in the sellar and suprasellar region (Falavigna and Kraemer, 2001). Large craniopharyngiomas that arise from this region and invade the third ventricle make the transcortical/transcallosal-transventricular approach inadequate when gross total resection is the goal. Multiple combined approaches have been recommended for this complicated situation and will be discussed in other chapters of this section. At our institution, the transcortical- or transcallosal-transventricular approach is most often combined with either the standard transnasal transsphenoidal approach or the extended transsphenoidal approach, when clival extension of the tumor is noted (Couldwell and Weiss, 1998; Chakrabarti et al., 2005).

COMPLICATIONS

Complications of Approach

The transcortical-transventricular and transcallosal-transventricular approaches to tumors require a disruption of neural tissue, by either a corticectomy or a callosotomy. Historically, the literature has reported post-operative seizure rates following the transcortical approach at 26–70% (Kobayashi et al., 1971; Fornari et al., 1981; Desai et al., 2002). Conventional wisdom has held that white matter (i.e., corpus callosum) and subcortical gray matter are not epileptogenic. The two most recent series on the transcortical approach to the lateral ventricle have reported post-operative epilepsy rates of 7% and 8% (Ellenbogen, 2001; Milligan and Meyer, 2010). Although the post-operative epilepsy rate following the transcallosal approach was first reported as 0% in a 47-patient cohort, a more recent study found the rate was 25% in a 75-patient cohort (Villani and Tomei, 2006; Milligan and Meyer, 2010). A possible explanation of this increased rate could be more comprehensive follow-up and reporting of post-operative complications, as no other factor was significant on multivariate analysis. With the advent of MRI and use of the neuronavigation allowing for a more focused trajectory, the violation of normal tissue has been minimized. Nevertheless, all patients at our institution who undergo a transcortical approach to access the ventricle are placed on post-operative antiepileptic medications until they are seen in clinic for post-operative follow-up.

Contralateral hemiparesis is a potential complication of the transcortical approach. Since the use of neuronavigation has become commonplace at our institution and great care is taken to plan the corticectomy well anterior to the motor strip, we have not had any cases of permanent post-operative hemiparesis at follow-up.

Both transcortical-transventricular and transcallosal-transventricular approaches are associated with memory deficits, although these are mostly transient. Published rates of memory deficit after surgery via the transcortical approach of 4–12% and after surgery via the transcallosal approach of 23–33% likely illustrate the importance of avoiding forniceal injury when accessing third ventricular craniopharyngiomas (Omay et al., 2006). Injury to any portion of the memory circuit, prevalent along the midline cortical and subcortical structures, can result in some form of memory deficit.

Anterior infarcts can be present post-operatively if venous drainage is compromised via the sagittal sinus directly or indirectly to an essential draining vein during the transcallosal approach. Rarely, an essential draining vein can be found draining into the anterior sagittal sinus. Retraction on the sagittal sinus should be minimized, and the surgeon should be cognizant of the amount of time that fixed retraction is in place. Additionally, significant care should be taken when tracing and dividing the callosomarginal and pericallosal vessels.

As noted above, craniopharyngiomas with intraventricular extension vary significantly in their vascularity. During the morcellation of the tumor and resection off of the ventricular wall, hemostasis should be maintained. Cottonoids and suction are used to control back-bleeding that may potentially block off the aqueduct of Sylvius and result in post-operative hydrocephalus.

SUMMARY

While craniopharyngiomas involving the third ventricle are complicated lesions to treat, they are accessible via the transcortical-transventricular and transcallosal-transventricular approaches. Advances in diagnostic capabilities, intra-operative navigation, and microsurgical technique have resulted in more extensive resections of these tumors with improved morbidity and mortality rates. Our transcortical-transventricular approach aims to minimize the corticectomy and cortical manipulation while maintaining adequate surgical control over the ventricular and suprasellar region.

Acknowledgments

The authors thank Kristin Kraus, M.Sc., for her assistance in the preparation of this chapter, Jennie Swensen, M.A., for her medical illustration, and Vance Mortimer for his audiovisual expertise.

References

Adamson, T.E., Wiestler, O.D., Kleihues, P., Yasargil, M.G., 1990. Correlation of clinical and pathological features in surgically treated craniopharyngiomas. J. Neurosurg. 73 (1), 12–17.

Barkhoudarian, G., Laws, E.R., 2013. Craniopharyngioma: history. Pituitary 16 (1), 1–8.

Chakrabarti, I., Amar, A.P., Couldwell, W., Weiss, M.H., 2005. Long-term neurological, visual, and endocrine outcomes following transnasal resection of craniopharyngioma. J. Neurosurg. 102 (4), 650–657.

Chamoun, R., Couldwell, W.T., 2013. Transcortical-transforaminal microscopic approach for purely intraventricular craniopharyngioma. Neurosurg. Focus 34 (Suppl. 1). Video 4.

Choux, M., Lena, G., 1998. Craniopharyngioma. In: Apuzzo, M. (Ed.), Surgery of the Third Ventricle. Williams & Wilkins, Baltimore.

Cohen-Gadol, A.A., 2013. Interhemispheric transcallosal route for resection of anterior third ventricular lesions. Neurosurg. Focus 34 (Suppl. 1). Video 7.

Couldwell, W., Weiss, M., 1998. The transnasal transsphenoidal approach. In: Apuzzo, M. (Ed.), Surgery of the Third Ventricle. Williams & Wilkins, Baltimore, pp. 553–574.

Cushing, H., 1932. Intracranial tumors. Notes upon a series of two thousand verified cases with surgical mortality percentages pertaining thereto. Charles C. Thomas, Springfield, p. 93–98.

Dandy, W., 1922. Diagnosis, localization, and removal of tumors of the third ventricle. Bull. Johns Hopkins Hosp. 33, 188–189.

Desai, K.I., Nadkarni, T.D., Muzumdar, D.P., Goel, A.H., 2002. Surgical management of colloid cyst of the third ventricle: a study of 105 cases. Surg. Neurol. 57 (5), 295–302, discussion 302–304.

Ehni, G., 1984. Interhemispheric and percallosal (transcallosal) approach to the cingulate gyri, intraventricular shunt tubes, and certain deeply placed brain lesions. Neurosurgery 14 (1), 99–110.

Ellenbogen, R.G., 2001. Transcortical surgery for lateral ventricular tumors. Neurosurg. Focus 10 (6), E2.

Erdheim, J., 1904. Uber hypophysengangges: chwulste und hirncholesteatome. Sitzungsber K Akad Wiss Mathnatrw CL 113, 537–726.

Falavigna, A., Kraemer, J.L., 2001. Infrasellar craniopharyngioma: case report. Arq. Neuropsiquiatr. 59 (2-B), 424–430.

Fornari, M., Savoiardo, M., Morello, G., Solero, C.L., 1981. Meningiomas of the lateral ventricles. Neuroradiological and surgical considerations in 18 cases. J. Neurosurg. 54 (1), 64–74.

Frazier, C., Alpers, B., 1931. Adamantinoma of the craniopharyngeal duct. Arch. Neurol. Psychiatry. 26, 905–965.

Hakuba, A., Nishimura, S., Inoue, Y., 1985. Transpetrosal-transtentorial approach and its application in the therapy of retrochiasmatic craniopharyngiomas. Surg. Neurol. 24 (4), 405–415.

Halstead, A., 1910. Remarks on the operative treatment of tumors of the hypophysis. With the report of two cases operated on by an oro-nasal method. Surg. Gynecol. Obstet. 10, 494–502.

Hoffman, H.J., Hendrick, E.B., Humphreys, R.P., Buncic, J.R., Armstrong, D.L., Jenkin, R.D., 1977. Management of craniopharyngioma in children. J. Neurosurg. 47 (2), 218–227.

Katz, E.L., 1975. Late results of radical excision of craniopharyngiomas in children. J. Neurosurg. 42 (1), 86–93.

Kobayashi, S., Okazaki, H., MacCarty, C.S., 1971. Intraventricular meningiomas. Mayo Clin. Proc. 46 (11), 735–741.

Liu, J.K., Das, K., Weiss, M.H., Laws Jr., E.R., Couldwell, W.T., 2001. The history and evolution of transsphenoidal surgery. J. Neurosurg. 95 (6), 1083–1096.

Love, J.G., Marshall, T.M., 1950. Craniopharyngiomas. Surg. Gynecol. Obstet. 90 (5), 591–601.

Milhorat, T.H., Baldwin, M., 1966. A technique for surgical exposure of the cerebral midline: experimental transcallosal microdissection. J. Neurosurg. 24 (3), 687–691.

Milligan, B.D., Meyer, F.B., 2010. Morbidity of transcallosal and transcortical approaches to lesions in and around the lateral and third ventricles: a single-institution experience. Neurosurgery 67 (6), 1483–1496; discussion 1496.

Omay, S., Baehring, J., Piepmeier, J., 2006. Approaches to lateral and third ventricular tumors. In: Schmidek, H., Roberts, D. (Eds.), Schmidek and Sweet's Operative Neurosurgical Techniques: Indications, Methods and Results. Saunders, Philadelphia, pp. 753–771.

Pascual, J.M., Prieto, R., Carrasco, R., Barrios, L., 2013. Displacement of mammillary bodies by craniopharyngiomas involving the third ventricle: surgical-MRI correlation and use in topographical diagnosis. J. Neurosurg. 119 (2), 381–405.

Ragel, B.T., Bishop, F.S., Couldwell, W.T., 2007. Recurrent infrasellar clival craniopharyngioma. Acta Neurochir. (Wien) 149 (7), 729–730; discussion 730.

Rougerie, J., 1979. What can be expected from the surgical treatment of craniopharyngiomas in children. Report of 92 cases. Childs Brain 5 (5), 433–449.

Samii, M., Bini, W., 1991. Surgical treatment of craniopharyngiomas. Zentralbl. Neurochir. 52 (1), 17–23.

Shibuya, M., Takayasu, M., Suzuki, Y., Saito, K., Sugita, K., 1996. Bifrontal basal interhemispheric approach to craniopharyngioma resection with or without division of the anterior communicating artery. J. Neurosurg. 84 (6), 951–956.

Suzuki, J., Katakura, R., Mori, T., 1984. Interhemispheric approach through the lamina terminalis to tumors of the anterior part of the third ventricle. Surg. Neurol. 22 (2), 157–163.

Suzuki, J., Mizoi, K., Yoshimoto, T., 1986. Bifrontal interhemispheric approach to aneurysms of the anterior communicating artery. J. Neurosurg. 64 (2), 183–190.

Sweet, W.H., 1976. Radical surgical treatment of craniopharyngioma. Clin. Neurosurg. 23, 52–79.
Villani, R., Tomei, G., 2006. Approach to tumors of the third ventricle. In: Schmidek, H., Roberts, D. (Eds.), Schmidek and Sweet's Operative Neurosurgical Techniques: Indications, Methods, and Results. Saunders, Philadelphia.
Yasargil, M.G., Curcic, M., Kis, M., Siegenthaler, G., Teddy, P.J., Roth, P., 1990. Total removal of craniopharyngiomas. Approaches and long-term results in 144 patients. J. Neurosurg. 73 (1), 3–11.

CHAPTER

14

Petrosal Approach for Retrochiasmatic Craniopharyngiomas

Osama Al-Mefty, Paulo Abdo do Seixo Kadri†*

*Department of Neurosurgery, Brigham and Women's Hospital, Boston, MA, USA;
†Department de Neurocirurgia, Universidade Federal de Mato Grosso do Sul, Campo Grande-Mato Grosso do Sul, Brasil

"The handling of a suprasellar tumor is one of the most difficult problems in neurosurgery, and no hard and fast rule can be laid down regarding the best way to deal with these cases." **Ernest Sachs, 1949**

INTRODUCTION

Craniopharyngiomas are controversial lesions to the neurosurgeon, both technically and philosophically. This histologically benign epithelial neoplasm arises from embryological remnants of squamous epithelium of the craniopharyngeal duct, intimately related with the hypothalamus, hypophysis, pituitary stalk, anterior aspect of the third ventricle, internal carotid, anterior cerebral, basilar arteries, and their perforators. Although such lesions present challenges in terms of their location and the difficulty of radical resection, and despite controversy (Cabezudo et al., 1981; Fisher et al., 1998; Kim et al., 2001; Merchant et al., 2002), total removal offers the best chance of cure (Garcia-Uria, 1978; Bhagwati et al., 1990; Yasargil et al., 1990; Hoffman et al., 1992; Samii et al., 1994; Maira et al., 1995; Villani et al., 1997; Fahlbusch et al., 1999; Kim et al., 2001; Van Effenterre and Boch, 2002; Rutka, 2002; Wang et al., 2002), and subtotal removal is reported to give higher recurrence rates (Duff and Levine, 1983; Fahlbusch et al., 1999; Duff et al., 2000).

The precise site of origin of the tumor related to the diaphragma sella determines the relationship of the expanding mass with the surrounding sellar structures, and sets the route of tumor extension. Because of different origins and extensions of craniopharyngiomas, several classification systems have been suggested (Yasargil et al., 1990; Hoffman et al., 1992; Samii et al., 1994; Van Effenterre and Boch, 2002) that have implications for the clinical findings, surgical approach, and outcome of patients with these tumors.

The tumor can be classified in terms of its relationship with the sella turcica and diaphragma sellae, the optic chiasm, the third ventricle, and also by its invasiveness

Craniopharyngiomas
http://dx.doi.org/10.1016/B978-0-12-416706-3.00014-3

(Van Effenterre and Boch, 2002). In relation to the optic chiasm, the tumor can be purely prechiasmatic, purely infrachiasmatic, purely retrochiasmatic, or a combination of these (Van Effenterre and Boch, 2002). Intrachiasmatic craniopharyngiomas have also been reported (Duff and Levine, 1983). Prechiasmatic craniopharyngiomas are thought to have a subdiaphragmatic origin, whereas retrochiasmatic craniopharyngiomas are believed to have a supradiaphragmatic origin (Wang et al., 2002). The origin and extension of the craniopharyngioma is implicated in its clinical presentation, choice of surgical approach, and patient outcome.

Retrochiasmatic craniopharyngiomas occur in 11–60% (Garcia-Uria, 1978; Ammirati et al., 1990; Hoffman et al., 1992; Lehrnbecher et al., 1998; Van Effenterre and Boch, 2002; Wang

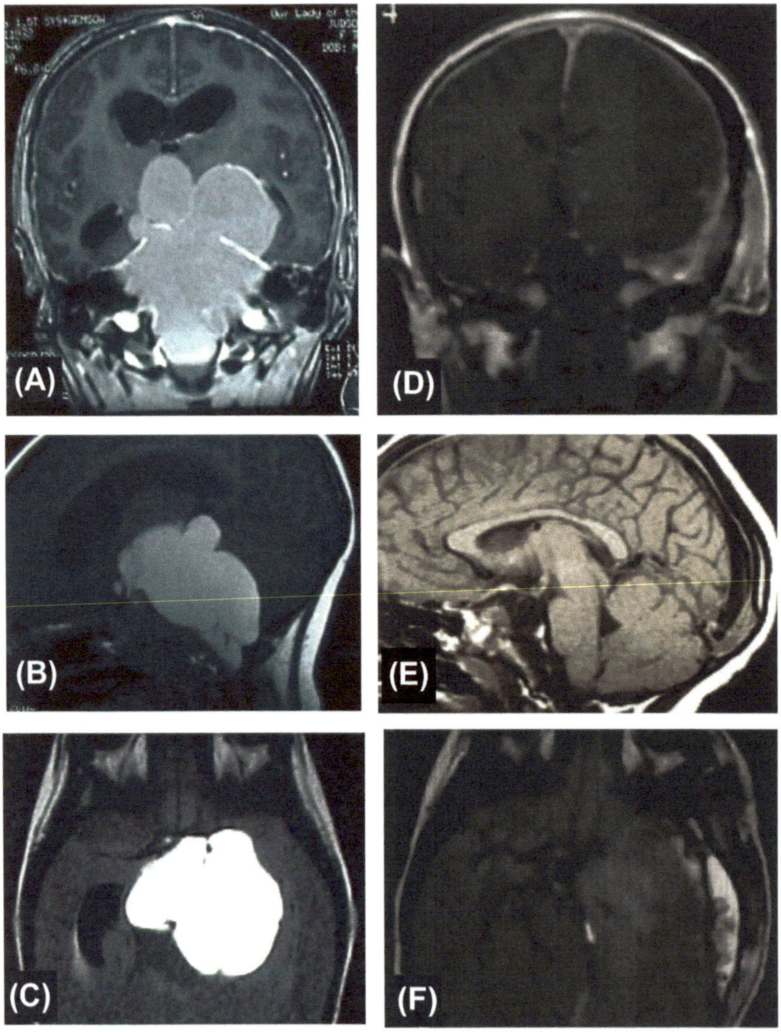

FIGURE 14.1 Imaging studies. **A–C**, Pre-operative coronal **A**, sagittal **B**, and axial **C**, MR images demonstrating the tumor's retrochiasmatic location and giant size with up- and downward extension. **D–F**, Post-operative coronal **D**, sagittal **E**, and axial **F**, MR images confirming total lesion removal.

et al., 2002) of cases. Because they are hidden behind the chiasm, and can extend upward into the third ventricle and downward in front of the brain stem (Figure 14.1), retrochiasmatic craniopharyngiomas remain among the most challenging to treat, and are associated with high surgical mortality (Maira et al., 1995); failure of total removal (Patterson Jr. and Danylevich, 1980; Fahlbusch et al., 1999; Van Effenterre and Boch, 2002); increased surgical complications, particularly hypothalamic complications (Maira et al., 1995; Fahlbusch et al., 1999; Wang et al., 2002); and higher recurrence rates.

Although total removal is the optimal procedure, this is not always possible for retrochiasmatic craniophryngiomas because of the risks to vital structures, namely the hypothalamus, the optic chiasm, the pituitary stalk, and blood vessels arising from the anterior communicating artery and posterior communicating artery (PCoA) (Maira et al., 1995; Villani et al., 1997; Fahlbusch et al., 1999; Van Effenterre and Boch, 2002; Wang et al., 2002).

Reported total removal in retrochiasmatic craniopharyngioma ranges from 31–100% (Ammirati et al., 1990; Bhagwati et al., 1990; Maira et al., 1995; Fahlbusch et al., 1999; Van Effenterre and Boch, 2002). The large size of the tumor (greater than 4 cm) affected the rate of total removal (Villani et al., 1997; Fahlbusch et al., 1999; Kaptain et al., 2001), although even larger tumors (up to 7 cm) have been removed (Al-Mefty et al., 1991, 2007, 2008) (Figures 14.1, 14.4, 14.6). The risk of permanent damage to hypothalamo-pituitary function is still of considerable concern in patients with craniopharyngioma (Inoue et al., 1997; Fahlbusch et al., 1999; Scott, 2005).

NEUROIMAGING EVALUATION

Recognizing a retrochiasmatic extension of the tumor is of paramount importance, because of the difficult exposure of these tumors and their association with high surgical morbidity, failure of total removal, increased surgical complications (primarily hypothalamic dysfunction), and higher recurrence rates (Rougerie, 1979). The various views provided by high-quality MRI precisely pinpoint the anatomical position of the tumor and its usual extension downward toward the posterior fossa and upward into the third ventricle, displacing the midbrain posteriorly and the optic chiasm anteriorly. Visualizing the anterior cerebral-anterior communicating artery complex by magnetic resonance (MR) angiography or digital subtraction angiograms is of supreme relevance to distinguish between pre- and retrochiasmatic lesions. In patients with retrochiasmatic lesions, the anterior cerebral arterial complex is not displaced upward, as it is in patients with prechiasmatic lesions. Computer tomography (CT) adds information about the type and extension of calcification (Figure 14.2).

SURGICAL APPROACHES

Several approaches have been used to achieve total removal of retrochiasmatic craniopharyngiomas (Patterson Jr. and Danylevich, 1980; Fujitsu and Kuwabara, 1985; Baskin and Wilson, 1986; Kanno et al., 1989; Ammirati et al., 1990; Yasargil et al., 1990; Al-Mefty et al., 1991, 2007, 2008; Hoffman, 1994; Samii et al., 1994; Maira et al., 1995; Inoue et al., 1997; Fahlbusch et al., 1999; Kaptain et al., 2001; Kim et al., 2001; Van Effenterre and Boch, 2002; Scott, 2005). Around 20% of craniopharyngiomas are located entirely behind the chiasm, and therefore were not

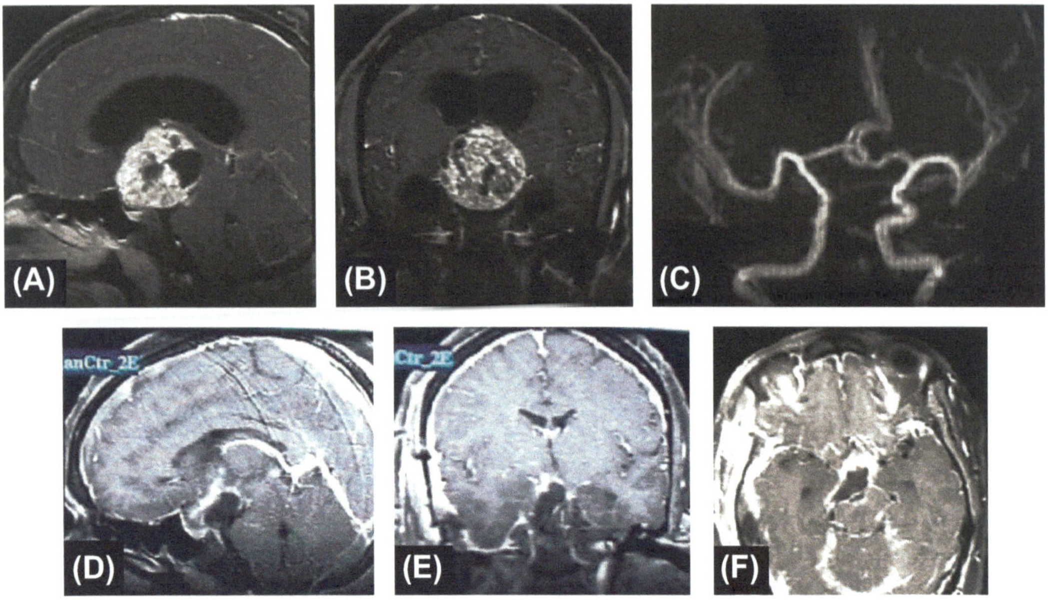

FIGURE 14.2 Imaging studies. Pre-operative axial **A**, sagittal **B**, and axial gadolinium-enhanced magnetic resonance image scans of a large retrochiasmatic craniopharyngioma showing extension into the third ventricle. **C**, magnetic resonance angiogram of a retrochiasmatic craniopharyngioma showing no upward displacement of the anterior cerebral artery. Post-operative sagittal **D**, coronal **E**, and sagittal **F**, MR images confirming total lesion removal.

accessible between the optic nerves at the beginning of the procedure (Van Effenterre and Boch, 2002). The hidden location of these craniopharyngiomas – behind an anteriorly displaced or prefixed chiasm – has led to the development of several approaches for their removal, most of them proceeding via the lamina terminalis. These include the pterional, frontopterional, subfrontopterional (Baskin and Wilson, 1986; Ammirati et al., 1990; Yasargil et al., 1990; Hoffman, 1994; Samii et al., 1994; Maira et al., 1995; Kim et al., 2001; Van Effenterre and Boch, 2002; Scott, 2005), bifrontal interhemispheric through the lamina terminalis, basal interhemispheric supra- or infrachiasmal (or both) (Inoue et al., 1997), zygomatic (Fujitsu and Kuwabara, 1985), and transsphenoidal approaches (Kaptain et al., 2001).

The surgical corridor in the pterional approach is narrow for retrochiasmatic craniopharyngiomas, and the lateral view through the optic carotid triangle is obstructed by perforating arteries (Fahlbusch et al., 1999). Approaches through the lamina terminalis require stripping away of the perforating vessels or mobilizing the anterior cerebral arteries and manipulation close to the chiasm (Kanno et al., 1989; Bhagwati et al., 1990; Fahlbusch et al., 1999). Apart from this obstruction, the tumor's upward extension into the third ventricle is not readily accessible via the horizontal projection of these approaches. In the interhemispheric translamina terminalis approach, the draining veins may need to be cut from the frontal lobe to the sagittal sinus. This maneuver, combined with retraction, may cause subcortical hemorrhaging or a reduction in the regional cerebral blood flow (Kanno et al., 1989). There is also considerable risk of post-operative obesity and other hypothalamic problems (Scott, 2005). The zygomatic approach requires elevating the PCoAs and optic tract

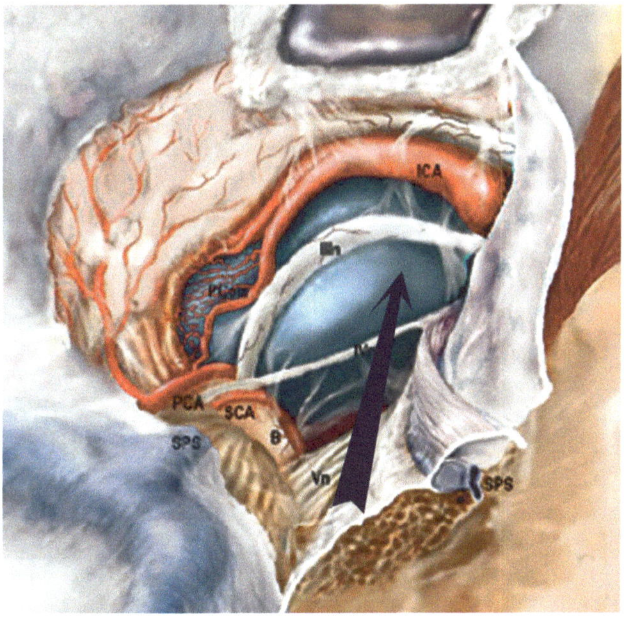

FIGURE 14.3 Illustration of a retrochiasmatic craniopharyngioma exposed via the petrosal approach. The tentorium is sectioned, allowing inferior-to-superior and posterior-to-anterior exposure of the tumor (arrow). B = BA; ICA = internal cerebral artery; PCA = PCoA; PCom = posterior communicating artery; SCA = superior cerebral artery SPS = superior petrosal sinus; IIIn = third cranial nerve; IVn = fourth cranial nerve; Vn = fifth cranial nerve.

(Fujitsu and Kuwabara, 1985), both of which present obstructions. The horizontal projection of the zygomatic approach also limits access to the tumor's upward extension into the third ventricle. The transsphenoidal approach has been used for total resection of posteriorly directed craniopharyngiomas, but visualization of larger tumors might be hindered (Kaptain et al., 2001). The petrosal approach, on the other hand, provides a direct avenue of attack, unobstructed by any vital organs, blood vessels, or perforating vessels (Figure 14.3) (Hakuba et al., 1985; Al-Mefty et al., 1991, 2007, 2008).

PATIENT SELECTION

The petrosal approach is indicated for large retrochiasmatic craniopharyngiomas, even in younger pediatric patients, who do not have fully developed mastoid air cells to perform mastoidectomy (Al-Mefty et al., 2007, 2008). This is diagnosed on pre-operative MRI scan (Lee et al., 2005). The anterior cerebral arteries are not displaced upward in these patients. This can be seen on magnetic resonance angiography (MRA) or DSA (digital subtraction angiogram) (Figure 14.2).

SURGICAL TECHNIQUE

Patient Positioning

The patient is placed supine on the operating table. The ipsilateral shoulder is elevated by placing an appropriate shoulder roll. The head and trunk are elevated by about 30 degrees.

The head is turned and tilted to the opposite side, inclined toward the floor, and fixed in a three-point headrest.

Intra-Operative Monitoring

Brain stem auditory potentials and median nerve somatosensory evoked potential are recorded continuously. Electromyogram is recorded for the third, sixth, and seventh cranial nerves. Other cranial nerves are monitored as required.

The Skin Flap

A reverse question mark incision is made, extending from the zygoma anterior to the tragus, circling 2 to 3 cm above the ear and descending medial to the mastoid process. The skin flap is raised sharply to the level of the external auditory meatus. A large triangular pericranial flap is elevated with its base at the base of the skin flap. This will be used at the end of the procedure for reconstruction.

The Bone Flap

The asterion, located at the junction of the lambdoidal, occipital-mastoid and parietal-mastoid sutures, is the key landmark in this approach. Four burr holes are drilled. The first, located medial and inferior to the asterion, opens into the posterior fossa below the transverse sigmoid sinus junction. The second, located at the squamal and mastoid junctions of the temporal bone along the projection of superior temporal line, opens into the supratentorial compartment. These two holes flank the sigmoid sinus. The other two holes are made medial to the first two on each side of the transverse sinus which runs along a line projecting along the zygomatic arch posteriorly. The temporal and occipital bones are incised between the burr holes, supra- and infratentorialy, using the foot attachment of the craniotome. For retrochiasmatic craniophayngiomas, the occipital part of the flap is somewhat smaller than the flap used for petroclival lesions. The foot attachment is not used to cross the sinus. The bone over the sinus is drilled carefully to expose the sinus between each of the holes flanking the sinus. The single bone flap is elevated, and carefully separated from the sinus and dura. The sinus might be tightly adhered to the sinus at the transverse sigmoid junction.

The Mastoidectomy

A small bony flap made of the cortices of the mastoid is elevated in one piece. This will be used at the end of the procedure to reconstruct the mastoid area. A complete mastoidectomy is performed. The sigmoid sinus is de-skeletonized down to the jugular bulb exposing the dura on both sides of the sinus. The dura anterior to the sigmoid sinus is exposed only enough to open and close the dura. The semicircular canals are carefully preserved to preserve hearing. Drilling continues along the pyramid to thin the petrous bone towards its apex.

Opening the Dura

The temporal dura is opened along the floor of the middle fossa, and the pre-sigmoid posterior fossa dura is then opened in turn. Insertions of the vein of Labbé and the posterior temporal veins are inspected, and then the superior petrosal sinus is coagulated and divided at a point that preserves the vein of Labbé and the posterior temporal veins.

Sectioning the Tentorium and Opening the Arachnoid

The tentorium is sectioned all the way through to the incisura, taking care to preserve the fourth nerve, rendering the sigmoid sinus free for posterior mobilization, while the posterior tentorial leaf together with the temporal lobe are supported with a brain spatula. The arachnoid membrane of the crural and ambient cisterns is opened identifying the third and fourth nerves, the posterior cerebral artery, and the superior cerebellar artery at the incisura.

At this point, the tumor is widely exposed under the chiasma, the hypothalamus and the retrosellar area; in front of the midbrain; and on top of the basilar artery. The exposure is thus superb indeed (Figures 14.4–14.7).

Exposing and Debulking the Tumor

The tumor is then identified anterior to the midbrain. A specimen is taken for immediate histological conformation. If there is a cystic portion, it is aspirated with cottonoids placed around the area to prevent spillage of the contents.

The tumor capsule is entered and the tumor is debulked internally. Solid calcification may require the use of an ultrasonic aspirator.

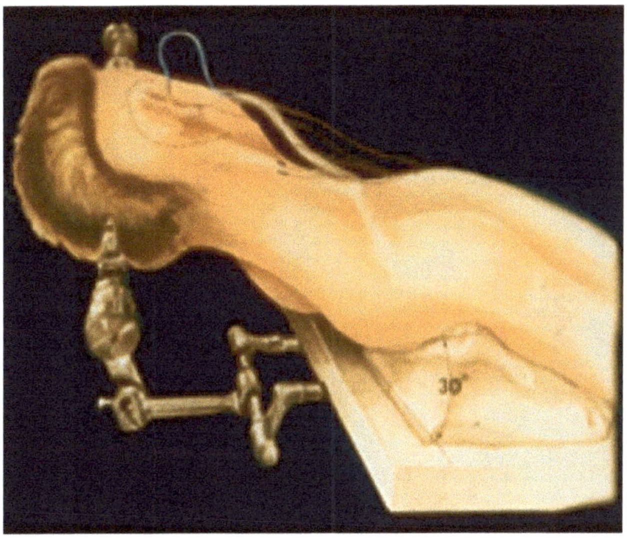

FIGURE 14.4 The patient's position is shown for the petrosal approach.

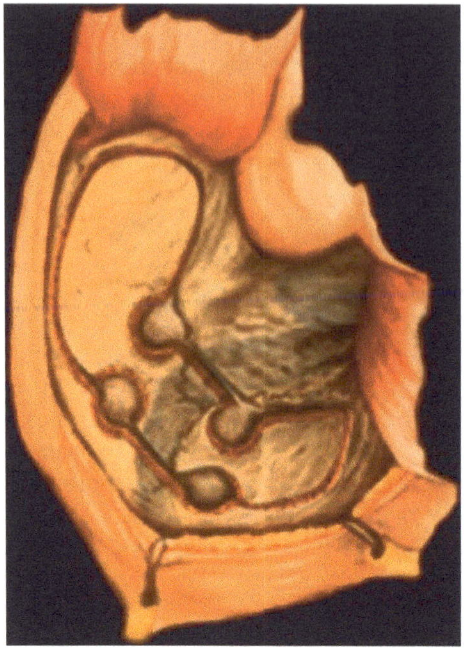

FIGURE 14.5 For the bone flap, four burr holes flank the transverse and sigmoid sinuses.

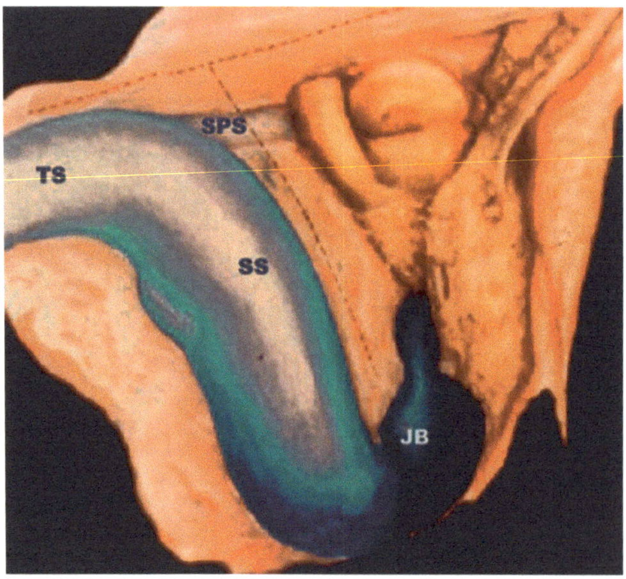

FIGURE 14.6 The mastoid is drilled away and the pre-sigmoid dura is exposed down to the jugular bulb. JB, jugular bulb; SPS, superior petrosal sinus; SS, sigmoid sinus; TS, transverse sinus. Dotted lines indicate sites of dural opening.

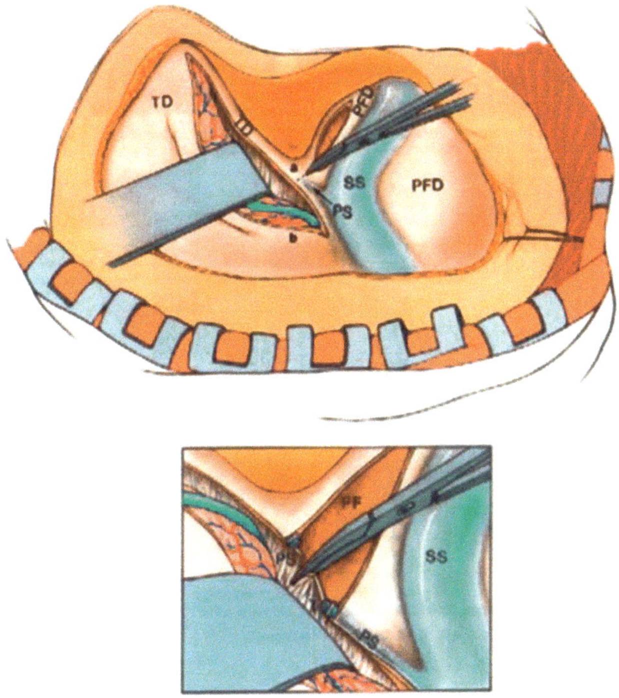

FIGURE 14.7 Opening the temporal dura is demonstrated. The vein of Labbé is identified and preserved and the pre-sigmoid dura is opened. The superior petrosal sinus is coagulated and divided anterior to the insertion of the vein of Labbé to preserve drainage from the temporal lobe (inset).

Dissection of the Tumor

After the tumor has been debulked, the capsule can be freed from the surrounding structures such as the third nerve, the fourth nerve, and the basilar artery and its perforators. The capsule in the interpeduncular fossa is separated from the anterior aspect of the brain stem, and the dissection progresses anteriorly towards the dorsum sella while the tumor descends free from the third ventricle giving way to a gliotic plane of dissection between the tumor capsule and the hypothalamic floor. The tumor is dissected off the inferior surface of the hypothalamus, by identifying the change in tissue appearance between the tumor and hypothalamus. The hypothalamus with its feeding perforators remains intact. As the dissection progresses anteriorly, the tumor is dissected off the carotid artery and the posterior communicating artery. The pituitary stalk is identified, preserved and followed into the sella, where the intrasellar portion of the tumor is removed, while preserving the gland itself. The gland is usually compressed but identifiable by its color and texture (Figures 14.5, 14.7).

Any tumor that lies beneath the optic nerves is dissected with care taken to avoid injury to these nerves. As the capsule extension of the tumor to the contralateral side is dissected, the contralateral third nerve and posterior cerebral artery can be identified. If the tumor extends into the third ventricle, it will come down as progressive tumor removal continues. This part of the tumor is removed in piecemeal fashion. The third ventricle is entered superior to the pituitary stalk and anterior to the mamillary bodies. When the tumor extends into the posterior fossa, it is dissected off the clivus and dorsum sella, the fifth, seventh, and eighth nerves, the lower cranial nerves, and the jugular foramen (Figures 14.8–14.11).

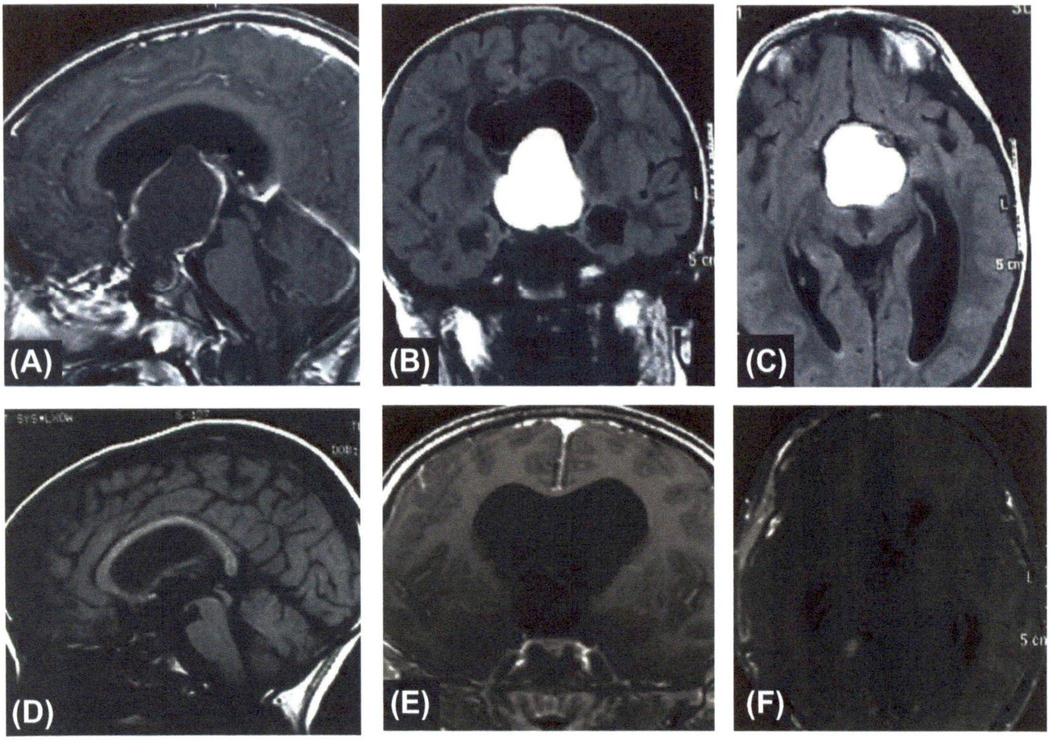

FIGURE 14.8 Imaging studies. A–C: Pre-operative sagittal **A,** coronal **B,** and axial **C,** MR images demonstrating the tumor's retrochiasmatic location and giant size with upward extension. D–F: Post-operative sagittal **D,** coronal **E,** and axial **F,** MR images confirming total lesion removal.

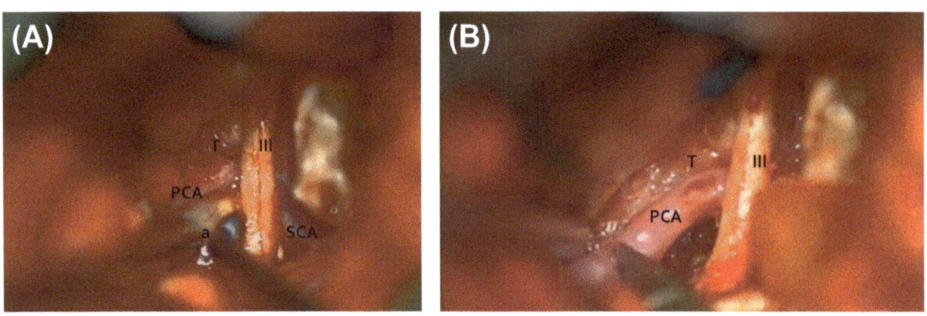

FIGURE 14.9 Intra-operative photographs (see pre- and post-operative MRs in Figure 14.4). **A,** Initial exposure of the tumor (T) capsule, separating it from the third nerve (III). **B,** Dissection of the tumor (T) from the hypothalamus.

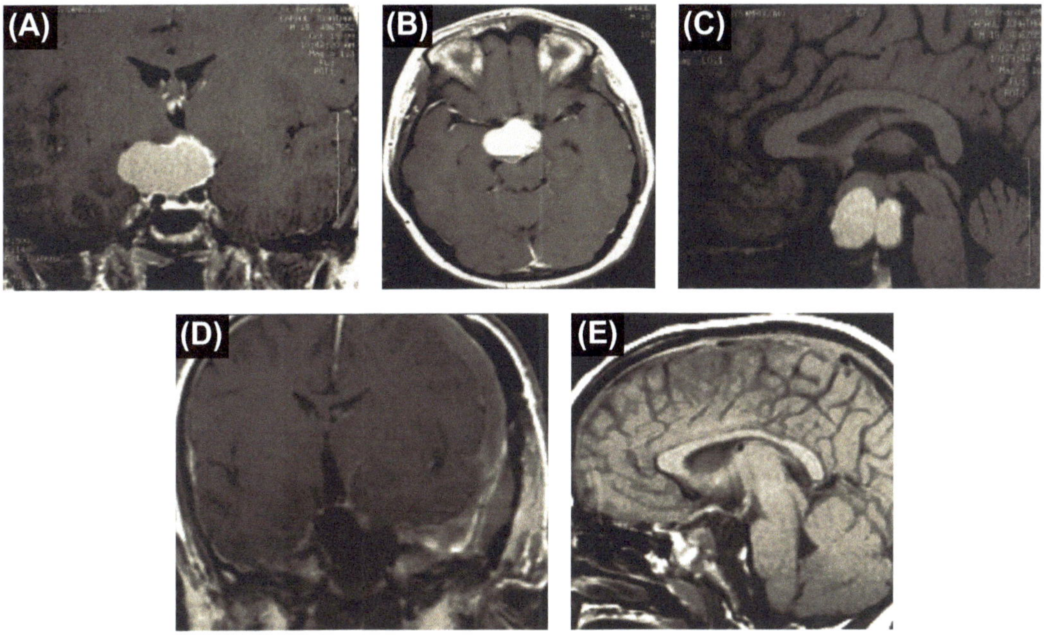

FIGURE 14.10 **A–C**: Pre-operative coronal **A**, sagittal **B**, and axial **C**, MR images demonstrating the tumor's retrochiasmatic location (see intra-operative pictures). **D,E**: Post-operative coronal **D**, sagittal **E**, MR images confirming total lesion removal.

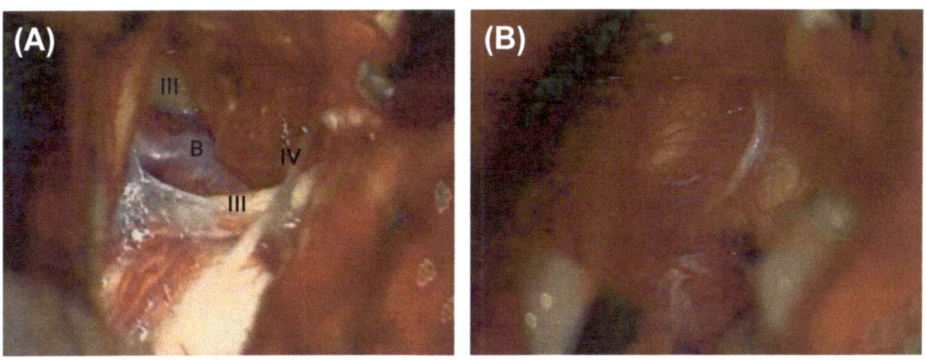

FIGURE 14.11 Intra-operative photographs (see pre- and post-operative MR in Figure 14.6). **A,** Dissection of the tumor at the BA tip (B in panel) between the third cranial nerve (III) on both sides, (IV, fourth cranial nerve). **B,** Preservation of the arachnoid plane with perforator arteries to the optic tract, hypothalamus, and brainstem.

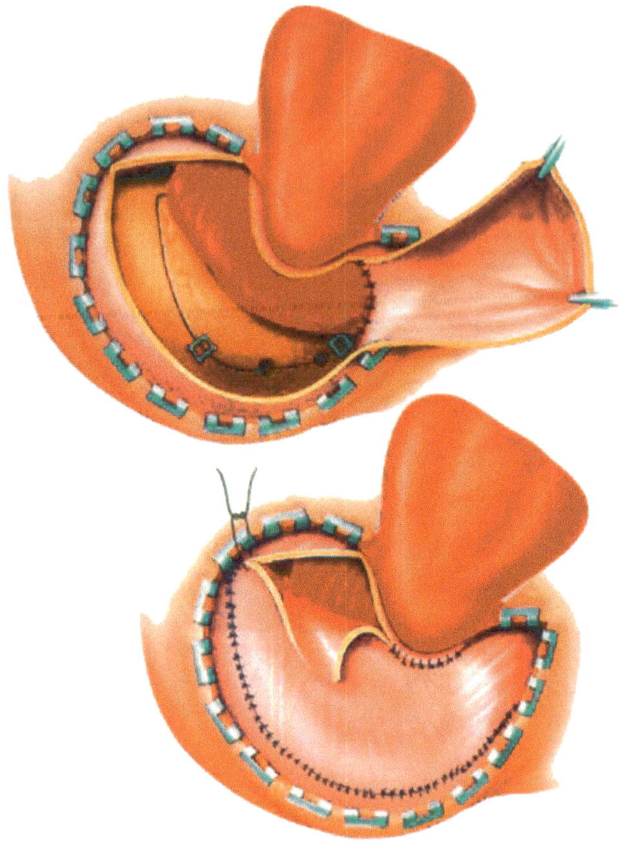

FIGURE 14.12 During closure, the temporal muscle is rotated over the defect and the temporal fascia is sutured.

Closure

The temporal and pre-sigmoid dura is closed watertight using 6/0 nylon and a pericranial free cranial graft if necessary. The drilled mastoid is sealed with bone substitute and the cavity is filled with fat. The triangular pericranial flap raised at the start of surgery is turned over the drilled surface. The temporal muscle is rotated over the defect and sutured to the sternomastoid muscle. The soft tissue and skin are closed in layers (Figure 14.12).

For retrochiasmatic craniophayngiomas, the occipital part of the flap is somewhat smaller than the flap used for petroclival lesions.

COMPLICATION MANAGEMENT

CSF Leak

Cerebrospinal fluid (CSF) leak can occur from the skin, or, more often in the form of rhinorrhea. Meticulous closure is very important for preventing such leaks. If leakage does occur, spinal drainage is carried out for 72 hours. If this continues, the wound is re-explored. If meningitis occurs as a result of CSF leak, it is treated with antibiotics and spinal drainage.

Diabetes Insipidus

Hourly fluid intake and fluid output are monitored immediately post-operatively. Electrolytes are measured in the blood. If urine output is more than 250 ml per hour for two consequent hours, or more than 500 ml per hour for any time and the sodium concentration in the blood is not low, then treatment with desmopressin - (1-desamino-8-D-arginine vasopressin) (DDAVP) is started. If sodium concentration is low, treatment is withheld until it is ascertained that polyuria is not due to fluid overload. If there is no polyuria in the first 24 hours, fluids (5% dextrose with half normal saline and added potassium) are given to equalize intake with output on hourly bases. If diabetes insipidus persists, DDAVP is given in scheduled doses.

Because the preoptic area and medial septal nucleus of the hypothalamus originate in the embryo from the medial ganglionic eminence, they receive their blood supply from the perforating branches of the recurrent artery of Heubner and the middle cerebral artery along the endonasal sulcus (Nunta-aree et al., 2001).

The posterior petrosal approach is uniquely advantageous in preserving the blood supply to the hypothalamus, the anterior cerebral arteries, and their perforating arteries (Al-Mefty et al., 1991, 2007, 2008). Despite surgical preservation of the pituitary stalk, diabetes insipidus – either temporary or permanent – can develop regardless of the surgical approach chosen (Al-Mefty et al., 1985, 2007, 2008; Hakuba et al., 1985; Bhagwati et al., 1990; Villani et al., 1997; Lehrnbecher et al., 1998; Honegger et al., 1999; Van Effenterre and Boch, 2002; Wang et al., 2002; Albright et al., 2005). In many cases, the pituitary stalk can be identified intra-operatively, dissected away from the tumor, and preserved. Preserving the pituitary stalk and gland is worthwhile, because anterior pituitary functions can be maintained intact (Honegger et al., 1999). In a few patients, however, the stalk might have to be sacrificed to achieve complete tumor removal (Honegger et al., 1999). If only part of the pituitary is invaded by tumor, it can be partially resected so that some of its function is preserved (Honegger et al., 1999).

The petrosal approach is a variable and useful option in the treatment of retrochiasmatic craniopharyngiomas. It provides direct projection to the tumor with no obstruction by any vital organ or blood vessels and perforators. Vascularization and function of the hypothalamus are thus preserved.

References

Albright, A.L., Hadjipanayis, C.G., Lunsford, L.D., Kondziolka, D., Pollack, I.F., Adelson, P.D., 2005. Individualized treatment of pediatric craniopharyngiomas. Childs Nerv. Syst. 21, 649–654.

Al-Mefty, O., Hassounah, M., Weaver, P., Sakati, N., Jinkins, J.R., Fox, J.L., 1985. Microsurgery for giant craniopharyngiomas in children. Neurosurgery 17, 585–595.

Al-Mefty, O., Ayoubi, S., Smith, R.R., 1991. The petrosal approach: indications, technique, and results. Acta Neurochir. Suppl. (Wien) 53, 166–170.

Al-Mefty, O., Ayoubi, S., Kadri, P.A., 2007. The petrosal approach for total removal of giant retrochiasmatic craniopharyngiomas in children. J. Neurosurg. 106 (Suppl.), 87–92.

Al-Mefty, O., Ayoubi, S., Kadri, P.A., 2008. The petrosal approach for the resection of retrochiasmatic craniopharyngiomas. Neurosurgery 62 (5 Suppl. 2), 331–335; discussion 335–336.

Ammirati, M., Samii, M., Sephernia, A., 1990. Surgery of large retrochiasmatic craniopharyngiomas in children. Childs Nerv. Syst. 6, 13–17.
Baskin, D.S., Wilson, C.B., 1986. Surgical management of craniopharyngiomas. A review of 74 cases. J. Neurosurg. 65, 22–27.
Bhagwati, S.N., Deopujari, C.E., Parulekar, G.D., 1990. Lamina terminalis approach for retrochiasmal craniopharyngiomas. Childs Nerv. Syst. 6, 425–429.
Cabezudo, J.M., Vaquero, J., Areitio, E., Martinez, R., de Sola, R.G., Bravo, G., 1981. Craniopharyngiomas: a critical approach to treatment. J. Neurosurg. 55, 371–375.
Duff, T.A., Levine, R., 1983. Intrachiasmatic craniopharyngioma. Case report. J. Neurosurg. 59, 176–178.
Duff, J.M., Meyer, F.B., Ilstrup, D.M., Laws Jr., E.R., Schleck, C.D., Scheithauer, B.W., 2000. Long-term outcomes for surgically resected craniopharyngiomas. Neurosurgery 46, 291–305.
Fahlbusch, R., Honegger, J., Paulus, W., Huk, W., Buchfelder, M., 1999. Surgical treatment of craniopharyngiomas: experience with 168 patients. J. Neurosurg. 90, 237–250.
Fisher, P.G., Jenab, J., Goldthwaite, P.T., Tihan, T., Wharam, M.D., Foer, D.R., et al., 1998. Outcomes and failure patterns in childhood craniopharyngiomas. Childs Nerv. Syst. 14, 558–563.
Fujitsu, K., Kuwabara, T., 1985. Zygomatic approach for lesions in the interpeduncular cistern. J. Neurosurg. 62, 340–343.
Garcia-Uria, J., 1978. Surgical experience with craniopharyngioma in adults. Surg. Neurol. 9, 11–14.
Hakuba, A., Nishimura, S.N., Inoue, Y., 1985. Transpetrosal-transtentorial approach and its application in the therapy of retrochiasmatic craniopharyngiomas. Surg. Neurol. 24, 405–415.
Hoffman, H.J., De Silva, M., Humphreys, R.P., Drake, J.M., Smith, M.L., Blaser, S.I., 1992. Aggressive surgical management of craniopharyngiomas in children. J. Neurosurg. 76, 47–52.
Hoffman, H.J., 1994. Surgical management of craniopharyngioma. Pediatr. Neurosurg. 21 (Suppl. 1), 44–49.
Honegger, J., Buchfelder, M., Fahlbusch, R., 1999. Surgical treatment of craniopharyngiomas: endocrinological results. J. Neurosurg. 90, 251–257.
Inoue, H.K., Fujimaki, H., Kohga, H., Ono, N., Hirato, M., Ohye, C., 1997. Basal interhemispheric supra- and/or infrachiasmal approaches via superomedial orbitotomy for hypothalamic lesions: preservation of the hypothalamo-pituitary functions in combination treatment with radiosurgery. Childs Nerv. Syst. 13, 250–256.
Kanno, T., Kasama, A., Shoda, M., Yamaguchi, C., Kato, Y., 1989. A pitfall in interhemispheric translamina terminalis approach for the removal of a craniopharyngioma. Significance of preserving draining veins. Part I. Clinical study. Surg. Neurol. 32, 111–115.
Kaptain, G.J., Vincent, D.A., Sheehan, J.P., Laws Jr., E.R., 2001. Transsphenoidal approaches for the extracapsular resection of midline suprasellar and anterior cranial base lesions. Neurosurgery 49, 94–101.
Kim, S.K., Wang, K.C., Shin, S.H., Choe, G., Chi, J.G., Cho, B.K., 2001. Radical excision of pediatric craniopharyngioma: recurrence pattern and prognostic factors. Childs Nerv. Syst. 17, 531–537.
Lee, D.H., Jun, B.C., Kim, D.G., Jung, M.K., Yeo, S.W., 2005. Volume variation of mastoid pneumatization in different age groups: a study by three-dimensional reconstruction based on computed tomography images. Surg. Radiol. Anat. 27, 37–42.
Lehrnbecher, T., Müller-Scholden, J., Danhauser-Leistner, I., Sorensen, N., von Stockhausen, H.B., 1998. Perioperative fluid and electrolyte management in children undergoing surgery for craniopharyngioma. A 10-year experience in a single institution. Childs Nerv. Syst. 14, 276–279.
Maira, G., Anile, C., Rossi, G.F., Colosimo, C., 1995. Surgical treatment of craniopharyngiomas: an evaluation of the transsphenoidal and pterional approaches. Neurosurgery 36, 715–724.
Merchant, T.E., Kiehna, E.N., Sanford, R.A., Mulhern, R.K., Thompson, S.J., Wilson, M.W., et al., 2002. Craniopharyngioma: the St. Jude Children's Research Hospital experience 1984–2001. Int. J. Radiat. Oncol. Biol. Phys. 53, 533–542.
Nunta-aree, S., Ohata, K., Soares Jr., S.B., Haque, M., Takami, T., Inoue, Y., et al., 2001. The morphological development of human basal ganglia. Congen. Anomal. 41, 177–186.
Patterson Jr., R.H., Danylevich, A., 1980. Surgical removal of craniopharyngioms by a transcranial approach through the lamina terminalis and sphenoid sinus. Neurosurgery 7, 111–117.
Rougerie, J., 1979. What can be expected from the surgical treatment of craniopharyngiomas in children. Report of 92 cases. Childs Brain 5, 433–449.
Rutka, J.T., 2002. Craniopharyngioma. J. Neurosurg. 97, 1–2.

Sachs, Ernest, 1949. Diagnosis and treatment of brain tumors and care of the neurosurgical patient. C.V. Mosby Company, St. Louis, p. 436.
Samii, M., Cheatham, M.L., Becker, D.P. (Eds.), 1994. Atlas of Cranial Base Surgery. WB Saunders, Philadelphia, pp. 176–179.
Scott, R.M., 2005. Craniopharyngioma: a personal (Boston) experience. Childs Nerv. Syst. 21, 773–777.
Van Effenterre, R., Boch, A.L., 2002. Craniopharyngioma in adults and children: a study of 122 surgical cases. J. Neurosurg. 97, 3–11.
Villani, R.M., Tomei, G., Bello, L., Sganzerla, E., Ambrosi, B., Re, T., et al., 1997. Long-term results of treatment for craniopharyngioma in children. Childs Nerv. Syst. 13, 397–405.
Wang, K.C., Kim, S.K., Choe, G., Chi, J.G., Cho, B.K., 2002. Growth patterns of caniopharyngioma in children: role of the diaphragm sellae and its surgical implication. Surg. Neurol. 57, 25–33.
Yasargil, M.G., Curcic, M., Kis, M., Siegenthaler, G., Teddy, P.J., Roth, P., 1990. Total removal of craniopharyngiomas. Approaches and long term results in 144 patients. J. Neurosurg. 73, 3–11.

CHAPTER

15

Endoscopic Transventricular Approach to Craniopharyngiomas

Konstantinos Margetis[*,†], *Mark Souweidane*[*,†]

[*]Department of Neurological Surgery, Weill Cornell Medical College, New York, New York; [†]Department of Neurological Surgery, Memorial Sloan-Kettering Cancer Center, New York, New York

"By the time these cases come to necropsy, the tumor has reached such a large size that it has often spread upward into the third ventricle, regardless of its point of origin." **CH Frazier and BJ Alpers, 1931**

INTRODUCTION

Intraventricular cystic tumors lend themselves to endoscopic intraventricular methods (Margetis and Souweidane, 2013b). The cystic nature of the tumor allows it to be decompressed and shrunk by aspirating the contents and thus making surgical manipulations more facile. Additionally, these tumors are in general less hemorrhagic than solid tumors, and their membranous walls are easier to recognize through endoscopic visualization than solid tumors. A cystic component is present in up to 90% of craniopharyngiomas (Fahlbusch et al., 1999), and very often they have an intraventricular component. It is hence easily conceivable that endoscopic intraventricular methods can be applied in craniopharyngiomas and offer a less invasive approach than traditional microsurgical approaches. Herein, we suggest the main indications for an endoscopic transventricular procedure in a craniopharyngioma patient, and we analyze the basic operative steps of such a procedure.

INDICATIONS

The endoscopic intraventricular approach can decompress a cystic craniopharyngioma (CP) (Figures 15.1, 15.2). The reduction in size offers a smaller target for radiation therapy and thus potentially minimizes the side effects of the radiation therapy (RT). The reduction in size can also provide symptomatic relief from obstructive hydrocephalus or compression of the optic apparatus. This symptomatic relief can prove a valuable temporizing measure in the very young

Craniopharyngiomas
http://dx.doi.org/10.1016/B978-0-12-416706-3.00015-5

patient population (< 5 years of age) as it means that radiation therapy can be postponed until an older age and thus protect the developing brain from the potential ill effects of RT. Further work is needed in order to clarify whether in older patients after symptomatic relief it is preferable to observe the tumor rather than administering upfront RT for the residual tumor.

Although a gross total resection (GTR) of a craniopharyngioma by an endoscopic intraventricular approach has been reported (Cinalli et al., 2006), a GTR or even a meaningful subtotal resection (STR) can rarely be achieved through a purely endoscopic route. The suprasellar and the infra-third ventricle floor components of the tumor are not frequently accessible in their entirety by this approach. Moreover, current endoscopic equipment does not provide the means for an effective and safe surgical dissection of the tumor tissue and is subject to significant limitations due to intra-operative vision obscuration by bleeding and suboptimal bimanual dissection capabilities (Qiao and Souweidane, 2011).

Puget et al. (2007) classified pediatric CPs into three categories on the basis of the degree of hypothalamic invasion, as evaluated by pre-operative MR imaging (Figure 15.3). In Grade

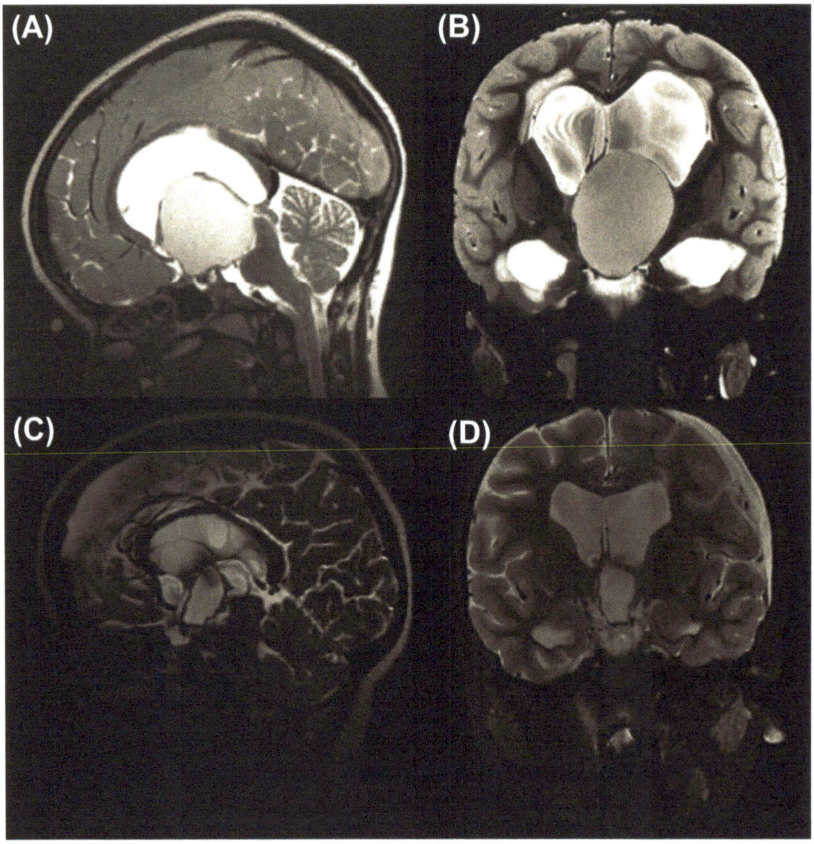

FIGURE 15.1 Pre-operative sagittal **A**, and coronal **B**, T2W MRI image of craniopharyngioma. In the post-operative sagittal **C**, and coronal **D**, T2W MRI image, following the endoscopic decompression of the cystic component of the tumor, the mass effect is alleviated and the hydrocephalus is addressed.

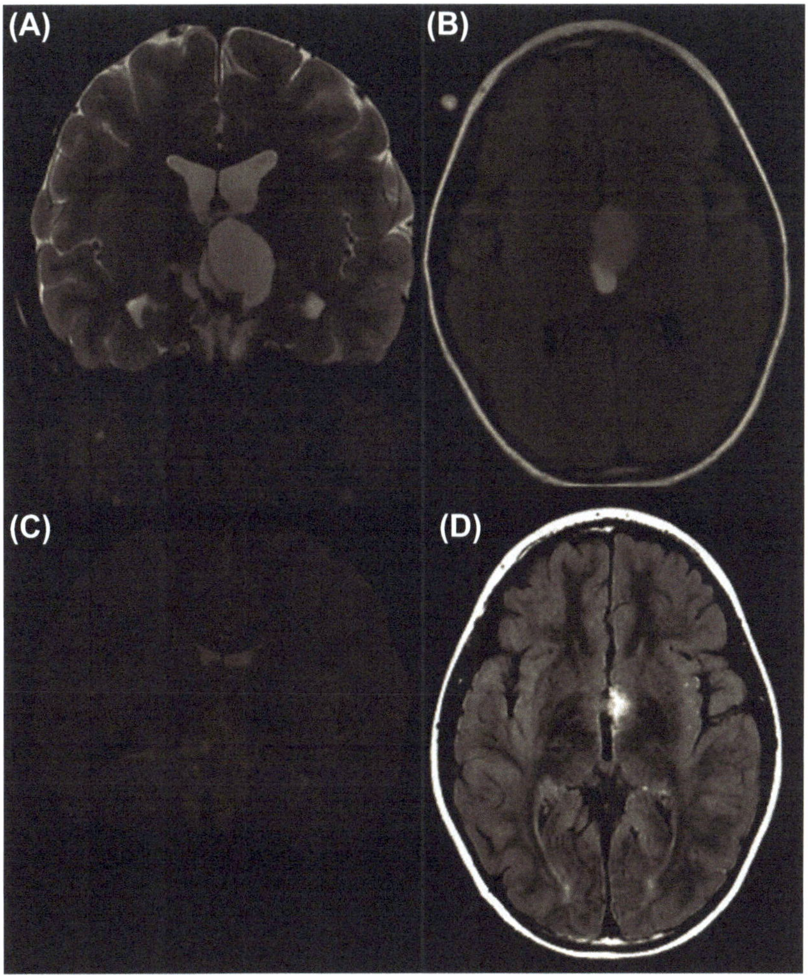

FIGURE 15.2 Another example of an endoscopic intraventricular subtotal resection of the cystic component of a craniopharyngioma. The pre-operative coronal T2W MRI **A,** and axial FLAIR MRI **B,** image and the post-operative coronal T2W MRI **C,** and axial FLAIR MRI **D,** images show the resection of the cystic component of the craniopharyngioma.

0 there was no hypothalamic involvement, in Grade 1 the tumor was displacing or abutting the hypothalamus, and in Grade 2 there was hypothalamic involvement. The endoscopic intraventricular approach is suitable for tumors that extend inside the third ventricle, so according to the Puget classification, it is suitable for either Grade 2 or Grade 1 that displace the floor of the third ventricle superiorly. Using the endoscopic transventricular approach, Grade 0 tumors can only be considered for biopsy after performing an endoscopic third ventriculostomy. Puget et al. (2007) proposed that subtotal resection and radiation therapy (RT) (for age >5 years) should be the preferred option for Grade 2 tumors. The increased rate of endocrinopathy and hypothalamic injury in the pediatric population with the GTR option compared with the STR+RT was also validated by a systematic review on the subject

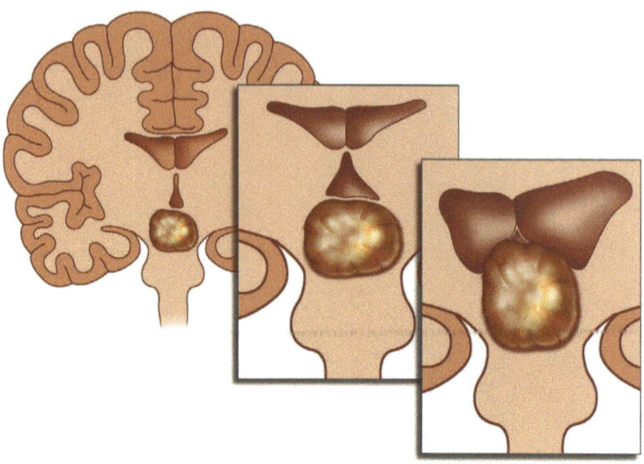

FIGURE 15.3 Craniopharyngioma classification with pre-operative MR imaging, according to Puget et al. (2007). A practical approach to this classification is to assess on sagittal or coronal images the location and the integrity of the third ventricular floor. An intact and in normal location third ventricular floor correlates to Grade 0 (left image); displacement with retention of the integrity correlates to Grade 1 (middle image); infiltration correlates with Grade 2 (right image).

(Clark et al., 2012). For Grade 1 CPs, the options are either STR+RT or an attempt at complete excision. The recommended treatments rely on the balance between operative morbidity and risk of recurrence. Reducing the grade of a CP from 2 or 3 to 1 offers the potential benefit of subsequent delayed complete excision; complete excision – if achieved – is preferable to subtotal resection in terms of recurrence risk (Yang et al., 2010; Mortini et al., 2011) and obviates the need for RT. Mallucci et al. (2012) showed that an initial neuroendoscopy procedure can reduce the cystic component of the tumor and lead to reclassification of the tumor from Grade 2 to Grade 1. The new grade changes the treatment strategy and allows complete excision to be attempted. Moreover, the reduction in size of the CP might make stereotactic radiosurgery possible (Nakahara et al., 2004), rather than conventional fractionated RT, an option that is felt to offer advantages for this WHO Grade 1 tumor (Veeravagu et al., 2010).

Another role for neuroendoscopy is the combined endoscopic-microsurgical resection of complex CPs (Filis et al., 2009). In this option, both approaches are performed under the same general anesthesia, or in two stages (Gangemi et al., 2009). Neuroendoscopy achieves cyst decompression and addresses the hydrocephalus. The microsurgical procedure that follows through a traditional pterional or subfrontal approach is more facile and safer, since the brain is more relaxed. Transventricular neuroendoscopy can be combined with endonasal, endoscopic techniques, in a similar manner to the combined endoscopic-microsurgical techniques. This combination integrates the less invasive merits of the transventricular neuroendoscopy with those of the endonasal neuroendoscopy (Schwartz et al., 2008; Komotar et al., 2012; Leng et al., 2012; Mascarenhas et al., 2013).

The minimal morbidity of the endoscopic procedure affords a more appealing concept of secondary procedures, should an indication for intervention (e.g., cyst recurrence) emerge (Delitala et al., 2004). The endoscopic intraventricular approach is also a minimally invasive method for the biopsy of the pathologic tissue (Constantini et al., 2013).

Another aspect of the initial endoscopic management of these tumors is the potential for a simultaneous endoscopic septum pellucidum fenestration. This procedure has great utility in the management of patients with craniopharyngioma owing to the frequency of bilateral obstruction of the foramen of Monro (Souweidane, 2005).

Neuroendoscopy may also be utilized for the accurate placement of intratumoral catheters (Pettorini et al., 2009). These catheters can be employed for sequential cyst aspiration or intracavitary ablative therapy (Cavalheiro et al., 2010).

Selection of the optimal treatment strategy for craniopharyngiomas is complex. Most importantly, therapy should be individualized on the basis of a multitude of features including patient age, degree of pre-existing pituitary dysfunction, amount of visual compromise, tumor composition, patient's access to long-term medical therapy, and hypothalamic approximation. Given the wide availability of legitimate options available, the patient and/or the patient's family should be integrated into this decision-making and informed consent process. The foremost consideration, however, in selecting a therapeutic strategy should be the lasting preservation of patient functional capacity. These tumors can be extremely indolent in their growth features and a transition in therapeutic philosophy to managing a "chronic ailment" can be justified in selected cases. With this emphasis in mind, endoscopic intraventricular methods should enter the decision-making process when appropriate, given the established tolerance and reduced risk profile associated with this type of surgical intervention. Given the advent of new promising therapies such as systemic pegylated interferon-a-2b (Yeung et al., 2012), minimizing the morbidity of any therapeutic intervention becomes a predominant criterion in the decision-making process.

SURGICAL TECHNIQUE

POSITIONING. The patient is positioned supine on a padded operating table with the head fixed on a three-pin Mayfield clamp and the arms tucked in at the side. The younger patient population requires a pin pressure lower than 60 lbs or a Sugitta head frame according to the surgeon's preferences. In rare situations when the child is less than two years of age, pin fixation might be avoided entirely and a horseshoe headrest might be best. The neck is slightly flexed and the head of the operating table is elevated to bring the incision to the highest level in order to minimize intra-operative cerebrospinal fluid (CSF) egress. When adjusting the head position, the surgeon should anticipate that the incision is usually close to the coronal suture. The frameless stereotactic system is registered with the pre-op MRI. It is standard practice for our group to use frameless stereotactic navigation in all elective cases of neuroendoscopy for CP. However, other authors in previous reports have successfully used a free hand technique (Delitala et al., 2004). Intravenous antibiotics (typically cefazolin) are administered. Dexamethasone is also preferred in an attempt to reduce any inflammatory potential from intraventricular spillage of cyst contents.

TRAJECTORY SELECTION. Once the stereotactic system is registered, a surgical trajectory is selected. The "inline" reconstructed views rather than the conventional sagittal/coronal/axial views are preferred for trajectory selection. The inline views show reconstructed images at the same plane as the pointer, and allow for easier recognition of any structures that need to be avoided as the endoscope is inserted. The trajectory should be through a gyrus and not through the sulci, in order to avoid the sulcal blood vessels. The paramedial approaches need special attention to avoid paths that encroach the pial interface of interhemispheric sulci, particularly the cingulate and callosal sulci. The next point of the linear path is the foramen of Monro. The trajectory should optimize a perpendicular approximation to the cystic tumor component for fenestration purposes. If a septum pellucidum fenestration is planned, then a more lateral trajectory should be chosen. A non-dominant side approach is usually selected, although sometimes the tumor might deform and displace foramina of Monro, making a dominant side approach advantageous. Following the trajectory selection, the entry point and the skin incision are marked. A self-adhesive, water-impermeable drape is placed on the forehead to keep the eyes and the endotracheal tube protected from any intra-operative fluid flow.

APPROACH. Standard prepping and draping of the surgical site is performed. Local anesthetic with epinephrine is injected along the linear incision line. The endoscopes are checked for proper white balance, orientation, and focus prior to ventricular cannulation. A stereotactic reference array is connected to the endoscopic sheath and the sheath is registered with the stereotactic system. Consideration needs to be given to avoiding crimping the sheath or using a reference array that will interfere with accessing the working portals. A burr hole is created and the dura is incised in a cruciate fashion. The cortex is inspected to verify that there is no sulcus or significant vein in the desired corticectomy site. A localized corticectomy is performed with the bipolar cautery and sharp dissection.

VENTRICULAR ACCESS. The vast majority of patients will have ventriculomegaly, and ventricular access should be straightforward, by advancing the endoscopic sheath under stereotactic guidance with the obturators in place. The endoscopic sheath has multiple channels for the optics, irrigation, CSF egress, and instrument insertion. The obturator blocks these channels all the way down to the tip of the endoscope to minimize disruption of brain tissue during the insertion process. Once ventricular access is achieved, the obturator is removed and the 0 degree endoscope is inserted into the endoscopic sheath. In patients with normal-sized ventricles, ventricular access is first achieved with a ventricular catheter that has been registered with the stereotactic system. The ventricular catheter is advanced under stereotactic guidance, until ventricular access is achieved. The stylet of the ventricular catheter is removed and the ventricular system is insufflated with 5 cc aliquots of normal saline (Margetis and Souweidane, 2013a) after making sure that the CSF egress portal is patent. Usually 2–3 aliquots are slowly injected with vigilant surveillance for any bradycardia or hypertension. The endoscopic sheath with the endoscope in place is advanced along the tract of the ventricular catheter under direct endoscopic view of the tract. In our procedures, we use a rigid endoscope (MINOP, B. Braun, Melsungen, Germany); other authors have used different scopes, such as the flexible endoscope (Delitala et al., 2004) or the rigid 3 mm fiberscope (Paediscope, B. Braun, Melsungen, Germany) (Gangemi et al., 2009). If there is any suspicion of a germ cell tumor, CSF should be collected and sent for analysis (cytology, tumor markers) once ventricular access is obtained.

PROCEDURE. Once confirmation of appropriate cannulation is made, free-flowing irrigation using lactated ringer's solution begins. Importantly, the egress portal must be patent at all times. The working portal should not be relied upon as the main egress portal owing to relative obstruction with the use of instruments. The safeguard to avoiding over-insufflation is to use a gravity-dependent system with the irrigation source no greater than 15 cm above the egress portal of the endoscope during use. Orientation inside the ventricular system is of paramount importance. The choroid plexus directs one to the foramen of Monro. The fornix is also readily recognized as the medial and superior border of the foramen of Monro. The thalamostriate vein follows a lateral to medial course to enter the foramen, and it is a structure that must be preserved. In most cases, the CP lies inside the third ventricle, beneath the level of the foramina of Monro but it may also protrude into the lateral ventricle. The tumor surface typically has speckled microcalcifications (Figures 15.4, 15.5). The positive identification of the tumor is followed by bipolar coagulation and perforation of a small area of the wall of its cystic component (Figure 15.6). The appearance of the cyst contents is variable. A 6-Fr pediatric suction catheter (Kendall, Safe-T-Vac, Tyco Healthcare Group LP, Mansfield, Massachusetts, USA) should be inserted immediately after the penetration of the cyst in order to aspirate the contents and minimize any spillage (Figure 15.7). If possible, the suction aspirator should be used to perforate the cyst wall to immediately allow aspiration of cyst contents. Once the cystic component is fenestrated, priority should be given to aspirating the contents that otherwise will diffuse into the CSF. The CSF tumor seeding potential of the cyst contents is considered low, if any. However, the spilled contents might lead to chemical meningitis or obstructive hydrocephalus. The use of a transparent catheter instead of a stainless steel version allows visualization of the aspirated material to help monitor the effectiveness of this stage of the procedure. Inadvertent aspiration of the choroid plexus into the catheter or stagnate transit of cyst material allows the surgeon to modulate the aspiration strength or change to a patent second catheter. Once the aspiration process is over, grasping forceps are used to manipulate the membranous wall. Depending on the tumor characteristics, scissors, grasping forceps, bipolar cautery, or tissue shaving device (NICO Myriad, Nico Corp., Indianapolis, Indiana) (Figure 15.8) are utilized in order to widen the fenestration or to achieve partial resection of the cyst wall. The goal is to minimize the risk of stoma occlusion and cyst recurrence. Tissue biopsy is performed either from the membranous wall, or ideally from the solid component of the tumor (Figure 15.9). When the primary pre-operative goal is to perform an intracavitary treatment with an agent, then the stoma dimensions should be as small as the diameter of the catheter that is intended to be inserted. Following stoma creation, the catheter is inserted into the cystic part of the tumor and

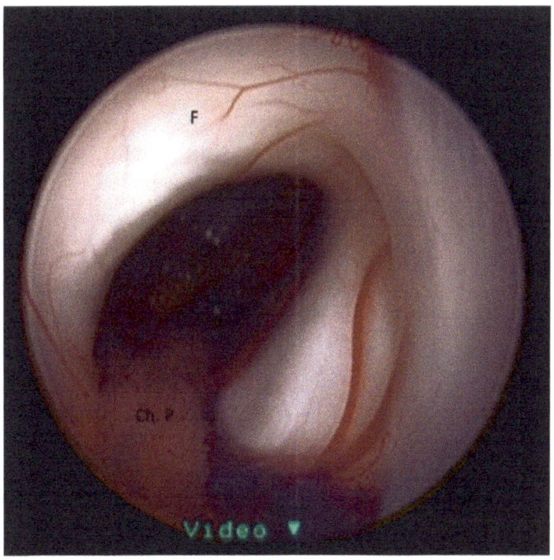

FIGURE 15.4 Intra-operative endoscopic view of the cystic component of a craniopharyngioma (CP) through the right foramen of Monro. The thalamostriate vein (Th.V.), the choroid plexus (Ch.P.) and the fornix (F) are visible.

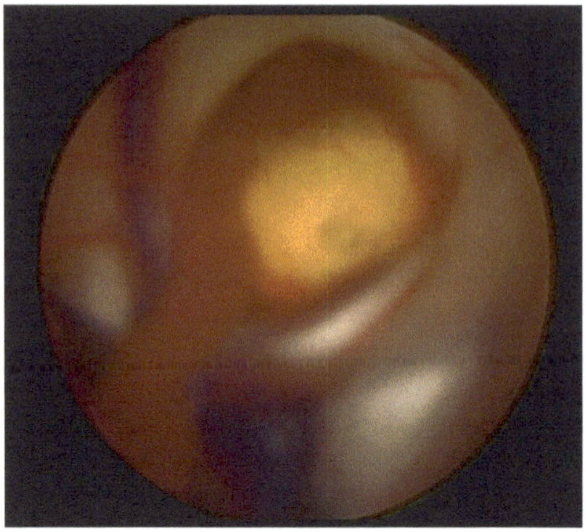

FIGURE 15.5 Intra-operative endoscopic view of the cystic component of a craniopharyngioma through the right foramen of Monro.

connected to a ventricular access device and reservoir. Depending on the location, the thickness of the tumor tissue, and its relation to critical nervous structure, an attempt at STR or coagulation of the tumor tissue by bipolar cautery might be employed as a means of minimizing the risk of recurrence. Another option is to perform a cysto-ventriculo-cisternostomy, and stent the stomas with a multi-holed catheter (Delitala et al., 2004). At the end of any endoscopic procedure, an inspection of the ventricular system will identify and allow removal of any clots or tumor fragments that might obstruct the circulation of the CSF (Figure 15.10). Based on the degree of intra-operative bleeding or the amount of spilled cyst contents, an externalized ventricular drain (EVD) might be indicated in the immediate post-operative period.

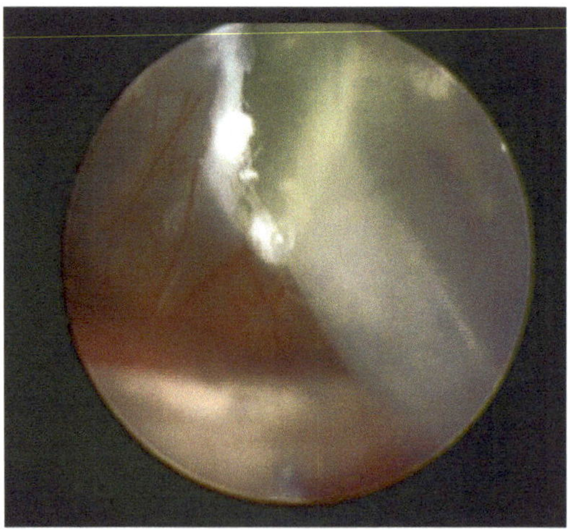

FIGURE 15.6 Following the fenestration of the wall of the cystic craniopharyngioma, a rapid flow of liquid cyst contents into the ventricular system is noted. This highlights the importance of the rapid insertion of the suction catheter following the cyst fenestration in order to minimize the spillage of the cyst contents into the ventricular system.

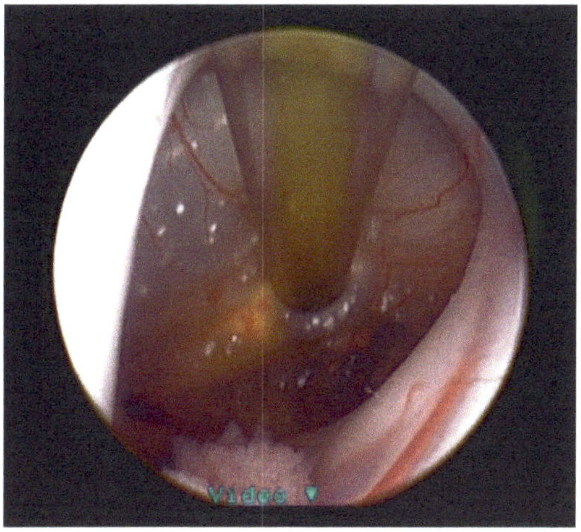

FIGURE 15.7 Aspiration of the cyst contents by utilizing a suction catheter.

CLOSURE. A semisolid hemostatic material is placed into the corticectomy site and immediate subcortical tissue immediately after the removal of the endoscope. This maneuver is intended to reduce the potential for persistent communication between the ventricle and the subdural compartment. A small titanium plate ("burr hole cover") is secured with screws over the burr hole and a layered closure is performed.

POST-OPERATIVE INSTRUCTIONS. The patient is transferred to an intensive care unit for at least 24 hours of observation with continuation of antibiotic prophylaxis for one day. Continuation of peri-operative steroids is used if there was a recognized spillage of cyst contents. The head of bed is elevated at 30 degrees. If an EVD is placed, then it is connected to a transducer for intracranial pressure (ICP) monitoring, and it is typically removed once normal pressures are recorded without CSF drainage. A baseline post-operative MRI is

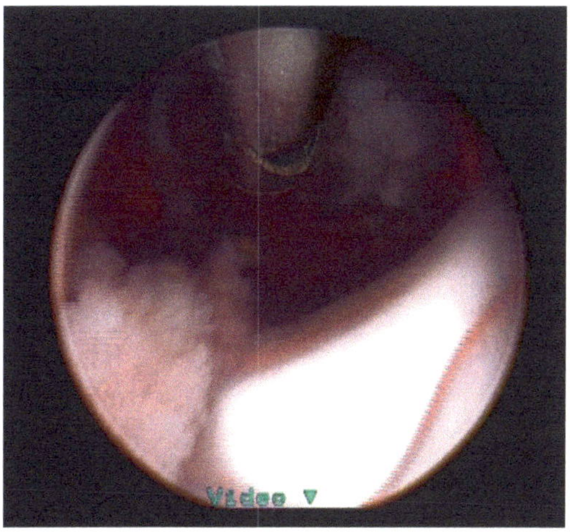

FIGURE 15.8 The tissue shaving device (NICO Myriad, Nico Corp., Indianapolis, Indiana) as it is being inserted into the third ventricle. The side opening at the tip is visible.

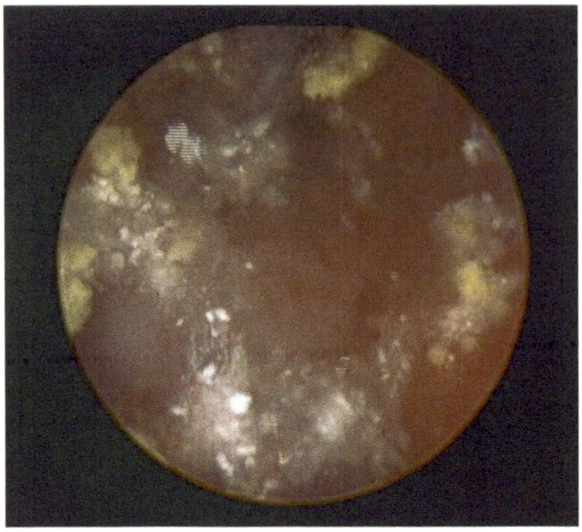

FIGURE 15.9 Intra-operative close up view of the solid component of a craniopharyngioma.

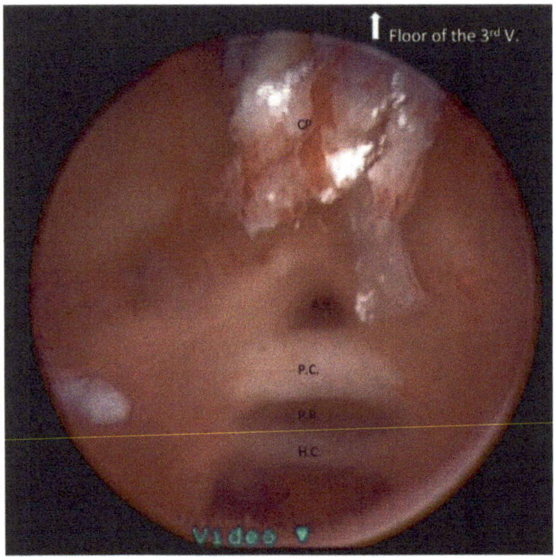

FIGURE 15.10 Intra-operative view of a craniopharyngioma inside the third ventricle, after a partial resection. The aqueduct of Sylvius (A.S.), the posterior commissure (P.C.), the pineal recess (P.R.) and the habenular commissure (H.C.) are also visible.

obtained prior to discharge. In asymptomatic patients, discharge to home typically takes place the first post-operative day.

COMPLICATIONS

The selection of a suboptimal trajectory is probably the most common cause of complications. A suboptimal trajectory might lead to undue torqueing of the endoscope against the brain parenchyma in order to access the tumor. Iatrogenic brain trauma can therefore result. The fornix and the thalamus define the foramen of Monro and are structures that are at risk of sustaining contusions from these manipulations. Dominant side fornix contusions can present as short-term memory deficits. A suboptimal trajectory might not allow access to the cystic part of the tumor or to the biopsy targets. Selecting a new trajectory and performing a new burr hole, or redirecting, are better options than using a suboptimal route, which could compromise the intended surgical goal and create injury to the brain parenchyma or unnecessary hemorrhage.

Since intraventricular endoscopy relies on the liquid medium of CSF for image transmission, small amounts of blood quickly lead to visualization impairment. Some bleeding sources can be controlled using bipolar coagulation. A useful tip for accurately locating the bleeding spot in an operative field obscured by bloody CSF is to approach the bleeding spot with the endoscope tip and increase the inflow of saline. The flow of the saline is higher near the endoscope tip where the irrigation channel ends. Therefore this increased local flow of irrigant helps in identification and hence in controlling the bleeding source. If hemorrhage is noted within a solid portion of the tumor or principally within the third ventricle, a temporarily inflated 3 French embolectomy catheter can be used for tamponade. If bleeding cannot be adequately controlled with the aforementioned methods, replacement of the endoscope with a ventricular catheter affords higher-volume irrigation. Re-inspection with the endoscope once the irrigation egress begins to clear should be instituted with clot removal if applicable.

The endoscopic intraventricular approach can lead to a post-operative subdural hygroma that is self-limited in most occasions. Intracranial hemorrhage, CSF leak, or infections are rarer complications of these procedures (Peretta et al., 2006).

CONCLUSION

Endoscopic intraventricular methods can prove useful in the treatment of craniopharyngiomas. Further work on the utility of intracavitary therapies, initial endoscopic decompression prior to any further therapeutic intervention, and the advent of new equipment that will facilitate resection might widen even further the role of endoscopic intraventricular procedures in this somewhat frustrating pathology.

References

Cavalheiro, S., Di Rocco, C., Valenzuela, S., Dastoli, P.A., Tamburrini, G., Massimi, L., Nicacio, J.M., Faquini, I.V., Ierardi, D.F., Silva, N.S., Pettorini, B.L., Toledo, S.R., 2010. Craniopharyngiomas: intratumoral chemotherapy with interferon-alpha: a multicenter preliminary study with 60 cases. Neurosurg. Focus 28. E12.

Cinalli, G., Spennato, P., Cianciulli, E., Fiorillo, A., Di Maio, S., Maggi, G., 2006. The role of transventricular neuroendoscopy in the management of craniopharyngiomas: three patient reports and review of the literature. J. Pediatr. Endocrinol. Metab. 19 (Suppl. 1), 341–354.

Clark, A.J., Cage, T.A., Aranda, D., Parsa, A.T., Auguste, K.I., Gupta, N., 2012. Treatment-related morbidity and the management of pediatric craniopharyngioma: a systematic review. J. Neurosurg. Pediatr. 10, 293–301.

Constantini, S., Mohanty, A., Zymberg, S., Cavalheiro, S., Mallucci, C., Hellwig, D., Ersahin, Y., Mori, H., Mascari, C., Val, J.A., Wagner, W., Kulkarni, A.V., Sgouros, S., Oi, S., 2013. Safety and diagnostic accuracy of neuroendoscopic biopsies: an international multicenter study. J. Neurosurg. Pediatr. 11, 704–709.

Delitala, A., Brunori, A., Chiappetta, F., 2004. Purely neuroendoscopic transventricular management of cystic craniopharyngiomas. Childs. Nerv. Syst. 20, 858–862.

Fahlbusch, R., Honegger, J., Paulus, W., Huk, W., Buchfelder, M., 1999. Surgical treatment of craniopharyngiomas: experience with 168 patients. J. Neurosurg. 90, 237–250.

Filis, A.K., Moon, K., Cohen, A.R., 2009. Synchronous ventriculoscopic and microsurgical resection of complex craniopharyngiomas. Pediatric. Neurosurg. 45, 434–436.

Frazier, C.H., Alpers, B.J., 1931. Adamantinoma of the craniopharyngeal duct. Arch. Neuro. Pysch. 26, 905–965.

Gangemi, M., Seneca, V., Mariniello, G., Colella, G., Magro, F., 2009. Combined endoscopic and microsurgical removal of a giant cystic craniopharyngioma in a six-year-old boy. Clin. Neurol. Neurosurg. 111, 472–476.

Komotar, R.J., Starke, R.M., Raper, D.M., Anand, V.K., Schwartz, T.H., 2012. Endoscopic endonasal compared with microscopic transsphenoidal and open transcranial resection of craniopharyngiomas. World Neurosurg. 77, 329–341.

Leng, L.Z., Greenfield, J.P., Souweidane, M.M., Anand, V.K., Schwartz, T.H., 2012. Endoscopic, endonasal resection of craniopharyngiomas: analysis of outcome including extent of resection, cerebrospinal fluid leak, return to preoperative productivity, and body mass index. Neurosurgery 70, 110–123, discussion 123–124.

Mallucci, C., Pizer, B., Blair, J., Didi, M., Doss, A., Upadrasta, S., Newman, W., Avula, S., Pettorini, B., 2012. Management of craniopharyngioma: the Liverpool experience following the introduction of the CCLG guidelines. Introducing a new risk assessment grading system. Childs. Nerv. Syst. 28, 1181–1192.

Margetis, K., Souweidane, M.M., 2013a. Endoscopic resection of colloid cyst in normal-sized ventricular system. Neurosurg. Focus 34. Video 8.

Margetis, K., Souweidane, M.M., 2013b. Endoscopic treatment of intraventricular cystic tumors. World Neurosurg. 79. S19 e1–11.

Mascarenhas, L., Moshel, Y.A., Bayad, F., Szentirmai, O., Salek, A.A., Leng, L.Z., Hofstetter, C.P., Placantonakis, D.G., Tsiouris, A.J., Anand, V.K., Schwartz, T.H., 2013. The transplanum transtuberculum approaches for suprasellar and sellar-suprasellar lesions: Avoidance of cerebrospinal fluid leak and lessons learned. World Neurosurg. pii: S1878–8750(13)00297-0. [Epub ahead of print].

Mortini, P., Losa, M., Pozzobon, G., Barzaghi, R., Riva, M., Acerno, S., Angius, D., Weber, G., Chiumello, G., Giovanelli, M., 2011. Neurosurgical treatment of craniopharyngioma in adults and children: early and long-term results in a large case series. J. Neurosurg. 114, 1350–1359.

Nakahara, Y., Koga, H., Maeda, K., Takagi, M., Tabuchi, K., 2004. Neuroendoscopic transventricular surgery for suprasellar cystic mass lesions such as cystic craniopharyngioma and Rathke cleft cyst. Neurol. Med. Chir. (Tokyo) 44, 408–413 discussion 414–5.

Peretta, P., Ragazzi, P., Galarza, M., Genitori, L., Giordano, F., Mussa, F., Cinalli, G., 2006. Complications and pitfalls of neuroendoscopic surgery in children. J. Neurosurg. 105, 187–193.

Pettorini, B.L., Tamburrini, G., Massimi, L., Caldarelli, M., Di Rocco, C., 2009. Endoscopic transventricular positioning of intracystic catheter for treatment of craniopharyngioma. Technical note. J. Neurosurg. Pediatr. 4, 245–248.

Puget, S., Garnett, M., Wray, A., Grill, J., Habrand, J.L., Bodaert, N., Zerah, M., Bezerra, M., Renier, D., Pierre-Kahn, A., Sainte-Rose, C., 2007. Pediatric craniopharyngiomas: classification and treatment according to the degree of hypothalamic involvement. J. Neurosurg. 106, 3–12.

Qiao, L., Souweidane, M.M., 2011. Purely endoscopic removal of intraventricular brain tumors: a consensus opinion and update. Minim. Invasive Neurosurg. 54, 149–154.

Schwartz, T.H., Fraser, J.F., Brown, S., Tabaee, A., Kacker, A., Anand, V.K., 2008. Endoscopic cranial base surgery: classification of operative approaches. Neurosurgery 62, 991–1002, discussion 1002–1005.

Souweidane, M.M., 2005. Endoscopic management of pediatric brain tumors. Neurosurg. Focus 18, E1.

Veeravagu, A., Lee, M., Jiang, B., Chang, S.D., 2010. The role of radiosurgery in the treatment of craniopharyngiomas. Neurosurg. Focus 28, E11.

Yang, I., Sughrue, M.E., Rutkowski, M.J., Kaur, R., Ivan, M.E., Aranda, D., Barani, I.J., Parsa, A.T., 2010. Craniopharyngioma: a comparison of tumor control with various treatment strategies. Neurosurg. Focus 28, E5.

Yeung, J.T., Pollack, I.F., Panigrahy, A., Jakacki, R.I., 2012. Pegylated interferon-alpha-2b for children with recurrent craniopharyngioma. J. Neurosurg. Pediatr. 10, 498–503.

CHAPTER

16

Surgical Approaches: Ommaya Reservoir for Cystic Craniopharyngiomas

Dominic Thompson, Kristian Aquilina

Department of Neurosurgery, Great Ormond Street Hospital for Children NHS Foundation Trust, London, UK

"With the evacuation of the cyst, the battle is only half won since in the majority of cases, the cyst will refill and all the symptoms, both local and general, will recur." ***RC Carpenter, GW Chamberlin, and CH Frazier, 1937***

INTRODUCTION

Craniopharyngiomas are typically solid-cystic lesions in the sellar and suprasellar region; cystic components occur in up to 90% of cases (Backlund, 1994). The cysts may constitute a significant proportion of the total mass effect exerted by the lesion, and may be directly responsible for some of the symptoms. Surgical approaches to craniopharyngiomas have changed over the last 20 years, as increasing awareness of the endocrine and hypothalamic morbidity associated with achieved or attempted gross total resection of large lesions, primary and recurrent, became apparent (De Vile et al., 1996; Kalapurakal et al., 2000; Stripp et al., 2004; Schoenfeld et al., 2012; Clark et al., 2012). This, together with an improved understanding of the efficacy of radiation therapy for craniopharyngioma, led to a trend towards more conservative, multimodal, surgery followed by radiotherapy (Wen et al., 1989; Fischer et al., 1990; Stripp et al., 2004; Thompson et al., 2005; Schoenfeld et al., 2012). While complete microsurgical resection of craniopharyngiomas that do not infiltrate the hypothalamus has been shown to be effective and safe in selected cases and will continue to have a place in treatment, a more tailored approach is required in that significant cohort of patients with more complex tumors (Puget et al., 2007).

In recognition of the morbidity associated with a policy of radical tumor resection for all cases we have attempted to risk-stratify patients according to their clinical and radiological features at presentation (Thompson et al., 2005). Children deemed to be at high risk (on the

Craniopharyngiomas
http://dx.doi.org/10.1016/B978-0-12-416706-3.00016-7

basis of previous studies) comprised those who had the following features: young age (less than 5 years), large multi-compartment tumors, severe hydrocephalus at presentation, and symptoms suggestive of hypothalamic dysfunction. For this group the risks attendant upon attempted radical resection were considered unacceptable and so treatment was modified. Less invasive surgical procedures, such as cyst drainage or subtotal resection followed by radiotherapy, would be offered to children old enough to safely undergo radiotherapy. For the younger children, these less invasive procedures were performed and repeated as necessary during a period of surveillance in an attempt to temporize until the child is old enough to receive radiotherapy. Large cystic components (a frequently observed feature of childhood craniopharyngioma) in particular lend themselves to a less invasive operative strategy with catheter drainage either in isolation or as part of a multimodality treatment plan.

Large cysts associated with craniopharyngiomas cause symptoms by compression of adjacent structures. These include the optic apparatus, the hypothalamus, and the third ventricle, where distortion leads to obstructive hydrocephalus. The endoscopic transnasal transphenoidal approach, in its standard or extended forms, is used for lesions predominantly below the diaphragma sellae. An associated cyst may be drained at the same time. We prefer to drain cysts related to lesions infiltrating the hypothalamus through an implanted catheter secured to a subgaleal Ommaya reservoir. This provides a direct way to reduce mass effect, improve symptoms and narrow the radiotherapy field. Occasionally, reduction of cyst size may change the assessment of resectability of the craniopharyngioma and allow consideration of an attempt at complete resection.

HISTORICAL OVERVIEW AND ROLE OF CYST DRAINAGE

The adaptation of an Ommaya reservoir to drain cystic tumors was first described in 1967, where the suprasellar cystic lesion described in this first study was probably a craniopharyngioma (Fox, 1967). The use of a subgaleal reservoir attached to a catheter placed within the cyst was subsequently described in four patients with large cystic craniopharyngiomas whose symptoms were improved by recurrent aspiration (Miles, 1977). This was considered a useful palliative procedure, superior to leaving the distal end of a cyst catheter free in the subcutaneous space. This technique was also better than one-off cyst drainage, performed through a precoronal burr hole under fluoroscopy after instillation of contrast medium (Taylor, 1971). Once computed tomography (CT) scanning became available, twist drill biopsy and aspiration of cystic craniopharyngiomas could be carried out more safely (Ignelzi and Squire, 1976). Drainage through the transsphenoidal route was also described in situations where an intracapsular resection of a craniopharyngioma below the diaphragma had been performed, ensuring that no communication with the subarachnoid space was present (Laws Jr, 1980).

A later publication, in 1980, described four patients where Pudenz catheters, connected to Ommaya reservoirs, were inserted into the cyst at operative debulking (Gutin et al., 1980). Repeated aspiration was an integral part of the management algorithm of these patients, together with subtotal surgical resection and radiotherapy; aspiration generally improved symptoms and even reversed visual deficits. Aspiration was unsuccessful on two occasions; in one, post mortem examination identified a solid recurrence obliterating the previous cyst, and in the second, the tube to the reservoir did not follow a straight course and was likely kinked (Gutin et al., 1980).

Particular difficulties with cyst drainage relate to multilocular cysts and tough cyst capsules. A tough capsule may allow a catheter to slide along its surface, with risk of injury to neurological and vascular structures adherent to it (Spaziante et al., 1989). The safety and effectiveness of the procedure have been recently reported. Moussa et al. published a series of 52 predominantly cystic craniopharyngiomas between 1990 and 2010, which were treated by insertion of an Ommaya reservoir (Moussa et al., 2013). Most of the patients were children. The reservoir was inserted stereotactically, using a Cosman-Roberts-Wells (CRW) frame, or free hand. In four patients, cyst fluid recollected early and bleomycin was injected weekly for 6 weeks after confirmation that the cyst did not communicate with the subarachnoid space. Surveillance imaging and trial aspiration showed that in 73% of 38 patients, cystic fluid did not re-accumulate. Ten required re-aspiration every 6 months. The authors were surprised by the low recurrence rate and suggest that, after aspiration and collapse of the cyst, the proximal holes along the catheter communicated with the subarachnoid space. This would have allowed free drainage of cyst fluid into the cerebrospinal fluid, allowing eventual absorption (Moussa et al., 2013). This reflected similar earlier experience, where an "extrathecal link" was purposefully established (Mokrusch et al., 1985; Spaziante et al., 1989). Dilution of craniopharyngioma fluid into the cerebrospinal fluid reduced cyst recurrence rates and did not lead to disturbance of fluid flow. There were no episodes of chemical meningitis, and no suggestion of tumor cell spread along the subarachnoid or intraventricular space (Spaziante et al., 1989). Direct opening of a craniopharyngioma cyst into the cerebellopontine cistern was also effective (Mokrusch et al., 1985).

The endoscopic approach is particularly useful when a craniopharyngioma cyst is also causing hydrocephalus. Intraventricular drainage of a cystic craniopharyngioma was initially described by Scarff in 1941 (Scarff, 1941). The standard endoscopic approach through a pre-coronal burr hole allows visualization of the cyst, usually in the lower third ventricle, as it displaces the foramina of Monro superiorly. In the two burr hole technique, a catheter is passed into the ventricle, under direct endoscopic vision, through a separate burr hole (Joki et al., 2002). Using a single burr hole and a transparent endoscopic sheath, the catheter may be been passed under direct vision by running it along the outside of the sheath (Mori et al., 2013). We have used a single port technique, with a peel-apart catheter (diameter 4.7 mm) that is able to accommodate a low-caliber rigid endoscope as well as the stylet-mounted ventricular catheter. This approach also allows biopsy of the deep part of the cyst wall at the same time and permits placement of the catheter under direct vision.

Although definitive histological diagnosis of craniopharyngioma is not possible from aspirated fluid, its color, consistency, and the presence of cholesterol are highly suggestive. The presence of beta human chorionic gonadotrophin (β-HCG) in cyst fluid is also highly suggestive of craniopharyngioma (Harris et al., 1988). Evaluation of β-HCG immunoreactivity in cyst fluid from 42 patients with cystic intracranial tumors demonstrated marked elevation in all the 17 craniopharyngiomas, whereas levels were only mildly elevated or absent in all other pathologies (Honegger et al., 1995). In addition, β-HCG immunoreactivity in the CSF was only found in two of the patients with craniopharyngioma.

Spillage of cyst fluid into the ventricles, spontaneous or related to intervention, may lead to chemical meningitis (Kumar et al., 2010; Rajput et al., 2012). This may be related to the concentration of cholesterol contents within the cyst fluid; in one case reporting spontaneous asymptomatic rupture of the cyst in a child, the cyst fluid was almost iso-intense to CSF (Kumar et al., 2010). In our series of endoscopic cyst drainage, where a small volume of cyst fluid inevitably escapes into the ventricular system, we have not seen any episodes of chemical meningitis.

Although radiotherapy is effective in controlling growth of residual tumor, the cystic component often enlarges during the course of treatment. In a phase II trial of conformal radiation therapy in pediatric craniopharyngioma, nearly half the patients demonstrated cystic enlargement during therapy; 13 of 28 patients required cyst aspiration at least once during treatment and in three the tumor change was significant enough to require revision of the treatment plan (Merchant et al., 2006). In another study evaluating tumor control after conformal and intensity-modulated radiation therapy using a reduced planning volume, cyst enlargement requiring a change in treatment plan occurred in 22 of 88 cases (Merchant et al., 2013). A change in the solid component was not observed in any patient. Regular and frequent MRI surveillance during radiation therapy of cystic tumors, with consideration of repeated cyst drainage, is required to prevent marginal failure, particularly if the volume irradiated is systematically reduced. It is recommended that children undergoing proton therapy for craniopharyngioma undergo surveillance imaging, with consideration of cyst aspiration, at least every 2 weeks during treatment (Winkfield et al., 2009).

An Ommaya reservoir may also be used to administer intracystic therapy. The first such therapy involved the use of beta-emitting radionuclides, particularly phosphorus (Kickingereder et al., 2012) or yttrium^{90}. This led to relatively effective reduction in cyst size, with low risk of new endocrinopathy. However, visual loss and hypothalamic radionecrosis occurred in up to 5% of cases (Julow et al., 2007). A more recent report on direct stereotactic injection of colloidal phosphorus has demonstrated more promising results (Kickingereder et al., 2012). Administration of bleomycin and interferon alpha through Ommaya reservoirs has also been described. Bleomycin has been reported to reduce cyst size by at least 25% in 90% of patients (Hukin et al., 2007). As bleomycin is toxic, it is important to ensure that all the catheter holes are placed within the cyst (Steinbok and Hukin, 2010). Evidence of leakage on MR imaging has been associated with extensive vasogenic edema and hypothalamic injury (Lafay-Cousin et al., 2007). There must be confirmation that contrast medium injected into the reservoir does not leak into the subarachnoid space, as seen on CT, prior to the first injection. Aspiration of the cyst before injection is minimized to reduce the risk of the most proximal holes exiting from the collapsing cyst. Unlike bleomycin, interferon alpha can enter the subarachnoid space without significant morbidity (Cavalheiro et al., 2010). Both agents provide short-term control of a cystic tumor and allow more definitive treatment, such as radiotherapy, to be delayed. This is particularly relevant in younger children in whom delayed radiotherapy carries a definite advantage.

OUR SERIES

Over the last 10 years, we have treated 20 children with craniopharyngiomas, aged 2 to 16 years, who underwent insertion of a catheter attached to an Ommaya reservoir into the cystic component of the tumor (Table 16.1). The principal indication was to reduce mass effect and associated symptoms within a short time interval, particularly when the cyst was large enough to threaten vision or cause hydrocephalus. We have also found that the technique facilitates formal microsurgical resection of large mixed cystic-solid craniopharyngiomas and reduces the radiotherapy field, and subsequent related long-term sequelae, in tumors with large cystic components.

TABLE 16.1 Patients Undergoing Insertion of Catheter and Ommaya Reservoir into Craniopharyngioma Cysts at Great Ormond Street Hospital Over the Last Ten Years

Patient	Age at diagnosis (yrs)	Primary procedure	Subsequent procedures	Radiation theraphy	Endocrine status	Follow-up (months)
1	15	Endoscopic catheter insertion	None	Yes	GH deficiency	26
2	13	Image-guided catheter insertion	Transphenoidal resection	Yes	Full hormone replacement	42
3	7	Endoscopic cyst drainage	Image-guided catheter insertion	Yes	No replacement	72
4	6	Endoscopic catheter insertion	None	No	No replacement	4
5	4	Endoscopic catheter insertion	None	No	No replacement	81
6	4	Image-guided catheter insertion	Craniotomy and STR; second craniotomy and GTR	No	Full hormone replacement	61
7	6	Craniotomy and catheter placement	None	Yes	No replacement	44
8	4	Craniotomy and catheter placement	Craniotomy and GTR	No	No replacement	30
9	3	Craniotomy and STR	Image-guided catheter insertion; second craniotomy	Yes	Full hormone replacement	100
10	10	Endoscopic cyst fenestration	Craniotomy and STR; endoscopic catheter insertion	Yes	Full hormone replacement	88
11	15	Image-guided catheter insertion	None	Yes	No replacement	58
12	15	Image-guided catheter insertion	None	Yes	No replacement	3
13	2	Image-guided catheter insertion	Craniotomy, GTR	No	Full hormone replacement	28
14	13	Endoscopic catheter insertion	None	Yes	Full hormone replacement	41
15	16	Image-guided catheter insertion	None	Yes	GH, ADH deficiency	24
16	2	Endoscopic fenestration	Craniotomy, STR, and open catheter insertion	Yes	Full hormone replacement	63
17	12	Endoscopic catheter insertion	None	Yes	No replacement	19

(*Continued*)

TABLE 16.1 Patients Undergoing Insertion of Catheter and Ommaya Reservoir into Craniopharyngioma Cysts at Great Ormond Street Hospital Over the Last Ten Years—cont'd

Patient	Age at diagnosis (yrs)	Primary procedure	Subsequent procedures	Radiation theraphy	Endocrine status	Follow-up (months)
18	15	Image-guided catheter insertion	None	Yes	Estrogen only	49
19	9	Endoscopic catheter insertion	None	Yes	No replacement	79
20	11	Image-guided catheter insertion	None	Yes	No replacement	10

In 15 cases, catheter insertion was the first procedure undertaken on presentation. In eight of these cases, the catheter was inserted through a burr hole under stereotactic frame-based or frameless guidance. Endoscopic insertion was used in five cases and, in two, insertion of the catheter was performed as part of an open microsurgical debulking procedure. In the five remaining cases, catheter insertion occurred later, in the course of treatment due to emergence of new, or progression of existing, tumor cysts. In our experience, insertion of catheters and repeated aspiration from the reservoir were safe and effective procedures. In one case, where the capsule was thick, image-guided catheter placement failed and an open microsurgical approach was undertaken. In another patient the reservoir became infected following multiple aspirations.

Currently, our preferred method of introducing a catheter into the tumor cyst is by means of frameless image guidance. A post-gadolinium high-resolution MRI data set is loaded into an image guidance system. Once a three-dimensional model is built from this data set, the optimum trajectory from a pre-coronal entry point is defined. As far as possible, the trajectory crosses only one pial surface and avoids the frontal horns of the lateral ventricles. Using electromagnetic guidance, the catheter (cut to pre-determined length as indicated on image guidance) is sheathed over the active electromagnetic probe. Through a pre-coronal burr hole on the appropriate side, the catheter is advanced along the pre-planned trajectory. Its track is followed on the image guidance system. A significant resistance, exerted by the tough capsule, is often felt at the point of entry into the cyst. Once into the cyst, the catheter is advanced for a further short distance, depending on cyst size, the electromagnetic probe is slowly withdrawn, and an Ommaya reservoir is attached to the catheter at the burr hole. The reservoir is then accessed with a 22G needle and fluid is aspirated until no more can be obtained. A post-operative MRI scan confirms reduction in size and appropriate placement of the catheter.

In cases where the craniopharyngioma cyst is causing distortion of the third ventricle with secondary hydrocephalus, an endoscopic approach is preferred. Nine of the 20 cases underwent endoscopy as a primary procedure; a reservoir was inserted at the same time in five of these. This is performed through a standard coronal burr hole, usually on the right side. Extensive distortion of the ventricular system is an indication for image guidance. A peel-apart cannula is passed into the lateral ventricle and a 0 degree endoscope is advanced through it. The primary endoscopic landmarks (the choroid plexus and the anterior septal and thalamostriate veins) are identified and the foramen of Monro is entered. The cyst

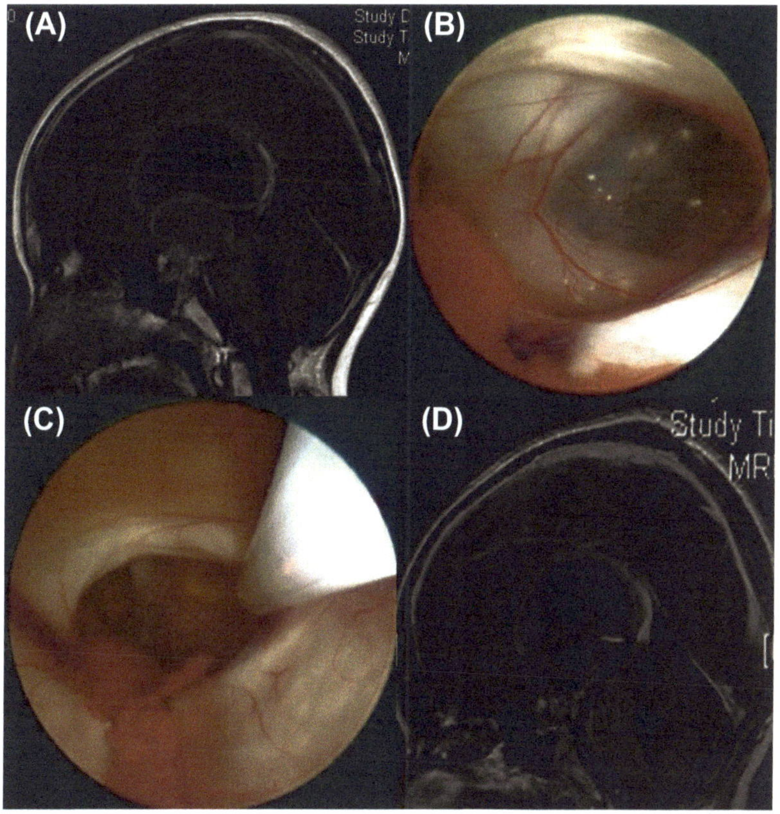

FIGURE 16.1 Post-contrast mid-sagittal MR image demonstrating large cystic craniopharyngioma with obstructive hydrocephalus, **A.** Endoscopy through the right frontal horn shows the foramen of Monro with the cyst extending through the floor of the third ventricle, **B.** A catheter is advanced through the sheath under direct vision and the cyst is drained, **C. D** demonstrates solid residual tumor after cyst drainage on post-contrast mid-sagittal MRI scan.

wall bulging into the third ventricle is now identifiable (Figure 16.1). It can be perforated with an ME2 electrode, releasing yellowish fluid of different consistency to CSF. The endoscope is then passed into the cyst and if any definite abnormal tissue is identified a biopsy may be taken. The cyst catheter can often be passed adjacent to the endoscope through the same peel-apart cannula. Its tip can then be directed into the cyst opening under direct vision. The superficial end of the catheter is then connected to an Ommaya reservoir after the endoscope and peel-apart cannula have been withdrawn.

CASE ILLUSTRATIONS

Case 1

An 11-year-old girl presented with a 3-month history of worsening headaches, later associated with nausea and vomiting. Over the 4 weeks prior to presentation, she complained of visual deterioration, with restriction of visual fields and reduced visual acuity, as well as ataxia. Goldman perimetry confirmed bitemporal hemianopia. Her visual acuity was log MAR 0.8 bilaterally. MR imaging showed a large cystic suprasellar lesion, with displacement and elevation of the optic chiasm and early obstructive hydrocephalus (Figure 16.2A, B). Some enhancement was evident in the cyst wall after gadolinium administration. Endocrinological investigations were normal.

The patient underwent insertion of a catheter and Ommaya reservoir into the cyst under frameless stereotactic guidance through a right pre-coronal burr hole. The procedure was uncomplicated and 12 ml of "machine oil" fluid, typical of craniopharyngioma, were aspirated. The fluid contained cholesterol crystals. Post-operative imaging confirmed satisfactory reduction in cyst size (Figure 16.2C, D).

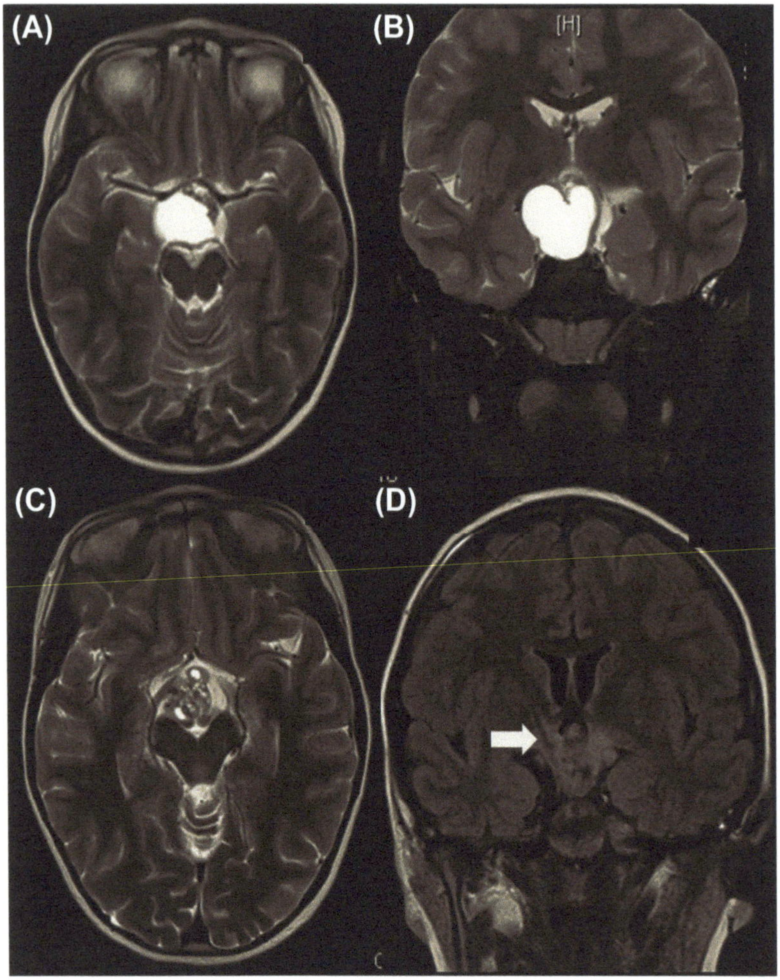

FIGURE 16.2 Pre-operative T2-weighted MR imaging, axial **A**, and coronal **B**, demonstrating large predominantly cystic suprasellar lesion. **C** and **D** demonstrate the solid components of the craniopharyngioma, on axial T2-weighted and coronal fluid attenuated inversion recovery (FLAIR) images, after aspiration through a catheter (white arrow in **D**) attached to an Ommaya reservoir.

The child recovered well and was discharged on the third post-operative day. Her headaches resolved and serial ophthalmological evaluation demonstrated progressive improvement in her visual acuity and fields. Her unsteady gait improved. She went on to have proton beam radiotherapy using a three-field three-dimensional conformal proton plan. During the 6-week radiotherapy program, she underwent weekly MRI to assess any cyst changes. There was a significant increase in cyst size 2 weeks into the program and further aspiration through the reservoir was undertaken.

Case 2

A 4-year-old boy presented with a 6-week history of left hemiparesis and facial weakness, associated with reduced vision in the left eye. Ophthalmological evaluation demonstrated left exotropia with visual acuity of log MAR 0.9 on the left and 0.85 on the right. There was a left hemianopia with a right infratemporal field defect. MR imaging showed a large solid-cystic mass in the suprasellar region with superior extension causing displacement of the chiasm and the left optic nerve (Figure 16.3A).

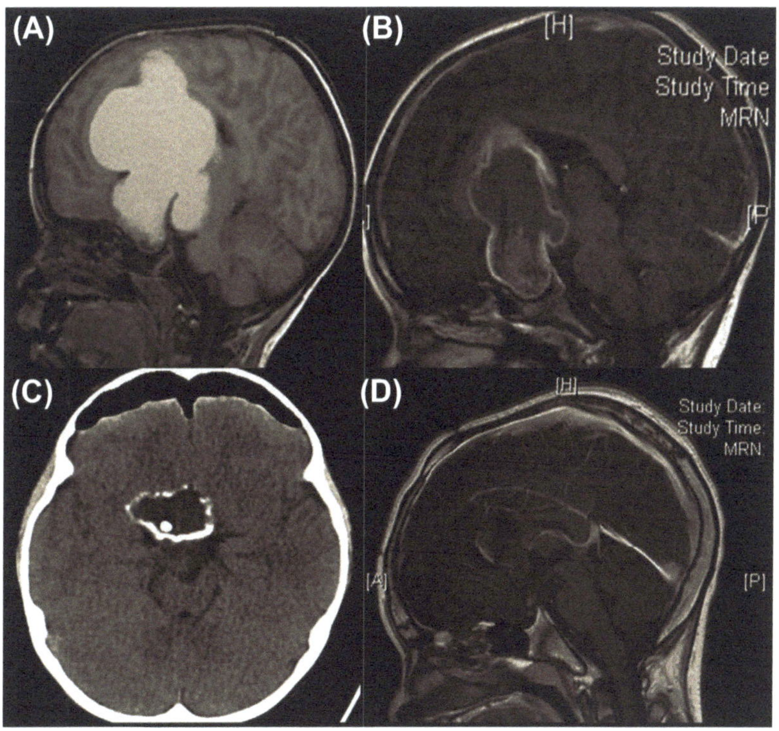

FIGURE 16.3 **A,** Pre-operative sagittal FLAIR image demonstrating a large complex lobulated suprasellar cystic lesion. The catheter is visible in the post-contrast T1-weighted MR image in **B,** where the cyst volume has been reduced by aspiration. **C** is a computed tomographic scan showing residual cystic tumor after partial resection through a bifrontal approach; gross total resection was obtained in the subsequent craniotomy – clear 5-year surveillance sagittal post-contrast T1-weighted MR image is shown in **D.**

A catheter attached to an Ommaya reservoir was inserted into the cyst under frameless image guidance. The cyst was successfully aspirated (Figure 16.3B), leading to consideration of surgical resection. Gross total resection of the craniopharyngioma was achieved in two procedures over the next 6 weeks, initially through a bifrontal approach and subsequently through a right pterional approach (Figure 16.3C, D). No radiotherapy has been administered, and his scans show no evidence of recurrent tumor at 5 years' follow-up (Figure 16.3D).

CONCLUSION

Cyst formation is a particularly prevalent feature of childhood craniopharyngoma, and insertion of a catheter attached to an Ommaya reservoir has a valuable role in the multimodality treatment of craniopharyngiomas. Catheter drainage may be used, either as a temporizing measure to improve mass effect, or as part of a definitive management plan that includes intracystic therapy. Contemporary techniques of image guidance and endoscopy now facilitate the safe and accurate placement of the catheter, and the incorporation of a reservoir allows intermittent long-term drainage as necessary.

Preliminary cyst drainage may change an initially high-risk tumor with perceived low chance of surgical cure into a lesion that is amenable to safe, complete resection. Moreover, given the potential morbidity of radical resection of craniopharyngioma and with increasing evidence of the efficacy of intracystic treatments such as interferon alpha, it is likely that there will become an increasing role for catheter placement as part of the armamentarium required to treat this formidable tumor.

The histologically benign nature of craniopharyngioma disguises the more malignant clinical course that so often typifies this disease. In recent years there has been an increasing acceptance of the role that treatment, particularly surgery, may play in adding to the burden of symptoms. At a time when neurosurgeons and oncologists are becoming increasingly cognizant of the quality of long-term outcomes, interventions that can be demonstrated to alleviate some of that burden while maintaining or improving disease control must surely be pursued.

References

Backlund, E.O., 1994. Treatment of craniopharyngiomas: the multimodality approach. Pediatr. Neurosurg. 21 (Suppl. 1), 82–89.

Carpenter, R.C., Chamberlin, G.W., Frazier, C.H., 1937. The treatment of hypophyseal stalk tumours by evacuation and irradiation. Am. J. Roent. 38, 162–167.

Cavalheiro, S., Di Rocco, C., Valenzuela, S., Dastoli, P., Tamburrini, G., Massimi, L., Nicacio, J., Faquini, I., Ierardi, D., Silva, N., Pettorini, B., Toledo, S., 2010. Craniopharyngiomas: intratumoral chemotherapy with interferon-alpha: a multicenter preliminary study with 60 cases. Neurosurg. Focus. 28 (4), E12.

Clark, A.J., Cage, T.A., Aranda, D., Parsa, A.T., Auguste, K.I., Gupta, N., 2012. Treatment-related morbidity and the management of pediatric craniopharyngioma: a systematic review. J. Neurosurg. Pediatr. 10 (4), 293–301.

De Vile, C.J., Grant, D.B., Kendall, B.E., Neville, B., Stanhope, R., Watkins, K., Hayward, R., 1996. Management of childhood craniopharyngioma: can the morbidity of radical surgery be predicted? J. Neurosurg. 85 (1), 73–81.

Fischer, E.G., Welch, K., Shillito Jr., J., Winston, K.R., Tarbell, N.J., 1990. Craniopharyngiomas in children. Long-term effects of conservative surgical procedures combined with radiation therapy. J. Neurosurg. 73 (4), 534–540.

Fox, J.L., 1967. Intermittent drainage of intracranial cyst via the subcutaneous Ommaya reservoir. Technical note. J. Neurosurg. 27 (3), 272–273.

Gutin, P.H., Klemme, W.M., Lagger, R.L., MacKay, A.R., Pitts, L.H., Hosobuchi, Y., 1980. Management of the unresectable cystic craniopharyngioma by aspiration through an Ommaya reservoir drainage system. J. Neurosurg. 52 (1), 36–40.

Harris, P.E., Perry, L., Chard, T., Chaudry, L., Cooke, B., Touzel, R., Coates, P., Lowe, D., Afshar, F., Wass, J., 1988. Immunoreactive human chorionic gonadotrophin from the cyst fluid and CSF of patients with craniopharyngioma. Clin. Endocrinol. (Oxf) 29 (5), 503–508.

Honegger, J., Mann, K., Thierauf, P., Zrinzo, A., Fahlbusch, R., 1995. Human chorionic gonadotrophin immunoactivity in cystic intracranial tumours. Clin. Endocrinol. (Oxf) 42 (3), 235–241.

Hukin, J., Steinbok, P., Lafay-Cousin, L., Hendson, G., Strother, D., Mercier, C., Samson, Y., Howes, W., Bouffet, E., 2007. Intracystic bleomycin therapy for craniopharyngioma in children: the Canadian experience. Cancer 109 (10), 2124–2131.

Ignelzi, R.J., Squire, L.R., 1976. Recovery from anterograde and retrograde amnesia after percutaneous drainage of a cystic craniopharyngioma. J. Neurol. Neurosurg. Psychiatry 39 (12), 1231–1235.

Joki, T., Oi, S., Babapour, B., Kaito, N., Ohashi, K., Ebara, M., Kato, M., Abe, T., 2002. Neuroendoscopic placement of Ommaya reservoir into a cystic craniopharyngioma. Childs. Nerv. Syst. 18 (11), 629–633.

Julow, J., Backlund, E.O., Lanyi, F., Hajda, M., Balint, K., Nyari, I., Szeifert, G., 2007. Long-term results and late complications after intracavitary yttrium-90 colloid irradiation of recurrent cystic craniopharyngiomas. Neurosurgery 61 (2), 288–295 discussion 295–286.

Kalapurakal, J.A., Goldman, S., Hsieh, Y.C., Tomita, T., Marymont, M.H., 2000. Clinical outcome in children with recurrent craniopharyngioma after primary surgery. Cancer J. 6 (6), 388–393.

Kickingereder, P., Maarouf, M., El Majdoub, F., Fuetsch, M., Lehrke, R., Wirths, J., Luyken, K., Schomaeker, K., Treuer, H., Voges, J., Sturm, V., 2012. Intracavitary brachytherapy using stereotactically applied phosphorus-32 colloid for treatment of cystic craniopharyngiomas in 53 patients. J. Neurooncol. 109 (2), 365–374.

Kumar, A., Kasliwal, M.K., Suri, A., Sharma, B.S., 2010. Spontaneous asymptomatic rupture of cystic craniopharyngioma in a child: case report and review of the literature. J. Child. Neurol. 25 (12), 1555–1558.

Lafay-Cousin, L., Bartels, U., Raybaud, C., Kulkarni, A., Guger, S., Huang, A., Bouffet, E., 2007. Neuroradiological findings of bleomycin leakage in cystic craniopharyngioma. Report of three cases. J. Neurosurg. 107 (Suppl. 4), 318–323.

Laws Jr, E.R., 1980. Transsphenoidal microsurgery in the management of craniopharyngioma. J. Neurosurg. 52 (5), 661–666.

Merchant, T.E., Kiehna, E.N., Kun, L.E., Mulhern, R., Li, C., Xiong, X., Boop, F., Sanford, R., 2006. Phase II trial of conformal radiation therapy for pediatric patients with craniopharyngioma and correlation of surgical factors and radiation dosimetry with change in cognitive function. J. Neurosurg. 104 (Suppl. 2), 94–102.

Merchant, T.E., Kun, L.E., Hua, C.H., Wu, S., Xiong, X., Sanford, R., Boop, F., 2013. Disease control after reduced volume conformal and intensity modulated radiation therapy for childhood craniopharyngioma. Int. J. Radiat. Oncol. Biol. Phys. 85 (4), e187–192.

Miles, J., 1977. Sump drainage: a palliative manoeuvre for the treatment of craniopharyngioma. J. Neurol. Neurosurg. Psychiatry 40 (2), 120–126.

Mokrusch, T., Schramm, J., Fahlbusch, R., 1985. Repeatedly reversible alteration of acoustic-evoked brainstem responses with a cystic craniopharyngioma. Surg. Neurol. 24 (5), 571–577.

Mori, R., Joki, T., Nonaka, Y., Ikeuchi, S., Abe, T., 2013. Parallel insertion endoscopic technique for precise catheter placement in cystic craniopharyngiomas. J. Neurol. Surg. A. Cent. Eur. Neurosurg.

Moussa, A.H., Kerasha, A.A., Mahmoud, M.E., 2013. Surprising outcome of ommaya reservoir in treating cystic craniopharyngioma: a retrospective study. Br. J. Neurosurg. 27 (3), 370–373.

Puget, S., Garnett, M., Wray, A., Grill, J., Habrand, J., Bodaert, N., Zerah, M., Bazerra, M., Renier, D., Pierre-Kahn, A., Sainte-Rose, C., 2007. Pediatric craniopharyngiomas: classification and treatment according to the degree of hypothalamic involvement. J. Neurosurg. 106 (Suppl. 1), 3–12.

Rajput, D., Srivastva, A., Kumar, R., Mahapatra, A., 2012. Recurrent chemical meningitis in craniopharyngioma without reduction in size of cyst: case report of two cases and review of the literature. Turk. Neurosurg. 22 (2), 233–236.

Scarff, J., 1941. A new method for treatment of cystic craniopharyngioma by intraventricular drainage. Acta. Neurol. Psychiatry 46, 843–867.

Schoenfeld, A., Pekmezci, M., Barnes, M.J., Tihan, T., Gupta, N., Lamborn, K., Banerjee, A., Mueller, S., Chang, S., Berger, M., Haas-Kogan, D., 2012. The superiority of conservative resection and adjuvant radiation for craniopharyngiomas. J. Neurooncol. 108 (1), 133–139.

Spaziante, R., De Divitiis, E., Irace, C., Cappabianca, P., Caputi, F., 1989. Management of primary or recurring grossly cystic craniopharyngiomas by means of draining systems. Topic review and 6 case reports. Acta. Neurochir. (Wien) 97 (3–4), 95–106.

Steinbok, P., Hukin, J., 2010. Intracystic treatments for craniopharyngioma. Neurosurg. Focus. 28 (4), E13.

Stripp, D.C., Maity, A., Janss, A.J., Belasco, J., Tochner, Z., Goldwein, J., Moshang, T., Rorke, L., Phillips, P., Sutton, L.N., Shu, H., 2004. Surgery with or without radiation therapy in the management of craniopharyngiomas in children and young adults. Int. J. Radiat. Oncol. Biol. Phys. 58 (3), 714–720.

Taylor, J.C., 1971. Crainopharyngioma – a radiological technique for outlining the anatomy of large cysts. J. Neurol. Neurosurg. Psychiatry 34 (1), 105.

Thompson, D., Phipps, K., Hayward, R., 2005. Craniopharyngioma in childhood: our evidence-based approach to management. Childs. Nerv. Syst. 21 (8–9), 660–668.

Wen, B.C., Hussey, D.H., Staples, J., Doornbos, J., Wen, B., Vigliotti, A., 1989. A comparison of the roles of surgery and radiation therapy in the management of craniopharyngiomas. Int. J. Radiat. Oncol. Biol. Phys. 16 (1), 17–24.

Winkfield, K.M., Linsenmeier, C., Yock, T.I., Grant, P., Yeap, B., Butler, W., Tarbell, N., 2009. Surveillance of craniopharyngioma cyst growth in children treated with proton radiotherapy. Int. J. Radiat. Oncol. Biol. Phys. 73 (3), 716–721.

CHAPTER

17

Endonasal Resection of Craniopharyngiomas: Post-operative Management

Leo F.S. Ditzel Filho, Daniel M. Prevedello*, Edward E. Kerr*, Ali O. Jamshidi*, Bradley A. Otto†, Ricardo L. Carrau†*

*Department of Neurological Surgery, The Ohio State University Wexner Medical Center, Columbus, OH, USA; †Department of Otolaryngology – Head and Neck Surgery, The Ohio State University Wexner Medical Center, Columbus, OH, USA

"Good postoperative care is an integral part of good surgery." **Ernest Sachs, 1949**

BACKGROUND

Craniopharyngiomas are formidable tumors; their predilection for the suprasellar space and ability to adhere to surrounding structures renders their safe removal a daunting challenge. Several approaches have been proposed for their surgical treatment, including pterional-transsylvian (Yasargil et al., 1990), fronto-lateral (Samii and Samii, 2000), supraorbital (Reisch and Perneczky, 2005; Fatemi et al., 2009), interhemispheric, subfrontal (Aryan et al., 2005), transsphenoidal (Halves and Bushe, 1979; Laws Jr., 1980, 1994; Honegger et al., 1992; Fahlbusch et al., 2000; Maira et al., 2004) and even transpetrosal approaches (Al-Mefty et al., 2007, 2008). Recent advances in technology and a more thorough understanding of skull base anatomy from a ventral perspective have allowed the addition of the endonasal corridor under endoscopic visualization (Frank et al., 2006; de Divitiis et al., 2007; Gardner et al., 2008; Kassam et al., 2008; Cavallo et al., 2009) to the armamentarium of the skull base surgeon who deals with these lesions.

The expanded endonasal approaches (EEAs), specifically the transsellar, transtuberculum, and transplanum modules (Kassam et al., 2005a), offer several advantages over their

Craniopharyngiomas
http://dx.doi.org/10.1016/B978-0-12-416706-3.00017-9

transcranial counterparts: direct visualization of the main tumor component and vital surrounding structures without the need for any brain or optic apparatus retraction is the main benefit over traditional techniques. The endonasal corridor grants ample access to the sellar and suprasellar compartments, as well as the anterior, middle, and posterior cranial fossae, when necessary. Direct visualization of the superior hypophyseal arteries, pituitary stalk and optic nerves and chiasm enables safe, microsurgical dissection of these structures from the tumor surface. Finally, the ventral perspective provides the surgeon with a superb view of the walls of the third ventricle, provided the tumor has violated them, a notoriously difficult area to safely access from a transcranial route.

These advantages come at a cost: the need for a partner who will "drive" the endoscope, the need for specialized training with a steep learning curve (Snyderman et al., 2007) and, more infamously, the possibility of cerebrospinal fluid (CSF) leakage are among the drawbacks of the technique. Given its peculiarities, it is only natural that complication prevention and post-operative management of patients submitted to this technique also requires specific measures. Thus, herein the authors present the post-operative strategies commonly employed after endonasal resection of craniopharyngiomas.

GENERAL MEASURES

All patients submitted to endonasal resection of a craniopharyngioma are sent to the neurological intensive care unit (ICU) for immediate post-operative care. Prior to that, they are awoken from anesthesia upon the completion of surgery and a neurological exam is performed to ensure that no gross focal abnormalities (vision loss, paresis) are present. Standard care and comfort measures are employed, including effective analgesia, hydration, and frequent neurological assessments. Though the vast majority of patients tolerate the procedure well, the ICU environment is still required for proper fluid and electrolyte monitoring, as these patients may present with new-onset *diabetes insipidus* (DI) post-operatively. Sodium levels, urine, and serum osmolality are routinely measured every six of the initial 24 post-operative hours; these assessments can be increased in frequency in the presence of DI.

The head of the bed is positioned at a 30 degree angle so as to facilitate venous return and CSF flow towards the spine. If the patient is awake and cooperative, oral nutrition is started and ambulation is encouraged as soon as possible. A Foley catheter is typically installed during anesthetic induction; this is kept in place for the first post-operative day but removed the following morning, in an attempt to further encourage ambulation and prevent urinary tract infections. If DI is suspected and there is a need for urinary output assessment, patients are oriented to utilize a specific container when voiding, so that urinary volume can be documented and analyzed.

Pain control is achieved with a combination of acetaminophen and narcotics; non-steroidal anti-inflammatory drugs (NSAIDs) are avoided due to the risk of nasal mucosal bleeding. Progressive headaches that do not respond to increasing doses of narcotic analgesics must be closely evaluated due to the risk of CSF leak and concomitant pneumocephalus. Conversely, narcotics may induce nausea/vomiting and constipation, which in turn may cause an increase in intracranial pressure (ICP), displacement of the skull base reconstruction and subsequent CSF leakage. Thus, the use of narcotic analgesia must be employed judiciously, using the lowest dosage possible needed for patient comfort. Furthermore, it is usually accompanied by anti-emetic drugs and pro-kinetics/laxatives, in order to prevent the aforementioned side effects.

Deep venous thrombosis is prevented initially by the use of intermittent lower extremity compressive devices; low-molecular-weight heparin may be initiated as early as post-operative day (POD) 2, though the majority of patients are fully ambulatory by then and do not require any additional prophylactic measures.

Patients are typically discharged from the ICU to a regular room on POD 1.

INFECTION PROPHYLAXIS

All patients submitted to an EEA receive prophylactic antibiotics during anesthetic induction, typically cefepime, a fourth-generation cephalosporin. If the patient is allergic to penicillins or even to cephalosporins, then cefepime is replaced by aztreonam. Both scenarios are complemented with vancomycin in case the pre-operative nasal swab detects meticillin-resistant (MRSA) *Staphylococcus aureus*. Whichever the regimen, it is continued for the initial 24 post-operative hours.

Reconstruction of the skull base utilizing a pedicled mucosal flap usually requires some degree of nasal packing to secure the multilayer construct in place whilst it heals. After the initial 24 post-operative hours, the prophylactic antibiotics started during anesthetic induction are replaced by either a second-generation cephalosporin, like cefuroxime, or the trimethoprim/sulfamethoxazole combination. These are kept in place until all nasal packing is removed, commonly on POD 5.

A common misconception is the belief that the use of the endonasal route with dural transgression, as seen in EEAs for craniopharyngioma resection, cause high rates of post-operative meningitis and brain abscess/subdural empyema formation. However, recent studies (Kassam et al., 2011; Kono et al., 2011) have demonstrated that this antibiotic scheme, coupled with continuous irrigation of the operative field with warm saline during surgery, together with early surgical management of CSF leaks actually yield surprisingly low rates of infectious complications after EEA.

POST-OPERATIVE IMAGING

All patients are submitted to imaging studies post-operatively. Typically, a non-contrast head computed tomography (CT) scan is performed within the first 3 hours after surgery; this aims to detect gross cerebral changes (hematomas, infarcts). This scan is also essential in establishing a baseline for future comparisons, especially when evaluating the patient for a potential CSF leak, as these tend to present with an increase in the amount of pneumocephalus when compared to the immediate post-operative scan (a minimal amount of air is commonly present within the basal cisterns).

A brain magnetic resonance imaging (MRI) scan is also performed within the first 24 hours after surgery, according to the patient's level of comfort. This study confirms the degree of resection, establishes a baseline for oncological comparisons, and detects ischemic complications that may have eluded the head CT performed earlier. It also confirms proper flap positioning and viability (a live nasoseptal flap will enhance upon contrast administration). If a gross total removal has been achieved, the MRI is repeated at 6 and 12 months and yearly after that. If a near total or subtotal resection was achieved, imaging follow-up is started at 3 months with varying intervals, based on the tumor's Ki-67 labeling and morphological features (cystic lesions are notorious for early or even sudden recurrences if complete removal of the tumor capsule was not possible).

CEREBROSPINAL FLUID LEAK PREVENTION AND MANAGEMENT

Perhaps the most notorious, though not necessarily the most lethal, complication after an expanded endonasal approach with dural transgression, CSF leakage has become increasingly less common with the advent of vascularized mucosal flaps (Kassam et al., 2011), especially the nasoseptal flap based on the posterior nasal artery (Kassam et al., 2005b, 2008; Hadad et al., 2006; Zanation et al., 2009). The majority of craniopharyngiomas approached endonasally will necessarily require entry into the suprasellar cistern, and may even provide communication with the third ventricle (Figure 17.1); these will translate into a high-flow CSF leak and must be dealt with accordingly. Thus, in all of these cases, the nasoseptal flap, when available, is raised at the beginning of the procedure and typically placed within the ipsilateral choana throughout resection. At the end, it is retrieved and placed to cover the defect in onlay fashion. Reconstruction techniques may vary from center to center, but they invariably rely on live, vascularized tissue to obtain effective, long-term closure.

Nevertheless, reconstruction is only one step in preventing a CSF leak. Although some authors defend the prophylactic use of lumbar drainage in high-flow CSF leaks, these authors

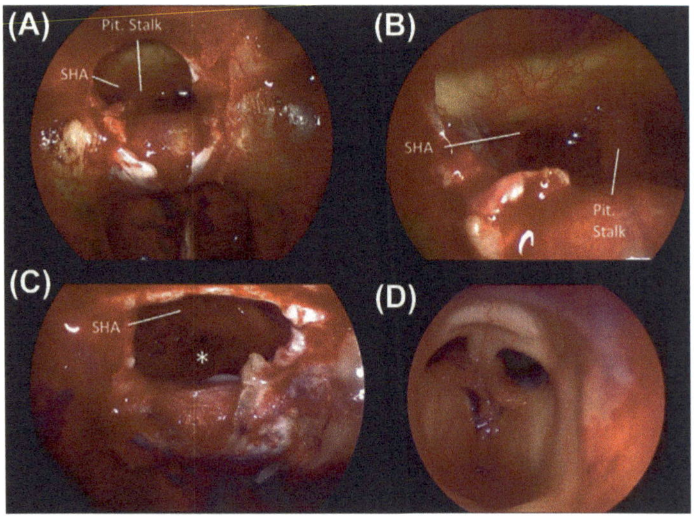

FIGURE 17.1 Skull base defects after endonasal resection of craniopharyngiomas. **A,** Suprasellar defect after resection of a Type I tumor, with entry into the suprasellar cistern. **B,** Close-up view of the defect shown in A; note the preservation of the superior hypophyseal arteries and pituitary stalk. **C,** Defect after resection of a Type III tumor, with entry into the suprasellar cistern and third ventricle (asterisk). **D,** Close-up anterior view of the third ventricle seen in C.

do not advocate its widespread use, as the majority of patients will progress satisfactorily provided certain steps are taken. These include:

- No use of straws;
- No incentive spirometry;
- Absolutely no transnasal canulas are allowed;
- Patients are oriented to cough and/or sneeze with the mouth open;
- The head of the bed is positioned at 30 degrees or higher;
- Early ambulation;
- No bending over or squatting;
- Routine use of anti-emetics;
- Routine use of stool softeners;
- Nasal packing is kept in place until POD 5.

These measures generally aim to prevent an increase in ICP and possible displacement of the skull base reconstruction, thus allowing the flap to heal at its borders and fuse with the surrounding mucosa.

If a patient presents with clear fluid drainage despite the aforementioned steps, physical examination with challenge of the reconstruction is required. This can be achieved by having the patient bend his or her head anteriorly, with assistance, towards the knees. If obvious, continuous clear fluid is observed, a CSF leak is presumably diagnosed and reoperation is indicated. If the amount of fluid is discrete or if no fluid is observed, despite previous reports (with or without witnesses), then additional investigation is necessary. This can be achieved by repeating a non-contrast head CT (new or increased pneumocephalus will confirm the leak), testing the nasal discharge for beta-2-transferrin or even direct bedside nasal endoscopic assessment.

Once confirmed, CSF leaks are always managed surgically with immediate transsphenoidal reoperation. In the vast majority of cases, the nasoseptal flap is found to be displaced, either due to improper placement or valsalva maneuvering. Simple repositioning of the flap and packing will usually suffice; occasionally the reconstruction is reinforced with abdominal fat, this being decided on a case-by-case basis, taking into account factors such as the difficulty of performing the reconstruction and defect size.

Although lumbar drainage is not routinely employed, it may be considered in the rare occasion of a recurrent CSF leak. Another option is the use of acetazolamide, which aims to decrease CSF production and, consequently, decrease the ICP, thus giving the reconstruction a chance to heal.

ADJUVANT THERAPIES

Residual tumors may be followed with serial imaging, submitted to reoperation, or to adjuvant radiotherapy. Although direct instillation of chemotherapeutic agents into cystic craniopharyngiomas has been shown to be effective, although with variable results (Julow et al., 1988; Rutka et al., 1992; Spaziante et al., 1993; Broggi and Franzini, 1996; Blackburn et al., 1999; Cavalheiro et al., 2005), systemic chemotherapy for solid residuals is yet to become a viable option (Hargrave, 2006).

Certain aspects must be taken into account when dealing with a solid residual, including size of the mass, its proximity to cranial nerves, the patient's age, and pituitary function status. In young patients with a small residual and a low Ki-67, the authors tend to favor serial imaging; if the remaining mass is large or if the tumor has aggressive pathological features then reoperation is considered, possibly through a different approach, given that the endonasal route did not allow a gross total resection. If the patient is already on hormonal replacement due to previous panhypopituitarism and the residual is not in close contact with the optic nerves or chiasm, radiation therapy has been shown to be an option for long-term control (Hoogenhout et al., 1984; Habrand et al., 1999; Laws Jr. and Vance, 1999; Chung et al., 2000; Barajas et al., 2002; Ulfarsson et al., 2002; Kobayashi et al., 2003; Kalapurakal, 2005). If gland function is preserved, or if the residual is in close proximity to the optic apparatus, or its size exceeds the permissible diameter for safe radiation planning, then radiation therapy is usually discarded in favor of observation or reoperation, again, based on patient's age and the pathological features of the tumor.

ENDOCRINE MANAGEMENT

The most feared complication (Yasargil et al., 1990; Pierre-Kahn et al., 2005) after surgical resection of craniopharyngiomas is new onset of endocrine dysfunction (De Vile et al., 1996; Fahlbusch et al., 1999; Duff et al., 2000; Karavitaki et al., 2005; Gardner et al., 2008). This is particularly true in Kassam's Type II lesions (Kassam et al., 2008), in which the pituitary stalk itself has become the tumor and resection is unlikely to be achieved without compromising the gland's function. Patients who already present with pre-operative hormonal deficits are not likely to recover; unfortunately, in a significant number of cases pituitary function is lost, regardless of the approach utilized (Koutourousiou et al., 2013).

Finding the balance between tumor removal and preservation of endocrine function is a challenging task. The authors believe that gross total resection should always be attempted, except for tumors which infiltrate the walls of the hypothalamus, even if this means incurring panhypopituitarism and a need for hormonal replacement.

If a patient already presents with endocrine dysfunction pre-operatively, hormonal replacement is maintained through surgery and the post-operative period, with special attention to steroidal stress dose and desmopressin supplementation for natremic control.

All patients with preserved pituitary function pre-operatively have their cortisol and prolactin levels tested in the morning of POD 1; this represents a direct assessment of maintenance of the gland's capacity. The prolactin level is ordered simply to ensure that the anterior hypophysis is functional because the lactotroph cells produce this hormone. Although prolactin was traditionally thought to only regulate reproduction, lactation, and libido, it is now considered to act on multiple targets and is responsible for osmoregulation, energy metabolism, growth, angiogenesis, brain function, and immune response. Therefore, the authors believe that it is crucial to ensure the health of the anterior gland with a confirmatory lab value; ensuring a normal prolactin level is vital in managing patients post-operatively. In addition, if the cortisol is decreased, supplementation with oral prednisone is initiated, provided the patient is awake and alert; IV steroid formulations can be employed if otherwise. Sodium levels, urine, and serum osmolalities are checked every 6 hours. If the patient is trending towards hypernatremia but is awake and alert, then fluid depletion is compensated by oral ingestion of water; desmopressin is withheld in the hope that a transient DI has ensued and that the gland will eventually pick up the pace and return to normal function. If in 48 hours there is no sign of function recovery, or if the patient is comatose and therefore cannot drink, desmopressin supplementation is initiated. In cases where preservation of the pituitary stalk was possible but the patient presented with hypopituitarism nonetheless, steroidal, and desmopressin can be slowly weaned off after 3 months of supplementation to challenge the gland's function. If the patient presents with increased diuresis and/or symptoms of hypocortisolism, replacement is resumed and function recovery is highly unlikely to ever take place.

Although panhypopituitarism can be effectively managed nowadays, the effects of hypothalamic dysfunction can be severe and less forgiving, particularly regarding changes in consciousness and induction of obesity. Hence, the hypothalamic components of the tumor must only be removed when a clear cleavage plain is present and dissection proves to be feasible.

CONCLUSIONS

The endoscopic endonasal resection of craniopharyngiomas is a safe and effective technique. Nonetheless, several measures must be taken in the post-operative period to prevent complications and to ensure a safe recovery, particularly in regards to CSF leak and pituitary dysfunction management.

References

Al-Mefty, O., Ayoubi, S., Kadri, P.A., 2007. The petrosal approach for the total removal of giant retrochiasmatic craniopharyngiomas in children. J. Neurosurg. 106 (Suppl. 2), 87–92.

Al-Mefty, O., Ayoubi, S., Kadri, P.A., 2008. The petrosal approach for the resection of retrochiasmatic craniopharyngiomas. Neurosurgery 62 (5 Suppl. 2), ONS331–335; discussion ONS335–336.

Aryan, H.E., Ozgur, B.M., Jandial, R., Levy, M.L., 2005. Subfrontal transbasal approach and technique for resection of craniopharyngioma. Neurosurg. Focus 18 (6A), E10.

Barajas, M.A., Ramirez-Guzman, G., Rodriguez-Vazquez, C., et al., 2002. Multimodal management of craniopharyngiomas: neuroendoscopy, microsurgery, and radiosurgery. J. Neurosurg. 97 (Suppl. 5), 607–609.

Blackburn, T.P., Doughty, D., Plowman, P.N., 1999. Stereotactic intracavitary therapy of recurrent cystic craniopharyngioma by instillation of 90yttrium. Br. J. Neurosurg. 13 (4), 359–365.

Broggi, G., Franzini, A., 1996. Bleomycin for cystic craniopharyngioma. J. Neurosurg. 84 (6), 1080–1081.

Cavalheiro, S., Dastoli, P.A., Silva, N.S., Toledo, S., Lederman, H., da Silva, M.C., 2005. Use of interferon alpha in intratumoral chemotherapy for cystic craniopharyngioma. Childs Nerv. Syst. 21 (8–9), 719–724.

Cavallo, L.M., Prevedello, D.M., Solari, D., et al., 2009. Extended endoscopic endonasal transsphenoidal approach for residual or recurrent craniopharyngiomas. J. Neurosurg. 111 (3), 578–589.

Chung, W.Y., Pan, D.H., Shiau, C.Y., Guo, W.Y., Wang, L.W., 2000. Gamma knife radiosurgery for craniopharyngiomas. J. Neurosurg. 93 (Suppl. 3), 47–56.

de Divitiis, E., Cappabianca, P., Cavallo, L.M., Esposito, F., de Divitiis, O., Messina, A., 2007. Extended endoscopic transsphenoidal approach for extrasellar craniopharyngiomas. Neurosurgery 61 (5 Suppl. 2), 219–227; discussion 228.

De Vile, C.J., Grant, D.B., Kendall, B.E., et al., 1996. Management of childhood craniopharyngioma: can the morbidity of radical surgery be predicted? J. Neurosurg. 85 (1), 73–81.

Duff, J.M., Meyer, F.B., Ilstrup, D.M., Laws Jr., E.R., Scleck, C.D., Scheithauer, B.W., 2000. Long-term outcomes for surgically resected craniopharyngiomas. Neurosurgery 46, 291–305.

Fahlbusch, R., Honneger, J., Buchfelder, M., 2000. Transsphenoidal microsurgery for craniopharyngiomas. In: Schmidek, H.H. (Ed.), Shmidek & Sweet, Operative neurosurgical techniques: Indications, methods, and results, vol 1. W.B. Saunders, Philadelphia, pp. 503–511.

Fahlbusch, R., Honegger, J., Paulus, W., Huk, W., Buchfelder, M., 1999. Surgical treatment of craniopharyngiomas: experience with 168 patients. J. Neurosurg. 90 (2), 237–250.

Fatemi, N., Dusick, J.R., de Paiva Neto, M.A., Malkasian, D., Kelly, D.F., 2009. Endonasal versus supraorbital keyhole removal of craniopharyngiomas and tuberculum sellae meningiomas. Neurosurgery 64 (5 Suppl. 2), 269–284; discussion 284–266.

Frank, G., Pasquini, E., Doglietto, F., et al., 2006. The endoscopic extended transsphenoidal approach for craniopharyngiomas. Neurosurgery 59 (Suppl. 1), ONS75–ONS83.

Gardner, P.A., Kassam, A.B., Snyderman, C.H., et al., 2008. Outcomes following endoscopic, expanded endonasal resection of suprasellar craniopharyngiomas: a case series. J. Neurosurg. 109 (1), 6–16.

Gardner, P.A., Prevedello, D.M., Kassam, A.B., Snyderman, C.H., Carrau, R.L., Mintz, A.H., 2008. The evolution of the endonasal approach for craniopharyngiomas. J. Neurosurg. 108 (5), 1043–1047.

Habrand, J.L., Ganry, O., Couanet, D., et al., 1999. The role of radiation therapy in the management of craniopharyngioma: A 25-year experience and review of the literature. Int. J. Radiat. Oncol. Biol. Phys. 44 (2), 255–263.

Hadad, G., Bassagasteguy, L., Carrau, R.L., et al., 2006. A novel reconstructive technique after endoscopic expanded endonasal approaches: vascular pedicle nasoseptal flap. Laryngoscope 116 (10), 1882–1886.

Halves, E., Bushe, K.A., 1979. Transsphenoidal operation on craniopharyngiomas with extrasellar extensions. The advantage of the operating endoscope [proceedings]. Acta Neurochir. Suppl. (Wien) 28 (2), 362.

Hargrave, D.R., 2006. Does chemotherapy have a role in the management of craniopharyngioma? J. Pediatr. Endocrinol. Metab. 19 (Suppl. 1), 407–412.

Honegger, J., Buchfelder, M., Fahlbusch, R., Daubler, B., Dorr, H.G., 1992. Transsphenoidal microsurgery for craniopharyngioma. Surg. Neurol. 37 (3), 189–196.

Hoogenhout, J., Otten, B.J., Kazem, I., Stoelinga, G.B., Walder, A.H., 1984. Surgery and radiation therapy in the management of craniopharyngiomas. Int. J. Radiat. Oncol. Biol. Phys. 10 (12), 2293–2297.

Julow, J., Lanyi, F., Hajda, M., et al., 1988. Further experiences in the treatment of cystic craniopharyngeomas with yttrium 90 silicate colloid. Acta Neurochir. Suppl. (Wien) 42, 113–119.

Kalapurakal, J.A., 2005. Radiation therapy in the management of pediatric craniopharyngiomas – a review. Childs Nerv. Syst. 21 (8–9), 808–816.

Karavitaki, N., Brufani, C., Warner, J.T., et al., 2005. Craniopharyngiomas in children and adults: systematic analysis of 121 cases with long-term follow-up. Clin. Endocrinol. (Oxf) 62 (4), 397–409.

Kassam, A.B., Gardner, P.A., Snyderman, C.H., Carrau, R.L., Mintz, A.H., Prevedello, D.M., 2008. Expanded endonasal approach, a fully endoscopic transnasal approach for the resection of midline suprasellar craniopharyngiomas: a new classification based on the infundibulum. J. Neurosurg. 108 (4), 715–728.

Kassam, A., Carrau, R.L., Snyderman, C.H., Gardner, P., Mintz, A., 2005a. Evolution of reconstructive techniques following endoscopic expanded endonasal approaches. Neurosurg. Focus 19 (1), E8.

Kassam, A., Snyderman, C.H., Mintz, A., Gardner, P., Carrau, R.L., 2005b. Expanded endonasal approach: the rostrocaudal axis. Part I. Crista galli to the sella turcica. Neurosurg. Focus 19 (1), E3.

Kassam, A.B., Thomas, A., Carrau, R.L., et al., 2008. Endoscopic reconstruction of the cranial base using a pedicled nasoseptal flap. Neurosurgery 63 (1 Suppl. 1), ONS44–52 discussion ONS52–43.

Kassam, A.B., Prevedello, D.M., Carrau, R.L., et al., 2011. Endoscopic endonasal skull base surgery: analysis of complications in the authors' initial 800 patients. J. Neurosurg. 114 (6), 1544–1568.

Kobayashi, T., Kida, Y., Hasegawa, T., 2003. Long-term results of gamma knife surgery for craniopharyngioma. Neurosurg. Focus (5), 14 e13.

Kono, Y., Prevedello, D.M., Snyderman, C.H., et al., 2011. One thousand endoscopic skull base surgical procedures demystifying the infection potential: incidence and description of post-operative meningitis and brain abscesses. Infect. Control Hosp. Epidemiol. 32 (1), 77–83.

Koutourousiou, M., Gardner, P.A., Fernandez-Miranda, J.C., Tyler-Kabara, E.C., Wang, E.W., Snyderman, C.H., 2013. Endoscopic endonasal surgery for craniopharyngiomas: surgical outcome in 64 patients. J. Neurosurg. 119 (5), 1194–1207.

Laws Jr., E.R., 1980. Transsphenoidal microsurgery in the management of craniopharyngioma. J. Neurosurg. 52 (5), 661–666.
Laws Jr., E.R., 1994. Transsphenoidal removal of craniopharyngioma. Pediatr. Neurosurg. Pediatr. Neurosurg. 21 (Suppl. 1), 57–63.
Laws Jr., E.R., Vance, M.L., 1999. Radiosurgery for pituitary tumors and craniopharyngiomas. Neurosurg. Clin. N. Am. 10 (2), 327–336.
Maira, G., Anile, C., Albanese, A., Cabezas, D., Pardi, F., Vignati, A., 2004. The role of transsphenoidal surgery in the treatment of craniopharyngiomas. J. Neurosurg. 100 (3), 445–451.
Pierre-Kahn, A., Recassens, C., Pinto, G., et al., 2005. Social and psycho-intellectual outcome following radical removal of craniopharyngiomas in childhood. A prospective series. Childs Nerv. Syst. 21 (8–9), 817–824.
Reisch, R., Perneczky, A., 2005. Ten-year experience with the supraorbital subfrontal approach through an eyebrow skin incision. Neurosurgery 57 (Suppl. 4), 242–255.
Rutka, J.T., Hoffman, H.J., Drake, J.M., Humphreys, R.P., 1992. Suprasellar and sellar tumors in childhood and adolescence. Neurosurg. Clin. N. Am. 3 (4), 803–820.
Sachs, E., 1949. Diagnosis and treatment of brain tumors and care of the neurosurgical patient. C.V. Mosby Company, St. Louis, p 13.
Samii, M., Samii, A., 2000. Surgical management of craniopharyngiomas. In: Schmidek, H.H. (Ed.), Schmidek & Sweet, Operative neurosurgical techniques: Indications, methods, and results, vol 1. W.B. Saunders, Philadelphia, pp. 489–502.
Snyderman, C., Kassam, A., Carrau, R., Mintz, A., Gardner, P., Prevedello, D.M., 2007. Acquisition of surgical skills for endonasal skull base surgery: a training program. Laryngoscope 117 (4), 699–705.
Spaziante, R., Irace, C., de Divitiis, E., 1993. Brachytherapy of cystic craniopharyngiomas. J. Neurosurg. 79 (6), 966–967.
Ulfarsson, E., Lindquist, C., Roberts, M., et al., 2002. Gamma knife radiosurgery for craniopharyngiomas: long-term results in the first Swedish patients. J. Neurosurg. 97 (Suppl. 5), 613–622.
Yasargil, M.G., Curcic, M., Kis, M., Siegenthaler, G., Teddy, P.J., Roth, P., 1990. Total removal of craniopharyngiomas. Approaches and long-term results in 144 patients. J. Neurosurg. 73 (1), 3–11.
Zanation, A.M., Carrau, R.L., Snyderman, C.H., et al., 2009. Nasoseptal flap reconstruction of high flow intra-operative cerebral spinal fluid leaks during endoscopic skull base surgery. Am. J. Rhinol. Allergy 23 (5), 518–521.

CHAPTER

18

Surgical Approaches: Complications of Surgical Management

Robert G. Louis[*,†], *Garni Barkhoudarian*[*], *Daniel F. Kelly*[*]

[*]**Brain Tumor Center, John Wayne Cancer Institute at Saint John's Health Center, Santa Monica, CA, USA;** [†]**Department of Anatomical Sciences, St George's University School of Medicine, Grenada**

"The hypothalamic-pituitary complex is essential for both endocrine and behavioral performance. Injury in this area, from tumor or treatment, will result in problems common among patients with craniopharyngioma." ***EG Fischer et al., 1990***

INTRODUCTION

Since Erdheim first described the histopathology of a craniopharyngioma in 1904 and A.E. Halstead first attempted resection in 1909, craniopharyngioma operations have challenged the skills of neurosurgeons (Erdheim, 1904; Halstead, 1910). Harvey Cushing described these tumors as "one of the most baffling problems to the neurosurgeon" (Elliott et al., 2011). Though characterized as benign, craniopharyngiomas are locally aggressive tumors of the sella and suprasellar region. Their location near numerous critical structures mediating visual, endocrinological, and behavioral functions makes their safe surgical removal one of the most formidable challenges in neurosurgery.

For many years, gross total resection (GTR) was felt to be the treatment of choice, owing to better rates of tumor control compared to subtotal resection (STR) alone. However, experience with aggressive surgical resection has led some to conclude that a goal of GTR in all patients can lead to unacceptable rates of morbidity. Instead, subtotal or near-complete resection followed by stereotactic conformal radiotherapy may be a more reasonable goal (Sughrue et al., 2011). However, the potential benefits of a less aggressive surgical approach that then mandates subsequent radiotherapy must be weighed against the relative risks of radiation to the optic apparatus, hypothalamic-pituitary axis, and surrounding brain and neurovascular structures as well as the potential for tumor recurrence. The balance of these risks and benefits must be considered in order to make an educated decision for each

Craniopharyngiomas
http://dx.doi.org/10.1016/B978-0-12-416706-3.00018-0

individual patient. The particular surgical approach and extent of resection is also highly dependent upon the tumor size, location, pre-operative visual and hormonal deficits, the degree of adhesions to critical neurovascular structures, and the surgical team's experience.

This chapter discusses the surgical complications associated with both transcranial and transsphenoidal approaches for craniopharyngiomas. Importantly, over the last 15 years, significant technical advances have been made in the endonasal endoscopic approach to midline skull base pathology, including craniopharyngiomas. Given that the majority of craniopharyngiomas are predominantly located in the retro-chiasmal and suprasellar space, they are increasingly being removed via the endonasal route. While this approach is not indicated for all craniopharyngiomas, this chapter will emphasize its relative advantages over transcranial approaches specifically as it relates to complications, and will stress when a transcranial route may offer a safer and potentially more effective route (Fatemi et al., 2009). Regardless of the surgical approach utilized, given the complex nature and potential treatment complications of craniopharyngiomas, a multidisciplinary team is strongly advocated, which includes neurosurgeons, head and neck surgeons, endocrinologists, neuro-ophthalmologists, radiation oncologists, and pathologists (McLaughlin et al., 2012).

ANATOMICAL CONSIDERATIONS

Surgical complications of craniopharyngioma removal are directly related to the anatomical surroundings of the parasellar, hypothalamic-pituitary region, and the specific approach used for surgical access. While suprasellar extension of craniopharyngiomas is most common, they may also involve the sella, anterior cranial fossa and middle fossa. An intricate knowledge of the relevant anatomy is critical to achieving safe tumor resection, as is a careful assessment of the pre-operative MRI. With the exception of purely intraventricular lesions, most craniopharyngiomas have involvement with the infundibulum which may be engulfed by the tumor, split by the tumor, or may be displaced anteriorly, posteriorly, or laterally (Kassam et al., 2008). They often may involve the circle of Willis vessels, compress the floor of the third ventricle, invade the hypothalamus, and extend to compress the cerebral peduncles, mesial temporal lobes, and basal frontal region. Craniopharyngiomas typically cause the optic chiasm to be displaced anteriorly (pre-fixed), while less frequently they displace the chiasm posteriorly (post-fixed) or may even engulf the optic chiasm. Pre-operative localization of the chiasm and optic nerves is essential in determining the best possible approach and ensuring safe and effective optic apparatus decompression. Whichever approach is used, successful resection of craniopharyngiomas amidst the confines of the optic apparatus, intracranial vessels, hypothalamus, pituitary gland, and cavernous sinuses presents a significant technical challenge.

VASCULAR COMPLICATIONS

Vascular complications in craniopharyngioma surgery may include injury to any of the major intracranial vessels and their branches; specifically, the carotid arteries, middle and anterior cerebral arteries, posterior communicating arteries, posterior cerebral arteries, and the basilar apex. Given the tendency of these tumors to encase or adhere to both larger and smaller vessels, careful identification and microdissection of the tumor away from vessels is one of the key challenges of craniopharyngioma surgery. Overly aggressive attempts to remove tumor capsule from major vessels, or inadvertent injury to smaller vessels such as the superior hypophyseal vessels, which irrigate the optic chiasm and pituitary gland, can have serious consequences (Blunt and Steele, 1956). In many instances, with dense tumor adhesions to vessels, the best approach is generally to accept a less than complete resection in order to avoid major vascular injury.

Whether using an endonasal or transcranial approach, pre-operative appreciation and intra-operative localization of major and minor vessels are critical to safe craniopharyngioma surgery. Although the use of intra-operative frameless navigation may help to localize the carotid arteries and other large vessels, Doppler ultrasonography may be more useful and potentially more accurate for localizing these vessels that may be hidden or engulfed by tumor (Dusick et al., 2007). Because the Doppler probe gives real-time feedback, it is less prone to inaccuracy, as frequently occurs with MRI or CT-based frameless navigation systems as tumor removal proceeds. The Doppler probe requires some subjective interpretation of the exact location from which the audible pulse is emanating. Nevertheless, it generally provides very useful and easily obtained information to help avoid inadvertent large vessel injury.

Vascular injury may include laceration, thrombosis, vasospasm, and delayed aneurysmal dilatation of the carotid artery or any of the major circle of Willis vessels (Sutton, 1994). Vascular injury to the carotid artery can be catastrophic and may require its sacrifice. While rare, this often can result in mortality or significant neurological morbidity including hemiplegia, aphasia, and vision loss. Komotar et al. report rates of vascular injury resulting in stroke in 2.9% of transcranial series and 2.7% of endoscopic transsphenoidal series (Komotar et al., 2012).

Fusiform dilation of the carotid artery is believed to result from possible adventitial damage that occurs when craniopharyngiomas are peeled off this vessel (Sutton, 1994; King, 2011). The clinical significance of this condition remains unknown. Sutton reported a 15.7% incidence of fusiform dilation of the carotid artery in a series of 57 patients who underwent surgery for craniopharyngioma over a 9-year period. According to their report, however, none of these patients suffered hemorrhage as a result of this vascular abnormality (Sutton, 1994). Based upon his experience, the author advocated that asymptomatic patients with fusiform dilatation of the carotid artery be simply observed, and that surgical exploration should be reserved for those patients who experience symptoms.

In addition to direct laceration and fusiform dilation, vasospasm to circle of Willis vessels can also occur post-operatively, leading to permanent neurological deficits. There are numerous case reports in the literature which describe vasospasm after surgery for craniopharyngiomas (Sutton, 1994; Macdonald and Hoffman, 1997; Salunke et al., 2013). Neurological sequelae of vasospasm typically appear in delayed fashion, usually within several days of surgery. These can range in severity and include visual, motor, language, or brainstem infarcts. New onset of neurological deficit several days after surgery should prompt immediate investigation, including digital subtraction or CT angiography. MRI can help to delineate completed infarcts (Figure 18.1). Judicious use of induced hypertension and hypervolemia may be appropriate in patients with documented and symptomatic vasospasm to prevent stroke and permanent neurological deficits (Deshaies et al., 2009).

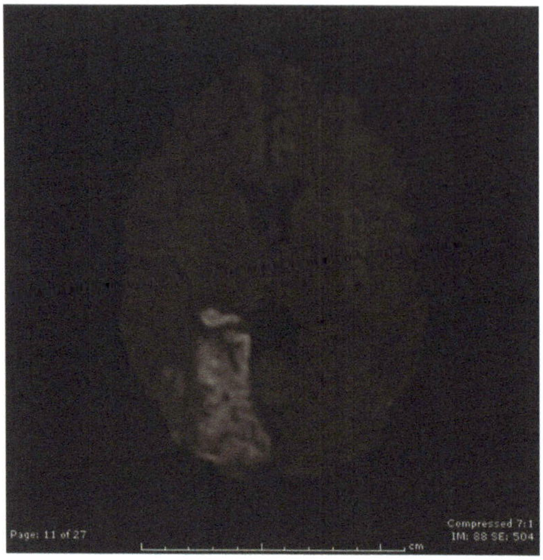

FIGURE 18.1 Axial diffusion weighted magnetic resonance image demonstrating a right posterior cerebral artery infarct from intra-operative manipulation and vasospasm.

VISUAL LOSS

Visual disturbances are the presenting complaint in the majority of cases of adult craniopharyngiomas, accounting for up to 80% of the initial presenting symptom in some series (Koutourousiou et al., 2013). Accordingly, one of the primary goals of surgery is to decompress and protect the optic apparatus. While improvement of visual symptoms is possible in the majority of cases, a significant number of patients experience visual deterioration as a result of surgical intervention. This can be one of the most devastating consequences of surgery, especially for patients with normal pre-operative vision. Visual loss can arise from direct surgical trauma, including aggressive traction and cautery, as well as from ischemia. (Figure 18.2A, B). Ischemia most commonly occurs while attempting to dissect tumor away from the optic chiasm and usually presents immediately post-operatively. Delayed visual loss can also occur and is usually the result of compression from post-operative hematoma but can also arise from vasospasm. Imaging should be performed promptly to rule out a hematoma (Figure 18.3) as early evacuation is essential to preservation and recovery of normal visual function. In cases where imaging does not demonstrate a hematoma, empiric hyperdynamic therapy for presumed vasospasm should be initiated (Deshaies et al., 2009).

The microvascular supply of the optic chiasm is relatively complex, and deep understanding of its anatomy may help to preserve vision during craniopharyngioma surgery. In general, vessels from the overlying pial network supply the chiasm. Inferiorly, the largest vessel contributing to this network is the superior hypophyseal artery, which gives off a recurrent branch along the inferomedial border of the proximal intracranial part of the optic nerve (Blunt and Steele, 1956; Abuzayed et al., 2010). These paired vessels are routinely encountered adherent to the tumor capsule in the endonasal endoscopic removal of

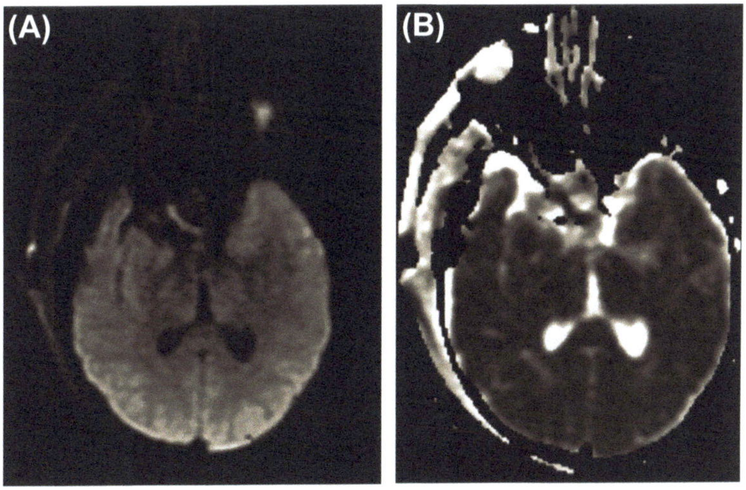

FIGURE 18.2 **A,** Axial diffusion weighted magnetic resonance image demonstrating restricted diffusion from a likely infarct of the right optic nerve. **B,** Apparent diffusion coefficient map of in the same patient, confirming infarction of the right optic nerve.

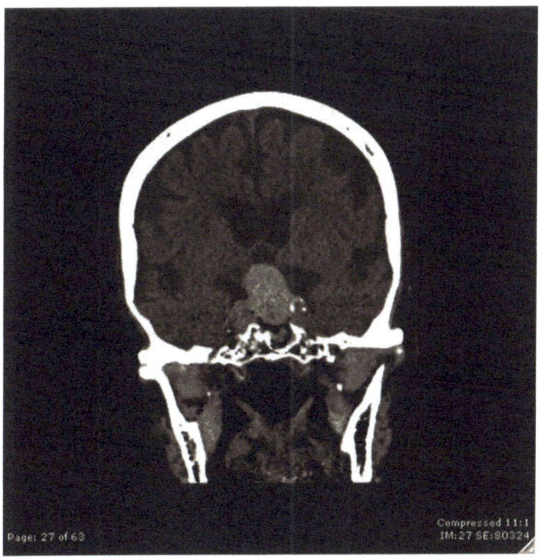

FIGURE 18.3 Coronal CT demonstrating a post-operative hematoma with suprasellar extension and pressure on the optic chiasm.

retro-chiasmal craniopharyngiomas, and every attempt must be made to preserve them using careful microsurgical technique and sharp dissection (Figure 18.4). Small branches from the internal carotid, anterior choroidal, and posterior communicating arteries also provide some additional blood supply to the optic chiasm and optic tracts. The pial plexus on the superior surface of the chiasm receives supply from the anterior cerebral and anterior

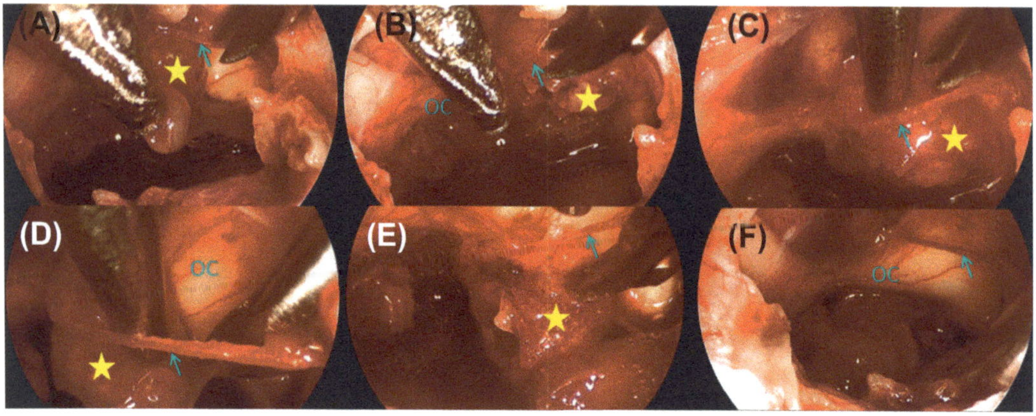

FIGURE 18.4 Intra-operative endonasal view with 30-degree endoscope, showing progressive sharp dissection of left superior hypophyseal artery (blue arrow) away from craniopharyngioma (yellow star) with preservation of arachnoid over optic chiasm (OC) **(A–F)**.

communicating arteries. Venous drainage of the anteroinferior surface of the chiasm is via the basal veins, whereas the superior surface is drained by the anterior cerebral veins (Blunt and Steele, 1956). During resection of craniopharyngiomas in close proximity to the optic chiasm, preservation of this pial vascular network is of paramount importance to prevent post-operative visual deficits. Limiting the use of electrocautery adjacent to the optic apparatus and small feeding vessels is strongly recommended. Use of sharp dissection over excessive mechanical traction is also preferred.

In our experience, we approached the majority of craniopharyngiomas via the endonasal route, as they were primarily retro-chiasmal in location (Fatemi et al., 2009). This common growth pattern of craniopharyngiomas displaces the chiasm into a pre-fixed or superior location creating a surgical avenue between the chiasm and pituitary gland ideal for the endonasal transsphenoidal approach. This approach is highly effective and allows even large retrochiasmal craniopharyngiomas to be removed with progressive internal debulking and endoscopic visualization (Figure 18.5). The endonasal approach also obviates the need to transgress the lamina terminalis, which is bordered by the optic tracts bilaterally and optic chiasm anteriorly, a requirement for transcranial removal of most retro-chiasmal tumors. Although the translamina terminalis approach for craniopharyngiomas is an effective route in experienced hands, it may pose greater risk to the optic apparatus than the endonasal approach. In contrast, craniopharyngiomas within the pre-chiasmatic space can be removed via a supraorbital or endonasal route, while tumors with lateral extensions or supra-chiasmatic extensions can be most effectively removed by a supra-orbital or lateral transcranial approach.

The rates of post-operative visual outcomes vary widely amongst surgical series. In a meta-analysis of large surgical series of transcranial resection of pediatric craniopharyngiomas, Elliott et al. reported that visual status improved in 47.7% of patients (454 of 1051) who had pre-operative deficits, whereas 13% of patients (263 of 2029) experienced new visual field (VF) and/or visual acuity (VA) deficits after treatment (Elliott et al., 2011). By comparison, their analysis of endonasal endoscopic surgical series demonstrated visual status improvement in 85.5% of patients who had pre-operative deficits (106 of 124), and only

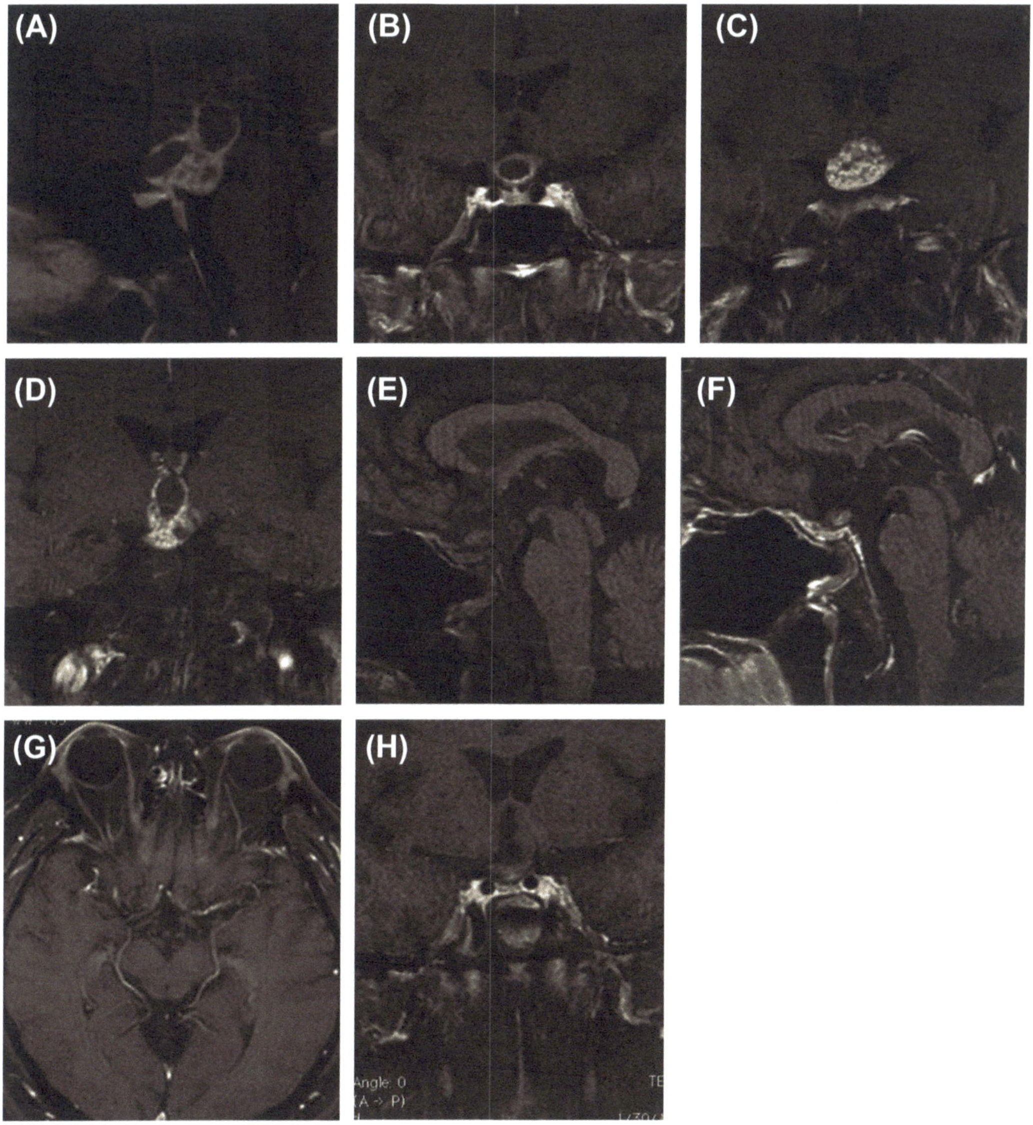

FIGURE 18.5 Pre-operative **(A–D)** and post-operative **(E–H)** MRI of large retro-chiasmal craniopharyngioma removed through endonasal endoscopic approach. The removal was accomplished by working entirely below chiasm and above the pituitary gland.

2.3% of patients experienced new VF and/or VA deficits after treatment (8 of 352) (Elliott et al., 2011). In the meta-analysis by Komotar et al., the respective rates of visual improvement and decline were 33.1% and 11.1% for transcranial series, 44% and 5.3% for microscopic transsphenoidal series, and 56.2% and 1.7% for endoscopic transsphenoidal series (Komotar et al., 2012).

According to Koutourousio et al., the published literature has shown that transcranial surgery is associated with somewhat worse visual outcomes in comparison with those for transsphenoidal surgery (Fernandez-Miranda et al., 2012; Koutourousiou et al., 2013). In a series of 168 patients with craniopharyngiomas, Fahlbusch et al. documented visual improvement in 73% of patients after transsphenoidal surgery, compared to 63% of patients undergoing transcranial surgery. Furthermore, visual deterioration was observed only in the transcranial group, affecting 14.3% of patients (Fahlbusch et al., 1999). Similarly, after managing 86 craniopharyngiomas, Chakrabarti et al. noticed visual improvement in 61% of the transcranial cases versus 87% of transsphenoidal cases; vision worsened postoperatively in 17% of the transcranial cohort versus 3% of the transsphenoidal cohort (Chakrabarti et al., 2005; Koutourousiou et al., 2013). Koutourousiou et al. documented normalization or improvement of vision in 86.4% of the patients undergoing transsphenoidal surgery, with only one post-operative visual deficit developed in a patient whose preoperative vision was intact (1.5%) (Koutourousiou et al., 2013).

Elliott et al. also endorse the transsphenoidal approach as being the most effective and safest route for lesions producing visual impairment by compression of the optic nerves and chiasm (Laws et al., 1977; Elliott et al., 2011). Approaching craniopharyngiomas from below, in most cases, allows for early decompression of the tumor while minimizing manipulation of the optic apparatus. In contrast, a transcranial approach often requires more manipulation of the optic apparatus and extracapsular dissection before decompression of the tumor (Elliott et al., 2010). This observation may account for the higher rates of visual improvement and lower rates of deterioration after transsphenoidal compared with transcranial resection of craniopharyngiomas.

Although relatively rare, ophthalmoplegia can also occur as a complication of transsphenoidal resection of sellar tumors, particularly with those lesions that invade into the cavernous sinus or into the subarachnoid space lateral to the optico-carotid cisterns. Shi and Wang reported a 2.7% incidence of new oculomotor paresis in 110 patients undergoing transcranial resection of craniopharyngiomas, although only one of these (0.9%) was permanent (Shi and Wang, 2001). By comparison, Konig et al. reported one case of transient oculomotor paresis in a series of 31 patients who underwent transsphenoidal resection (3.2%). Other large transsphenoidal series have reported no incidence of new oculomotor palsies. Overall, the incidence of new ophthalmoplegia in craniopharyngioma series is less than one percent.

NEUROENDOCRINE COMPLICATIONS

Endocrinopathy is a common presenting problem in patients with craniopharyngioma, with more than 75% of patients having deficiency of at least one adenohypophyseal hormone axis at presentation; most commonly hypogonadal hypogonadism or growth hormone deficiency (Sklar, 1994; Paja et al., 1995; Honegger et al., 1999). Although not quite as prevalent, diabetes insipidus is also a common presenting symptom, occurring in 12% to 32% of patients (Honegger et al., 1999; Komotar et al., 2012).

Injury to the anterior or posterior pituitary gland, infundibulum, or hypothalamus during surgical removal may exacerbate hypothalamic-pituitary dysfunction or create new permanent endocrine deficits. Although these injuries usually occur from direct surgical insults, they can also arise from post-operative hemorrhage or ischemia. Some authors argue that some level of endocrinopathy should be accepted as a nearly universal sequela to craniopharyngioma treatment (Duff et al., 2000; Elliott et al., 2010). In some cases, the pituitary stalk is deliberately transected to preserve hypothalamic function by reducing traction. Given that hormonal dysfunction is so common with craniopharyngioma surgery, close collaboration with an endocrinologist is essential for all such patients. As described in Chapter 5, a complete pre-operative anterior and posterior pituitary hormonal assessment should be performed for all patients with a presumed craniopharyngioma to allow essential hormone replacement, including possible thyroid and glucocorticoid therapy as well as treatment of DI. In the immediate post-operative period, the two critical hormonal deficiencies that must be carefully monitored are diabetes insipidus and adrenal insufficiency. In patients with pre-operative DI and/or hypocortisolism, ongoing replacement therapy with desmopressin (DDAVP) and stress dose glucocorticoids should continue. For patients who preoperatively have an intact adrenocortical axis and no DI, careful post-operative monitoring of cortisol levels, serum sodium and urine specific gravity is essential to provide timely and appropriate replacement. For those patients who undergo stalk transection or hypophysectomy, stress dose glucocorticoids should begin intraoperatively with a gradual taper to maintenance replacement, as dictated by the patient's clinical condition. Administration of DDAVP in the immediate post-operative period should initially be on an as-needed basis (typically every 12 hours) to avoid iatrogenic hyponatremia, then transitioned to a standard daily dosing over the next several days. A morning–evening schedule should be considered to help patients reach a reasonable cycle compatible with their circadian rhythm.

A key consideration for the extent of tumor removal is the degree of pre-existing endocrinopathy and the location of the infundibulum. In general, for patients with no preoperative endocrinopathy or only one anterior hormonal deficit with an identifiable stalk on MRI, an attempt to save the infundibulum and the hypothalamic–pituitary structures is warranted. However, in patients with pre-operative DI and/or additional pituitary dysfunction, a more aggressive approach in tumor removal may be reasonable, given the likelihood that such endocrine deficits will not be reversible. A careful review of the preoperative MRI to identify the infundibulum and intraoperative confirmation of its location are the essential first steps in preserving the hypothalamic–pituitary function in patients with a craniopharyngioma. Use of sharp dissection to remove tumor along the stalk is also critical and, in some instances, leaving densely adherent tumor along the stalk may be a necessary compromise to preserve hormonal and hypothalamic function postoperatively (Figure 18.6A, B, C).

Diabetes insipidus: DI is one of the most common complications arising from surgical treatment of craniopharyngiomas, with some series reporting post-operative rates as high as 100% (Kalapurakal et al., 2003; Mottolese et al., 2005). Surprisingly, however, Honegger et al. reported that only 4.9% of patients with craniopharyngiomas sought medical attention for DI as the presenting complaint (Honegger et al., 1999). Following endocrine evaluation, the same authors reported a 16.1% incidence of pre-operative DI, indicating that many cases of DI go unrecognized by both patients and physicians.

The reported incidences of post-operative DI in major surgical series for craniopharyngioma range from "rare", or 4%, to 100% (Fatemi et al., 2009; Elliott et al., 2011;

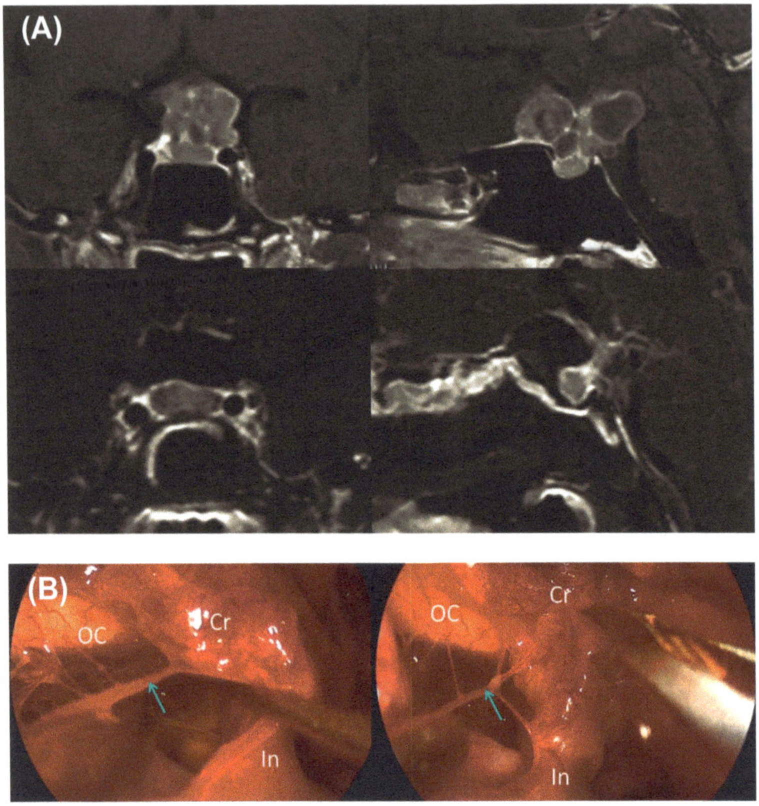

FIGURE 18.6 **A,** Pre-operative (top row) and Day 1 post-operative MRI (T1 post-gadolinium images) of suprasellar pre- and post-chaismatic craniopharyngioma in a 33-year-old woman with normal pituitary hormonal function who desired preservation of gland function. **B,** Intra-operative endonasal endoscopic view of infundibulum (In) engulfed by craniopharyngioma (Cr) necessitating subtotal removal. OC – optic chisam; right superior hypophyseal artery (blue arrow).

Komotar et al., 2012). This variability is, in part, due to the lack of a defined time-period for persistent post-operative DI. As with visual outcomes, there appears to be a significant trend toward a lower incidence of DI in transsphenoidal (36%) as compared to transcranial (69%) cases (Elliott et al., 2010; Komotar et al., 2012). The underlying explanation may lie in the improved visualization of the pituitary gland and stalk that allows a more controlled and sharp dissection of the tumor from the stalk. Moreover, anatomical differences may be partially responsible, given the more distal involvement of the stalk in intrasellar tumors (trend toward transsphenoidal approach) compared with primarily suprasellar tumors (trend toward transcranial approach) that intimately involve the tuber cinereum and proximal infundibulum (Elliott et al., 2011). In their meta-analysis, Komotar et al. reported rates of permanent DI of 54.8% in transcranial series, 31.7% in microscopic transsphenoidal series, and 27.7% in endoscopic transsphenoidal series (Komotar et al., 2012). In contrast to these data, however, other authors have reported similar rates of new post-operative DI in transcranial (66.3%) and transsphenoidal (68.6%) groups (Honegger et al., 1999). In their transcranial series, Honegger et al. reported no difference in endocrine results between the group of patients in whom the pituitary stalk was identified and preserved intraoperatively and the group in whom the stalk was not identified during transsphenoidal surgery. In transsphenoidal cases, the results were more favorable when the pituitary stalk was not identified, with new DI observed in 90.9% of cases where the stalk was identified and "preserved", compared to 56.5% in cases where the stalk was not identified (Honegger et al., 1999). This is likely due to the fact that removal of tumor adherent to the infundibulum requires identification, manipulation, and dissection of the stalk, placing this structure at greater functional risk post-operatively. Whereas, when the tumor either does not involve the infundibulm or attempts are not made at tumor resection from this region, post-operative DI is less likely.

Based upon their observations and review of the literature, Elliott et al. concluded that, given the high rates of DI with radical resection, regardless of pituitary stalk integrity, that attempted stalk preservation should not preclude GTR (Elliott et al., 2011). Long-term management of post-operative DI does not appear to have a negative impact on overall survival or quality of life.

Anterior pituitary dysfunction: Craniopharyngiomas typically arise from the corridor along the floor of the third ventricle and infundibulum toward the sella. As a result, the adenohypophysis is often found inferior and anterior to the tumor. This has been reported in as many as 50–60% of cases (Maira et al., 1995; Fahlbusch et al., 1999; Fatemi et al., 2009). In order to gain sufficient access to a dorsally located tumor through a transsphenoidal approach, various authors have reported the successful mobilization of the gland using a vertical incision, with a low incidence of post-operative iatrogenic hypopituitarism (Maira et al., 1995; Fahlbusch et al., 1999; Honegger et al., 1999).

As with DI, rates of post-operative adenohypophyseal dysfunction vary widely among surgical series, depending on the approach chosen and the goals of resection. In a series of 143 adult and pediatric craniopharyngioma patients, Honegger et al. reported that symptoms related to endocrine deficiency prompted medical consultation in 28.7% of patients (Honegger et al., 1999). Pre-operatively, delayed puberty and growth retardation dominated among presenting endocrinological symptoms. On pre-operative endocrine evaluation, the rates of secondary hypogonadism, secondary adrenal insufficiency, and secondary hypothyroidism were 77.4%, 31.5%, and 24.5% of patients, respectively. Hyperprolactinemia was found in 41.3% of patients at initial presentation in that series. Overall, only 16.1% of 124 patients presented with completely normal pituitary function, prior to surgery (Honegger et al., 1999).

Most transsphenoidal series reported new anterior pituitary dysfunction in approximately one third of patients (Elliott et al., 2010). By comparison, average rates approach 50% in transcranial series. However, Komotar et al. report rates of new hypopituitarism from their meta-analysis as 48.1% in transcranial series and 47.1% in endoscopic transsphenoidal series. In general, new anterior gland failure is seen less frequently than DI. Deterioration of an endocrine axis that was partially deficient pre-operatively is relatively common, and recovery of pre-operative anterior pituitary deficits is relatively rare. In their series of 124 patients with careful endocrine evaluation and follow-up, Honegger et al. compared rates in transsphenoidal and transcranial patients with new post-operative adrenal insufficiency (2.9% vs. 35.9%), hypothyroidism (5.7% vs. 20%), and hypogonadism (3.3% vs. 2.6%). The same authors report a significantly higher rate of new panhypopituitarism in transcranial patients (23.9%) compared to transsphenoidal patients (2.9%) (Honegger et al., 1999). A comparison of pre-operative and post-operative endocrine function in transsphenoidal and transcranial patients is summarized in Table 18.2. Other series have compared endocrinological outcomes in transcranial and transsphenoidal approaches. Chakrabarti et al. compared the endocrinological outcomes of patients who underwent transsphenoidal or transcranial resection of their craniopharyngiomas. They reported higher rates of new post-operative growth hormone deficiency (57% vs. 22%), hypothyroidism (79% vs. 22%), and adrenal insufficiency (53% vs. 17%) in the transcranial group (Chakrabarti et al., 2005). As with visual complications, there is also a trend towards a higher rate of new endocrine dysfunction in patients undergoing more aggressive surgery.

Hypothalamic injury: Beyond regulating adenohypophyseal and neurohypophyseal functions, the medial region of the hypothalamus is responsible for thermoregulation, hunger and satiety, circadian rhythm, and some aspects of behavior and memory. As many craniopharyngiomas extend into the suprasellar space and floor of the third ventricle, these structures are subject to direct injury during attempted resection. Injury to the ventromedial nucleus can result in obesity and hyperphagia, particularly in children. Injury to the dorsomedial nucleus can result in sham rage, whereas lesions to the anterior hypothalamic nucleus can result in difficulty with thermoregulation (Hardy, 2002). The supraoptic and paraventricular nuclei contribute to vasopressin synthesis. When injured, osmoregulation can occur, particularly adipsic diabetes insipidus. This condition results in polyuria without increased thirst and can be very difficult to manage (Crowley, 2007). If the posterior nucleus and mammillary bodies are injured, poikilothermia and memory problems can occur, respectively. These behavioral and homeostatic complications have been described in many surgical series of craniopharyngiomas in both adults and children (Yasargil et al., 1990; Elliott et al., 2010, 2011; Komotar et al., 2012).

Of these behavioral complications, hyperphagia and obesity have the largest propensity to affect quality of life. The reported ranges of post-operative obesity range from 0–70% (Elliott et al., 2011; Park et al., 2013). Obesity rates in children with craniopharyngiomas vary from 6–30% at diagnosis and increase to 40–60% after surgery (Park et al., 2013). When comparing transcranial and transsphenoidal series by meta-analysis, obesity rates are very similar, averaging 32.2% and 32.1%, respectively (Elliott et al., 2011).

Some authors have identified pre-operative risk factors that can predict hypothalamic morbidity and serve as a guide to limit aggressive resection. Puget et al. advocated an MRI-based grading scale that evaluated hypothalamic involvement by the tumor in pediatric patients, and recommend stratifying treatment strategy accordingly (Puget et al., 2007). Similarly, De Vile et al. reported a vertical tumor height of 3.5 cm, the presence of pre-operative hypothalamic disturbance, and intra-operative adherence of the tumor to the floor of the third ventricle to be predictive of hypothalamic morbidity in pediatric patients (De Vile et al., 1996; Elliott et al., 2011). They recommend limited resection plus radiation in those instances. Other authors have reported higher rates of obesity and hyperphagia with suprasellar tumors (Gonc et al., 2004; Lee et al., 2008). Based upon their own observations and those of other centers, Elliott et al. conclude that tumor location at presentation was the largest predictor of hypothalamic morbidity both before and after surgery, and that injury to the hypothalamus is more likely a consequence of involvement of the tumor with the walls of the third ventricle,

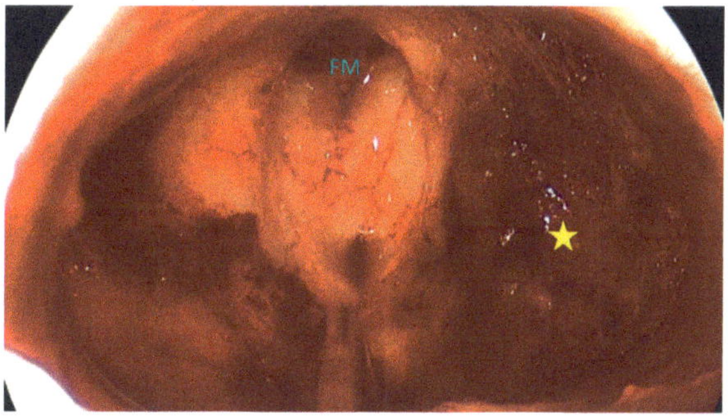

FIGURE 18.7 Intra-operative endonasal 0-degree endoscopic view into retro-chiasmal space and third ventricle after near-complete tumor removal with residual rind of craniopharyngioma adherent to left hypothalamic wall (star). FM – foramina of Monro.

rather than being dependent on the approach chosen (Elliott et al., 2011). In a univariate regression analysis, Park et al. reported that pre-operative and post-operative hypothalamic involvement as well as pre-operative body mass index Z-scores predicted post-operative hyperphagia and obesity (Park et al., 2013). Furthermore, their data indicated that obesity outcomes were unaffected by gender, age at diagnosis, gross total removal, pituitary stalk preservation, tumor recurrence, reoperations, radiotherapy, and the number of hormone deficiencies (among ACTH, TSH, GH) or DI.

Hypothalamic morbid obesity is poorly responsive to diet, physical activity, and most pharmacological therapies (Lee and Korner, 2009). Accordingly, recognition of hyperphagia, leading to early prophylactic and therapeutic interventions is recommended during the critical period of rapid weight gain. According to Park et al., the first post-operative year was the critical period for rapid increase in BMI, and most patients with craniopharyngioma experience a major increase in weight and BMI during the early post-operative period (Park et al., 2013). Peri-operative dexamethasone administration and GH deficiency may exacerbate post-operative weight gain (Muller et al., 2003). The effects of the hyperphagia can be so severe that some authors have advocated bariatric surgical procedures to help with long-term weight management. Bretault et al. performed a meta-analysis that demonstrated the efficacy of gastric bypass or banding in treating obesity in craniopharyngioma patients, with a mean weight loss of 20.9 kg after 6 months (Bretault et al., 2013).

As indicated with other causes of morbidity, surgical strategies to preserve hypothalamic integrity by experienced surgeons are mandatory for the prevention of severe obesity caused by craniopharyngiomas and treatment should be confined to experienced multidisciplinary teams. In many, if not most, large retro-chiasmal craniopharyngiomas, tumor compression of the walls of the hypothalamus is common. Over-aggressive attempts to remove such tumors that are densely adherent to the hypothalamus carry high risk of long-term hypothalamic dysfunction. Leaving a rind of tumor along the hypothalamus may be the best compromise to avoid this serious and debilitating complication (Figure 18.7). In addition, early changes to lifestyle should be emphasized during the early post-operative period, especially in patients with greater hypothalamic damage (Figure 18.8) (Muller et al., 2001; Park et al., 2013).

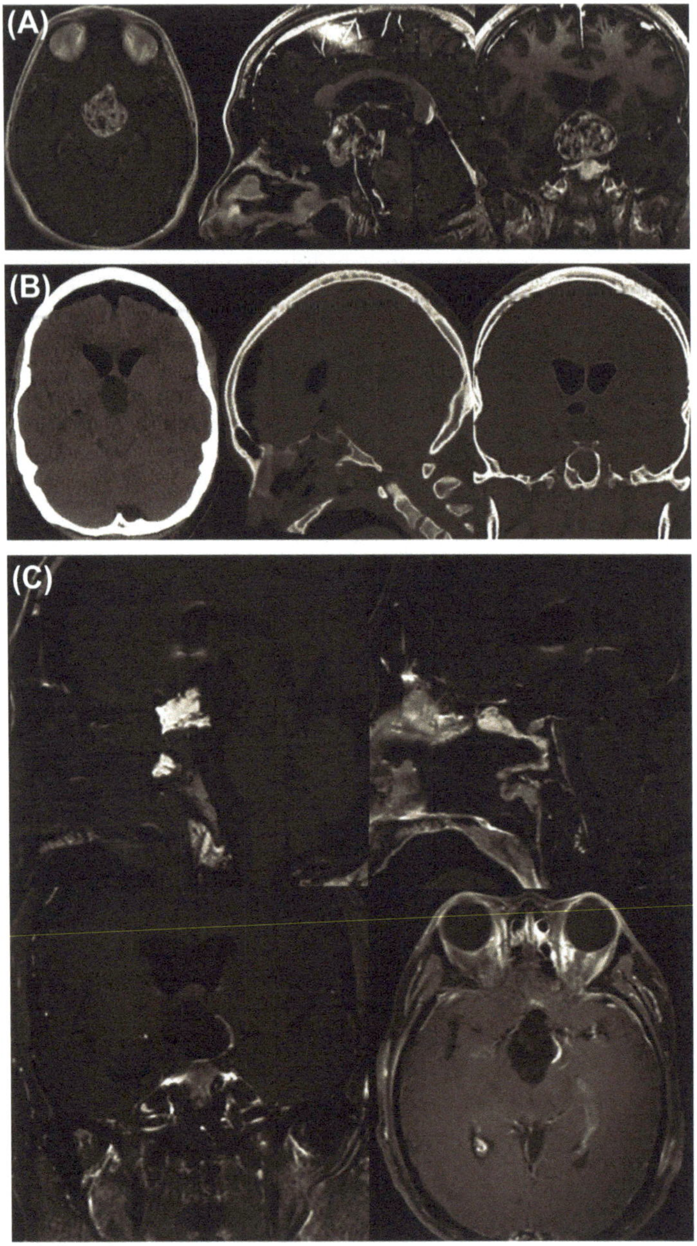

FIGURE 18.8 Pre-operative MRI (**A**), immediate post-operative CT (**B**) with sagittal and coronal reconstructions after and post-operative day 1 MRI after endonasal endoscopic near-complete removal of retro-chiasmal craniopharyngioma. The immediate post-operative CT provides a baseline view of skull base reconstruction with fat graft, bone graft sellar buttress, quantifies degree of initial pneumocephalus and evaluates for possible early hemorrhage. The post-operative day 1 MRI (**C**) shows fat graft positioning (upper left image T1-weighted), enhancing naso-septal flap and minimal residual tumor along left hypothalamus.

APPROACH-SPECIFIC COMPLICATIONS

CSF Leak and Meningitis

Although post-operative cerebrospinal fluid (CSF) leaks can occur after transcranial approaches for craniopharyngiomas, this complication is more frequently observed as a complication in transsphenoidal series. In a meta-analysis by Komotar et al., the reported incidences of post-operative CSF leak after operations for craniopharyngioma were 2.6% for open transcranial, 9.0% for transsphenoidal microscopic and 18.4% for endoscopic transsphenoidal (Komotar et al., 2012). By comparison, Elliott et al. reported a CSF leak rate of 9.4% after endoscopic transsphenoidal cases, but CSF leak was not included as a complication after transcranial cases (Elliott et al., 2011). In a direct comparison of the endoscopic transsphenoidal approach and the supra-orbital transcranial approach, Fatemi et al. reported a higher rate of CSF leak in the transsphenoidal series (16% vs. 0%) (Fatemi et al., 2009). In fact, frequent post-operative CSF leaks have been considered as the major limitation of the transsphenoidal approach, with rates as high as 58% reported in some series (Gardner et al., 2008). However, as techniques have evolved, experienced teams have had significant success, both in reducing these rates and in managing the patients in whom leaks do occur. As experience has grown, reconstruction techniques have advanced over time; from simple bone and fascia overlays to sophisticated multilayer closure techniques with both inlay and overlay fascial or synthetic grafts, bony reconstruction, and pedicled rotational flaps. With these advances, more recent series have reported significantly lower rates of post-operative CSF leak, ranging from 0–4% (Jane et al., 2010; Komotar et al., 2012; Leng et al., 2012). In particular, the introduction of the nasoseptal flap has been instrumental in reducing rates of post-operative CSF leakage. For example, Koutourousiou et al. reported that the incidence of post-operative CSF leak decreased from 23.4% with standard reconstructive techniques to 10.6% with the pedicled nasoseptal flap (Koutourousiou et al., 2013). Additional therapies including post-operative acetazolamide or lumbar drain CSF diversion can decrease CSF pressure and allow the skull base reconstruction to solidify.

For the endonasal endoscopic approach described in Chapter 8, the use of a pedicled nasoseptal flap is strongly advocated for this problem. Eloy et al. demonstrated the efficacy of this technique in repairing post-operative leaks, with a 0% reoperation rate (Eloy et al., 2012).

Meningitis

Meningitis can occur as a complication of either transcranial or transsphenoidal surgery for craniopharyngioma. Both bacterial and chemical meningitis have been reported. Bacterial meningitis is observed more frequently and can present in a hyperacute, acute, subacute, or chronic fashion. Kotomar et al. reported bacterial meningitis rates of 2.3% for transcranial series and 5.1% for endoscopic transsphenoidal series, but the difference was not statistically significant (Komotar et al., 2012). Elliott et al. reported an overall incidence of meningitis of 2.9% in transsphenoidal series. Other transsphenoidal series have reported incidences of bacterial meningitis as high as 7.8% (Koutourousiou et al., 2013). In cases of suspected bacterial meningitis, a diagnostic lumbar puncture is performed and broad-spectrum empiric antibiotic coverage is initiated. Results of the CSF culture and sensitivity testing can help to tailor the antibiotic regimen. Although variable at some centers, duration of treatment is typically 3 weeks. Chemical meningitis is a rare phenomenon due to rupture of a craniopharyngioma cyst that develops because of presence of cholesterol crystals secreted by the squamous epithelium lining the cyst. Chemical meningitis should be considered as a possibility in the post-operative period after craniopharyngioma surgery. Once bacterial sources have been rules out, treatment is achieved with corticosteroids.

Seizures

Seizures have also been reported as a complication of craniopharyngioma surgery, typically following transcranial resection. The rate of post-operative seizures has been reported by several authors. On meta-analysis, the incidence of seizures after transcranial resection of craniopharyngioma was found to be 8.5%, whereas no seizures were reported in the transsphenoidal group (Komotar et al., 2012). Visser et al. reported seizures as a cause of late mortality in two pediatric craniopharyngioma patients (Visser et al., 2010). Although seizures can occur as a presenting symptom of craniopharyngioma, post-operative, iatrogenic seizures have not been reported after endoscopic transsphenoidal resection. In patients who do suffer from seizures, standard management involves treatment with anti-epileptic drugs such as levetiracetam or phenytoin.

Hydrocephalus

Because of their location of origin near the floor of the third ventricle, craniopharyniogmas have a propensity to cause hydrocephalus and increased intracranial pressure. Hydrocephalus can occur as a result of direct obstruction by the tumor or from breakdown products after surgical resection. The incidence of pre-operative hydrocephalus ranges from 5.1% to 41.7% (Elliott et al., 2011). Komotar et al. reported incidences of hydrocephalus of 10.1% and 15.8%, in transcranial and endoscopic transsphenoidal series, respectively. This difference was not statistically significant, however (Komotar et al., 2012). Treatment of hydrocephalus is with CSF diversion and, ultimately, shunting, as needed.

Transcranial resection of craniopharyngiomas is also subject to the same complications of wound infection and breakdown and bone flap infection as other craniotomies. Transsphenoidal resection is subject to sinonasal complications, such as sinusitis and chronic inflammation. A detailed discussion of these complications is beyond the scope of this chapter.

PERI-OPERATIVE MORTALITY

Fortunately, the mortality rate associated with craniopharyngioma surgery has decreased dramatically over the last 50 years. Initial attempts at resection were met with mortality rates as high as 41% in some series, prompting many surgeons to argue that the operative risks were prohibitive (Hoff and Patterson, 1972). With the introduction of steroid therapy in the 1950s, Matson and Crigler demonstrated the capacity to remove craniopharyngiomas safely and completely (Matson and Crigler, 1969). More recently, advances in technique and technology have allowed us to further reduce the mortality risk. Modern series of craniopharyngiomas report mortality rates from 1.7% to 5.4% (Hoff and Patterson, 1972; Honegger et al., 1999; Elliott et al., 2010; King, 2011; Mortini et al., 2011), although Yasargil et al. reported an operative mortality rate of 16.7% in a series of 144 patients (Yasargil et al., 1990).

Some authors have reported a lower mortality risk in transsphenoidal than in transcranial resection. A meta-analysis of 2955 pediatric patients treated with transcranial surgery yielded an operative mortality of 0–12% with an average of 2.6% (Elliott et al., 2011). By comparison, the same report yielded an overall mortality of 1.3% in patients undergoing endoscopic transsphenoidal resection (Elliott et al., 2011). Mortality is most often associated with infection, hypothalamic injury, vascular injury, or coexisting medical conditions. Some authors have reported an increased risk of mortality in patients undergoing reoperation as compared with primary operation. In a series of 121 patients, Karavitaki et al. found that the peri-operative mortality of the patients who had any type of neurosurgical intervention due to recurrence was higher than that observed after primary surgery (24% vs. 1.8%) (Karavitaki et al., 2005). Di Rocco also found significantly increased mortality during reoperation (11%) compared to initial operation (3.7%) (Di Rocco et al., 2006). However, other series have reported no differences (Elliott et al., 2010). Other factors associated with increased risk of mortality include larger tumor size, advanced or very young patient age, and medical comorbidities. In a series of 144 patients (adult and pediatric) Yasargil et al. (1990) observed an overall peri-operative mortality of 16.7%, and categorized peri-operative deaths into three categories: operative, early post-operative, and late post-operative. The rate of operative mortality (from hemorrhage) was found to be 2.1%. Early post-operative mortality (6.9%) resulted from infection, pulmonary emboli, pneumonia, and endocrinological complications, whereas late post-operative mortality (7.6%) resulted from either endocrinological or shunt-related complications. In that series, seven out of eight (87.5%) patients with giant tumors (> 6 cm) died peri-operatively; underscoring the risks of aggressive resection of giant tumors, even in experienced hands. Zhao found that peri-operative hyperpyrexia was the most significant risk factor for peri-operative mortality (Zhao et al., 2012).

Overall, for purposes of patient counseling, the rate of peri-operative mortality approaches 1–3%. In general, radical excision and larger tumors have been associated with higher mortality, and there is a trend toward lower mortality in patients undergoing transsphenoidal as compared to transcranial resection. Tables 18.1 and 18.2 provide a summary comparison of morbidity and mortality data from major transcranial and transsphenoidal series of craniopharyngiomas (Table 18.3).

TABLE 18.1 Summarizes Operative Comparison from the Meta-Analysis Performed by Elliott et al., Comparing Transsphenoidal and Transcranial Series of Pediatric Craniopharyngiomas (Elliott et al., 2011)

	Transcranial series % (number)	**Transsphenoidal series % (number)**	***P* Value**
Operative mortality	2.6 (68 of 2622)	1.3 (5 of 373)	.21
Neurological morbidity	9.4 (200 of 2140)	3.1 (10 of 325)	.001
Diabetes insipidus	69.1 (1437 of 2076)	23.9 (76 of 318)	.001
Vision improvement	47.7 (454 of 1051)	85.5 (106 of 124)	.001
Vision deterioration	13 (263 of 2029)	2.3 (8 of 352)	.001
Obesity or hyperphagia	32.2 (439 of 1363)	32.1 (35 of 109)	1.00

TABLE 18.2 Summarizes Operative Outcomes from the Meta-Analysis Performed by Komotar et al., Comparing Open Transcranial, Microscopic Transsphenoidal and Endoscopic Transsphenoidal Series of Adult and Pediatric Craniopharyngiomas (Komotar et al., 2012)

	Open transcranial		Microscopic transsphenoidal		Endoscopic transsphenoidal	
Complication	**Occurrence/ Total patients**	**Percentage**	**Occurrence/ Total patients**	**Percentage**	**Occurrence/ Total patients**	**Percentage**
Visual outcome						
Improved	410/1238	33.1%	107/243	44%	68/121	56.2%
Stable	461/1241	37.1%	32/208	15.4%	13/121	10.7%
Deteriorated	199/1758	11.3%	8/151	5.3%	2/121	1.7%
Complications						
Permanent DI	925/1689	54.8%	88/278	31.7%	13/47	27.7%
Hypopituitarism	396/823	48.1%	10/78	12.8%	16/34	47.1%
CSF leak	15/582	2.2%	22/245	9%	25/136	18.4%
Meningitis	10/430	2.3%	3/170	1.8%	5/98	5.1%
Seizure	51/600	8.5%	0/380	0	0/183	0
Hydrocephalus	20/198	10.1%	0/1	0	3/19	15.8%
Stroke	21/723	2.9%	0/1	0	1/37	2.7%
Wound infection	5/232	2.2%	0	0	0	0
Mortality	39/1221	3.2%	2/60	3.3%	1/54	1.9%

TABLE 18.3 Endocrine Outcomes in Patients Undergoing Transcranial vs. Transsphenoidal Resection of Craniopharyngiomas from (Honegger et al. 1999)

	Transsphenoidal		Transcranial	
Condition	**Preop**	**Postop**	**Preop**	**Postop**
Adrenal insufficiency	60%	62.9%	22.8%	58.7%
Hypothyroidism	45.7%	51.4%	18.5%	38.0%
Hypogonadism	90.0%	93.3%	75.9%	78.5%
Hyperprolactinemia	54.3%	8.6%	39.1%	39.1%

CONCLUSIONS – PRIMUM NON NOCERE

Surgical resection of craniopharyngiomas amidst the confines of the optic apparatus, circle of Willis, hypothalamus, and brainstem presents a technical challenge even to experienced surgeons. Overall, thanks to advances in technique and technology, surgical morbidity and mortality have significantly decreased in recent years. In part, this can be attributed to the recognition that in many cases, the aggressive approach of ensuring a gross total resection has been replaced with a more judicious and conservative resection. While complete resection should always be considered, our combined experience suggests that it may be preferable to leave a small residua rather than risk significant visual, hypothalamic, or vascular morbidity. As experience with the endoscope continues to grow, many of the advantages of this approach may become even more apparent. Regardless of the approach, it is recommended that larger, complex craniopharyngiomas be referred to experienced, multidisciplinary teams in order to achieve the best possible outcome with the lowest risk of harm to the patient.

References

Abuzayed, B., Tanriover, N., Akar, Z., Eraslan, B.S., Gazioglu, N., 2010. Extended endoscopic endonasal approach to the suprasellar parachiasmatic cisterns: anatomic study. Childs Nerv. Syst. 26, 1161–1170.

Blunt, M.J., Steele, E.J., 1956. The blood supply of the optic nerve and chiasma in man. J. Anat. 90, 486–493.

Bretault, M., Boillot, A., Muzard, L., Poitou, C., Oppert, J.M., Barsamian, C., Gatta, B., Muller, H., Weismann, D., Rottembourg, D., Inge, T., Veyrie, N., Carette, C., Czernichow, S., 2013. Clinical review: Bariatric surgery following treatment for craniopharyngioma: a systematic review and individual-level data meta-analysis. J. Clin. Endocrinol. Metab. 98, 2239–2246.

Chakrabarti, I., Amar, A.P., Couldwell, W., Weiss, M.H., 2005. Long-term neurological, visual, and endocrine outcomes following transnasal resection of craniopharyngioma. J. Neurosurg. 102, 650–657.

Crowley, R.K., Sherlock, M., Agha, A., Smith, D., Thompson, C.J., 2007. Clinical insignts into adipsic diabetes insipidus: a large case series. Clin. Endocrinol. (Oxf) 66, 475–482.

De Vile, C.J., Grant, D.B., Kendall, B.E., Neville, B.G., Stanhope, R., Watkins, K.E., Hayward, R.D., 1996. Management of childhood craniopharyngioma: can the morbidity of radical surgery be predicted? J. Neurosurg. 85, 73–81.

Deshaies, E.M., Boulos, A.S., Popp, A.J., 2009. Peri-operative medical management of cerebral vasospasm. Neurol. Res. 31, 644–650.

Di Rocco, C., Caldarelli, M., Tamburrini, G., Massimi, L., 2006. Surgical management of craniopharyngiomas – experience with a pediatric series. J. Pediatr. Endocrinol. Metab. 19 (Suppl. 1), 355–366.

Duff, J., Meyer, F.B., Ilstrup, D.M., Laws Jr., E.R., Schleck, C.D., Scheithauer, B.W., 2000. Long-term outcomes for surgically resected craniopharyngiomas. Neurosurgery 46, 291–302 discussion 302–305.

Dusick, J.R., Esposito, F., Malkasian, D., Kelly, D.F., 2007. Avoidance of carotid artery injuries in transsphenoidal surgery with the Doppler probe and micro-hook blades. Neurosurgery 60, 322–328 discussion 328–329.

Elliott, R.E., Hsieh, K., Hochm, T., Belitskaya-Levy, I., Wisoff, J., Wisoff, J.H., 2010. Efficacy and safety of radical resection of primary and recurrent craniopharyngiomas in 86 children. J. Neurosurg. Pediatr. 5, 30–48.

Elliott, R.E., Jane Jr., J.A., Wisoff, J.H., 2011. Surgical management of craniopharyngiomas in children: meta-analysis and comparison of transcranial and transsphenoidal approaches. Neurosurgery 69, 630–643 discussion 643.

Eloy, J.A., Kuperan, A.B., Choudhry, O.J., Harirchian, S., Liu, J.K., 2012. Efficacy of the pedicled nasoseptal flap without cerebrospinal fluid (CSF) diversion for repair of skull base defects: incidence of postoperative CSF leaks. Int. Forum. Allergy. Rhinol. 2, 397–401.

Erdheim, J., 1904. Uber hypophysenganggeschwwuste und hirncholesteatome, Gerold.

Fahlbusch, R., Honegger, J., Paulus, W., Huk, W., Buchfelder, M., 1999. Surgical treatment of craniopharyngiomas: experience with 168 patients. J. Neurosurg. 90, 237–250.

Fatemi, N., Dusick, J.R., De Paiva Neto, M.A., Malkasian, D., Kelly, D.F., 2009. Endonasal versus supraorbital keyhole removal of craniopharyngiomas and tuberculum sellae meningiomas. Neurosurgery 64, 269–284, discussion 284–286.

Fernandez-Miranda, J.C., Gardner, P.A., Snyderman, C.H., Devaney, K.O., Strojan, P., Suarez, C., Genden, E.M., Rinaldo, A., Ferlito, A., 2012. Craniopharyngioma: a pathologic, clinical, and surgical review. Head Neck 34, 1036–1044.

Fischer, E.G., Welch, K., Shillito Jr, J., Winston, K.R., Tarbell, N.J., 1990. Craniopharyngiomas in children: long term effects of conservative surgical procedures combined with radiation therapy. J. Neurosurg. 73, 534–540.

Gardner, P.A., Kassam, A.B., Snyderman, C.H., Carrau, R.L., Mintz, A.H., Grahovac, S., Stefko, S., 2008. Outcomes following endoscopic, expanded endonasal resection of suprasellar craniopharyngiomas: a case series. J. Neurosurg. 109, 6–16.

Gonc, E.N., Yordam, N., Ozon, A., Alikasifoglu, A., Kandemir, N., 2004. Endocrinological outcome of different treatment options in children with craniopharyngioma: a retrospective analysis of 66 cases. Pediatr. Neurosurg. 40, 112–119.

Halstead, A.E., 1910. Remarks on the operative treatment of tumors of the hypophysis. Trans. Am. Surg. Assoc. 28, 73–93.

Hardy, S.G.P., Chronister, R.B., Parent, A.D., 2002. The Hypothalamus. In: Haines, D.E. (Ed.), Fundamental Neuroscience, Second. ed. Churchill Livingstone, Philadelphia, Pennsylvania.

Hoff, J.T., Patterson Jr., R.H., 1972. Craniopharyngiomas in children and adults. J. Neurosurg. 36, 299–302.

Honegger, J., Buchfelder, M., Fahlbusch, R., 1999. Surgical treatment of craniopharyngiomas: endocrinological results. J. Neurosurg. 90, 251–257.

Jane Jr., J.A., Kiehna, E., Payne, S.C., Early, S.V., Laws Jr., E.R., 2010. Early outcomes of endoscopic transsphenoidal surgery for adult craniopharyngiomas. Neurosurg. Focus 28, E9.

Kalapurakal, J.A., Goldman, S., Hsieh, Y.C., Tomita, T., Marymont, M.H., 2003. Clinical outcome in children with craniopharyngioma treated with primary surgery and radiotherapy deferred until relapse. Med. Pediatr. Oncol. 40, 214–218.

Karavitaki, N., Brufani, C., Warner, J.T., Adams, C.B., Richards, P., Ansorge, O., Shine, B., Turner, H.E., Wass, J.A., 2005. Craniopharyngiomas in children and adults: systematic analysis of 121 cases with long-term follow-up. Clin. Endocrinol. (Oxf) 62, 397–409.

Kassam, A.B., Gardner, P.A., Snyderman, C.H., Carrau, R.L., Mintz, A.H., Prevedello, D.M., 2008. Expanded endonasal approach, a fully endoscopic transnasal approach for the resection of midline suprasellar craniopharyngiomas: a new classification based on the infundibulum. J. Neurosurg. 108, 715–728.

King, J.A.F., Mehta, V., Black, P.M., 2011. Craniopharyngioma. In: Winn, H.R. (Ed.), Youman's Neurological Surgery, Sixth. ed. Elsevier, Philadelphia, Pennsylvania.

Komotar, R.J., Starke, R.M., Raper, D.M., Anand, V.K., Schwartz, T.H., 2012. Endoscopic endonasal compared with microscopic transsphenoidal and open transcranial resection of craniopharyngiomas. World Neurosurg. 77, 329–341.

Koutourousiou, M., Gardner, P.A., Fernandez-Miranda, J.C., Tyler-Kabara, E.C., Wang, E.W., Snyderman, C.H., 2013. Endoscopic endonasal surgery for craniopharyngiomas: surgical outcome in 64 patients. J. Neurosurg 119 (5), 1194–1207.

Laws Jr., E.R., Trautmann, J.C., Hollenhorst Jr., R.W., 1977. Transsphenoidal decompression of the optic nerve and chiasm. Visual results in 62 patients. J. Neurosurg. 46, 717–722.

Lee, M., Korner, J., 2009. Review of physiology, clinical manifestations, and management of hypothalamic obesity in humans. Pituitary 12, 87–95.

Lee, Y.Y., Wong, T.T., Fang, Y.T., Chang, K.P., Chen, Y.W., Niu, D.M., 2008. Comparison of hypothalamopituitary axis dysfunction of intrasellar and third ventricular craniopharyngiomas in children. Brain Dev. 30, 189–194.

Leng, L.Z., Greenfield, J.P., Souweidane, M.M., Anand, V.K., Schwartz, T.H., 2012. Endoscopic, endonasal resection of craniopharyngiomas: analysis of outcome including extent of resection, cerebrospinal fluid leak, return to preoperative productivity, and body mass index. Neurosurgery 70, 110–123 discussion 123–124.

Macdonald, R.L., Hoffman, H.J., 1997. Subarachnoid hemorrhage and vasospasm following removal of craniopharyngioma. J. Clin. Neurosci. 4, 348–352.

Maira, G., Anile, C., Rossi, G.F., Colosimo, C., 1995. Surgical treatment of craniopharyngiomas: an evaluation of the transsphenoidal and pterional approaches. Neurosurgery 36, 715–724.

Matson, D.D., Crigler Jr., J.F., 1969. Management of craniopharyngioma in childhood. J. Neurosurg. 30, 377–390.

Mclaughlin, N., Laws, E.R., Oyesiku, N.M., Katznelson, L., Kelly, D.F., 2012. Pituitary centers of excellence. Neurosurgery 71, 916–924 discussion 924–926.

Mortini, P., Losa, M., Pozzobon, G., Barzaghi, R., Riva, M., Acerno, S., Angius, D., Weber, G., Chiumello, G., Giovanelli, M., 2011. Neurosurgical treatment of craniopharyngioma in adults and children: early and long-term results in a large case series. J. Neurosurg. 114, 1350–1359.

Mottolese, C., Szathmari, A., Berlier, P., Hermier, M., 2005. Craniopharyngiomas: our experience in Lyon. Childs Nerv. Syst. 21, 790–798.

Muller, H.L., Bueb, K., Bartels, U., Roth, C., Harz, K., Graf, N., Korinthenberg, R., Bettendorf, M., Kuhl, J., Gutjahr, P., Sorensen, N., Calaminus, G., 2001. Obesity after childhood craniopharyngioma–German multicenter study on pre-operative risk factors and quality of life. Klin. Padiatr. 213, 244–249.

Muller, H.L., Heinrich, M., Bueb, K., Etavard-Gorris, N., Gebhardt, U., Kolb, R., Sorensen, N., 2003. Peri-operative dexamethasone treatment in childhood craniopharyngioma – influence on short-term and long-term weight gain. Exp. Clin. Endocrinol. Diabetes 111, 330–334.

Paja, M., Lucas, T., Garcia-Uria, J., Salame, F., Barcelo, B., Estrada, J., 1995. Hypothalamic-pituitary dysfunction in patients with craniopharyngioma. Clin. Endocrinol. (Oxf) 42, 467–473.

Park, S.W., Jung, H.W., Lee, Y.A., Shin, C.H., Yang, S.W., Cheon, J.E., Kim, I.O., Phi, J.H., Kim, S.K., Wang, K.C., 2013. Tumor origin and growth pattern at diagnosis and surgical hypothalamic damage predict obesity in pediatric craniopharyngioma. J. Neurooncol. 113, 417–424.

Puget, S., Garnett, M., Wray, A., Grill, J., Habrand, J.L., Bodaert, N., Zerah, M., Bezerra, M., Renier, D., Pierre-Kahn, A., Sainte-Rose, C., 2007. Pediatric craniopharyngiomas: classification and treatment according to the degree of hypothalamic involvement. J. Neurosurg. 106, 3–12.

Salunke, P., Sodhi, H.B., Aggarwal, A., Ahuja, C.K., 2013. Delayed cerebral vasospasm following surgery for craniopharyngioma. J. Neurosci. Rural. Pract. 4, 107–109.

Shi, X., Wang, Z., 2001. Experience in surgical treatment of 110 patients with craniopharyngiomas. Zhonghua Wai Ke Za Zhi 39, 608–610.

Sklar, C.A., 1994. Craniopharyngioma: endocrine abnormalities at presentation. Pediatr. Neurosurg. 21 (Suppl. 1), 18–20.

Sughrue, M.E., Yang, I., Kane, A.J., Fang, S., Clark, A.J., Aranda, D., Barani, I.J., Parsa, A.T., 2011. Endocrinologic, neurologic, and visual morbidity after treatment for craniopharyngioma. J. Neurooncol. 101, 463–476.

Sutton, L.N., 1994. Vascular complications of surgery for craniopharyngioma and hypothalamic glioma. Pediatr. Neurosurg. 21 (Suppl. 1), 124–128.

Visser, J., Hukin, J., Sargent, M., Steinbok, P., Goddard, K., Fryer, C., 2010. Late mortality in pediatric patients with craniopharyngioma. J. Neurooncol. 100, 105–111.

Yasargil, M.G., Curcic, M., Kis, M., Siegenthaler, G., Teddy, P.J., Roth, P., 1990. Total removal of craniopharyngiomas. Approaches and long-term results in 144 patients. J. Neurosurg. 73, 3–11.

Zhao, X., Yi, X., Wang, H., Zhao, H., 2012. An analysis of related factors of surgical results for patients with craniopharyngiomas. Clin. Neurol. Neurosurg. 114, 149–155.

SECTION IV

RADIOTHERAPY

CHAPTER

19

Radiotherapy and Radiosurgery for Craniopharyngiomas

Cheng-Chia Lee, Dale Ding, Jason P. Sheehan

Lars Leksell Gamma Knife Center, Department of Neurological Surgery, University of Virginia Health System, Charlottesville, VA, USA

"Precisely as for all other intracranial tumors, there is but one treatment for hypophyseal tumors. Recourse to radium and x-ray treatments has, in my experience, been entirely futile." **Walter Dandy, 1945**

OVERVIEW

Craniopharyngiomas are benign parasellar tumors that arise from residual epithelial cells of Rathke's pouch. They are characterized by a propensity to involve and densely adhere to surrounding vital neural and vascular structures (Karavitaki and Wass, 2008; Lindholm and Nielsen, 2009). Although the mainstay therapeutic approach is surgical gross tumor resection (GTR), the intimate association of the tumor with surrounding neurovascular structures can make resection challenging. Even though advances in microsurgical and endoscopic techniques have improved surgical outcomes, specifically increased rates of GTR and improved success of repeat resection, the current rates of operative morbidity and mortality continue to pose formidable challenges to long-term remission of craniopharyngiomas (Adler Jr. et al., 2006; Jang et al., 2009; Komotar et al., 2009; Campbell et al., 2010). Therefore, adjuvant therapies such as radiation therapy have been considered since as early as 1904 (Lindholm and Nielsen, 2009).

The concept of using radiation to treat craniopharyngiomas arose from experience with treating acromegaly (Lindholm and Nielsen, 2009). The procedure, described by Gramegna, would deliver a total of 200 roentgens to the sella over a period of one month with sessions lasting one hour twice per week. On the other hand, Belere introduced the idea of rotating the patient so that "the hypophysis was treated by cross-fire through four or five different areas on the fronto-temporal region" (Beclere, 1909; Gramegna, 1909). The first systematic report on radiotherapy of a craniopharyngioma was published in 1937 (Carpenter and Frazier, 1937). The results were unsatisfactory, and the authors concluded that the hypophyseal stalk tumors may be resistant to radiation therapy (Carpenter and Frazier, 1937).

Craniopharyngiomas
http://dx.doi.org/10.1016/B978-0-12-416706-3.00019-2

TABLE 19.1 Comparison of Several Radiation Facilities Used For the Treatment of Craniopharyngioma

Radiation facilities	Source	Immobilization	Fractionation
Conventional radiotherapy	X-rays (LINAC)	Mask	Multiple (25–30)
Intensity modulated RT (IMRT)	X-rays (LINAC)	Mask	Multiple (25–30)
Stereotactic radiosurgery (SRS)/fractionated stereotactic radiotherapy (FSRT)			
Gamma-Knife	Gamma-rays (^{60}Co)	Stereotactic fixed frame or relocatable frame	1 fraction *
Cyberknife	X-rays (compact linac)	Mask	1–5 fractions
LINAC-based	X-rays (LINAC)	Stereotactic fixed frame, relocatable frame, or mask	1–5 fractions
Proton beam			
Proton radiosurgery	Proton beam (Cyclotron)	Stereotactic fixed frame or mask	1–5 fractions
Proton radiotherapy	Proton beam (Cyclotron)	Mask	Multiple (25–30)

** Most GKS was performed with single fraction, however, hypofractionated GKS (3–5 fractions) can be performed by the newly released Extend system®.*

With advances in neuroimaging and radiotherapy systems, the dose delivery is more accurate and focused, resulting in decreasing complication rates over time. Radiation treatment options for craniopharyngiomas include conventional external beam radiation therapy (RT), intensity-modulated radiation therapy (IMRT), single fraction stereotactic radiosurgery (SRS) (e.g., Gamma Knife), fractionated stereotactic radiotherapy (FSRT), and proton beam radiotherapy (Table 19.1). In this chapter, we introduce the different modalities and compare their outcomes, including complications and prognostic factors for craniopharyngioma treatment.

GENERAL CONSIDERATIONS

Radiation biology allows one to decipher the relationship between a delivered radiation dose and the consequent biological response. In most cases, both favorable and unfavorable radiation-induced effects are intimately related. Such dose–response curves have a sigmoid shape, with the incidence of radiation effects approaching zero at lower doses and the incidence of radiation effects approaching 100% at higher doses. The ratio of tumor response to normal tissue damage is defined as the therapeutic ratio or therapeutic index. The therapeutic index may be manipulated by varying the dose and fractionation scheme or by using medications that preferentially increase tumor response. After radiation delivery, most tumor cells die a mitotic death: that is, they die in attempting the next or a subsequent mitosis. In some tissues, tumor cells die by apoptosis: that is, programmed cell death.

The biological effect of radiation on cells may be summarized by the "4 R's":

- Repair of sublethal damage
- Reassortment of cells within the cell cycle
- Repopulation
- Re-oxygenation.

Based on the tissue responses of radiation initially described in animal models, dividing a dose into several fractions relatively spares normal tissue due to repair of sublethal damage and cellular repopulation between dose fractions. In contrast, dose fractionation increases damage to tumor tissues secondary to re-oxygenation and reassortment of cells into varying radiosensitive phases of the cycle between dose fractions. The advantages of treatment prolongation are sparing adverse injury to slowly dividing normal cells and maximizing toxicity to rapidly dividing tumor cells.

In the past, it was believed that dose fractionation resulted in better tumor control for a given level of normal tissue toxicity than a single, large dose. More recently, Leksell introduced the concept of stereotactic radiosurgery (SRS), specifically Gamma Knife radiosurgery (GKS). GKS delivers focused, high-dose radiation in a single fraction with a high therapeutic ratio which optimizes irradiation of the target while minimizing toxicity to surrounding normal tissue.

CONVENTIONAL RADIOTHERAPY

Large studies of conventional radiotherapy for craniopharyngiomas were not published until the 1960s. At the time, many neurosurgeons were reluctant to believe in the therapeutic benefits of radiation therapy for craniopharyngiomas, although the very first recorded case had tumor control for 2.5 years (Carpenter and Frazier, 1937). Love and Marshall introduced the policy of combining intentional subtotal resection with radiotherapy using a relatively high dose of radiation immediately following surgery. They recruited ten patients and reported promising results (Love, 1950). Subsequently, the use of fractionated radiotherapy became more routine in craniopharyngioma patients.

Indications

Currently, radiotherapy is used in instances when the risk of surgical complications is high (Yasargil et al., 1990; Hoffman et al., 1992; Fahlbusch et al., 1999; Minniti et al., 2009; Schoenfeld et al., 2011), or it is used following resection when residual or recurrent tumor is seen (Hetelekidis et al., 1993; Rajan et al., 1993; Habrand et al., 1999). Compared to SRS, radiotherapy is preferred for large tumors (typically greater than 3 cm in diameter or 15 cc in volume), cystic tumors, and tumors abutting radiation-sensitive structures such as the optic apparatus or hypothalamus.

Radiation Technique

Radiation delivery has evolved from 2-D to 3-D; 3-D conformal external beam radiotherapy is the current standard treatment that is comprised of photons delivered by a linear accelerator. Precise immobilization, accurate tumor neuroimaging, and computerized 3-D treatment planning are necessary. Immobilization is achieved by an individually molded thermoplastic mask with a relocation accuracy of 2–4 mm. A high-quality, contrast-enhanced magnetic resonance imaging (MRI) scan may be co-registered with a computed tomography (CT) planning scan performed with the mask on in the treatment position. The combination of macroscopically visible tumor on neuroimaging and presumed microscopic extension is defined as the gross tumor volume (GTV). An additional 3–5 mm margin is added to account for relocation accuracy in the mask and the technical uncertainties associated with target localization, computer planning, and treatment delivery. The GTV combined with the additional margin is defined as the planning target volume (PTV).

Radiation therapy is targeted to the tumor, encompassing all its components. A coronal arc configuration of treatment is recommended. The goal of 3-D conformal radiotherapy is to deliver the same dose (dose homogeneity to within 7% of the maximum dose) to the entire tumor. This is achieved with 3–4 equally spaced radiation beams that are shaped with multi-leaf collimators (MLCs). Computer planning determines the beam position that will achieve dose homogeneity within the PTV, and allows for optimum avoidance of surrounding critical neurovascular structures such as the optic apparatus, internal carotid arteries, hypothalamus, and pituitary stalk.

With advances in delivery devices, the relocation accuracy and intensity modulation of radiation have improved significantly. The GTV–PTV margin can be reduced with better immobilization, thereby exposing a smaller amount of normal tissue to high radiation doses. Intensity-modulated radiotherapy (IMRT) allows more individualized beam shaping, particularly for avoidance of normal structures within concave target volumes. However, there is no clear evidence that IMRT results in better treatment outcomes for craniopharyngiomas.

The optimal total dose and fractionation scheme for craniopharyngiomas has not been standardized. In general, the total dose is 50–60 Gy separated into 28–30 fractions. Regine et al. reported recurrence risks of 44% versus 16% using total doses less than or greater than a dose cut off of 54 Gy (Regine et al., 1993). In a series of 24 patients, Varlotto et al. did not note any treatment failures with a dose of at least 60 Gy (Varlotto et al., 2002), Habrand et al. demonstrated improved tumor control with a dose of at least 55 Gy (Habrand et al., 1999). There are several additional reports of 5-year tumor control rates of over 90% utilizing doses of 50–54 Gy in fractions of 1.7–1.8 Gy (Rajan et al., 1993; Merchant et al., 2002, 2006; Combs et al., 2007; Minniti et al., 2007). It is important to note that total doses over 60 Gy in 1.8–2 Gy fractions delivered to the optic apparatus may result in an unacceptably high risk of optic neuropathy and brain necrosis (Mayo et al., 2010).

Cystic craniopharyngiomas can be treated with stereotactic cyst aspiration of the cyst to decrease the PTV or stereotactically delivered, intracystic, colloidal yttrium-90 or phosphorus-32. Brachytherapy doses are typically higher than fractionated radiotherapy doses. However, the penetration of these radioisotopes is relatively low. For patients who have undergone prior brachytherapy, dose reduction with subsequent fractionated radiotherapy should be considered.

Recent Advances

The use of beam shaping and IMRT have been refined so that both the shape and intensity modulation of the radiation beam can be carried out as the linear accelerator is moving in a circle around the target this is known as arcing IMRT which is a faster means of delivering complex 3-D conformal RT or IMRT. commercially, arcing IMRT goes by the names RapidArc® or VMAT® when using a standard linear accelerator, or tomotherapy when using a dedicated linear accelerator which only delivers coplanar beams along an arc.

A major advance in radiotherapy in the last decade has been the introduction of imaging during the course of treatment. This ensures that radiation is being accurately delivered to the predefined target throughout the course of treatment. This can be done using X-rays either mounted separately in the treatment room (e.g., Novalis ExacTrac) or directly on the linear accelerator as orthogonal planar or CT imaging. A CT scanner mounted on the linear accelerator is known as cone beam CT (CBCT).

Efficacy

GTR can be achieved in 45–90% of craniopharyngiomas (Van Effenterre and Boch, 2002; Shirane et al., 2002; Zuccaro, 2005; Chakrabarti et al., 2005; Minamida et al., 2005; Shi et al., 2008). with 5-year tumor control rates of 70–90% (Hoffman et al., 1992; Fahlbusch et al., 1999; Van Effenterre & Boch, 2002). Rate of tumor progression increased significantly, up to 85%, in cases where only subtotal resection is acheived (Fahlbusch et al., 1999; Shirane et al., 2002; Van Effenterre and Boch, 2002; Zuccaro, 2005; Shi et al., 2008). The surgical mortality rate for craniopharyngiomas is 0–4% (Fahlbusch et al., 1999; Van Effenterre and Boch, 2002; Shi et al., 2008). Although some reported rates are as high as 10–17% when aggressive attempts are made at GTR (Yasargil et al., 1990). Surgical morbidity rates vary widely between 20–80% when complications, including pituitary dysfunction, hypothalamic dysregulation, visual deficits, and neurocognitive deterioration, are present (Hoffman et al., 1992; Fahlbusch et al., 1999; Honegger et al., 1999; Van Effenterre and Boch, 2002).

Despite the best microsurgical efforts, clear limitations remain on what may be achieved with resection. Residual or recurrent craniopharyngiomas are the most common targets for adjuvant radiation therapy, with the primary goal of longitudinal tumor control. Most long-term reports demonstrate 10-year tumor control rates of 75–90% (Hetelekidis et al., 1993; Rajan et al., 1993; Habrand et al., 1999; Van Effenterre and Boch, 2002; Aggarwal et al., 2013). which is superior to subtotal surgical resection alone (30–50%) (Hetelekidis et al., 1993; Van Effenterre and Boch, 2002; Aggarwal et al., 2013). Furthermore, the application of radiotherapy following incomplete resection of craniopharyngiomas significantly limits the need for repeat surgery, which has been associated with higher rates of morbidity and mortality than initial resection (Hoffman et al., 1992; Fahlbusch et al., 1999; Aggarwal et al., 2013).

Stripp et al. (2004) compared 57 patients treated with surgery alone to 18 patients treated with subtotal resection followed by radiotherapy. The 10-year tumor control rate was 42% after surgery alone compared to 84% after subtotal resection and radiotherapy. Hetelekidis et al. (1993) reported a 10-year progression-free survival of 31% for pediatric craniopharyngioma patients treated with surgery alone, versus 86% following combined surgery and radiotherapy. The superior rates of tumor control for adjuvant radiotherapy after surgical resection compared to resection alone are echoed by several similar series in the literature (Wen et al., 1989, 1992; Honegger et al., 1999; Merchant et al., 2002; Scott, 2005; Tomita and Bowman, 2005). Overall, the data for the use of radiotherapy in conjunction with surgical resection suggest that tumor control following subtotal resection bolstered by subsequent radiotherapy is better than subtotal resection alone and comparable to GTR alone. The long-term efficacy of conventional radiotherapy has been confirmed by a number of large series, with reported 10- and 20-year local control rates of 53–91% and 54–79%, respectively (Hetelekidis et al., 1993; Rajan et al., 1993; Regine et al., 1993; Habrand et al., 1999; Merchant et al., 2002; Varlotto et al., 2002; Stripp et al., 2004; Moon et al., 2005) (Table 19.2).

STEREOTACTIC RADIOSURGERY (SRS)

SRS is another radiotherapeutic option for treating craniopharyngiomas, which can be delivered with modified linear accelerators or the Gamma Knife. In 1951, Leksell published a description of focused radiation delivery using a stereotaxic method (Leksell, 1951). The name "Gamma Knife" is based on collimated photon radiation derived from the radioactive isotope Cobalt-60 (Park et al., 2011). Through the use of a stereotactic frame, SRS is delivered using tightly focused beams of gamma radiation with high precision from multiple directions at intracranial lesions such as craniopharyngiomas. The beam paths converge at the target volume, delivering a single, large cumulative dose of radiation while sparing adjacent healthy tissue from significant levels of irradiation.

Indication

Similarly to conventional fractionated radiotherapy, SRS is intended to treat residual or recurrent craniopharyngiomas. In patients with mixed-type tumors, especially those with large cystic lesions adjacent to a solid nodular component, SRS has largely been reserved for treating only the solid portion in conjunction with instillation of radioisotopes for the cystic portion. Occasionally, radiosurgical treatment of the solid portion of a cystic craniopharyngioma may shrink the cyst, although this phenomenon does not occur reliably.

Gamma Knife Technique

At the University of Virginia, the Leksell G frame is placed under monitored anesthesia for all adult patients. Pediatric patients under 14 years of age are given general anesthesia for frame placement which is maintained throughout the GKS procedure. Stereotactic MRI is then performed for treatment planning. If the patient cannot tolerate MRI due to incompatible implants, CT is used to define the target. Prior to 1994, dose planning was performed with the Kula software, which was subsequently replaced with the Gamma Plan software after 1994. For craniopharyngiomas, the goal of GKS dose planning is to cover the solid component of the tumor with one or more isocenters while limiting irradiation of surrounding normal structure as much as possible, especially radiation-sensitive tissue such as the optic apparatus, hypothalamus, and brainstem.

A margin dose of 8–16 Gy is delivered to the 50% isodose line, which is most commonly used to define the borders of the target. Craniopharyngiomas in close proximity to the optic apparatus are treated with relatively low doses, such that the maximum dose to the visual pathway structures is 10–12 Gy (Leber et al., 1998; Aggarwal et al., 2013). The target volume

TABLE 19.2 Conventional Radiotherapy/3D Conformal Radiotherapy/IMRT For Craniopharyngioma (Selected From the Reports That Provide Actuarial 10-Year Overall Survival and Tumor Control Rate)

Author	N	Mean age (yrs)	Prior Resect	Intracavitary Isotope Tx		Bleomycin Tx		Mean FU (yrs)	Mean Total Dose (Gy)	Mean TV (mL)	10 year Tumor Control				10-year overall survival
				Pre RT	Post RT	Pre RT	Post RT				Sol	Cyst	Mix	Total	
Lin, 2008	11	9	11	0%	9%	0%	0%	6.5	4600	3.6	NA	NA	NA	58%	96%
Merchant, 2006	28	7.3	28	NA	NA	NA	NA	3	5400 or 5580	NA	NA	NA	NA	90% (3 yr)*	96% (3 yr)*
Moon, 2005	50	< 20:15 > 20:35	49	NA	NA	NA	NA	12.8	5400	12	NA	NA	NA	91%	91%
Pemberto, 2005	87	< 15:28 > 15:59	87	NA	NA	NA	NA	8	4250	NA	NA	NA	NA	78%	86%
Stripp, 2004	76	8.5	76	NA	NA	NA	NA	7.6	5500	NA	NA	NA	NA	53%	85%
Varlotto, 2002	24	29	22	NA	NA	NA	NA	12	6000	NA	NA	NA	NA	89%	100%
Habrand, 1999	37	7.4	36	NA	NA	NA	NA	> 5	5000	NA	NA	NA	NA	57%	65%
Regine, 1993	58	< 16:19 > 16:39	56	NA	NA	NA	NA	17	5588 −6243	NA	NA	NA	NA	79%	NA
Rajan, 1993	173	< 16:77 > 16:96	103	NA	NA	NA	NA	12	5000	NA	NA	NA	NA	83%	77%
Hetelekidis 1993	46	7.5	37	NA	NA	NA	NA	10	5464	NA	NA	NA	NA	86%	94%

FU: follow-up, Gy: gray, mL: milliliter, N/A: not available, RT: radiotherapy, Sol: solid, TV: tumor volume, Tx: treatment, yr: years

* *Mechant's report only provided 3-year tumor control rate and overall survival.*

encompasses the solid component of the tumor. The cystic component may be treated with stereotactic aspiration followed by intracavitary radioactive phosphorous-32, or chemotherapeutically with bleomycin implantation (Park et al., 2011; Higuchi et al., 2012; Liu et al., 2012).

Advances in GKS

In the earlier model of the Leksell Gamma Knife (LGK, Elekta, Norcross, GA), 201 ^{60}CO sources were placed in a nearly complete hemispherical arrangement in order that the radiation beams would converge on a single point; the size of the high-dose volume delivered by one shot was determined by one of four possible helmets with collimators ranging in size from 4–18 mm in diameter. The latest model of the GKS system, Perfexion™ PFX, adopts eight, independent, position-controlled source module sectors and a stationary, built-in collimator system with three apertures for each source corresponding to 4, 8, and 16 mm beam sizes. This new technology has led to an improvement in efficiency in treatment planning, delivery, and workflow.

In 2009, the release of the Extend system for the Gamma Knife Perfexion (Elekta AB) enabled multi-session GKS treatments using a non-invasive, vacuum-assisted, immobilization system. This frameless system makes fractionated GKS possible (Sayer et al., 2011; Schlesinger et al., 2012). Hypofractionated treatment regimens can improve the therapeutic ratio, which may be especially useful for suprasellar tumors. However, the efficacy and safety of multi-session GKS has yet to be fully defined.

Efficacy

GKS results for craniopharyngioma patients have been described in 14 published reports (Prasad et al., 1995; Mokry, 1999; Chung et al., 2000; Yu et al., 2000; Chiou et al., 2001; Ulfarsson et al., 2002; Amendola et al., 2003; Barua et al., 2003; Albright et al., 2005; Kobayashi et al., 2005a, 2005b; Niranjan et al., 2009; Yomo et al., 2009; Xu et al., 2010; Jeon et al., 2011). There are four reports which include long-term follow-up: the 5-year progression-free survival rates are 52–68%, and 5-year overall survival rates are 86–97% (Table 19.3). Xu et al. (2010) reported a series of 37 patients who underwent GKS for craniopharyngiomas, and these authors reported 5-year overall survival and in-field progression-free survival rates of 75.6% and 67%, respectively. Hasegawa et al. (2010) demonstrated 5- and 10-year progression-free survival rates of 62% and 52%, respectively, in 100 craniopharyngiomas patients. Niranjan et al. (2009) reported a 97.5% overall survival rate at 5 years following GKS and a 91.6% 5-year progression-free survival in 46 patients with long-term follow-up (mean 62.2 months). A potential explanation for the discrepancies in overall survival and progression-free survival among different craniopharyngioma radiosurgery series is the relatively small number of patients and shorter follow-up periods compared to similar data from conventional radiotherapy series (Table 19.3).

Factors prognostic for improved in-field, progression-free survival are absence of visual field deficits prior to GKS, solid tumor volume less than 1.6 cm^3, and margin dose greater than 14.5 Gy (Xu et al., 2010). The magnitude of the margin dose is considerably dependent upon tumor volume and its proximity to critical structures (Chung et al., 1998; Hasegawa et al., 2010). Pre-treatment absence of visual field deficits may be a surrogate indicator of

TABLE 19.3 Gamma Knife Surgery for Craniopharyngioma (Selected From the Reports that Provide Actuarial 5-Year or 10-Year Overall Survival and Tumor Control Rate)

				Intracavitary Isotope Tx		Bleomycin Tx					Actuarial Tumor Control				
Author	N	Mean age (years)	Prior Resect	Pre GKS	Post GKS	Pre GKS	Post GKS	Mean FU (yrs)	Median Margin Dose (Gy)	Median TV (mL)	Sol	Cyst	Mix	Total	Overall Survival
Xu, 2010	37	36	83%	27%	0%	0%	0%	4.2	14.5	1.6	NA	NA	NA	67% (5 yr)	86% (5 yr)
Hasegawa, 2010	100	40< 15 yo 60> 15 yo	96%	NA	NA	NA	NA	5.7	11.4	3.3	NA	NA	NA	52% (10 yr)	88% (10 yr)
Niranjan, 2009	46	24	100%	24%	0%	0%	0%	5.2	13.0	1.0	78%	100%	59%	68% (5 yr)	97% (5 yr)
Kobayashi 2009	98	38< 15 yo 60> 15 yo	100%	0%	0%	3%	0%	5.5	11.5	3.5	NA	NA	NA	54% (10 yr)	91% (10 yr)

FU: follow-up, Gy: gray, mL: milliliter, N/A: not available, RT: radiotherapy, Sol: solid, TV: tumor volume, Tx: treatment, yr: years.

tumor separation from the optic apparatus such that it may be treated with a higher margin dose, thereby increasing the likelihood of prolonged progression-free survival. Optimal GKS outcomes are therefore achieved in small tumors (Xu et al., 2010).

Additional factors associated with a favorable response to GKS are non-cystic tumor composition, fewer previous interventions, and lower tumor volume. For cases of significant tumor recurrence, cytoreductive surgery may be considered prior to treatment with SRS.

FRACTIONATED STEREOTACTIC RADIOTHERAPY (FSRT)

As a blending of conventional radiotherapy and stereotactic radiosurgery, fractionated stereotactic radiotherapy (FSRT) has been shown to be effective in treating craniopharyngiomas, although its outcomes are not as well defined as conventional radiotherapy or SRS. FSRT is not as constrained by tumor volume or proximity to critical structures as stereotactic radiosurgery, and it therefore provides a further degree of versatility.

Efficacy

From the few available reports, it can be seen that FSRT provides favorable results in terms of local tumor control and overall survival. Minniti et al. treated 39 craniopharyngioma patients with FSRT and reported progression-free survival at 3 and 5 years of 97% and 92%, respectively, overall survival at 5 years of 100%, and endocrine and visual complication rates similar to SRS after a median follow-up of 40 months (Minniti et al., 2007). A retrospective analysis by Combs et al. demonstrated 100% local tumor control at 10 years, and overall survival rates at 5 and 10 years of 97% and 89%, respectively (Combs et al., 2007). Although further investigation is warranted to confirm the effectiveness and safety of FSRT, the current literature shows promising benefit for craniopharyngioma patients.

PROTON BEAM

Radiation Techniques

Protons and other charged particles have recently become an increasingly attractive source for radiation therapy due to their physical dose distribution. The relative biological effectiveness of protons is indistinguishable from that of 250 kV X-rays. The oxygen enhancement ratio for protons is also indistinguishable from that of X-rays, which is approximately 2.5–3.0. These biological characteristics are consistent with the physical features of high-energy proton beams – they are sparsely ionizing except for a very short region at the end of the particle's range.

The theoretical advantage of protons and other heavy charged particles with the same radiobiological effect as photons is the deposition of energy at a defined point along its path (Bragg peak) with little radiation beyond that point. The beam has sharp edges with little side-scatter, and the dose falls to zero after the Bragg peak at the end of the particle's range. The possibility of precisely confining a high radiation dose to the target with little effect on surrounding normal tissue is inherently attractive to the radiotherapist. Dosimetric evaluation of 3-D conformal proton therapy in pediatric craniopharyngiomas has shown a reduction in the volume of irradiated brain parenchyma along with improved target dose distribution compared to photon radiotherapy (Beltran et al., 2012; Boehling et al., 2012).

Proton beam technology has made it possible to deliver a large radiation dose to a craniopharyngioma without causing significant damage to nearby structures. These treatments have been performed for several years at medical centers in Berkeley, Harvard, Europe, and Japan. Hospital-based, high-energy cyclotrons with isocentric mounts are now being used to treat a broader spectrum of cancer patients with proton beam radiotherapy.

Efficacy

Early results of small case series of proton therapy report similar results to those achieved with fractionated 3-D CRT and SRS, with 5-year, progression-free survival rates of over 90% (Fitzek et al., 2006). The potential advantage of lower doses to normal tissues beyond the irradiated target (Beltran et al., 2012) has not yet been translated to a lower reported toxicity. Currently, it is the perception of improved outcomes that drives the implementation of proton radiotherapy, particularly in pediatric patients, where any avoidance of normal tissue irradiation is considered important.

There are two large craniopharyngioma proton beam series. Winkfield et al. from Massachusetts General Hospital (Winkfield et al., 2009) reported a series of 24 pediatric patients from 2001–2007 and demonstrated no local failures over a median follow-up period of 40.5 months. However, cystic growth beyond the initial treatment fields was found in six patients during radiation course, requiring subsequent enlargement of the treatment plan. One patient underwent cyst drainage to avoid treatment field adjustment. The authors suggested that routine imaging should be performed during treatment at 2-week intervals.

Luu et al. (2006) reported another series of 16 craniopharyngioma patients which were treated with prescription doses of 50.4–59.4 cobalt gray equivalents. The local tumor control rate was 93%, and the overall survival rate was 80%. Long-term follow-up and larger, prospective series are necessary to fully define the outcomes and complications of proton beam therapy for craniopharyngiomas.

COMPLICATIONS OF RADIATION THERAPY

The side effects of radiation therapy are classified as acute (within days), early delayed (within weeks), and late delayed toxicities (within months to years). The risk of radiation injury depends on the dose (either total dose or per fraction), duration of treatment, and volume of normal brain irradiated (Regine et al., 1993; Chung et al., 1998; Chakrabarti et al., 2005; Kobayashi et al., 2005; Adler Jr. et al., 2006; Liu et al., 2009; Campbell et al., 2010; Hasegawa et al., 2010).

Acute Radiation Injury

Acute radiation toxicity occurs infrequently but may result in significant clinical manifestations in those who are afflicted. Approximately 10–20% of patients develop cystic enlargement of the craniopharyngiomas, leading to compression of the optic apparatus (Rajan et al., 1993, 1997). Occasionally, the development of cystic enlargement can cause acute hydrocephalus. Early intervention and drainage are necessary when cysts result in neurological deterioration. Other acute radiation injuries include transient diabetes insipidus (DI), skin changes, and hair loss.

Early Delayed Radiation Injury

Early delayed radiation injuries include radiation necrosis, visual deterioration, hypopituitarism, hypothalamic dysfunction, and cognitive dysfunction or dementia. Complications resulting from radiation therapy vary with patient age, tumor size, and radiation doses (Kalapurakal, 2005). However, several authors have found that SRS allows effective tumor control with minimal post-treatment morbidity or mortality (Mokry, 1999; Chung et al., 2000; Chiou et al., 2001; Amendola et al., 2003; Albright et al., 2005; Kobayashi et al., 2005).

Radiation Necrosis

Radiation necrosis occasionally occurs after radiation treatment for craniopharyngiomas. The neurological deterioration due to radiation necrosis is often delayed, occurring several weeks to several months, even several years, after radiation therapy. For craniopharyngioma patients, radiation necrosis usually occurs in the hypothalamus, which causes hypothalamic dysfunction including hypopituitarism (see the section "Hypopituitarism and hypothalamic dysfunction"). Temporal lobe necrosis is rare in contemporary radiation therapy or radiosurgery practice.

Visual deterioration, optic neuritis, and optic compression neuropathy

Optic neuritis occurs in 1–2% of patients who received doses of 50 Gy with conventional radiotherapy and is mostly confined to those with visual impairment prior to radiotherapy (Brada and Thomas, 1993; Rajan et al., 1993). Patients who received higher doses (> 55 Gy) were at greater risk of developing optic neuritis (Regine et al., 1993; Varlotto et al., 2002). This risk is related to the total dose, dose per fraction, and pre-treatment damage to the optic chiasm. For a total dose of 50–55 Gy administered in daily doses of 1.8 Gy, the rate of damage to the optic chiasm is $< 3\%$. However, this complication rate increases significantly for doses between 55 and 60 Gy (Regine et al., 1993; Varlotto et al., 2002).

Only a single case of optic neuritis following SRS has been reported (Chiou et al., 2001). The discrepancy between the rates of optic neuritis in conventional radiotherapy and SRS may result from:

1) Most patients having some degree of visual impairment prior to radiation,
2) Visual deterioration after SRS is usually caused by tumor progression rather than radiation injury,
3) SRS is typically used for smaller craniopharyngiomas,

4) A single SRS dose to the optic apparatus is virtually always kept under 10–12 Gy, and
5) Compared to conventional radiotherapy, the duration of post-SRS follow-up is, on average, shorter.

Hypopituitarism and hypothalamic dysfunction

Hypothalamic–pituitary dysfunction is the most common late complication of radiation therapy regardless of the radiation technique utilized. Most craniopharyngioma patients of already have some degree of hypopituitarism before irradiation. Approximately 30–50% of patients develop a new hormone deficiency, and most require some degree of hormone replacement 5–10 years after radiation (Hetelekidis et al., 1993; Rajan et al., 1993; Habrand et al., 1999). Very few patients develop new-onset DI after radiation therapy, and the occurrence of DI after radiotherapy is strictly related to changes in tumor anatomy that mechanically affect the pituitary. At doses higher than 60 Gy, the incidence of hypopituitarism may be up to 80% versus 36% at doses of less than 60 Gy (Regine et al., 1993).

Based on our institutional GKS experience in more commonly treated sellar lesions, such as pituitary adenomas, 30% of patients developed delayed-onset hypopituitarism within 3 years. The thyroid function was affected most, followed by gonadotrophic hormone, adrenocorticotrophic hormone, and growth hormone (Xu et al., 2013). Higher margin dose and suprasellar extension were independent predictors of post-radiosurgery hypopituitarism (Xu et al., 2013).

Other manifestations of hypothalamic dysfunction include poor control of body temperature and alterations in sleep and appetite regulation. Similar to hypopituitarism, most patients had some degree of pre-treatment hypothalamic dysfunction.

Cognitive dysfunction and dementia

Cognitive decline has been observed following radiation therapy for sellar and parasellar tumors (Grattan-Smith et al., 1992; Peace et al., 1997). While conventional radiotherapy to large volumes of normal brain is associated with neurocognitive dysfunction, the frequency of neurocognitive decline after low-volume irradiation is not well known, particularly in a situation in which the disease itself and surgical intervention may also exert independent effects (Rajan et al., 1993; Regine et al., 1993). As radiation therapy has become more conformal, resulting in reduced doses to normal brain tissue, pediatric patients are tolerating radiotherapy without appreciable treatment-related decline (Regine et al., 1993; Rajan et al., 1997; Merchant et al., 2002, 2006; Stripp et al., 2004; Moon et al., 2005; Pemberton et al., 2005). Kiehna et al. reported that post-radiation IQ remains stable for 5 years and then begins to decline. Negative prognostic factors include age less than 7 years, hydrocephalus requiring CSF diversion, large cystic tumors requiring multiple aspirations, extensive resection, and DI (Merchant et al., 2006). Jalali et al. also demonstrated that IQ remains stable over a 2-year period following treatment, and that age less than 15 years and higher dose to the temporal lobe were significant causes of neurocognitive decline (Jalali et al., 2009).

Late delayed radiation effects

Late delayed radiation complications include stroke from radiation-induced vascular occlusion and radiation-induced secondary brain tumors (Brada et al., 1992, 1999, 2002; Minniti et al., 2005). Liu et al. observed development of vasculopathy on neuroimaging in six out of 20 patients after receiving radiation therapy for craniopharyngiomas (Liu et al., 2009). One study of radiation therapy to the parasellar region demonstrated a 21% incidence of cerebrovascular events (Keene et al., 2006). The risk of developing moyamoya syndrome has been estimated to increase by 7% for every 100 cGy increase in radiation dose above 5000 cGy, with a delay in occurrence of approximately 5–12 years (Hetelekidis et al., 1993; Ullrich et al., 2007).

The risk of a radiation-therapy-induced secondary malignancy, including high-grade gliomas, meningiomas, and central nervous system (CNS) lymphomas, is approximately 1.9% at 10 years (Kalapurakal, 2005). Out of 626 craniopharyngioma patients who underwent radiation therapy reviewed by Kahn et al. (Kiehna and Merchant, 2010), only four developed secondary malignancies. However, in the modern era, in which more conformal radiation modalities are used to restrict the dose to normal tissue, the rate of secondary tumor malignancy may be lower (Figures 19.1 and 19.2).

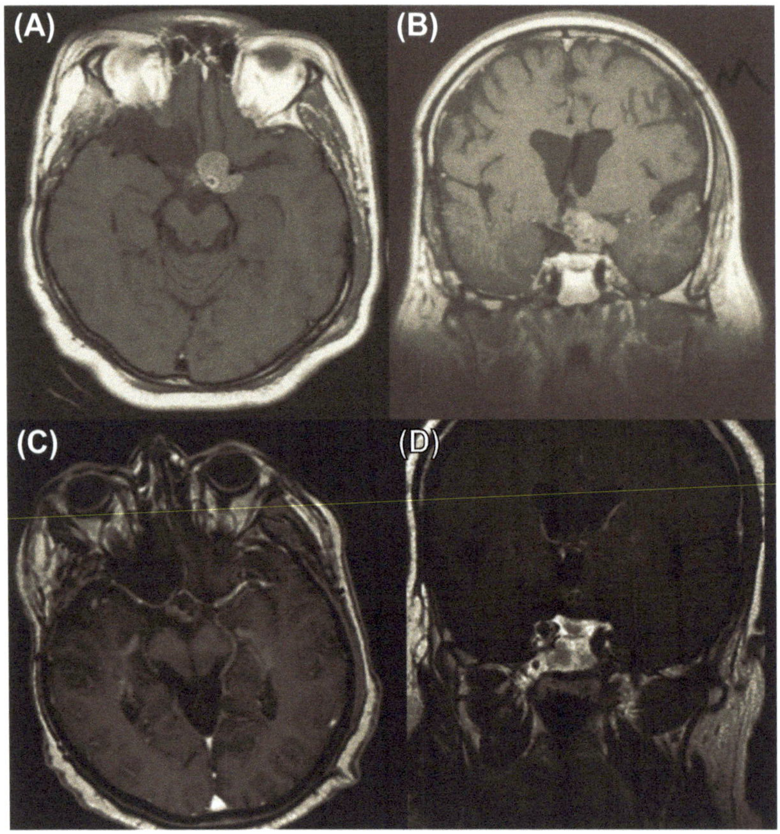

FIGURE 19.1 A 37-year-old male patient had a mixed-type craniopharyngioma status post two surgical resections. Bitemporal hemianipsia and panhypopituitarism had developed before GKS. **A, B**, axial and coronal images showing a 33 mm x 29 x 19 mm tumor, which was treated with 8 Gy to the tumor margin via two isocenters. **C, D**, Images revealing a small residual tumor attaching the optic chasm 94 months after GKS with stable ophthalmological condition and consistent panhypopituitarism under hormone replacement therapy. *From Dr. Xu: Outcomes of Gamma Knife Surgery for Craniopharyngioma.*

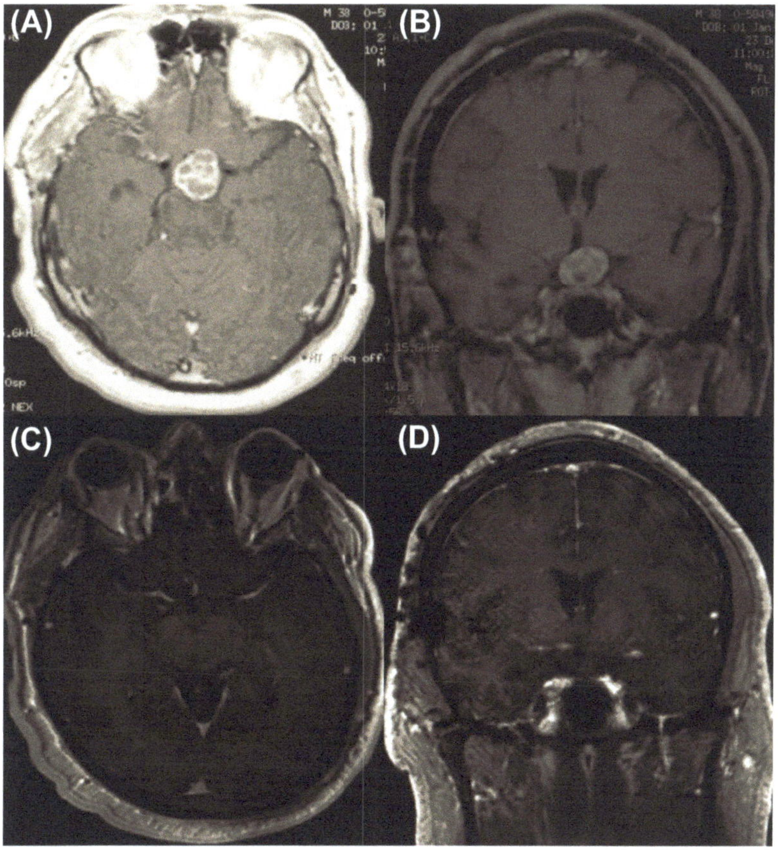

FIGURE 19.2 A 40-year-old male patient had a mixed-type craniopharyngioma status after two surgical resections and conventional radiotherapy with 35 Gy. Before GKS, he already had blurred vision and pan-hypopituitarism. **A, B**, Axial and coronal images revealing a 22 x 22 x 12 mm tumor. Ten Gy was delivered to the tumor margin via five isocenters. **C, D**, At 107 months after GKS, the tumor appeared as a tiny ill-defined suprasellar spot with mild enhancement, no cyst visualized. His neuroendocrine and ophthalmological status was stable at the last follow-up. *From Dr. Xu: Outcomes of Gamma Knife Surgery for Craniopharyngioma.*

SPECIAL CONSIDERATIONS AND DEBATES

Cyst development and enlargement during radiation therapy

The cystic component of a craniopharyngioma commonly presents a problem for radiation therapy and radiosurgery. Cyst re-accumulation is not equal to tumor recurrence, and shrinkage of the tumor's solid component is not always accompanied by cyst regression. The solid component of the tumor can usually be controlled by radiation, but the cyst may require surgical decompression. Tumor growth and cyst enlargement are sometimes independent. According to this principle, several approaches are also useful for managing patients with cystic craniopharyngiomas, either at initial presentation or recurrence. The following treatments are commonly used to decrease cyst size: intermittent aspiration by stereotaxic puncture or placement of an Ommaya reservoir, sclerosis of the cyst wall by chemotherapeutic drugs, and internal irradiation (i.e., brachytherapy) with implanted radioisotopes.

Percutaneous aspiration of cyst contents has been used to alleviate cyst-related symptoms, and intermittent aspiration may be recommended for patients who are poor surgical candidates. An alternative is placement of an Ommaya reservoir for intermittent aspiration of cysts that cannot be completely resected. Recently, several case reports have demonstrated that stereotactic cyst aspiration in conjunction with same-day SRS may be a successful strategy for achieving tumor control (Park et al., 2011; Higuchi et al., 2012; Liu et al., 2012) (Figure 19.3).

When repeated cyst aspirations are not feasible, intralesional radiotherapy or chemotherapy can be utilized. Several reports have described minimal cyst excision with intermittent intralesional bleomycin through an Ommaya reservoir in pediatric patients with cystic craniopharyngiomas. Another alternative in patients with solitary or multicystic tumors is intracavitary irradiation via stereotactically applied radioisotopes. Beta-emitting isotopes,

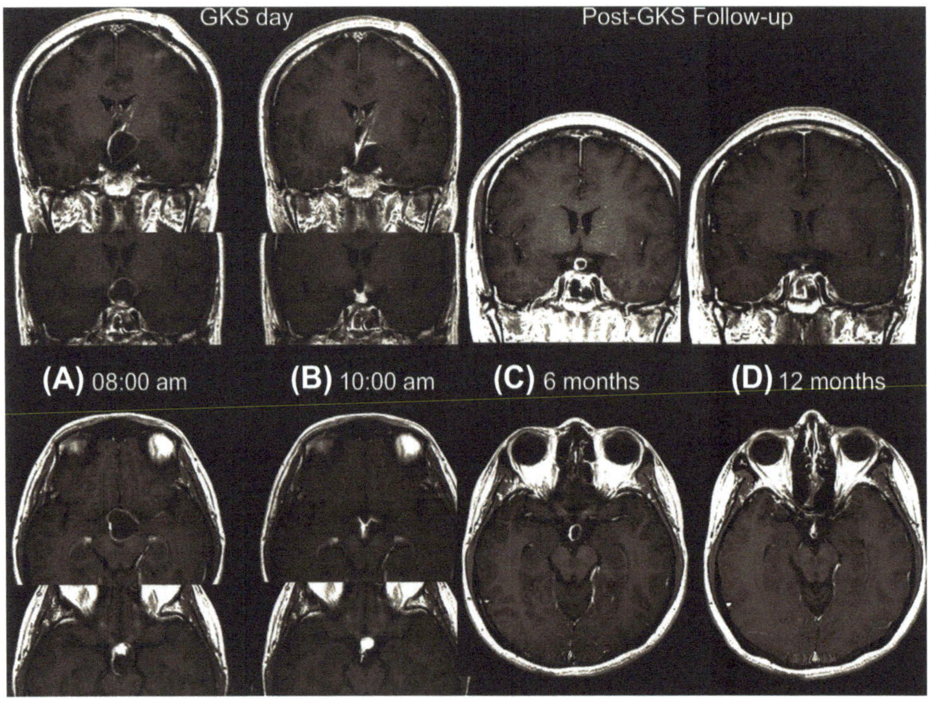

FIGURE 19.3 A 35-year-old female patient had a cyst-type craniopharyngioma status post stereotactic aspiration with Ommaya shunt implantation. **A,** The initial cyst was 2.8 cm in diameter with optic apparatus compression. **B,** Two hours before GKS, the patient underwent aspiration via Ommaya reservoir. The cyst was decompressed and showed a small solid, enhanced part of tumor. A radiosurgery dose of 12 Gy was delivered to the tumor margin via 11 isocenters. **C, D,** After 6 and 12 months follow-up, the trend of shrinkage was significant and the tumor was controlled. The patient is currently free from visual field deficits and pituitary dysfunction. *Courtesy of Prof. David HC Pan, Prof. WY Chung, and Prof. WY Guo, Taipei Veteran General Hospital, Taiwan.*

such as ^{90}Yt (yttrium-90), ^{186}Rh (rhenium-196) (Jeon et al., 2011), and ^{32}P (phosphorus-32), are preferred due to the limited penetration of the emitted energy and relative ease of handling. The reported results are similar to those achieved with microsurgery.

Debates

Although the effect of radiation on craniopharyngiomas has been proven, two critical issues remain sources of significant controversy:

1) The merits of GTR versus subtotal resection followed by radiation given the surgical morbidity and mortality associated with aggressive resection, and
2) The role of radiotherapy immediately following surgical resection without first monitoring for tumor progression and the role of radiotherapy in the absence of resection.

Several authors recommend subtotal resection and radiation as an acceptable alternative to total resection, on the basis of the complications associated with aggressive surgical resection and the proven efficacy of radiation for craniopharyngiomas. Although clinicians can often mitigate the effects of neurological deficits and endocrine dysfunction, the psychosocial deficits associated with radical resection are now recognized as a major limiting factor on quality of life as pediatric patients grow into adulthood. Thus, minimization of surgical hypothalamic injury is crucial for optimizing post-operative quality of life for craniopharyngioma patients, especially those who are younger. In order to limit significant neurological, endocrine, and psychosocial morbidities that may accompany radical resection, some physicians prefer less aggressive resection with subsequent radiotherapy.

Some pediatric series indicate that radiotherapy given immediately after surgery (upfront) may be preferable to radiotherapy at recurrence (salvage) with lower rates of morbidity and improved tumor control (Weiss et al., 1989; Regine et al., 1993; Habrand et al., 1999; Moon et al., 2005). In contrast, for adult craniopharyngioma patients there is no significant difference in either tumor control or overall survival when comparing upfront to salvage radiotherapy (Rajan et al., 1993; Varlotto et al., 2002; Combs et al., 2007; Minniti et al., 2007). Therefore, some clinicians advocate early post-operative radiotherapy or SRS for partially resected tumors (Minniti et al., 2009).

Due to the steep dose fall-off of SRS compared to conventional radiotherapy, some physicians use SRS as a primary treatment for craniopharyngiomas. In a study of five pediatric craniopharyngioma patients in which SRS was the primary treatment for the solid portion of mixed tumors after intracavitary ^{32}P was used to treat the cystic portion, two patients experienced tumor regression and another two had tumor control (Albright et al., 2005) Additional studies have shown higher tumor control rates in single-type tumors, solid or cystic, compared to mixed-type tumors. Chung et al. (2000) found single-type tumors were more responsive to primary radiosurgical treatment than mixed-type tumors. It is also believed that solid-type tumors and the solid portions of mixed tumors are less responsive than cystic tumors to intracavitary irradiation (Julow et al., 2007a, 2007b). As a result, Prasad et al. (1995) recommended that mixed-type tumors should be treated with a combination of radioisotope instillation and SRS. The combination of SRS and intracavitary radiation has been advocated as a primary treatment for mixed cystic-solid tumors (Yu et al., 2000; Albright et al., 2005).

CONCLUSION

Without regard to the design differences among conventional radiotherapy, SRS, FSRT, and proton beam, all treatment modalities share the same fundamental concepts of radiobiology and treatment goals. Selection of the appropriate radiation technique and delivery device must be done by a multidisciplinary team comprised of neurosurgeons and radiation oncologists. Radiation therapy and radiosurgery play important roles in the treatment of recurrent or residual craniopharyngiomas. The use of upfront radiation treatment may be reasonable for carefully selected craniopharyngioma patients. Long-term follow-up of craniopharyngioma patients should be performed to assess for tumor response, neurological changes, and neuroendocrine dysfunction.

References

Adler Jr., J.R., Gibbs, I.C., Puataweepong, P., Chang, S.D., 2006. Visual field preservation after multi-session cyberknife radiosurgery for perioptic lesions. Neurosurgery 59, 244–254 discussion 244–254.

Aggarwal, A., Fersht, N., Brada, M., 2013. Radiotherapy for craniopharyngioma. Pituitary 16, 26–33.

Albright, A.L., Hadjipanayis, C.G., Lunsford, L.D., Kondziolka, D., Pollack, I.F., Adelson, P.D., 2005. Individualized treatment of pediatric craniopharyngiomas. Childs Nerv. Syst. 21, 649–654.

Amendola, B.E., Wolf, A., Coy, S.R., Amendola, M.A., 2003. Role of radiosurgery in craniopharyngiomas: a preliminary report. Med. Pediatr. Oncol. 41, 123–127.

Barua, K.K., Ehara, K., Kohmura, E., Tamaki, N., 2003. Treatment of recurrent craniopharyngiomas. Kobe. J. Med. Sci. 49, 123–132.

Beclere, A., 1909. The radiotherapeutic treatment of tumours of the hypophysis, gigantism and acromegaly. Arch. Roentgen. Ray 14, 142–150.

Beltran, C., Roca, M., Merchant, T.E., 2012. On the benefits and risks of proton therapy in pediatric craniopharyngioma. Int. J. Radiat. Oncol. Biol. Phys. 82, e281–287.

Boehling, N.S., Grosshans, D.R., Bluett, J.B., Palmer, M.T., Song, X., Amos, R.A., Sahoo, N., Meyer, J.J., Mahajan, A., Woo, S.Y., 2012. Dosimetric comparison of three-dimensional conformal proton radiotherapy, intensity-modulated proton therapy, and intensity-modulated radiotherapy for treatment of pediatric craniopharyngiomas. Int. J. Radiat. Oncol. Biol. Phys. 82, 643–652.

Brada, M., Thomas, D.G., 1993. Craniopharyngioma revisited. Int. J. Radiat. Oncol. Biol. Phys. 27, 471–475.

Brada, M., Ford, D., Ashley, S., Bliss, J.M., Crowley, S., Mason, M., et al., 1992. Risk of second brain tumour after conservative surgery and radiotherapy for pituitary adenoma. BMJ 304, 1343–1346.

Brada, M., Burchell, L., Ashley, S., Traish, D., 1999. The incidence of cerebrovascular accidents in patients with pituitary adenoma. Int. J. Radiat. Oncol. Biol. Phys. 45, 693–698.

Brada, M., Ashley, S., Ford, D., Traish, D., Burchell, L., Rajan, B., 2002. Cerebrovascular mortality in patients with pituitary adenoma. Clin. Endocrinol. (Oxf) 57, 713–717.

Campbell, P.G., McGettigan, B., Luginbuhl, A., Yadla, S., Rosen, M., Evans, J.J., 2010. Endocrinological and ophthalmological consequences of an initial endonasal endoscopic approach for resection of craniopharyngiomas. Neurosurg. Focus 28, E8.

Carpenter, R.C.C.G., Frazier, C.H., 1937. The treatment of hypophyseal stalk tumors by evacuation and irradiation. Am. J. Roentgenol. 38, 162–177.

Chakrabarti, I., Amar, A.P., Couldwell, W., Weiss, M.H., 2005. Long-term neurological, visual, and endocrine outcomes following transnasal resection of craniopharyngioma. J. Neurosurg. 102, 650–657.

Chiou, S.M., Lunsford, L.D., Niranjan, A., Kondziolka, D., Flickinger, J.C., 2001. Stereotactic radiosurgery of residual or recurrent craniopharyngioma, after surgery, with or without radiation therapy. Neuro. Oncol. 3, 159–166.

Chung, W.Y., Pan, H.C., Guo, W.Y., Shiau, C.Y., Wang, L.W., Wu, H.M., et al., 1998. Protection of visual pathway in gamma knife radiosurgery for craniopharyngiomas. Stereotact. Funct. Neurosurg. 70 (Suppl. 1), 139–151.

Chung, W.Y., Pan, D.H., Shiau, C.Y., Guo, W.Y., Wang, L.W., 2000. Gamma knife radiosurgery for craniopharyngiomas. J. Neurosurg. 93 (Suppl. 3), 47–56.

Combs, S.E., Thilmann, C., Huber, P.E., Hoess, A., Debus, J., Schulz-Ertner, D., 2007. Achievement of long-term local control in patients with craniopharyngiomas using high precision stereotactic radiotherapy. Cancer 109, 2308–2314.

Dandy, Walter E., 1945. Surgery of the Brain. W. F. Prior Company, Inc, Hagerstown. Print, p. 554.

Fahlbusch, R., Honegger, J., Paulus, W., Huk, W., Buchfelder, M., 1999. Surgical treatment of craniopharyngiomas: experience with 168 patients. J Neurosurg 90, 237–250.

Fitzek, M.M., Linggood, R.M., Adams, J., Munzenrider, J.E., 2006. Combined proton and photon irradiation for craniopharyngioma: long-term results of the early cohort of patients treated at Harvard Cyclotron Laboratory and Massachusetts General Hospital. Int. J. Radiat. Oncol. Biol. Phys. 64, 1348–1354.

Gramegna, A., 1909. Un cas d'acromégalie traité par la radiothérapie. Rev. Neurol. (Paris) 17, 15–17.

Grattan-Smith, P.J., Morris, J.G., Shores, E.A., Batchelor, J., Sparks, R.S., 1992. Neuropsychological abnormalities in patients with pituitary tumours. Acta Neurol. Scand. 86, 626–631.

Habrand, J.L., Ganry, O., Couanet, D., Rouxel, V., Levy-Piedbois, C., Pierre-Kahn, A., Kalifa, C., 1999. The role of radiation therapy in the management of craniopharyngioma: a 25-year experience and review of the literature. Int. J. Radiat. Oncol. Biol. Phys. 44, 255–263.

Hasegawa, T., Kobayashi, T., Kida, Y., 2010. Tolerance of the optic apparatus in single-fraction irradiation using stereotactic radiosurgery: evaluation in 100 patients with craniopharyngioma. Neurosurgery 66, 688–694 discussion 694–685.

Hetelekidis, S., Barnes, P.D., Tao, M.L., Fischer, E.G., Schneider, L., Scott, R.M., et al., 1993. 20-year experience in childhood craniopharyngioma. Int. J. Radiat. Oncol. Biol. Phys. 27, 189–195.

Higuchi, F., Kawamoto, S., Abe, Y., Kim, P., Ueki, K., 2012. Effectiveness of a 1-day aspiration plus Gamma Knife surgery procedure for metastatic brain tumor with a cystic component. J. Neurosurg. 117 (Suppl.), 17–22.

Hoffman, H.J., De Silva, M., Humphreys, R.P., Drake, J.M., Smith, M.L., Blaser, S.I., 1992. Aggressive surgical management of craniopharyngiomas in children. J. Neurosurg. 76, 47–52.

Honegger, J., Buchfelder, M., Fahlbusch, R., 1999. Surgical treatment of craniopharyngiomas: endocrinological results. J. Neurosurg. 90, 251–257.

Jalali, R., Mallick, I., Dutta, D., Goswami, S., Gupta, T., Munshi, A., et al., 2009. Factors influencing neurocognitive outcomes in young patients with benign and low-grade brain tumors treated with stereotactic conformal radiotherapy. Int. J. Radiat. Oncol. Biol. Phys. 77, 974–979.

Jang, W.Y., Lee, K.S., Son, B.C., Jeun, S.S., Hong, Y.K., Lee, S.W., et al., 2009. Repeat operations in pediatric patients with recurrent craniopharyngiomas. Pediatr. Neurosurg. 45, 451–455.

Jeon, C., Kim, S., Shin, H.J., Nam, D.H., Lee, J.I., Park, K., et al., 2011. The therapeutic efficacy of fractionated radiotherapy and gamma knife radiosurgery for craniopharyngiomas. J. Clin. Neurosci. 18, 1621–1625.

Julow, J., Backlund, E.O., Lanyi, F., Hajda, M., Balint, K., Nyary, I., et al., 2007a. Long-term results and late complications after intracavitary yttrium-90 colloid irradiation of recurrent cystic craniopharyngiomas. Neurosurgery 61, 288–295 discussion 295–286.

Julow, J., Lanyi, F., Hajda, M., Szeifert, G.T., Viola, A., Balint, K., et al., 2007b. Stereotactic intracavitary irradiation of cystic craniopharyngiomas with yttrium-90 isotope. Prog. Neurol. Surg. 20, 289–296.

Kalapurakal, J.A., 2005. Radiation therapy in the management of pediatric craniopharyngiomas – a review. Childs Nerv. Syst. 21, 808–816.

Karavitaki, N., Wass, J.A., 2008. Craniopharyngiomas. Endocrinol. Metab. Clin. North Am. 37, 173–193 ix–x.

Keene, D.L., Johnston, D.L., Grimard, L., Michaud, J., Vassilyadi, M., Ventureyra, E., 2006. Vascular complications of cranial radiation. Childs Nerv. Syst. 22, 547–555.

Kiehna, E.N., Merchant, T.E., 2010. Radiation therapy for pediatric craniopharyngioma. Neurosurg. Focus 28, E10.

Kobayashi, T., Kida, Y., Mori, Y., Hasegawa, T., 2005a. Long-term results of gamma knife surgery for the treatment of craniopharyngioma in 98 consecutive cases. J. Neurosurg. 103, 482–488.

Kobayashi, T., Mori, Y., Tsugawa, T., Hashizume, C., Takahashi, H., 2005b. Prognostic factors for tumor recurrence after gamma knife radiosurgery of partially resected and recurrent craniopharyngiomas. Nagoya. J. Med. Sci. 74, 141–147.

Komotar, R.J., Roguski, M., Bruce, J.N., 2009. Surgical management of craniopharyngiomas. J. Neurooncol. 92, 283–296.

Leber, K.A., Bergloff, J., Pendl, G., 1998. Dose-response tolerance of the visual pathways and cranial nerves of the cavernous sinus to stereotactic radiosurgery. J. Neurosurg. 88, 43–50.
Leksell, L., 1951. The stereotaxic method and radiosurgery of the brain. Acta Chir. Scand. 102, 316–319.
Lindholm, J., Nielsen, E.H., 2009. Craniopharyngioma: historical notes. Pituitary 12, 352–359.
Liu, A.K., Bagrosky, B., Fenton, L.Z., Gaspar, L.E., Handler, M.H., McNatt, S.A., et al., 2009. Vascular abnormalities in pediatric craniopharyngioma patients treated with radiation therapy. Pediatr. Blood Cancer 52, 227–230.
Liu, X., Yu, Q., Zhang, Z., Zhang, Y., Li, Y., Liu, D., et al., 2012. Same-day stereotactic aspiration and Gamma Knife surgery for cystic intracranial tumors. J. Neurosurg. 117 (Suppl.), 45–48.
Love, J.G., 1950. MT: Craniopharyngiomas (pituitary adamantinomas). Surg. Gynecol. Obstet. 90, 591–601.
Luu, Q.T., Loredo, L.N., Archambeau, J.O., Yonemoto, L.T., Slater, J.M., Slater, J.D., 2006. Fractionated proton radiation treatment for pediatric craniopharyngioma: preliminary report. Cancer J. 12, 155–159.
Mayo, C., Martel, M.K., Marks, L.B., Flickinger, J., Nam, J., Kirkpatrick, J., 2010. Radiation dose-volume effects of optic nerves and chiasm. Int. J. Radiat. Oncol. Biol. Phys. 76, S28–35.
Merchant, T.E., Kiehna, E.N., Sanford, R.A., Mulhern, R.K., Thompson, S.J., Wilson, M.W., et al., 2002. Craniopharyngioma: the St. Jude Children's Research Hospital experience 1984–2001. Int. J. Radiat. Oncol. Biol. Phys. 53, 533–542.
Merchant, T.E., Kiehna, E.N., Kun, L.E., Mulhern, R.K., Li, C., Xiong, X., et al., 2006. Phase II trial of conformal radiation therapy for pediatric patients with craniopharyngioma and correlation of surgical factors and radiation dosimetry with change in cognitive function. J. Neurosurg. 104, 94–102.
Minamida, Y., Mikami, T., Hashi, K., Houkin, K., 2005. Surgical management of the recurrence and regrowth of craniopharyngiomas. J. Neurosurg. 103, 224–232.
Minniti, G., Traish, D., Ashley, S., Gonsalves, A., Brada, M., 2005. Risk of second brain tumor after conservative surgery and radiotherapy for pituitary adenoma: update after an additional 10 years. J. Clin. Endocrinol. Metab. 90, 800–804.
Minniti, G., Saran, F., Traish, D., Soomal, R., Sardell, S., Gonsalves, A., et al., 2007. Fractionated stereotactic conformal radiotherapy following conservative surgery in the control of craniopharyngiomas. Radiother. Oncol. 82, 90–95.
Minniti, G., Esposito, V., Amichetti, M., Enrici, R.M., 2009. The role of fractionated radiotherapy and radiosurgery in the management of patients with craniopharyngioma. Neurosurg. Rev. 32, 125–132 discussion 132.
Mokry, M., 1999. Craniopharyngiomas: A six year experience with Gamma Knife radiosurgery. Stereotact. Funct. Neurosurg. 72 (Suppl. 1), 140–149.
Moon, S.H., Kim, I.H., Park, S.W., Kim, I., Hong, S., Park, C.I., et al., 2005. Early adjuvant radiotherapy toward long-term survival and better quality of life for craniopharyngiomas – a study in single institute. Childs Nerv. Syst. 21, 799–807.
Niranjan, A., Kano, H., Mathieu, D., Kondziolka, D., Flickinger, J.C., Lunsford, L.D., 2009. Radiosurgery for craniopharyngioma. Int. J. Radiat. Oncol. Biol. Phys. 78, 64–71.
Park, K.J., Niranjan, A., Kondziolka, D., Kano, H., Castillo, P., Matchett, J.C., et al., 2011. Combining brain diagnosis and therapy in a single strategy: the safety, reliability, and cost implications using same-day versus separate-day stereotactic procedures. Stereotact. Funct. Neurosurg. 89, 346–356.
Peace, K.A., Orme, S.M., Sebastian, J.P., Thompson, A.R., Barnes, S., Ellis, A., et al., 1997. The effect of treatment variables on mood and social adjustment in adult patients with pituitary disease. Clin. Endocrinol. (Oxf) 46, 445–450.
Pemberton, L.S., Dougal, M., Magee, B., Gattamaneni, H.R., 2005. Experience of external beam radiotherapy given adjuvantly or at relapse following surgery for craniopharyngioma. Radiother. Oncol. 77, 99–104.
Prasad, D., Steiner, M., Steiner, L., 1995. Gamma knife surgery for craniopharyngioma. Acta Neurochir. (Wien) 134, 167–176.
Rajan, B., Ashley, S., Gorman, C., Jose, C.C., Horwich, A., Bloom, H.J., et al., 1993. Craniopharyngioma – a long-term results following limited surgery and radiotherapy. Radiother. Oncol. 26, 1–10.
Rajan, B., Ashley, S., Thomas, D.G., Marsh, H., Britton, J., Brada, M., 1997. Craniopharyngioma: improving outcome by early recognition and treatment of acute complications. Int. J. Radiat. Oncol. Biol. Phys. 37, 517–521.
Regine, W.F., Mohiuddin, M., Kramer, S., 1993. Long-term results of pediatric and adult craniopharyngiomas treated with combined surgery and radiation. Radiother. Oncol. 27, 13–21.
Sayer, F.T., Sherman, J.H., Yen, C.P., Schlesinger, D.J., Kersh, R., Sheehan, J.P., 2011. Initial experience with the eXtend System: a relocatable frame system for multiple-session gamma knife radiosurgery. World Neurosurg. 75, 665–672.

Schlesinger, D., Xu, Z., Taylor, F., Yen, C.P., Sheehan, J., 2012. Interfraction and intrafraction performance of the Gamma Knife Extend system for patient positioning and immobilization. J. Neurosurg. 117 (Suppl.), 217–224.

Schoenfeld, A., Pekmezci, M., Barnes, M.J., Tihan, T., Gupta, N., Lamborn, K.R., Banerjee, A., Mueller, S., Chang, S., Berger, M.S., Haas-Kogan, D., 2011. The superiority of conservative resection and adjuvant radiation for craniopharyngiomas. J. Neurooncol. 108, 133–139.

Scott, R.M., 2005. Craniopharyngioma: a personal (Boston) experience. Childs Nerv. Syst. 21, 773–777.

Shi, X.E., Wu, B., Fan, T., Zhou, Z.Q., Zhang, Y.L., 2008. Craniopharyngioma: surgical experience of 309 cases in China. Clin. Neurol. Neurosurg. 110, 151–159.

Shirane, R., Ching-Chan, S., Kusaka, Y., Jokura, H., Yoshimoto, T., 2002. Surgical outcomes in 31 patients with craniopharyngiomas extending outside the suprasellar cistern: an evaluation of the frontobasal interhemispheric approach. J. Neurosurg. 96, 704–712.

Stripp, D.C., Maity, A., Janss, A.J., Belasco, J.B., Tochner, Z.A., Goldwein, J.W., et al., 2004. Surgery with or without radiation therapy in the management of craniopharyngiomas in children and young adults. Int. J. Radiat. Oncol. Biol. Phys. 58, 714–720.

Tomita, T., Bowman, R.M., 2005. Craniopharyngiomas in children: surgical experience at Children's Memorial Hospital. Childs Nerv. Syst. 21, 729–746.

Ulfarsson, E., Lindquist, C., Roberts, M., Rahn, T., Lindquist, M., Thoren, M., et al., 2002. Gamma knife radiosurgery for craniopharyngiomas: long-term results in the first Swedish patients. J. Neurosurg. 97, 613–622.

Ullrich, N.J., Robertson, R., Kinnamon, D.D., Scott, R.M., Kieran, M.W., Turner, C.D., et al., 2007. Moyamoya following cranial irradiation for primary brain tumors in children. Neurology 68, 932–938.

Van Effenterre, R., Boch, A.L., 2002. Craniopharyngioma in adults and children: a study of 122 surgical cases. J. Neurosurg. 97, 3–11.

Varlotto, J.M., Flickinger, J.C., Kondziolka, D., Lunsford, L.D., Deutsch, M., 2002. External beam irradiation of craniopharyngiomas: long-term analysis of tumor control and morbidity. Int. J. Radiat. Oncol. Biol. Phys. 54, 492–499.

Weiss, M., Sutton, L., Marcial, V., Fowble, B., Packer, R., Zimmerman, R., et al., 1989. The role of radiation therapy in the management of childhood craniopharyngioma. Int. J. Radiat. Oncol. Biol. Phys. 17, 1313–1321.

Wen, B.C., Hussey, D.H., Staples, J., Hitchon, P.W., Jani, S.K., Vigliotti, A.P., et al., 1989. A comparison of the roles of surgery and radiation therapy in the management of craniopharyngiomas. Int. J. Radiat. Oncol. Biol. Phys. 16, 17–24.

Wen, D.Y., Seljeskog, E.L., Haines, S.J., 1992. Microsurgical management of craniopharyngiomas. Br. J. Neurosurg. 6, 467–474.

Winkfield, K.M., Linsenmeier, C., Yock, T.I., Grant, P.E., Yeap, B.Y., Butler, W.E., et al., 2009. Surveillance of craniopharyngioma cyst growth in children treated with proton radiotherapy. Int. J. Radiat. Oncol. Biol. Phys. 73, 716–721.

Xu, Z., Yen, C.P., Schlesinger, D., Sheehan, J., 2010. Outcomes of Gamma Knife surgery for craniopharyngiomas. J. Neurooncol. 104, 305–313.

Xu, Z., Lee Vance, M., Schlesinger, D., Sheehan, J.P., 2013. Hypopituitarism after stereotactic radiosurgery for pituitary adenomas. Neurosurgery 72, 630–637; 636–637.

Yasargil, M.G., Curcic, M., Kis, M., Siegenthaler, G., Teddy, P.J., Roth, P., 1990. Total removal of craniopharyngiomas. Approaches and long-term results in 144 patients. J. Neurosurg. 73, 3–11.

Yomo, S., Hayashi, M., Chernov, M., Tamura, N., Izawa, M., Okada, Y., et al., 2009. Stereotactic radiosurgery of residual or recurrent craniopharyngioma: new treatment concept using Leksell gamma knife model C with automatic positioning system. Stereotact. Funct. Neurosurg. 87, 360–367.

Yu, X., Liu, Z., Li, S., 2000. Combined treatment with stereotactic intracavitary irradiation and gamma knife surgery for craniopharyngiomas. Stereotact. Funct. Neurosurg. 75, 117–122.

Zuccaro, G., 2005. Radical resection of craniopharyngioma. Childs Nerv. Syst. 21, 679–690.

CHAPTER

20

Stereotactic Radiosurgery as Part of Multimodality Craniopharyngioma Management

Irene Kim, Eugenia Shekhtman, Jeffrey H. Wisoff, Douglas Kondziolka

Department of Neurosurgery, NYU Langone Medical Center, New York, NY, USA

"It would therefore seem feasible to replace the needle by narrow beams of radiant energy directed at the target in the brain and thereby produce a local destruction of the lesion." **Lars Leksell, 1951**

INTRODUCTION

Craniopharyngiomas are slow-growing neuroepithelial tumors arising from the remnants of Rathke's pouch within the sellar and suprasellar space. They occur in a bimodal age distribution, occurring in children from 5–15 years old and adults from 50–75 years of age. Tumors can be solid, cystic, or mixed. Given their benign histology, gross total resection is the optimal treatment for a cure if it can be performed safely. However, the location of these tumors can make complete resection difficult without incurring debilitating endocrine, visual, and cognitive deficits. The tumor can also surround the cerebral arteries, further increasing the risk of pursuing gross total resection (GTR). When GTR is not possible without unacceptable patient risk, irradiation is an effective option for improving survival and slowing the rate of tumor progression.

Residual craniopharyngioma tends to recur and leads to increased morbidity and mortality over several years. Radiation can be used as an adjuvant to treat residual tumor after subtotal resection (STR), as primary therapy, or to treat recurrence which is not amenable to surgery. Many surgeons now favor a multimodal approach, consisting of a combination of surgical resection with adjuvant radiation for any remaining tumor. The extent of tumor surgery varies along the spectrum from biopsy and/or cyst aspiration to subtotal resection, depending on multiple factors including the patient's age, comorbidities, and tumor characteristics

Craniopharyngiomas
http://dx.doi.org/10.1016/B978-0-12-416706-3.00020-9

(Veeravagu et al., 2010). The radiation options include conformal fractional irradiation, stereotactic radiosurgery (SRS), fractionated stereotactic radiotherapy, and intracavitary irradiation.

RADIATION THERAPY

Fractionated radiation therapy (RT) was the first radiation modality to be used for the treatment of craniopharyngioma, beginning in the 1950s. Kramer et al. treated ten patients with high-voltage radiation consisting of 55–70 gray (Gy), depending on patient age, over the course of 6–7 weeks, after only minimal surgical treatment consisting of cyst aspiration and/or biopsy. They obtained good results, with nine out of ten patients alive at 7-year follow-up (one patient died of unrelated causes), and with only one patient showing evidence of recurrence (Kramer et al., 1961). Regine et al. evaluated 58 patients from 1958 to 1982 who were treated with external beam radiation of 55–65 Gy, with 40 of those patients undergoing radiation as their primary treatment. Recurrence rates were low; 26% for adults and 18% for children at 17-year follow-up. They noted fewer recurrences with higher doses of radiation (44% recurrence for < 54 Gy vs. 16% for > 54 Gy), but more complications with doses > 61 Gy, proposing 55 Gy as the optimal dose for treatment (Regine et al., 1993).

Subsequent studies looked at using RT as an adjuvant therapy along with STR. With STR alone, the tumor progression rate has been shown to be 55–85% (Amacher, 1980; Weiss et al., 1989; Wen et al., 1989; Rajan et al., 1993; Stripp et al., 2004). The use of RT in conjunction with varying amounts of tumor resection decreases the rate of recurrence to 15–30% (Lichter et al., 1977; Wen et al., 1989; Hetelekidis et al., 1993; Regine et al., 1993; Merchant et al., 2002; Stripp et al., 2004). In a 24-patient series by Varlotto et al., most of which were treated with RT following STR, survival rate was 100% at 10 years and 92% at 20 years, with the optimum outcome-free survival noted at doses between 55–63 Gy (Varlotto et al., 2002). Habrand et al. also observed improvement in survival in patients who underwent adjuvant RT following resection or after recurrence, with the best results noted with 55 Gy or greater (Habrand et al., 1999). However, other studies did not show a difference in tumor control response based on the dose of radiation. Wen et al. showed that 50–55 Gy was as effective as higher doses (55–60 and 60–70 Gy), and had fewer associated complications (Wen et al., 1989); this was also supported later by Mark et al. in their series of 49 post-resection patients (Mark et al., 1995). While it is unclear whether there is a definite dose–response correlation, 54–56 Gy at 180 centigray (cGy) per fraction appears to be the optimum range for maximizing tumor control and minimizing patient morbidity.

The target in RT is defined as the imaging-defined tumor with an additional margin of 5–10 mm, including any cystic components. The first use of RT in the 1950s involved parallel opposed portals, which resulted in a high dose of radiation to the temporal lobes. Increasingly, modern linear accelerators allow the radiation to be distributed through two or more 180 degree or one 360 degree arcs in order to minimize radiation to the surrounding brain. In the 1960s this was done by placing a plaster cap onto a patient's head and using it to map the distance to the site of the tumor (Kramer et al., 1961). As use of MRI became widespread, three-dimensional conformal radiation became possible, with more accurate visualization of the tumor and better avoidance of surrounding structures, such as the pituitary gland and optic nerves.

Since most centers use RT as an adjunct to surgery, it is difficult to determine how many of the adverse events can be attributed to just RT alone as opposed to treatment in general, or even the natural progression of the disease. Furthermore, it is possible that very long-term effects and/or complications are under-reported given the relative dearth of such outcome data in the craniopharyngioma literature. SRS with RT is generally shown to have improved survival, and several studies have shown that the multimodality treatment had similar or fewer side effects than surgery alone (Weiss et al., 1989; Brada and Thomas, 1993; Hetelekidis et al., 1993; Rajan et al., 1993; Merchant et al., 2002). The most common complication was pituitary dysfunction, seen in 20–80% of patients, and varying from mild diabetes insipidus (DI) and/or growth hormone (GH) insufficiency to panhypopituitarism (Hetelekidis et al., 1993; Regine et al., 1993; Habrand et al., 1999; Stripp et al., 2004; Niranjan et al., 2010). Visual problems including visual field deficits were seen in 10–15% of patients, some of which was secondary to hydrocephalus or enlargement of the cystic component of the tumor (Minniti et al., 2009). Optic neuropathy was found in 2–8% at higher doses; these decreased to 1–1.5% with doses of 55 Gy or lower (Mark et al., 1995; Varlotto et al., 2002; Niranjan et al., 2010). Changes in IQ did not demonstrate a statistically significant difference between the surgery and the multiple modality treatment groups (Merchant et al., 2002).

Vascular injury and secondary malignancy are always a concern in radiation treatment. Moyamoya syndrome following irradiation to vascular locations, such as the sellar and parasellar regions, has been recognized in the past. The incidence of Moyamoya vasculopathy following radiation is 2–4% in the craniopharyngioma literature (Hetelekidis et al., 1993; Varlotto et al., 2002). Secondary malignancy is an uncommonly seen event, but is nonetheless a concern for the overall prognosis, especially in young children. In a literature review from 1989, Weiss et al. noted one patient who developed sarcoma after high-dose RT (144 Gy over 3 years), two patients developed malignant astrocytomas after 60 Gy, and one patient was found to have glioblastoma multiforme (GBM) after 54 Gy (Weiss et al., 1989). Habrand et al. noted one in-field GBM at 9 years (Habrand et al., 1999). In a series of 334 patients treated with surgery and RT for pituitary adenoma, the rate of secondary malignancy was 1.3% over the first 10 years, and 1.9% over 20 years. Two of the patients developed astrocytoma, two had meningioma, and one had meningeal sarcoma (Brada et al., 1992).

STEREOTACTIC RADIOSURGERY

More recently, SRS has been used as an adjunctive in the treatment of craniopharyngiomas. In SRS, multiple beams are utilized to deliver a high dose of radiation to a very focal, stereotactically targeted volume, usually in a single dose and typically in no more than five doses (Veeravagu et al., 2010). The use of multiple beams allows a very steep radiation dose fall-off beyond the planned targeted field (Tarbell et al., 1994; Gopalan et al., 2008).

Gamma Knife (GK) radiosurgery is the predominant form of SRS for which details have been published on craniopharyngiomas. Developed by Lars Leksell in 1968, the GK unit contains 192–201 cobalt-60 (^{60}Co) gamma radiation-emitting sources arranged in a hemisphere (Wu et al., 1990; Minniti et al., 2009). It was originally designed for functional neurosurgical procedures to treat movement disorders, pain, and refractory behavioral disorders (Wu et al., 1990). It was subsequently used for the treatment of tumors, and Leksell was among the first to use GK in the treatment of craniopharyngiomas (Kobayashi et al., 2005). GK is best suited for smaller tumors (< 3 cm in diameter) with a predominant solid component, and ideally, is at least a few millimeters away from the optic apparatus; smaller cystic or mixed tumors near the optic apparatus are also appropriate targets (Kobayashi et al., 1994; Suh and Gupta, 2006; Veeravagu et al., 2010).

GK radiosurgery requires application of the Leksell stereotactic headframe. This is usually placed under local anesthesia for adolescents and adults and under general anesthesia for children (Mokry, 1999; Xu et al., 2011). High-resolution gadolinium-enhanced MR images are obtained with the head frame in place, which are then used to plan the radiosurgery. The enhancing tumor serves as the target for the procedure, including both solid and cystic components. However, many centers report that in certain tumors where there is a large cystic component, particularly near the optic apparatus, only the solid tumor is targeted (Mokry, 1999; Chiou et al., 2001; Kobayashi et al., 2005; Niranjan et al., 2010; Xu et al., 2011). Only one treatment session is required for GK.

There is no definitive consensus on the treatment dose for craniopharyngiomas, although the mean marginal dose appears to be approximately 12 Gy in many studies. In the largest described series to date, Kobayashi et al. treated 98 patients with a mean maximum dose of 21.8 Gy and a mean tumor margin dose of 11.5 Gy (Kobayashi et al., 2005). Similarly, in their series of 31 patients, Chung et al. reported a mean maximum dose of 24.2 Gy with a mean margin dose of 12.2 Gy (Chung et al., 2000). One review of ten case series reported a mean marginal dose of 12.3 Gy, while another review of eight studies noted a median marginal dose of 12 Gy (Gopalan et al., 2008; Minniti et al., 2009).

The treatment dose for GK is limited primarily because of its location adjacent to structures that are less tolerant of radiation, namely the optic apparatus. It had generally been believed that the limiting dose to the optic apparatus was 8 Gy in a single fraction (Tishler et al., 1993). Leber et al. subsequently demonstrated that up to 10 Gy could be tolerated without risk of optic neuropathy (Leber et al., 1998). More recently, Hasegawa et al. suggested that the optic apparatus may be even more tolerant than previously thought, and able to tolerate up to 14 Gy in specific circumstances (Hasegawa et al., 2010).

Craniopharyngiomas appear to be relatively radiosensitive, especially the solid components of these tumors (see Figure 20.1). Serial imaging demonstrates that in response to GK, there is an initial progressive loss of central enhancement followed by cystic changes and tumor regression (Chung et al., 2000). Kobayashi noted a 79.6% tumor control rate with complete response in 19.4% of patients at a mean follow-up period of 65.5 months (Kobayashi et al., 2005). Chung et al. reported a tumor control rate of 87.2%, with complete response in 32.7% of patients (Chung et al., 2000). In their review of ten case series, Gopalan et al. found the mean tumor control rate was 75%, with a 90% control rate in solid tumors and a 58.6% control rate in mixed tumors (Gopalan et al., 2008). Another review of eight studies by Minniti et al. demonstrated similar results with an overall tumor control rate of 69% at a median follow-up of 57 months, with control rates of 90% in solid tumors, 88% in cystic tumors, and 60% in mixed tumors (Minniti et al., 2009).

In general, GK is well tolerated in properly selected patients. Gopalan et al. reported an overall morbidity rate of 4% and mortality rate of 0.5% (Gopalan et al., 2008). Kobayashi et al. reported a morbidity rate of 6.1% in their large series (Kobayashi et al., 2005). In their series of 46 patients, Niranjan et al. reported an overall 5-year survival rate of 97.1%. Of the

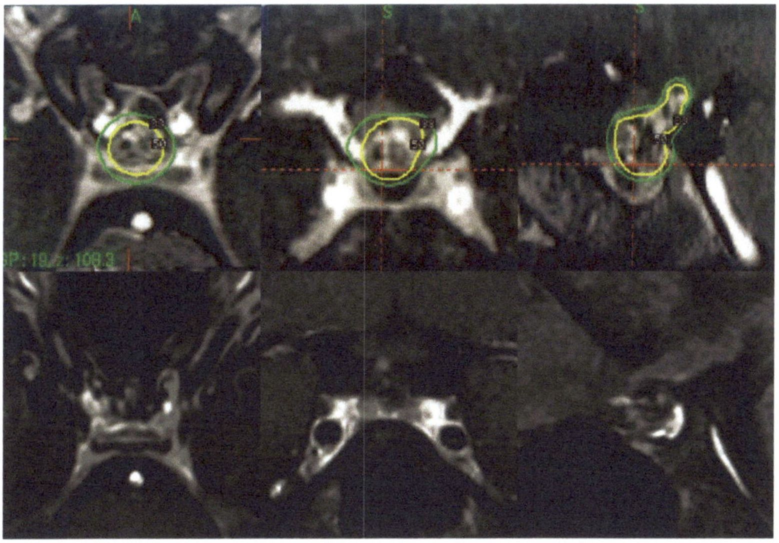

FIGURE 20.1 Axial, coronal, and sagittal MR images at radiosurgery (top) and 12 years later (bottom) for a 5-year-old boy who had stereotactic ^{32}P intracavitary irradiation for two tumor cysts with complete regression, and then GK radiosurgery to a solid tumor nodule (shown). Significant regression of the tumor remnant was maintained. Normal vision was preserved.

five patient deaths in their series, three were due to tumor progression of unresectable tumors with brainstem infiltration, one was secondary to status epilepticus, and one was from an unidentified etiology (Niranjan et al., 2010). The most common morbidities from GK are secondary to visual deterioration and endocrine dysfunction, most commonly DI. In their series, Niranjan et al. noted that 8% of patients with normal visual fields developed homonymous hemianopsias from tumor progression after GK. Of patients with visual field defects prior to the procedure, 26.3% had progression of their visual field defects secondary to tumor progression despite GK, while 10.5% had resolution of their visual defects in conjunction with their tumor regression. With respect to pituitary function, they noted that all patients with normal pituitary function and all patients with panhypopituitarism prior to GK radiosurgery remained unchanged after the procedure. Of 15 patients with anterior lobe hypopituitarism, one patient noted improvement and one patient progressed to panhypopituitarism without tumor progression after GK radiosurgery (Niranjan et al., 2010).

CyberKnife (CK) is another form of SRS. CK is a linear accelerator attached to a robotic arm with six degrees of freedom of movement (Veeravagu et al., 2010; Kortmann, 2011; Iwata et al., 2012). Instead of fixating a headframe to the patient, patients are immobilized in a custom-molded thermoplastic mask, which can be used over multiple sessions (Minniti et al., 2009; Iwata et al., 2012). This is utilized in combination with a frameless, image-guided, target-locating system, which can be adjusted for patient movement. Treatment with CK usually requires multiple sessions, typically 3–5 sessions, but as many as ten sessions have been described (Lee et al., 2008; Iwata et al., 2012).

Far fewer studies have been performed using CK for the treatment of craniopharyngiomas than GK, but these studies indicate that tumors are responsive to CK. In one small study of 11 patients, Lee et al. reported a 91% tumor control rate at a mean follow-up of 15.4 months (Lee et al., 2008). In another series of 43 patients, Iwata et al. reported a local control rate of 85% at 3 years and 65% at 5 years (Iwata et al., 2012).

Proton beam SRS is another form of SRS, which will be discussed in another chapter.

INTRACAVITARY IRRADIATION

In addition to SRS, the use of intracavitary or intracystic irradiation, also sometimes referred to as intracavitary brachytherapy, has been explored in the treatment of predominantly cystic craniopharyngiomas. First described by Leksell and Liden in the 1950s, the procedure is performed by using a fine needle to puncture the cyst or cysts under stereotactic guidance. The amount of radionuclide to be delivered is calculated using a standard formula based on the cyst volume. This calculation can be difficult for very small cysts. An equivalent volume of cyst fluid is first aspirated, before the radionuclide is then injected into the cysts. It is important not to alter the size and shape of the cyst, as this ensures even distribution of the radioisotope over the entire internal cyst wall without wall collapse or "wrinkling" (Backlund, 1994; Lunsford et al., 1994; Pollock et al., 1995; Voges et al., 1997).

The first radioisotope described in the literature was phosphorus-32 (^{32}P), a pure beta-emitting radionuclide with an effective radiation range of 0.9 mm, thereby minimizing the radiation dose to the adjacent normal tissues, and a half-life of 14 days (Backlund, 1994; Lunsford et al., 1994). Yttrium-90 (^{90}Y), which has a much shorter half-life of 3 days, was also tried with good results (Lunsford et al., 1994). However, studies comparing ^{32}P and ^{90}Y are limited, because ^{32}P is the only radioisotope approved for use in the United States, while ^{90}Y is much more widely used throughout Europe and Japan (Pollock et al., 1995). A variety of other beta-emitting radioisotopes have been trialed for intracavitary radiation, including gold, bismuth, and rhenium, and determined to be unsuitable (Lunsford et al., 1994).

An ideal dose of beta irradiation induces gradual, progressive shrinkage of the cyst over the course of weeks to months (Backlund, 1994). Most studies indicate that a minimum dose of 200 Gy to the inside of the cyst wall is necessary for effective treatment with intracystic irradiation (Van den Berge et al., 1992; Backlund, 1994; Pollock et al., 1995; Voges et al., 1997). In their series of 62 patients treated with beta-emitting radioisotopes, Voges et al. noted a 79.5% tumor response rate; 83% of cysts treated with ^{90}Y and 87.5% of cysts treated with ^{32}P responded to treatment; four cysts treated with rhenium-186 (^{186}Re) did not respond to treatment (Voges et al., 1997). Van den Berge et al. noted a 90% tumor control rate in 31 patients treated with ^{90}Y (Van den Berge et al., 1992). Lunsford et al. reported a 96% cyst control rate with ^{32}P in 26 patients at a median follow-up of 31 months (Lunsford et al., 1994). Pollock et al. noted an 88% cyst regression rate in their series of 32 cysts treated with ^{32}P. However, 33% of their patients required additional surgical intervention for tumor resection (Pollock et al., 1995). Intracystic irradiation is generally well tolerated. Pollock et al. noted no cyst leakage in their patients (Pollock et al., 1995). Voges et al. noted cyst leakage in 10.2% of patients, with no subsequent sequelae noted (Voges et al., 1997). Intracavitary irradiation and radiosurgery can often be used together in patients with tumors that have a larger cystic component and a smaller residual solid component.

CONCLUSION

While radiation can be used as a stand-alone therapy to treat craniopharyngiomas, it is especially valuable as an adjuvant option in combination with other modalities, namely surgery. The availability of radiation options makes it possible to obtain good results with STR, while minimizing peri-operative morbidity. The surgeon can choose to incorporate post-resection RT, SRS, or intracystic irradiation as a proven method of increasing patient survival and quality of life. The use of radiation as monotherapy or as adjuvant therapy in the overall treatment plan for a patient is one that must be determined by the surgeon and radiation oncologist in discussion with the patient and his/her family as it requires balancing the acute morbidities associated with surgery against the delayed consequences associated with radiation. In the future, randomized trials and further research may lead to the development of standardized algorithms of combined surgery and radiation treatment for craniopharyngiomas.

References

Amacher, A.L., 1980. Craniopharyngioma: the controversy regarding radiotherapy. Childs Brain 6, 57–64.

Backlund, E.O., 1994. Treatment of craniopharyngiomas: the multimodality approach. Pediatr. Neurosurg. 21, 82–89.

Brada, M., Ford, D., Ashley, S., Bliss, J.M., Crowley, S., Mason, M., Rajan, B., Traish, D., 1992. Risk of second brain tumour after conservative surgery and radiotherapy for pituitary adenoma. BMJ 304, 1343–1346.

Brada, M., Thomas, D.G., 1993. Craniopharyngioma revisited. Int. J. Radiat. Oncol. Biol. Phys. 27, 471–475.

Chiou, S.M., Lunsford, L.D., Niranjan, A., Kondziolka, D., Flickinger, J.C., 2001. Stereotactic radiosurgery of residual or recurrent craniopharyngioma, after surgery, with or without radiation therapy. Neuro. Oncol. 3, 159–166.

Chung, W.Y., Pan, D.H., Shiau, C.Y., Guo, W.Y., Wang, L.W., 2000. Gamma knife radiosurgery for craniopharyngiomas. J. Neurosurg. 93 (Suppl. 3), 47–56.

Gopalan, R., Dassoulas, K., Rainey, J., Sherman, J.H., Sheehan, J.P., 2008. Evaluation of the role of Gamma Knife surgery in the treatment of craniopharyngiomas. Neurosurg. Focus 24, E5.

Habrand, J.L., Ganry, O., Couanet, D., Rouxel, V., Levy-Piedbois, C., Pierre-Kahn, A., Kalifa, C., 1999. The role of radiation therapy in the management of craniopharyngioma: a 25-year experience and review of the literature. Int. J. Radiat. Oncol. Biol. Phys. 44, 255–263.

Hasegawa, T., Kobayashi, T., Kida, Y., 2010. Tolerance of the optic apparatus in single-fraction irradiation using stereotactic radiosurgery: evaluation in 100 patients with craniopharyngioma. Neurosurgery 66, 688–694 discussion 694–5.

Hetelekidis, S., Barnes, P.D., Tao, M.L., Fischer, E.G., Schneider, L., Scott, R.M., Tarbell, N.J., 1993. 20-year experience in childhood craniopharyngioma. Int. J. Radiat. Oncol. Biol. Phys. 27, 189–195.

Iwata, H., Tatewaki, K., Inoue, M., Yokota, N., Baba, Y., Nomura, R., Shibamoto, Y., Sato, K., 2012. Single and hypofractionated stereotactic radiotherapy with CyberKnife for craniopharyngioma. J. Neuro. Oncol. 106, 571–577.

Kobayashi, T., Kida, Y., Mori, Y., Hasegawa, T., 2005. Long-term results of gamma knife surgery for the treatment of craniopharyngioma in 98 consecutive cases. J. Neurosurg. Pediatr. 103, 482–488.

Kobayashi, T., Tanaka, T., Kida, Y., 1994. Stereotactic gamma radiosurgery of craniopharyngiomas. Pediatr. Neurosurg. 21 (Suppl. 1), 69–74.

Kortmann, R.D., 2011. Different approaches in radiation therapy of craniopharyngioma. Front. Endocrinol. 2, 1–2.

Kramer, S., Mckissock, W., Concannon, J.P., 1961. Craniopharyngiomas. Treatment by combined surgery and radiation therapy. J. Neurosurg. 18, 217–226.

Leber, K.A., Bergloff, J., Pendl, G., 1998. Dose-response tolerance of the visual pathways and cranial nerves of the cavernous sinus to stereotactic radiosurgery. J. Neurosurg. 88, 43–50.

Lee, M., Kalani, M.Y., Cheshier, S., Gibbs, I.C., Adler, J.R., Chang, S.D., 2008. Radiation therapy and CyberKnife radiosurgery in the management of craniopharyngiomas. Neurosurg. Focus 24, E4.

Leksell, L., 1951. The stereotaxic method and radiosurgery of the brain. Acta Chir. Scand. 102, 316–319.

Lichter, A.S., Wara, W.M., Sheline, G.E., Townsend, J.J., Wilson, C.B., 1977. The treatment of craniopharyngiomas. Int. J. Radiat. Oncol. Biol. Phys. 2, 675–683.

Lunsford, L.D., Pollock, B.E., Kondziolka, D.S., Levine, G., Flickinger, J.C., 1994. Stereotactic options in the management of craniopharyngioma. Pediatr. Neurosurg. 21 (Suppl. 1), 90–97.

Mark, R.J., Lutge, W.R., Shimizu, K.T., Tran, L.M., Selch, M.T., Parker, R.G., 1995. Craniopharyngioma: treatment in the CT and MR imaging era. Radiology 197, 195–198.

Merchant, T.E., Kiehna, E.N., Sanford, R.A., Mulhern, R.K., Thompson, S.J., Wilson, M.W., Lustig, R.H., Kun, L.E., 2002. Craniopharyngioma: the St. Jude Children's Research Hospital experience 1984–2001. Int. J. Radiat. Oncol. Biol. Phys. 53, 533–542.

Minniti, G., Esposito, V., Amichetti, M., Enrici, R.M., 2009. The role of fractionated radiotherapy and radiosurgery in the management of patients with craniopharyngioma. Neurosurg. Rev. 32, 125–132.

Mokry, M., 1999. Craniopharyngiomas: A six year experience with Gamma Knife radiosurgery. Stereotact. Funct. Neurosurg. 72, 140–149.

Niranjan, A., Kano, H., Mathieu, D., Kondziolka, D., Flickinger, J.C., Lunsford, L.D., 2010. Radiosurgery for craniopharyngioma. Int. J. Radiat. Oncol. Biol. Phys. 78, 64–71.

Pollock, B.E., Lunsford, L.D., Kondziolka, D., Levine, G., Flickinger, J.C., 1995. Phosphorus-32 intracavitary irradiation of cystic craniopharyngiomas: current technique and long-term results. Int. J. Radiat. Oncol. Biol. Phys. 33, 437–446.

Rajan, B., Ashley, S., Gorman, C., Jose, C.C., Horwich, A., Bloom, H.J., Marsh, H., Brada, M., 1993. Craniopharyngioma – long-term results following limited surgery and radiotherapy. Radiother. Oncol. 26, 1–10.

Regine, W.F., Mohiuddin, M., Kramer, S., 1993. Long-term results of pediatric and adult craniopharyngiomas treated with combined surgery and radiation. Radiother. Oncol. 27, 13–21.

Stripp, D.C., Maity, A., Janss, A.J., Belasco, J.B., Tochner, Z.A., Goldwein, J.W., Moshang, T., Rorke, L.B., Phillips, P.C., Sutton, L.N., Shu, H.K., 2004. Surgery with or without radiation therapy in the management of craniopharyngiomas in children and young adults. Int. J. Radiat. Oncol. Biol. Phys. 58, 714–720.

Suh, J.H., Gupta, N., 2006. Role of radiation therapy and radiosurgery in the management of craniopharyngiomas. Neurosurg. Clin. N. Am. 17, 143–148, vi–vii.

Tarbell, N.J., Barnes, P., Scott, R.M., Goumnerova, L., Pomeroy, S.L., Black, P.M., Sallan, S.E., Billett, A., Lavally, B., Helmus, A., et al., 1994. Advances in radiation therapy for craniopharyngiomas. Pediatr. Neurosurg. 21 (Suppl. 1), 101–107.

Tishler, R.B., Loeffler, J.S., Lunsford, L.D., Duma, C., Alexander 3rd, E., Kooy, H.M., Flickinger, J.C., 1993. Tolerance of cranial nerves of the cavernous sinus to radiosurgery. Int. J. Radiat. Oncol. Biol. Phys. 27, 215–221.

Van Den Berge, J.H., Blaauw, G., Breeman, W.A., Rahmy, A., Wijngaarde, R., 1992. Intracavitary brachytherapy of cystic craniopharyngiomas. J. Neurosurg. 77, 545–550.

Varlotto, J.M., Flickinger, J.C., Kondziolka, D., Lunsford, L.D., Deutsch, M., 2002. External beam irradiation of craniopharyngiomas: long-term analysis of tumor control and morbidity. Int. J. Radiat. Oncol. Biol. Phys. 54, 492–499.

Veeravagu, A., Lee, M., Jiang, B., Chang, S.D., 2010. The role of radiosurgery in the treatment of craniopharyngiomas. Neurosurg. Focus 28, E11.

Voges, J., Sturm, V., Lehrke, R., Treuer, H., Gauss, C., Berthold, F., 1997. Cystic craniopharyngioma: long-term results after intracavitary irradiation with stereotactically applied colloidal beta-emitting radioactive sources. Neurosurgery 40, 263–269 discussion 269–70.

Weiss, M., Sutton, L., Marcial, V., Fowble, B., Packer, R., Zimmerman, R., Schut, L., Bruce, D., D'angio, G., 1989. The role of radiation therapy in the management of childhood craniopharyngioma. Int. J. Radiat. Oncol. Biol. Phys. 17, 1313–1321.

Wen, B.C., Hussey, D.H., Staples, J., Hitchon, P.W., Jani, S.K., Vigliotti, A.P., Doornbos, J.F., 1989. A comparison of the roles of surgery and radiation therapy in the management of craniopharyngiomas. Int. J. Radiat. Oncol. Biol. Phys. 16, 17–24.

Wu, A., Lindner, G., Maitz, A.H., Kalend, A.M., Lunsford, L.D., Flickinger, J.C., Bloomer, W.D., 1990. Physics of gamma knife approach on convergent beams in stereotactic radiosurgery. Int. J. Radiat. Oncol. Biol. Phys. 18, 941–949.

Xu, Z., Yen, C.P., Schlesinger, D., Sheehan, J., 2011. Outcomes of Gamma Knife surgery for craniopharyngiomas. J. Neurooncol. 104, 305–313.

CHAPTER

21

Linear Accelerator-Based Fractionated Radiotherapy

Arif N. Ali, Walter J. Curran

Department of Radiation Oncology and Winship Cancer Institute, Emory University, Atlanta, GA, USA

"I feel sure that certain brain tumors, which today are treated inadequately, will be removed successfully or, if not removed, will be destroyed by other means." **Ernest Sachs, 1949**

PRINCIPLES OF FRACTIONATED RADIOTHERAPY (FRT)

The benefit of fractionated radiation therapy lies primarily in its ability to preferentially reduce tumor cell populations while sparing normal tissue. The energies of the photons produced by modern linear accelerators (LINACs) are generally between 4 MV and 18 MV. At these energies, the photons interact with water to produce ionic radicals according to the following equation:

$$H_2O \rightarrow H_2O^+ + e^-$$

These radicals then react further with water to produce hydroxyl radicals according to the following:

$$H_2O^+ + H_2O \rightarrow H_3O^+ + OH$$

The hydroxyl radicals then diffuse into the nucleus and react with deoxyribonucleic acid (DNA) resulting in strand breaks within the double helix structure. This type of indirect action is believed to be responsible for approximately two-thirds of the cellular damage caused by ionizing radiation at LINAC energies, while the remaining one-third is believed to be due to direct action on DNA (Hall and Giaccia, 2006).

Given the fact that normal tissue is in close proximity to tumor, a typical radiation field will initially deliver equivalent damage to both tumor cells and adjacent normal cells. However, normal cells proliferate at a much slower rate than do tumor cells, and therefore they will have more time to repair the DNA damage prior to replication than tumor cells

Craniopharyngiomas
http://dx.doi.org/10.1016/B978-0-12-416706-3.00021-0

(Elkind et al., 1965; Bernier et al., 2004). If cells (normal or tumor) try to undergo cellular division with inherently damaged DNA, they will fail and ultimately die through mitotic catastrophe (Castedo et al., 2004). Thus, with every given fraction of radiation, proportionally more tumor cells will die than normal cells if enough time is allowed between fractions for normal tissue to repair sublethal damage, but not enough time for tumor cells to be able to repopulate. This preferential sparing of normal tissue over tumor tissue has been termed the therapeutic ratio.

One caveat to the therapeutic ratio advantages of fractionated radiation is that there must be a greater cell death response of tumor tissue to radiation than normal tissue at any given radiation fraction dose. If the two tissue types respond similarly with nearly equal cellular lethality, then there will be reduced benefit in the use of fractionated radiation.

A mathematical model, termed the linear-quadratic model, has been developed to predict the surviving fraction of cells as a function of radiation fraction dose (Douglas and Fowler, 1976; Fowler, 1989; Jones et al., 2001). This model is represented by the equation:

$$SF = e^{-\left(\alpha D + \beta D^2\right)}$$

where SF is the surviving fraction, D is the radiation fraction dose, and α and β are derived coefficients.

The ratio of the two coefficients, α and β, has been found to be a useful measure for comparing dose effect curves (Williams et al., 1985). Generally, a low α/β ratio corresponds to rather slowly proliferating, late responding tissue that is greatly spared when using the low individual fraction doses of conventionally fractionated radiation therapy (2 Gy). A high α/β ratio, however, corresponds to rapidly proliferating, acutely responding tissue that will preferentially die with conventionally fractionated radiation therapy. In general, normal tissue tends to have α/β ratios of around 1.5 to 5 Gy, whereas tumors that are highly responsive to fractionated radiation have α/β ratios from 6 to 14 Gy. Although the exact α/β ratio of craniopharyngiomas is unknown, it is generally believed to be low (Varlotto et al., 2002; Veeravagu et al., 2010). Even though craniopharyngiomas have a low α/β ratio, they still proliferate at a faster rate than normal brain tissue and therefore the therapeutic ratio benefits of fractionated radiation therapy should still theoretically be applicable.

In addition to exploiting the differences in sublethal repair to increase the therapeutic ratio, fractionated radiation also offers the potential benefit of delivering radiation during the most optimal, radiosensitive part of the cell cycle (redistribution). Cell cycle regulation has been proposed by some researchers as perhaps the most important determinant of sensitivity to radiation (Pawlik and Keyomarsi, 2004). The mechanism by which ionizing radiation causes cell death is primarily DNA damage resulting in mitotic catastrophe during cellular division. Due to the various types of DNA repair checkpoints, located at various time points during the cell cycle, there are some phases of the cell cycle that are inherently more sensitive to ionizing radiation than others (Withers, 1975). Specifically, the G_2-M phase is the most sensitive, while the G_1 and latter part of the S phase are the least sensitive (Pawlik and Keyomarsi, 2004). The administration of ionizing radiation can slow the progression of cells through the cell cycle and cause an accumulation of cells in the G_2 phase. Thus, an advantage of multiple fraction radiation over single fraction stereotactic radiosurgery is that an initial dose of radiation is given which results in a redistribution of a previously asynchronous cellular population to one that favors the G_2 phase. A second fraction of radiation is then given just as the cellular population has optimally redistributed to the more radiosensitive G_2-M phase (Marks, 1993; Elkind, 1997; Pawlik and Keyomarsi, 2004).

While fractionated radiation offers advantages over single fraction radiation regimens in terms of increased therapeutic ratio due to the cellular effects of sublethal repair and cell cycle redistribution, it also theoretically capitalizes on the effects of tumor re-oxygenation during the fractionated radiation course (Marks, 1993). In general, tumors contain a significant portion of hypoxic cells, usually within the central portions of the tumor, due to immature or ineffective intratumoral vasculature and/or transient closing of tumor blood vessels (Hall and Brenner, 1993; Hall and Giaccia, 2006). Multiple experiments have shown that the biological effect of ionizing radiation at energies typical of modern LINACs is highly dependent on the presence of oxygen (Railton et al., 1974). In fact, there may be up to a three-fold increase in biological effect in an oxygenated environment compared to hypoxic conditions, depending on the dose level (Dasu and Denekamp, 1998). Thus, a single fraction of X-ray (LINAC) radiation will kill proportionally more oxygenated cells than hypoxic cells. After a given fraction of radiation, re-oxygenation of previously hypoxic cells is believed to occur due to tumor reduction and opening of transiently closed blood vessels, thus allowing previously hypoxic cells to be aerated and killed by subsequent fractions of radiation (Hall and Brenner, 1993). However, it is currently unclear how much, if any, re-oxygenation occurs during a craniopharyngioma fractionated radiation course.

EVOLUTION OF FRACTIONATED RADIOTHERAPY TECHNOLOGY

For most of radiation oncology's history, the technology for the delivery of therapeutic radiation has remained rather stagnant, with developmental advances remaining few and far between. It has only been with the last 20–30 years that we have seen exponential growth and a series of quantum leaps made in the available radiation delivery technology, mostly due to previously unimaginable advances in computing technology and capability (Bernier et al., 2004).

Current radiation therapy machines (LINACs) are based on the principle of a traveling electromagnetic wave within the microwave range that carries and accelerates electrons. This results in higher-energy electrons, which then translates to higher-energy photons (X-rays) once they interact with a tungsten target. Modern commercial LINACs are capable of producing X-rays with energies in the range of 4 MV to 18 MV, compared to cobalt-60 teletherapy units which produce lower-energy γ-rays (1.17 MeV and 1.33 MeV). The higher energy of the LINACs allows more efficient penetration of dose, less surface dose (and thus less skin fibrosis), and a smaller penumbra. The drawback of LINACs is that they are more mechanically and electronically complex and thus require more maintenance and highly skilled maintenance personnel than cobalt units.

With the advent of modern computing technology came the capability to perform highly complex and exhaustive radiation dose calculations within fractions of a second. This allowed for a change in the paradigm of radiation treatment planning, from forward planning to inverse or automated planning. Forward planning involves the clinician first defining a target and then defining a radiation field arrangement and aperture geometry to cover the target. Once the fields have been defined, relatively simplistic calculations are performed to determine the amount of radiation to deliver (monitor units) through the field in order to sufficiently cover the target. Inverse planning, however, involves a radiation oncologist first defining a target and associated critical normal structures. Then, a sophisticated computer program utilizing modern radiation dosimetric prediction models (pencil beam, Monte Carlo, convolution-superposition, etc.) are implemented to optimize all aspects of the radiation delivery including such factors as field angles, field shape, intensity modulation within the field, dose delivery rate, etc. (Galvin et al., 2004).

The primary advantage of inverse planning is the ability to fully optimize an intensity modulated radiation therapy (IMRT) plan. IMRT delivery, as compared to three-dimensional conformal radiation therapy (3D-CRT), utilizes various hardware and software techniques to create variations in beam intensity within any given field. This results in highly conformal radiation plans with radiation dose regions that tightly embrace the irregular three-dimensional geometric shape of tumors, including surface invaginations (Teh et al., 1999; Intensity Modulated Radiation Therapy Collaborative Working Group, 2001; Galvin et al., 2004). Such a highly conformal plan theoretically allows for maximal delivery of radiation to the tumor with minimal radiation to normal structures, thus increasing the therapeutic ratio.

Other advances in radiation delivery for craniopharyngiomas stem from improvements in magnetic resonance imaging (MRI) and its incorporation into the treatment planning process with registration software from companies such as Velocity Medical Solutions (Atlanta, GA), Varian Medical Systems (Palo Alto, CA), or Mim Software Inc (Cleveland, OH) (Harwood-Nash, 1994; Choi et al., 2007; Schreibmann et al., 2009; Schreibmann et al., 2012). Prior to the availability of registration software, computed tomography (CT) simulation images were primarily used to define the boundaries of the craniopharyngioma. However, in comparison with a CT, MRI has been found to be vastly superior for the detection of the various cystic and solid tissue components of a craniopharyngioma (see Figure 21.1) (Pigeau et al., 1988). The incorporation of MRI into the treatment planning process offers a radiation

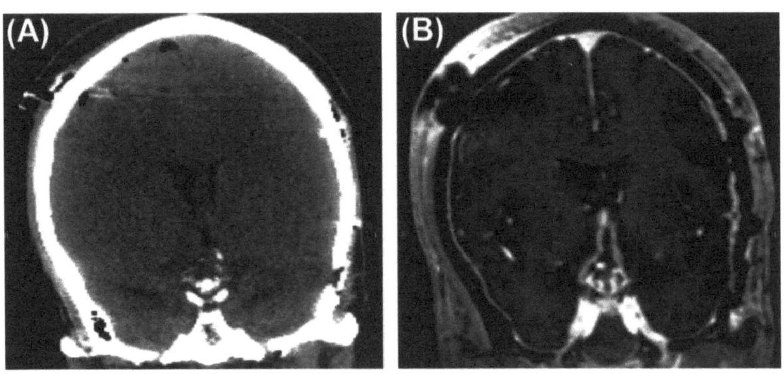

FIGURE 21.1 Comparison of post-op craniopharyngioma in **A,** helical CT and **B,** T1 post-contrast MRI. It is seen that though some of the calcified portion of the main tumor is identifiable on the CT image, the cystic wall and tumor boundaries are only able to be effectively visualized on MRI.

oncologist greater confidence in the tumor boundary, thus potentially allowing for a reduction in margin and a theoretical increase in the therapeutic ratio.

In addition to the use of MRI in the treatment planning process, advanced registration software has also allowed for an increase in the positional accuracy of frameless cranial fixation systems. Previously, in order to obtain the maximum possible positional accuracy, an external stereotactic headframe in direct contact with the patient's cranium was required. However, with the use of on-board cone beam CT scans, equivalent or near-equivalent positional accuracy may be obtained with frameless systems utilizing a non-invasive thermoplastic mask (Tryggestad et al., 2011). These systems involve placing the patient in a thermoplastic mask, performing a cone beam CT prior to every treatment, and then using registration software to match the CT simulation to the cone beam CT. The translational and rotational shifts generated by the matching algorithm are then physically applied to the treatment couch to further refine the target alignment, achieving millimeter to sub-millimeter accuracy (Tryggestad et al., 2011; Ohtakara et al., 2012; Rosenfelder et al., 2013; Ruschin et al., 2013).

Future technological directions to improve both positional accuracy and radiation target definition include the elimination of the CT to MRI registration process altogether with the use of an MRI simulator. Such an MRI simulator would allow direct target definition on the simulation image, but requires more complex dosimetric calculations and post-processing to account for image distortion (Stanescu et al., 2008, 2009; Devic, 2012; Rank et al., 2013).

CURRENT FRACTIONATED RADIOTHERAPY TECHNIQUE

The planning process for fractionated radiotherapy begins with a CT-based simulation. During the CT simulation, the patient is placed supine on the CT simulator couch and a thermoplastic mask or other, highly accurate, immobilization system is fitted to the patient. A CT scan with slice thickness varying from 0.5 mm to 2.5 mm is then performed with the patient immobilized and wearing the thermoplastic mask in the treatment planning position.

The use of MRI in the treatment planning process is, for the most part, a requirement in order to effectively delineate the tumor and define normal structures. A high-resolution (1.0 mm to 2.0 mm thick slices) axial MRI with and without gadolinium contrast is generally performed either a few days before or after a CT simulation and then registered to the CT simulation using specialized software.

The gross tumor volume (GTV) is defined on the MRI, as are the critical and relevant normal structures, including (but not limited to) the optic nerves, chiasm, lenses, globes, and brainstem. The GTV is then expanded by a certain margin to create the clinical tumor volume (CTV). The exact GTV to CTV margin expansion is at the discretion of the treating radiation oncologist and varies depending on the anatomy and specifics of each patient's tumor, but generally falls within the range of 3 mm to 10 mm. The CTV is then cropped anatomically to account for microscopic tumor spread and then expanded by an additional margin to create the planning tumor volume (PTV). The PTV will vary depending on the positional accuracy of the equipment used, but generally falls within the range of 3 mm to 5 mm with modern cranial fixation systems and daily on-board imaging.

The PTV is then treated to a prescription dose of 50–54 Gray (Gy) in standard fractionation (1.8–2.0 Gy per fraction). Given the generally young age of patients and proximity to critical structures, it is recommended that a high conformality radiation delivery technique be employed, including, but not limited to, IMRT, tomotherapy, or volumetric modulated arc therapy (VMAT). In rare instances in which such modern techniques are not available, three-dimensional conformal radiation therapy (3D-CRT) could be used but would be considered by many radiation oncologists to be sub-optimal. Margins, of course, would need to be adjusted for 3D-CRT.

Standard normal tissue constraints are used to minimize the risk of late toxicity (Mayo et al., 2010a, 2010b). While there is certainly some institutional variation in the normal tissue constraints implemented, common parameters include an optic nerve maximum radiotherapy (RT) dose less than 54 Gy, chiasm maximum dose less than 54 Gy, globe maximum dose less than 40 Gy, lens maximum dose less than 5 Gy, and brainstem maximum dose less than 54 Gy. Generally, there is very little difficulty in achieving these constraints with a conformal radiation delivery technique and standard treatment dose.

It has commonly been found that the cystic and/or solid component of a craniopharyngioma may temporarily expand during the 5–6-week fractionated radiotherapy course (Hamamoto et al., 2002; Winkfield et al., 2009; Beltran et al., 2010). Thus, given the reduced margins commonly implemented as part of modern IMRT or VMAT planning, it is possible for the tumor to grow beyond the high-dose treatment region during the radiation course. In order to account for this, many radiation oncologists will routinely order one or more MRIs during the radiation course and adjust the treated tumor volumes as necessary. If the cystic component of the tumor is large, due to medical or surgical inoperability, and clearly visible on CT, then weekly cone beam CTs could also be considered as an additional measure to ensure adequate target coverage (see Figure 21.2). Daily image-guided radiation therapy (IGRT) techniques utilizing two-dimensional kilovoltage (KV) imaging or other similar systems should be used, if available, to ensure optimal positional accuracy.

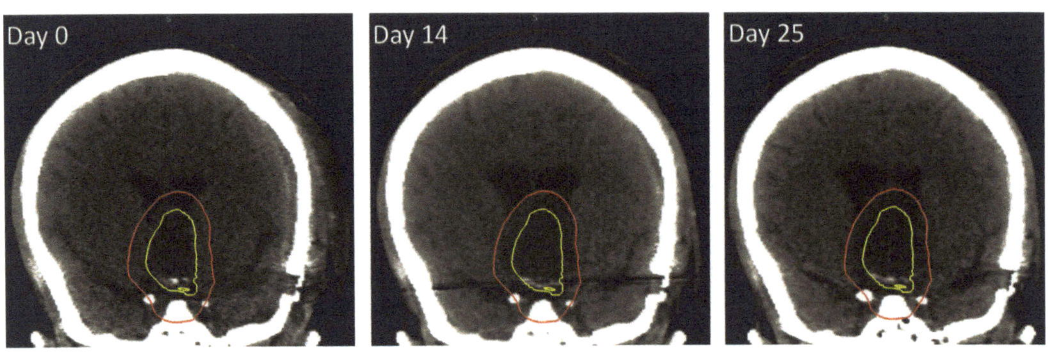

FIGURE 21.2 Selected serial CT images taken at the time of simulation (Day 0) and during treatment (Days 14 and 25). The GTV is delineated in yellow and the PTV is delineated in red. It can be seen that even though the cystic wall is not visible on CT, the hypodense fluid within the cystic component of the craniopharyngioma tumor is identifiable by CT imaging and continues to progress such that a re-plan is required mid-treatment.

LONG-TERM OUTCOMES WITH FRACTIONATED RADIOTHERAPY

Extent of Surgical Resection

Multiple retrospective series have evaluated the effect of adjuvant radiation on the local control, progression-free survival, and overall survival of craniopharyngioma patients (Sung et al., 1981; Wen et al., 1989; Hetelekidis et al., 1993; Rajan et al., 1993; Habrand et al., 1999; Stripp et al., 2004; Karavitaki et al., 2005; Schoenfeld et al., 2012; Masson-Cote et al., 2013). Many of these series simply compared patients that received only surgery of any extent with those that received surgery and radiation. These series concluded that, in general, the addition of radiation to surgery results in an improvement in progression-free survival (PFS) (Sung et al., 1981; Hetelekidis et al., 1993; Stripp et al., 2004).

However, some series looked more closely at the extent of surgical resection by stratifying patients into the various subcategories of gross total resection, subtotal resection, and biopsy only or no surgery (Wen et al., 1989; Rajan et al., 1993; Karavitaki et al., 2005; Schoenfeld et al., 2012). An older series by Wen et al. evaluated 52 craniopharyngioma patients treated between 1961 and 1986. They found that initial tumor control was worse for those patients that received an incomplete resection but no adjuvant radiation. The initial tumor control for those patients treated with complete resection was 50% and for those patients with incomplete resection and radiation was 100%. However, for those patients who received an incomplete resection without adjuvant radiation, their initial tumor control was only 15% (Wen et al., 1989).

Similarly, another older but larger series by Rajan et al. evaluated 173 craniopharyngioma patients treated at their institution between 1950 and 1986. All patients in this series had fractionated radiation, but there was variation in the extent of surgical resection. Specifically, four patients had a GTR + FRT, 99 patients had a STR + FRT, 14 patients had biopsy only + FRT, 34 patients had aspiration only + FRT, and 22 patients had only FRT without any surgery. They found that the actuarial PFS was not statistically different between the surgical groups with a 10-year PFS of 100% for the GTR + FRT patients, 88% for the STR + FRT patients, 77% for the biopsy or aspiration only + FRT patients, and 77% for those patients which received only radiation without any surgery. When those same patients were evaluated at a 20-year time point, they found that 84% of the STR + FRT patients remained free of progression, 74% of the biopsy or aspiration only + FRT patients remained free of progression and 71% of the patients that received only radiation without any surgery remained free of progression (Rajan et al., 1993).

A recent study by Karavitaki et al. looked at 121 pediatric and adult craniopharyngioma patients with a mean follow-up period of 103 months. The patients were divided into six groups: gross total resection (16 patients), gross total resection + FRT (three patients), subtotal resection (51 patients), subtotal resection + FRT (33), cyst evacuation alone (six patients) and cyst evacuation + FRT (three patients). They found that the patients with only a subtotal resection (STR) had a significantly reduced recurrence-free survival rate at 10 years of only 38% compared to a 100% recurrence-free survival for gross total resection (GTR) and 77% for STR + FRT (Karavitaki et al., 2005).

Another recent series from the University of California San Francisco (UCSF) evaluated 122 craniopharyngioma patients treated between 1980 and 2009 (Schoenfeld et al., 2012).

At a median follow-up time of 56.4 months, they found that STR alone resulted in a significantly worse progression-free survival (hazard ratio 4.152) and overall survival (hazard ratio 4.880) than STR combined with radiation. As might be expected, they also found that patients with a GTR had better PFS (hazard ratio 0.299) than patients with a STR. Notably, they did not see any statistically significant difference in the PFS or OS between patients that received a GTR and those that had a STR combined with adjuvant radiation (Schoenfeld et al., 2012).

Fractionated Radiation Timing after Surgery

A nearly universal conclusion of the previously discussed studies is that a subtotal resection without any adjuvant radiation will result in higher recurrence rates than a subtotal resection with the addition of radiation. Most series also found that a GTR alone has comparable recurrence rates with a subtotal resection and adjuvant radiation. The main area of debate, however, is whether to offer radiation immediately after surgery or at the time of recurrence as a salvage therapy.

Currently, in the literature, there are conflicting results among various retrospective series. The series by Pemberton et al. looked at 87 patients treated between 1976 and 2002. They found that the 10-year and 20-year OS were 86% and 76%, respectively. They also found that the 10- and 20-year PFS were 78% and 66%, respectively. When the patients were analyzed by timing of radiation, they found that there was no statistical difference in the 10-year or 20-year OS between the patients treated with adjuvant radiation and those receiving radiation at relapse (89% vs. 80% and 76% vs. 66%, $P = 0.25$). Similarly, they found no difference in the 10-year or 20-year PFS between adjuvant radiation and salvage radiation (79% vs. 77% and 73% vs. 60%, $P = 0.34$) (Pemberton et al., 2005).

The older Royal Marsden series by Jose et al. considered 25 patients that received radiation at the time of recurrence. They found the 10-year PFS for those patients to be 72% and the 10-year OS to be 77%, which was comparable to their larger series of 173 patients that received radiation at the time of diagnosis (83% and 77%, respectively). Although their evidence indicated comparable results with delayed radiation as with immediate adjuvant radiation, they did acknowledge that selection bias is a possible issue with most retrospective series, including their own. They ultimately argued for a policy of immediate adjuvant radiation for incompletely resected tumors due to the high probability of recurrence and morbidity risk associated with a second or third salvage surgery (Jose et al., 1992).

In contrast to Pemberton et al. and Jose et al., the series by Regine et al. found a substantial and statistically significant difference in the survival of children treated with radiation in the adjuvant setting compared to those treated in the salvage setting. Specifically, this study found that the 20-year survival for children treated at the time of presentation was 78%, compared to only 25% for children treated with radiation at the time of recurrence. However, Regine et al. did not find a difference in the outcome between adults treated at the time of presentation and adults treated at the time of recurrence (Regine and Kramer, 1992). Wen et al. looked at both adults and children combined and found that there was a difference in local control between patients treated with radiation as part of the initial course (90% local control) and those that were treated with radiation at the time of recurrence (69%) (Wen et al., 1989).

Pediatric vs. Adult Patients

Most series that have compared the outcomes of pediatric and adult patients with a craniopharyngioma have found that the pediatric patients have tended to do better. Regine et al. found that the 10-year OS for pediatric patients in their study was 72%, but the 10-year OS for adults was only 51% (Regine and Kramer, 1992). Similarly, Sung et al. found that the 10-year OS was 72% for pediatric patients, but only 40% for adult patients (Sung et al., 1981). Rajan et al. also found statistically worse survival for patients older than or aged 40 years compared to patients less than age 16 or between the ages of 16 and 39 on both univariate analysis and multivariate analysis (Rajan et al., 1993).

Effect of Radiation Dose

The effect of escalating radiation dose has been investigated by several groups. Regine et al. found that 44% of patients treated to a fractionated radiation therapy dose of less than or equal to 54 Gy recurred compared to only 16% of patients treated with over 54 Gy (Regine and Kramer, 1992). Habrand et al. found a statistically improved event-free survival with doses of radiation greater than or equal to 55 Gy, but did not detect a statistically significant difference in overall survival (Habrand et al., 1999). Sung et al., using older radiation techniques, compared patients with doses of less than 50 Gy, 55–57 Gy and 60–70 Gy. They found recurrence rates of 46.7%, 16%, and 22%, respectively (Sung et al., 1981). Wen et al. also stratified patients into three radiation dose groups: 50–55 Gy, 55–60 Gy, and 60–70 Gy. They found that 50–55 Gy was just as effective as the higher doses (Wen et al., 1989). Thus, most institutions currently treat patients using a dose of around 54 Gy as this dose seems to offer the best balance between tumor control and potential toxicity.

FOLLOW-UP RECOMMENDATIONS

Many of the previously mentioned craniopharyngioma series have reported median times to failure after surgery or radiation within the first couple years (Stripp et al., 2004; Karavitaki et al., 2005; Pemberton et al., 2005). The shortest time to failure was reported in the Stripp et al. series, which had a median time to regrowth of only 3.5 months, and all patients failed before 9 months (Stripp et al., 2004). However, the failure times seem to be longer after radiation as reported by Karavitaki et al. and Pemberton et al. (Karavitaki et al., 2005; Pemberton et al., 2005). In fact, Habrand et al. reported failures as long as 9 years after treatment (Habrand et al., 1999). Given these results, a follow-up schedule of every 3 months for the first couple of years and every 6 months thereafter should be considered. However, as with any tumor, the follow-up schedule should ultimately be based on clinical judgment and individual patient considerations.

One point of caution, however, is that it has been found by a recently published study that up to 52.4% of patients may develop some transient tumor enlargement (usually of the cystic component) on serial MRI evaluation after the completion of radiation (Shi et al., 2012). The median time to tumor or cyst expansion in this investigation was reported to be 1.5 months. Thereafter, the tumor or cyst would begin to contract and a median time to maximal response post-radiation was found to be approximately 9.5 months. Given the transient nature of this tumor enlargement, the authors advised against a rapid, reactionary salvage surgery during the early period post-radiation (Shi et al., 2012).

Should a tumor genuinely fail radiation, however, the next step should be surgery. Although it is commonly believed that a failure after radiation is unlikely to be effectively salvaged, there is a small amount of data to suggest that such a situation is not completely hopeless. The series by Habrand et al., reports that a total of eight children failed after radiation. Four of these eight children underwent salvage surgery. Three of these were alive without any evidence of disease at follow-up times ranging from 42–216 months (Habrand et al., 1999). Thus, unless there are other issues involved, any patient who fails radiation should be quickly referred back to an experienced neurosurgeon.

References

Beltran, C., Naik, M., Merchant, T.E., 2010. Dosimetric effect of target expansion and setup uncertainty during radiation therapy in pediatric craniopharyngioma. Radiother. Oncol. 97 (3), 399–403.

Bernier, J., Hall, E.J., Giaccia, A., 2004. Radiation oncology: a century of achievements. Nat. Rev. Cancer. 4 (9), 737–747.

Castedo, M., Perfettini, J.-L., Roumier, T., Andreau, K., Medema, R., Kroemer, G., 2004. Cell death by mitotic catastrophe: a molecular definition. Oncogene 23 (16), 2825–2837.

Choi, S.H., Kwon, B.J., Na, D.G., Kim, J.H., Han, M.H., Chang, K.H., 2007. Pituitary adenoma, craniopharyngioma, and Rathke cleft cyst involving both intrasellar and suprasellar regions: differentiation using MRI. Clin. Radiol. 62 (5), 453–462.

Dasu, A., Denekamp, J., 1998. New insights into factors influencing the clinically relevant oxygen enhancement ratio. Radiother. Oncol. 46 (3), 269–277.

Devic, S., 2012. MRI simulation for radiotherapy treatment planning. Medical Physics 39, 6701.

Douglas, B., Fowler, J., 1976. The effect of multiple small doses of X-rays on skin reactions in the mouse and a basic interpretation. Radiat. Res. 66 (2), 401–426.

Elkind, M.M., Sutton-Gilbert, H., Moses, W.B., Alescio, T., Swain, R.W., 1965. Radiation response of mammalian cells grown in culture. V. Temperature dependence of the repair of X-ray damage in surviving cells (aerobic and hypoxic). Radiat. Res. 25, 359–376.

Elkind, M.M., 1997. Cell-cycle sensitivity, recovery from radiation damage and a new paradigm for risk assessment. Int. J. Radiat. Biol. 71 (6), 657–665.

Fowler, J.F., 1989. The linear-quadratic formula and progress in fractionated radiotherapy. Br. J. Radiol. 62 (740), 679–694.

Galvin, J.M., Ezzell, G., Eisbrauch, A., et al., 2004. Implementing IMRT in clinical practice: a joint document of the American Society for Therapeutic Radiology and Oncology and the American Association of Physicists in Medicine. Int. J. Radiat. Oncol. Biol. Phys. 58 (5), 1616–1634.

Habrand, J.-L., Ganry, O., Couanet, D., et al., 1999. The role of radiation therapy in the management of craniopharyngioma: A 25-year experience and review of the literature. Int. J. Radiat. Oncol. Biol. Phys. 44 (2), 255–263.

Hall, E.J., Brenner, D.J., 1993. The radiobiology of radiosurgery: rationale for different treatment regimes for AVMs and malignancies. Int. J. Radiat. Oncol. Biol. Phys. 25 (2), 381–385.

Hall, E.J., Giaccia, A.J., 2006. Radiobiology for the radiologist, 6th. ed. Lippincott Williams & Wilkins, Philadelphia.

Hamamoto, Y., Niino, K., Adachi, M., Hosoya, T., 2002. MR and CT findings of craniopharyngioma during and after radiation therapy. Neuroradiology 44 (2), 118–122.

Harwood-Nash, D.C., 1994. Neuroimaging of childhood craniopharyngioma. Pediatr. Neurosurg. 21 (Suppl. 1), 2–10.

Hetelekidis, S., Barnes, P.D., Tao, M.L., et al., 1993. 20-year experience in childhood craniopharyngioma. Int. J. Radiat. Oncol. Biol. Phys. 27 (2), 189–195.

Intensity Modulated Radiation Therapy Collaborative Working Group, 2001. Intensity-modulated radiotherapy: current status and issues of interest. Int. J. Radiat. Oncol. Biol. Phys. 51 (4), 880–914.

Jones, L., Hoban, P., Metcalfe, P., 2001. The use of the linear quadratic model in radiotherapy: a review. Australas. Phys. Eng. Sci. Med. 24 (3), 132–146.

Jose, C.C., Rajan, B., Ashley, S., Marsh, H., Brada, M., 1992. Radiotherapy for the treatment of recurrent craniopharyngioma. Clin. Oncol. (R Coll Radiol) 4 (5), 287–289.

Karavitaki, N., Brufani, C., Warner, J., et al., 2005. Craniopharyngiomas in children and adults: systematic analysis of 121 cases with long-term follow-up. Clinic. Endocrinol. 62 (4), 397–409.

Marks, L.B., 1993. Conventional fractionated radiation therapy vs. radiosurgery for selected benign intracranial lesions (arteriovenous malformations, pituitary adenomas, and acoustic neuromas). J. Neurooncol. 17 (3), 223–230.

Masson-Cote, L., Masucci, G.L., Atenafu, E.G., et al., 2013. Long-term outcomes for adult craniopharyngioma following radiation therapy. Acta. Oncol. 52 (1), 153–158.

Mayo, C., Martel, M.K., Marks, L.B., Flickinger, J., Nam, J., Kirkpatrick, J., 2010a. Radiation dose–volume effects of optic nerves and chiasm. Int. J. Radiat. Oncol. Biol. Phys. 76 (3), S28–S35.

Mayo, C., Yorke, E., Merchant, T.E., 2010b. Radiation associated brainstem injury. Int. J. Radiat. Oncol. Biol. Phys. 76 (3), S36–S41.

Ohtakara, K., Hayashi, S., Tanaka, H., et al., 2012. Clinical comparison of positional accuracy and stability between dedicated versus conventional masks for immobilization in cranial stereotactic radiotherapy using 6-degree-of-freedom image guidance system-integrated platform. Radiother. Oncol. 102 (2), 198–205.

Pawlik, T.M., Keyomarsi, K., 2004. Role of cell cycle in mediating sensitivity to radiotherapy. Acta. Oncol. 59 (4), 928–942.

Pemberton, L.S., Dougal, M., Magee, B., Gattamaneni, H.R., 2005. Experience of external beam radiotherapy given adjuvantly or at relapse following surgery for craniopharyngioma. Radiother. Oncol. 77 (1), 99–104.

Pigeau, I., Sigal, R., Halimi, P., Comoy, J., Doyon, D., 1988. MRI features of craniopharyngiomas at 1.5 Tesla. A series of 13 cases. Journal of neuroradiology. J. Neuroradiol. 15 (3), 276–287.

Railton, R., Porter, D., Lawson, R.C., Hannan, W.J., 1974. The oxygen enhancement ratio and relative biological effectiveness for combined irradiations of Chinese hamster cells by neutrons and γ-rays. J. de Neuroradiologie 25 (2), 121–127.

Rajan, B., Ashley, S., Gorman, C., et al., 1993. Craniopharyngioma – long-term results following limited surgery and radiotherapy. Radiother. Oncol. 26 (1), 1–10.

Rank, C.M., Hünemohr, N., Nagel, A.M., Röthke, M.C., Jäkel, O., Greilich, S., 2013. MRI-based simulation of treatment plans for ion radiotherapy in the brain region. Radiother. Oncol.

Regine, W.F., Kramer, S., 1992. Pediatric craniopharyngiomas: long term results of combined treatment with surgery and radiation. Int. J. Radiat. Oncol. Biol. Phys. 24 (4), 611–617.

Rosenfelder, N.A., Corsini, L., McNair, H., et al., 2013. Achieving the relocation accuracy of stereotactic frame-based cranial radiotherapy in a three-point thermoplastic shell. Clin. Oncol. 25 (1), 66–73.

Ruschin, M., Komljenovic, P.T., Ansell, S., et al., 2013. Cone beam computed tomography image guidance system for a dedicated intracranial radiosurgery treatment unit. Int. J. Radiat. Oncol. Biol. Phys. 85 (1), 243–250.

Sachs, Ernest, 1949. Diagnosis and treatment of brain tumors and care of the neurosurgical patient. C.V. Mosby Company, 1949, St. Louis, p. 537.

Schoenfeld, A., Pekmezci, M., Barnes, M., et al., 2012. The superiority of conservative resection and adjuvant radiation for craniopharyngiomas. J. Neurooncol. 108 (1), 133–139.

Schreibmann, E., Elder, E., Fox, T., 2009. Automated quality assurance for image-guided radiation therapy. J. Appl. Clin. Med. Phys. 10 (1).

Schreibmann, E., Pantalone, P., Waller, A., Fox, T., 2012. A measure to evaluate deformable registration fields in clinical settings. J. Appl. Clin. Med. Phys. 13 (5).

Shi, Z., Esiashvili, N., Janss, A.J., et al., 2012. Transient enlargement of craniopharyngioma after radiation therapy: pattern of magnetic resonance imaging response following radiation. J. Neurooncol. 109 (2), 349–355.

Stanescu, T., Jans, H., Pervez, N., Stavrev, P., Fallone, B., 2008. A study on the magnetic resonance imaging (MRI)-based radiation treatment planning of intracranial lesions. Phys. Med. Biol. 53 (13), 3579.

Stanescu, T., Kirkby, C., Wachowich, K., Fallone, B., 2009. Developments in MRI-based radiation treatment planning. Paper presented at: World Congress on Medical Physics and Biomedical Engineering, September 7–12, 2009. Germany, Munich.

Stripp, D.C., Maity, A., Janss, A.J., et al., 2004. Surgery with or without radiation therapy in the management of craniopharyngiomas in children and young adults. Int. J. Radiat. Oncol. Biol. Phys. 58 (3), 714–720.

Sung, D.I., Chang, C.H., Harisiadis, L., Carmel, P.W., 1981. Treatment results of craniopharyngiomas. Cancer 47 (5), 847–852.

Teh, B.S., Woo, S.Y., Butler, E.B., 1999. Intensity Modulated Radiation Therapy (IMRT): A new promising technology in radiation oncology. Oncologist 4 (6), 433–442.

Tryggestad, E., Christian, M., Ford, E., et al., 2011. Inter- and intrafraction patient positioning uncertainties for intracranial radiotherapy: A study of four frameless, thermoplastic mask-based immobilization strategies using daily cone-beam CT. Int. J. Radiat. Oncol. Biol. Phys. 80 (1), 281–290.

Varlotto, J.M., Flickinger, J.C., Kondziolka, D., Lunsford, L.D., Deutsch, M., 2002. External beam irradiation of craniopharyngiomas: long-term analysis of tumor control and morbidity. Int. J. Radiat. Oncol. Biol. Phys. 54 (2), 492–499.

Veeravagu, A., Lee, M., Jiang, B., Chang, S.D., 2010. The role of radiosurgery in the treatment of craniopharyngiomas. Neurosurg. Focus 28 (4), E11.

Wen, B., Hussey, D.H., Staples, J., et al., 1989. A comparison of the roles of surgery and radiation therapy in the management of craniopharyngiomas. Int. J. Radiat. Oncol. Biol. Phys. 16 (1), 17–24.

Williams, M.V., Denekamp, J., Fowler, J.F., 1985. A review of αβ ratios for experimental tumors: Implications for clinical studies of altered fractionation. Int. J. Radiat. Oncol. Biol. Phys. 11 (1), 87–96.

Winkfield, K.M., Linsenmeier, C., Yock, T.I., et al., 2009. Surveillance of Craniopharyngioma Cyst Growth in Children Treated With Proton Radiotherapy. Int. J. Radiat. Oncol. Biol. Phys. 73 (3), 716–721.

Withers, H.R., 1975. Cell cycle redistribution as a factor in multifraction irradiation. Radiology 114 (1), 199–202.

CHAPTER

22

The Role of Proton Therapy in the Treatment of Craniopharyngioma

Julie A. Bradley, Daniel J. Indelicato

University of Florida Proton Therapy Institute, Jacksonville, FL, USA

"Until some method is devised whereby the usually multilocular epithelial lesion can be destroyed or inactivated in situ, the mortality will doubtless remain high." - ***Harvey Cushing, 1932***

Proton therapy is often discussed as a new radiation modality, although Robert R. Wilson recognized its physical properties and clinical advantages in 1946 (Halperin, 2006). The clinical use of protons began at Harvard University (Boston, MA) in the 1950s. Since 2007, over 137 pediatric patients have been treated on 12 different Children's Oncology Group (COG) protocols, most of which now have proton-specific guidelines for radiation design and delivery. Protons deposit their maximum energy in tissue shortly before they come to rest (Durante and Loeffler, 2010), whereas photons deposit most of their energy superficially, decreasing the dose as the depth in tissue increases. The distance over which any specified proton energy is released, called the Bragg peak, is narrow, thus a variety of energies are used to allow the dose to be deposited over a greater length of tissue, producing a spread-out Bragg peak (SOBP; Figure 22.1). Photons continue to deposit energy beyond the target volume, yet protons come to rest abruptly after reaching the depth of their maximum deposition, thereby eliminating the "exit dose" of photon-based radiation, or the radiation dose deposited distal to the target volume (Figure 22.2). Protons, like photons, are an ionizing radiation with a low linear energy transfer (LET). The relative biological effectiveness (RBE) of protons is 1.1; therefore, unlike heavy ion therapy, which also eliminates the exit dose but carries a high LET, protons and photons have a similar and predictable impact on normal tissue.

Owing to these unique physical properties, the primary clinical advantages of proton therapy include decreased radiation dose to normal tissue and reduced late radiation toxicity. These benefits are particularly relevant in treating craniopharyngiomas, which are always located in the central aspect of the brain, close to critical structures like the optic pathway, pituitary, hypothalamus, temporal lobes, and circle of Willis. The tumor itself can cause functional disruption of these cranial structures, as can biopsy or surgical resection. Radiotherapy plays an important role in achieving local control in subtotally resected or unresectable craniopharyngiomas. Current chemotherapy options are not curative.

Craniopharyngiomas
http://dx.doi.org/10.1016/B978-0-12-416706-3.00022-2

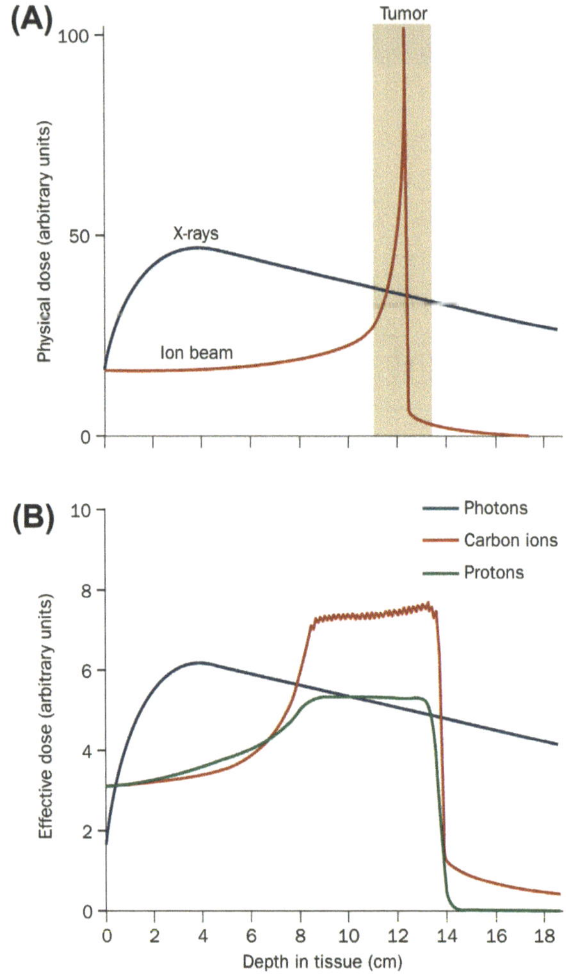

FIGURE 22.1 **A,** Depth-dose distributions for X-rays and high-energy charged particles. **B,** Depth-dose distributions of a spread-out Bragg peak (SOBP) in comparison to photons and carbon ions. *Reprinted with permission from Durante M., Loeffler J.S., 2010. Charged particles in radiation oncology. Nat. Rev. Clin. Oncol. 7(1), 37–43.*

Patients with craniopharyngioma who are treated with modern radiation doses have a good prognosis and often achieve long-term survival. Craniopharyngiomas most commonly arise in the pediatric population, with a peak incidence between the ages of 5 and 14 years, and young patients represent the most radiosensitive population. Therefore, late effects of radiotherapy, which can permanently affect function and quality of life, are a highly relevant survivorship issue. These tumors that lie adjacent to multiple radiosensitive and critical structures and have high control rates derive the greatest relative benefit from proton therapy. Accordingly, despite its low incidence, craniopharyngioma was the sixth most common pediatric tumor treated with proton therapy in the United States in 2012. Of the 694 pediatric patients treated with proton therapy, 5.8% had craniopharyngiomas (Figure 22.3).

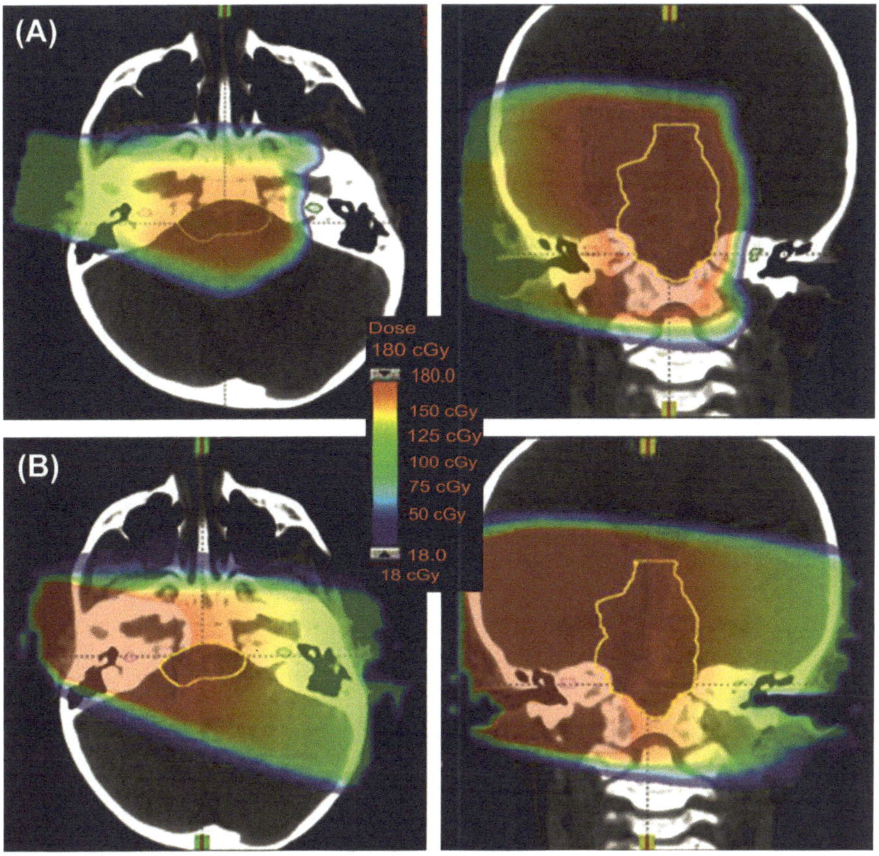

FIGURE 22.2 **A,** Dose distribution from a single proton beam (axial and coronal) compared to **B,** a single photon beam (axial and coronal). Note the difference in entrance dose (higher for photon beams compared to proton beams) and exit dose. This dose profile for the proton beam allows for a reduction in the integral dose to the patient.

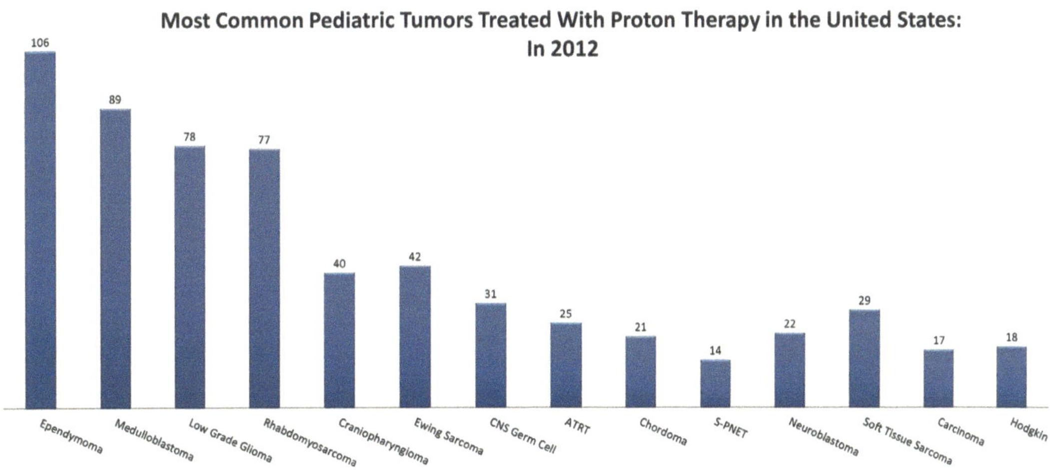

FIGURE 22.3 Numbers of pediatric patients treated with proton therapy in 2012 by type of malignancy. Craniopharyngioma was the sixth most common pediatric cancer to be treated with proton therapy in 2012.

DOSIMETRIC RATIONALE FOR PROTON THERAPY

Multiple dosimetric studies suggest proton therapy offers an advantage over conventional photon radiation, including intensity-modulated radiation therapy (IMRT), for patients with craniopharyngioma (Figure 22.4). Boehling et al. (2012) performed a dosimetric study on ten pediatric patients with craniopharyngioma, and compared three-dimensional (3D) conformal proton radiotherapy, IMRT, and intensity-modulated proton therapy (IMPT) (Boehling et al., 2012). All plans utilized the same beam orientation, which consisted of a vertex beam and two symmetric lateral beams, with the primary dosimetric goal of hippocampal avoidance. While adequate planning target volume (PTV) coverage was achieved with all radiation techniques, both proton techniques decreased the dose to normal tissues and structures, including the hippocampi, dentate gyri, subventricular zones, major vascular structures, infratentorial and supratentorial brain, and brainstem. Another dosimetric study from St Jude Children's Research Hospital (Memphis, TN) on 14 patients with craniopharyngioma compared double-scatter proton therapy, IMPT, and IMRT (Beltran et al., 2012). IMPT offered the highest conformality index. Double-scatter proton therapy was superior to IMRT in minimizing the dose to the cochlea, optic chiasm and brain, as well as the scanned body dose, but IMRT had a higher conformality index and lower optic nerve dose. The authors of these dosimetric studies predict that the reduced integral dose with proton therapy and reduced dose to many surrounding critical structures will translate into fewer late effects for patients treated with this radiation modality.

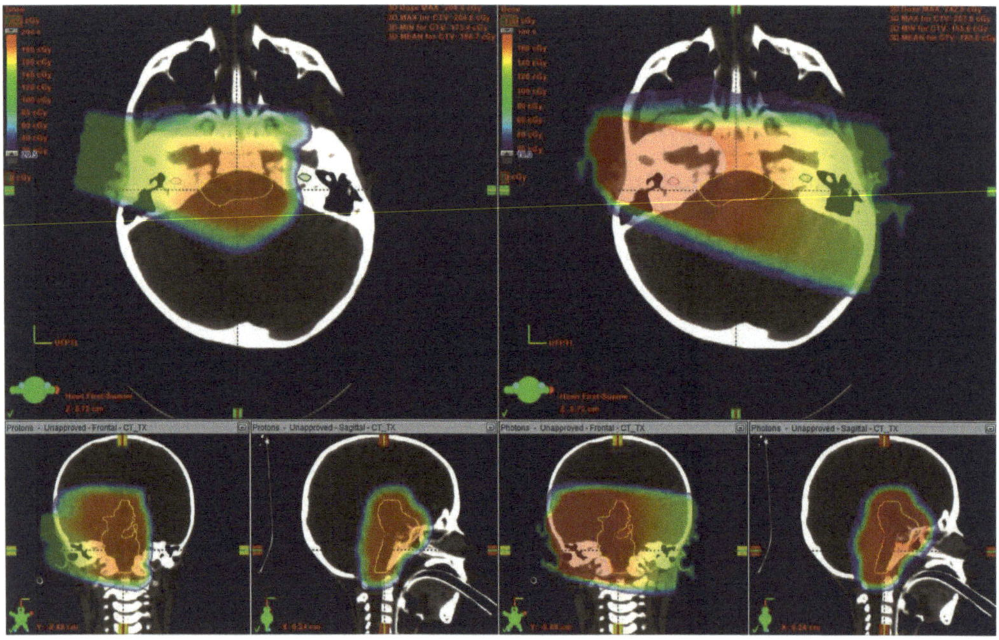

FIGURE 22.4 Dosimetry plans comparing double-scatter proton therapy to IMRT for a 5-year-old child with a craniopharyngioma.

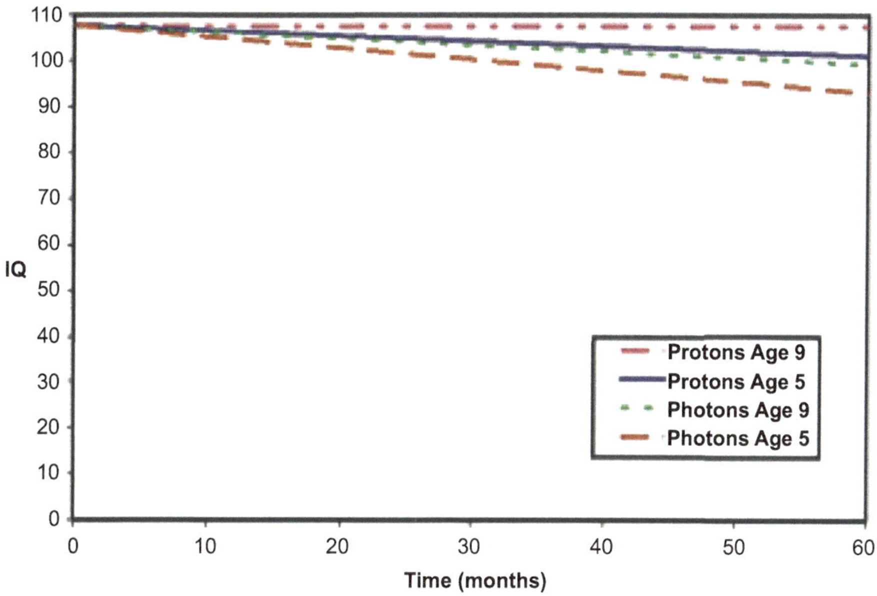

FIGURE 22.5 Change in IQ over time after radiotherapy according to age at the time of radiotherapy and radiation modality. *Reprinted with permission from Merchant T.E., Hua C.H., Shukla, H., Ying X., Nill S., Oelfke U. Proton versus photon radiotherapy for common pediatric brain tumors: comparison of models of dose characteristics and their relationship to cognitive function. Pediatr. Blood Cancer. 51, 110–117.*

The potential benefit of proton therapy is also evident from indirect dosimetric data. A model to estimate IQ based on patient age, mean dose to the supratentorium and time since irradiation has been developed for patients with craniopharyngioma (Merchant et al., 2008). Based on this longitudinal model, differences in IQ were detected based on the type of radiotherapy (double-scattered protons versus photons) and patient age (Figure 22.5). Merchant et al. also demonstrated a significantly reduced cochlea dose with proton therapy. In a prospective study of craniopharyngioma patients treated with 3D conformal photon therapy and IMRT, 70 patients underwent cognitive testing at baseline, 6 months after radiotherapy and then annually for a maximum of 10 years. Longitudinal IQ was associated with mean whole-brain radiation dose and time at a rate of 0.00227 points/cGy/year, as estimated for an average patient based on linear mixed-effects models (Merchant et al., 2013). These cognitive dose models allow predictive comparisons of expected outcomes following proton therapy and illustrate that, by further reducing the low-dose regions with proton therapy, the mean whole-brain dose will be decreased, mitigating the decline in IQ over time.

In addition to neurocognitive changes, childhood cancer survivors are at risk of developing second malignancies. By using proton therapy to decrease the integral dose, survivors should experience fewer radiation-induced second tumors. According to the Childhood Cancer Survivor Study, which assessed all types of tumors, the cumulative incidence of second malignancy at 30 years after diagnosis is 7.9% (Friedman et al., 2010). For patients who received radiotherapy, the relative risk of a second malignancy is 2.7 (Friedman et al., 2010).

Modeling for other primary tumors treated with proton therapy demonstrates a two- to 15-fold decrease in the rate of second malignancies with proton therapy compared to photon radiotherapy (Miralbell et al., 2002).

CLINICAL EXPERIENCE AND OUTCOMES

In one of the first published outcomes studies on the clinical use of proton therapy for craniopharyngioma, Fitzek et al. reported on 15 patients treated between 1981 and 1988, including five children and ten adults (Fitzek et al., 2006). These patients were treated over 20 years ago, allowing for long-term follow-up, which, for this slow-growing tumor, is critical for obtaining accurate knowledge of tumor control and treatment toxicity. One-third of the patients were treated with proton therapy alone and two-thirds with a combined proton-photon technique. A change in the calibration technique occurred for proton dosimetry in 1997; the dose delivered was recalculated and a 6.5% increase from the prescribed dose was identified. The delivered doses were higher than the prescribed doses, with a median dose of 55.6 CGE for the pediatric patients and 62.7 CGE for the adult patients. Patients treated with a combination of protons and photons received a median proton dose of 26.9 CGE, or 47% of the total dose. The primary aim of the study was to assess safety and efficacy. The investigators observed 5- and 10-year actuarial local control rates of 93% and 85%, respectively. No pediatric patients experienced tumor progression. Four patients died, all 5 years or more after completing radiotherapy. Tumor recurrence was the cause of death in two patients (5.0 and 9.1 years after radiotherapy); treatment toxicity was the cause of death in the other two (5.6 and 6.9 years after radiotherapy). Further toxicity data are presented in the following section.

Of note, both patients with tumor progression had an interruption in their radiation course of more than 20 consecutive days. Nevertheless, the local control rates compare favorably with those published for 79 pediatric patients treated with conventional radiotherapy from 1976 to 2003 at the same institution, with 5- and 10-year actuarial local control rates of 74% and 69%, respectively (Winkfield et al., 2011). Winkfield et al. published the next series of this cohort from the same institution, with 24 children treated between 2001 and 2007 (Winkfield et al., 2009). No tumor progression has occurred over a median follow-up of 40.5 months.

A retrospective review of 16 patients with craniopharyngioma also reported high rates of local control with proton therapy, achieved in 14 of 15 patients (one patient was lost to follow-up) with a mean follow-up of 60.2 months (range, 12–121 months) (Luu et al., 2006). Twelve of these patients were undergoing treatment for progressive disease after surgery alone. The sole relapse occurred 80 months after radiotherapy, and the patient ultimately succumbed to the disease. Actuarial rates of tumor control were not reported in this study. Two other patients died from treatment-related complications: one from sepsis and one from a right middle cerebral artery infarct.

Alapetite et al. presented their data in 2012 on the treatment of 49 children with craniopharyngioma, 10 having received mixed photon-proton beams and 39 protons alone, between 1994 and 2009 (Alapetite et al., 2012). The V20 for the temporal lobes was less than 10%. Nevertheless, neurocognitive dysfunction was still reported, including altered short-term memory, social and emotional functioning, school difficulties and behavioral disorders, which allude to the multifactorial nature of neurocognitive decline in craniopharyngioma patients. Over a median follow-up of 53 months, five patients experienced disease progression. Survival rates were not addressed in this abstract. No patients developed radiation-induced optic neuropathy. Chang et al. presented retrospective data on 14 patients with craniopharyngioma treated between 2004 and 2008. Local control was 100% with a median follow-up of 16.5 months and stabilization or improvement of vision was observed in all patients (Chang et al., 2009). In another cohort of 19 pediatric patients with craniopharyngioma treated with proton therapy between 2007 and 2012, the 5-year actuarial overall survival rate was 93% and the 5-year progression-free survival rate was 91% (Bishop et al., 2013). One patient died due to complications of diabetes insipidus, the diagnosis of which preceded the radiation therapy. The actuarial rate of tumor control was not reported. Table 22.1 summarizes local control rates reported in the literature on proton therapy for patients with craniopharyngioma.

TOXICITY OUTCOMES

Available clinical data suggest that acute toxicity for central nervous system malignancies is low in patients treated with proton therapy. In a retrospective review of 48 pediatric patients (four with craniopharyngioma), fatigue was the most common acute symptom (Suneja et al., 2013). Approximately two-thirds of the cohort developed grade 1 fatigue, 10% developed grade 2 fatigue and 0% developed grade 3 fatigue or higher. Alopecia and dermatitis were the other most common acute toxicities, with 73% experiencing grade 1 or 2 alopecia and 63% grade 1 or 2 dermatitis. Another retrospective review of 13 patients treated with proton therapy for craniopharyngioma reported no grade 3 acute toxicities and one grade 2 headache (Confer et al., 2012). Acute toxicity data collected on 40 patients supports the retrospective data, with no grade 3 toxicities (Indelicato et al., 2012). Grade 2 toxicities in this cohort included emesis ($n=10$), headache ($n=1$), and pre-syncope ($n=2$). Nine patients required antiemetics; none required steroids.

Late effects are of greater concern, as the toxicity from radiotherapy can develop months to years after the completion of RT, and can persist for a lifetime. One study reported that children treated with photons for craniopharyngioma remained at risk of death related to treatment toxicity up to 10 and even 20 years after the completion of therapy (Visser et al., 2010). Deaths were attributed to multiple factors, including uncontrolled diabetes insipidus, panhypopituitarism and cerebrovascular disease. Table 22.1 summarizes toxicity rates of proton therapy from the current literature.

Two patients in the study by Fitzek et al. experienced optic injury: one with hemianopsia 10 months after radiotherapy (optic chiasm dose, 64 CGE) and one with unilateral blindness 5 months after radiotherapy (optic chiasm dose, 55.3 CGE). In the absence of tumor progression, the remaining patients experienced stable or improved vision. In 11 of the 15 patients, the optic chiasm dose was constrained to 56 CGE or less. Prior to radiotherapy, 100% of the children and 80% of the adults required medical supplementation for endocrine deficiencies. Following radiotherapy, all patients required endocrine supplementation. Treatment-related deaths occurred in the two patients who suffered visual sequela; they died more than 5 years after radiotherapy. One of these patients developed memory loss, hemianopsia and hypothalamic syndrome, with a non-malignant necrotic mass resected without symptom

TABLE 22.1 Literature Review of Outcomes Following Proton Therapy for Patients with Craniopharyngioma

Study	No. of Patients	Median Follow-up (y)	Treatment Modality	5-year Actuarial Local Control	10-year Actuarial Local Control	Acute Toxicity, No. of Patients	Late Toxicity, No. of Patients	Absolute Number of Deaths due to Tumor Progression	Absolute Number of Deaths due to Treatment Toxicity
Fitzek et al., 2006	15	13.1	Surgery/biopsy + proton-photon	93%	85%	None, 7; nausea, 1; fatigue, 3; headaches, 4	Visual deficits, 2; endocrinopathy, 15 neurocognitive, 1	2 (5 and 9.1 years after RT)	2 (5.6 and 6.9 years after RT)
Luu et al., 2006	16	5	Surgery + proton or proton alone (n = 12 being treated for progression after surgery)	94%^	NR	NR	Vasculopathy, 2; second tumor, 1; endocrinopathy, 14; sepsis, 1	1	2
Chang et al., 2009*	14	1.4	Surgery/ biopsy + proton	100%^	NR	NR	Endocrinopathy, 11 (of 11 with endocrine results)	0	0
Alapetite et al., 2012*	49	4.4	Surgery + proton-photon (n = 10); Surgery + proton (n = 39)	90%^	NR	NR	Neuropsychological dysfunction (altered short-term memory, social and emotional functioning, school difficulties, behavioral disorders), no. pts. NR	NR	NR
Confer et al., 2012*	13	0.7	Surgery/ biopsy + proton	85^	NR	Headache, 1	NR	0	0
Indelicato et al., 2012*	40	0.7	Surgery/biopsy + proton	100%^	NR	Emesis, 1; headache, 1; pre-syncope, 2; nausea, 9	None to date	0	0
Bishop et al., 2013*	19	2.7	Surgery/biopsy + proton (n = 15); Proton alone (n = 4)	91%	NR	NR	Vasculopathy, 2; endocrinopathy, 17	0	1

NR = not reported; RT = radiation therapy.
* *abstract only.*
^ *Crude rate at time reported.*

improvement. He spent 3 years in a nursing home before his death. The other patient developed unilateral blindness and died from vascular causes. As explained above, most patients in this study received less than half of the dose with protons, and years after treatment, the administered dose was discovered to be higher than the prescribed dose due to a change in calibration.

In the series by Bishop et al., with a median follow-up of 31.8 months, neuroendocrine dysfunction was common: 89% of patients required hormone replacement therapy and 42% had panhypopituitarism (n = 8; six diagnosed before and two after radiotherapy). Following radiation, 10.5% of patients (two out of 19) developed vasculopathy (Bishop et al., 2013). Luu et al. report that only three of the 12 living patients endured a new toxicity after radiotherapy: panhypopituitarism at 26 months after RT, cerebrovascular accident at 34 months after RT with complete neurologic recovery, and posterior fossa meningioma at 59 months after radiotherapy in a patient who had previously received external-beam radiotherapy before salvage proton therapy (Luu et al., 2006). In these studies, no radionecrosis was reported. Neurovascular and neuroendocrine toxicity attributable to proton therapy was rare. For critical organs within the PTV and immediately adjacent to the PTV, such as the circle of Willis, optic chiasm and hypothalamus–pituitary axis, there is no indication that proton therapy is associated with increased toxicity.

We know that radiation therapy can induce secondary tumors in the radiation field years after primary therapy. In a retrospective cohort study with a median follow-up of 6.7 years, the rate of second malignancies was lower in patients treated with proton therapy than those who received photon therapy (5.2% vs. 7.5% respectively; hazard ratio, 0.52; 95% CI, 0.32–0.85; $P = 0.009$, Chung et al., 2013). There was an approximately 3% difference in the 10-year cumulative incidence rates for second malignancies: 5.4% for proton patients versus 8.6% for photon patients (Chung et al., 2013). Fewer than 10% of the participants in both the proton and photon cohorts were pediatric patients, and none of these patients developed a second malignancy during the follow-up period. Adding more pediatric patients and increasing the length of follow-up may reveal a more pronounced difference in cumulative incidence rates for second malignancies among children than adults.

Neurocognitive dysfunction is a common late effect of radiotherapy in pediatric brain tumors such as craniopharyngioma. These changes in cognition occur through various mechanisms, including radiation dose to the temporal lobes and hippocampi. Demyelination and axonal degradation are also postulated to contribute to this late effect of radiotherapy on the brain (Khong et al., 2006). Diffusion tensor imaging (DTI) can assess white matter demyelination through parameters such as fractional anisotropy (FA) and radial diffusivity (RD). In a study of ten patients with craniopharyngioma treated with proton therapy, FA decreased and RD increased at 3 months after radiation compared to baseline, but by 6 months these parameters returned to baseline levels (Figure 22.6) (Uh et al., 2013), suggesting that white matter demyelination after proton therapy is mild and transient. In contrast, after photon therapy, FA decreased and RD increased linearly over time (Figure 22.7) (Nagesh et al., 2008). The clinical manifestation of these changes remains to be determined, but it is plausible that the mild and transient changes seen after proton therapy will result in improved neurocognitive function. Data to support this hypothesis include a study by Chapman et al., in which changes in diffusivity in the parahippocampal cingulum correlated linearly with a

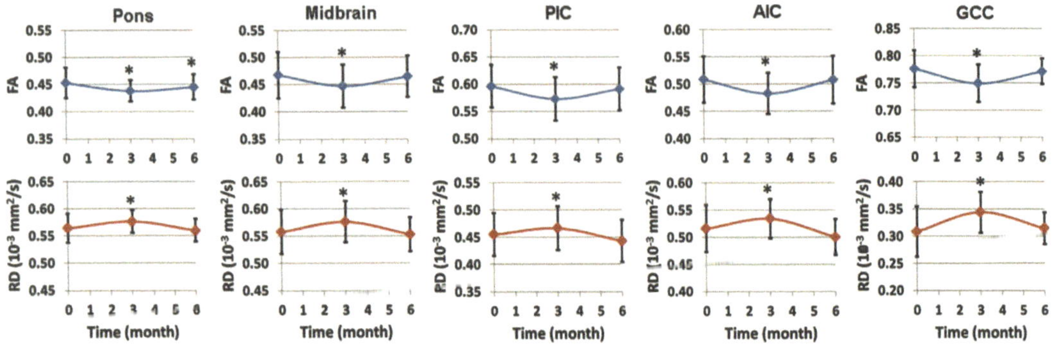

FIGURE 22.6 Mean fractional anisotropy and radial diffusivity values as a function of time after radiotherapy. A change in these parameters is seen at 3 months, but they return to baseline at 6 months. The standard deviation of the ten patients is indicated by the error bar and the asterisk denotes a statistically significant difference from baseline. *Reprinted with permission from Uh, J., Hua, C., Lam, M., Indelicato, D.J., Merchant, T.E., Assessment of structural integrity of normal brain tissues in craniopharyngioma patients after proton therapy. International Society for Magnetic Resonance in Medicine Annual Meeting 2013; Salt Lake City, UT: abstr. 3639.*

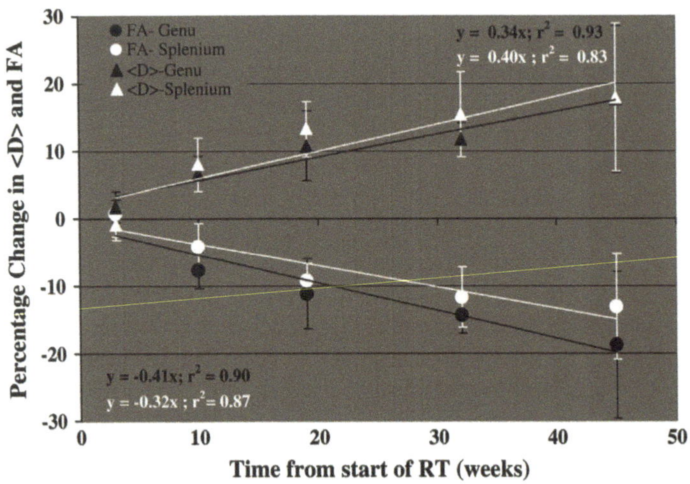

FIGURE 22.7 Percent change in fractional anisotropy and mean diffusivity as a function of time, beginning at the start of radiotherapy. These values show a linear change over time with no return to baseline. *Reprinted with permission from Nagesh, V., Tsien, C.I., Chenevert, T.L., Ross, B.D., Lawrence, T.S., Junick, L., Cao, Y., 2008. Radiation-induced changes in normal-appearing white matter in patients with cerebral tumors: a diffusion tensor imaging study. Int. J. Radiat. Oncol. Biol. Phys. 15;70(4):1002–1010.*

decline in verbal recall (Chapman et al., 2012). Further, the score from neurocognitive testing correlated with results of the quality of life survey.

In the Fitzek et al. study, all five children completed high school and three attended college. All were able to live independently and support themselves. One of the five had some learning difficulties (in verbal, math and writing) but was able to pass college courses despite these impediments. The patients treated in adulthood all resumed their previous professional duties.

Survivor quality of life is indefinitely altered by toxicities that can develop years after treatment, by the common need for lifelong medication, and by the permanence of numerous side effects. In one study of 29 families with a child treated with proton therapy for craniopharyngioma, the overall quality of life self-report was in the normal range with a mean follow-up period of approximately 6 years (minimum, 1 year) (Laffond et al., 2012). The mean age at diagnosis was 7 years and 10 months. Depression and executive function comprised the most common symptoms and corresponded with lower quality of life scores. Initiation, working memory and organization were reported as common areas of difficulty, in addition to shift and emotional control. Of the survivors included in this study, 78% reported daily fatigue and 41% had received psychological or psychiatric care, with two patients on medication for anxiety or depression. Isolation, frustration, and helplessness were common descriptors used by the families. Moreover, 26 children attended mainstream school, with 34% repeating a year of school. Of the five patients aged 18 years or older, two graduated from high school. This study highlights that quality of life and survivorship care are critical in all patients treated for craniopharyngioma, regardless of the radiation treatment modality. In a different cohort of 29 patients treated with conventional radiation, 79% reported impairment in one or more quality-of-life categories, most frequently emotion and pain (with 41% reporting an impairment in each) (Merchant et al., 2002). Self-care was compromised in 14%, cognition in 35%, sensation in 38% and mobility in 38%. "Normal" functionality was seen in six of the 29 patients. While differences in quality of life with proton therapy versus photon therapy cannot be directly compared between these two studies, they provide essential information to help physicians address survivorship issues and serve as a benchmark to compare future investigations.

PREPARATION FOR PROTON THERAPY

Patient position and tumor localization must be carefully considered when using proton therapy to treat pediatric brain tumors like craniopharyngiomas, given their location amid various critical structures. Daily image guidance is recommended to minimize the setup uncertainty and thus the PTV margin. Cone-beam computed tomography (CT) is not typically available for use with proton therapy, although widespread adaptation of this technology to the proton vault is in progress. Therefore, daily image guidance is usually performed with orthogonal kV X-rays, most often aligned to bony landmarks of the skull. In prepubertal children, however, bone development is incomplete and therefore bony landmarks may be suboptimal for daily patient alignment (Aldana et al., 2010). Instead, some institutions recommend placement of four small titanium fiducial markers prior to proton radiotherapy in young patients with cranial tumors such as craniopharyngiomas. Existing surgical hardware can also be used for daily setup alignment.

CT simulation may be performed in the standard fashion with the patient lying supine wearing a base-of-skull frame, facemask, and bite plate for immobilization to minimize intra- and interfraction motion. As with conventional radiation, young children may require anesthesia for this planning session and for daily radiotherapy administration. A slice thickness of 1 mm is recommended for the planning CT to generate the detailed formation digital radiographic reconstructions (DRRs) used for daily setup (equivalent to the DRR in standard radiotherapy; Figure 22.8). Prior CTs and magnetic resonance images (MRIs) are fused to facilitate accurate delineation of normal structures and the target volume. Provocative early data suggest that carbon-11 methionine positron emission tomography (PET) may be useful in target delineation of craniopharyngioma (Laser et al., 2013), but this is not commonplace.

As with other radiotherapy techniques, target volumes and normal tissue structures are contoured. The normal structure volumes are typically comprehensive to prioritize and maximize the benefit of proton therapy by avoiding as many of the critical organs and brain structures as possible for each case. These avoidance targets may include the optic chiasm, optic nerves, brainstem surface, brainstem core, retinae, lens, bilateral cochlea, lacrimal glands, temporal lobes, hippocampal head and tail bilaterally, pituitary, hypothalamus, bilateral mastoid air cells, posterior nasopharynx, scalp, supratentorial brain, and non-target brain. With a dose of 54 Gy, the optic chiasm and proximal optic nerves are near the tolerance dose, and every effort is made to avoid a hot spot on these critical structures and the brainstem. A 5- to 10-mm clinical target volume (CTV) is utilized, with weekly MRI of the tumor to monitor for cyst growth (Beltran et al., 2012). Prior data from St. Jude Children's Research Hospital suggest a 10-mm margin is adequate for tumor control and infrequent replanning is required owing to this relatively generous CTV (Merchant et al., 2006). The University of Florida and St Jude Children's Research Hospital are currently collaborating on an open phase II protocol (RT2CR) to examine the efficacy of limited surgery, proton therapy, and a 5-mm margin for craniopharyngiomas. A 3- to 5-mm CTV-to-PTV margin is used for image-guided proton therapy of the brain in the beam's eye view (Figure 22.9).

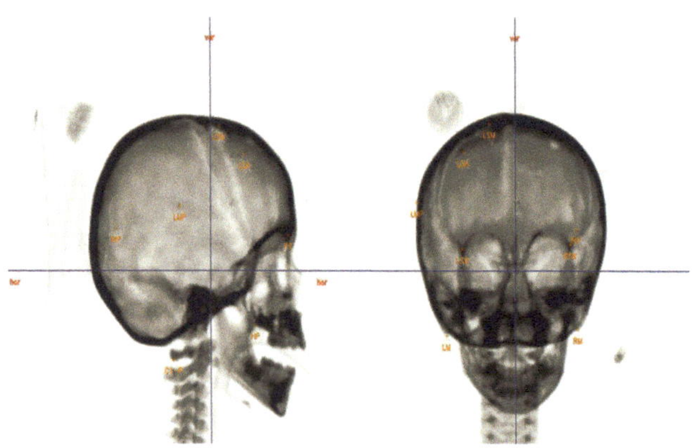

FIGURE 22.8 Orthogonal images used for daily patient alignment. Setup points include fiducial markers and bony landmarks.

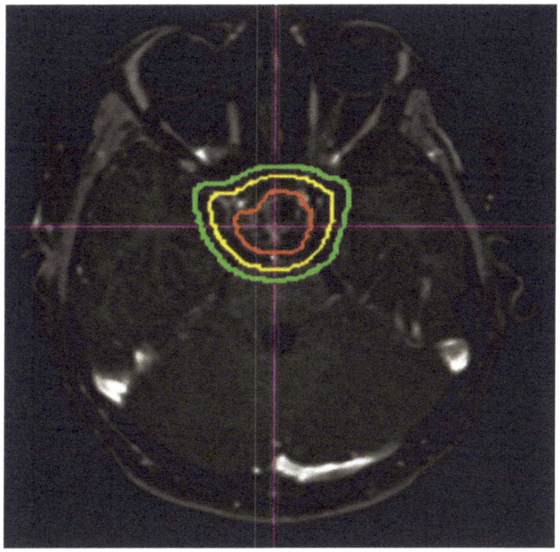

FIGURE 22.9 Representative slice of craniopharyngioma target definition. Gross tumor volume (GTV) = red; clinical target volume (CTV) = yellow; planning target volume (PTV) = green. In this patient, a 5-mm margin was applied to the GTV to create the CTV. A 3-mm expansion of the CTV formed the PTV.

PROTON THERAPY TECHNIQUES

With all types of proton therapy, beam arrangements must be selected thoughtfully. A higher RBE occurs at the distal end of the proton beam (Robertson et al., 1975), which is the region of range uncertainty, necessitating multiple beams that do not stop at the same location in the normal tissue outside of the PTV.

In most cases, proton therapy techniques allow for fewer beams than IMRT and stereotactic body radiotherapy (SBRT). For craniopharyngiomas treated with double-scatter proton therapy, three beams are typical, but a four-field technique is occasionally employed. In the craniopharyngioma series by Fitzek et al. (2006), all patients (proton only and combined proton-photon) were treated with a three-field technique consisting of two lateral fields and a superior oblique field. The most common technique in the subsequent series published by the Harvard group (Winkfield et al., 2009) consisted of a four-field approach including opposed lateral fields, an anterosuperior field and a posterior field. Paired alternate beams were used daily. Luu et al. report that most of the patients in their cohort were treated with right and left lateral beams in addition to a vertex (Luu et al., 2006).

Variations in tumor size and sporadic locations of cystic components make it impossible to universally apply the same beam arrangement to all patients. In addition, air cells, metallic devices, and tissue that may change size or shape, such as a seroma, should be avoided in the beam path, if possible, to minimize range uncertainty.

The most widely used technique in proton therapy remains 3D conformal passive double scattering. For craniopharyngioma treatments, forward planning is used and beam energies

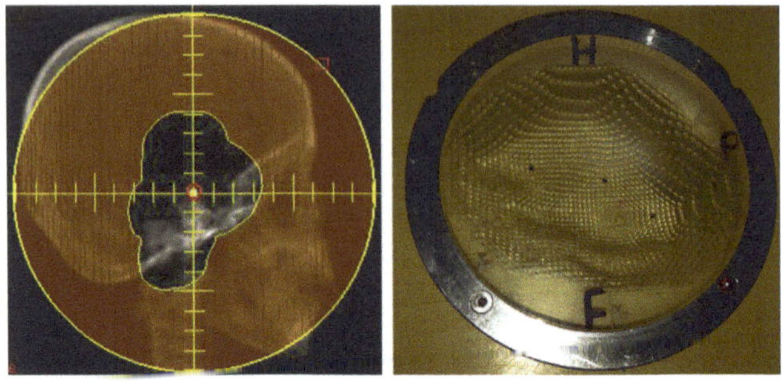

FIGURE 22.10 Custom brass apertures and Lucite compensators are designed for each field for each patient.

typically range from 140 MeV to 180 MeV. Custom brass apertures and Lucite compensators are designed for each field for each patient (Figure 22.10). Compensator smearing helps to correct range and setup uncertainty. Uniform scanning is another form of 3D conformal proton therapy. Apertures and compensators are also required to define the lateral and distal margins; however, rather than a scattering device, a scanning magnet is used to expand the pencil beam laterally (Farr et al., 2008). The PTV is used to determine the aperture, but the proximal and distal margins are typically determined by the CTV. Distal and proximal margins are used along the beam's axial direction and are institution-specific. For example, at the University of Florida, the current practice for calculating the distal and proximal margin is [0.025 x (CTV maximum/minimum range) + 1.5 mm], where the first term is an estimate of CT-Hounsfield units relative to proton relative linear stopping power conversion uncertainties; and the second term of 1.5 mm is an estimate of the delivered beam-range uncertainty. Daily image guidance is used with an institution-specific tolerance (commonly $\leq$1 to 2 mm).

Spot scanning proton therapy is a newer technique that employs active scanning to increase dose conformality compared to the passive techniques. The conformality is related to the spot size of the proton beam: a smaller spot size allows tighter conformality at the cost of increased treatment time and thus susceptibility to target motion. Spot scanning plans can be optimized based on a single field or multiple fields. With single-field optimization, the entire target is covered by the prescribed dose for each field. In multiple-field optimization (MFO), partial target coverage is achieved with each beam, and the sum of the beams results in full target coverage by the prescription dose. While this technique improves conformality and normal tissue sparing, it is the most sensitive of all the techniques to variations in daily setup and change in tumor volume (Lomax, 2008a, 2008b). With increasing depth, spot scanning proton therapy has a larger penumbra compared to the double-scatter technique; therefore, in some cases, the compromise may be a more conformal high-dose distribution but increased regions of low dose. This is further compromised by the common use of more than three beams. This trade-off needs to be considered on a case-by-case basis.

Several dosimetric studies have compared IMPT to 3D conformal proton radiotherapy. In a study by Boehling et al. (2012), IMPT was superior to 3D conformal proton therapy in the dose delivered to the vascular structures and subventricular zone; but 3D conformal proton therapy was superior in the dose delivered to the infratentorial brain and brainstem. Beltran et al. found that IMPT afforded the highest conformality, but double-scatter proton therapy was less sensitive to changes in target volume due to cyst growth. In a clinical case study, Yeung et al. created IMPT plans for eight patients who had been treated with double-scatter proton therapy (Yeung et al., 2014). IMPT increased the therapeutic ratio through improved target coverage conformality and normal tissue avoidance, while MFO better avoided normal tissue compared to the single-field uniform dose (Figure 22.11). In a pediatric craniopharyngioma case report by Amsbaugh et al., the authors advocate spot scanning with single-field optimization because it "creates highly conformal plans yet is less sensitive to

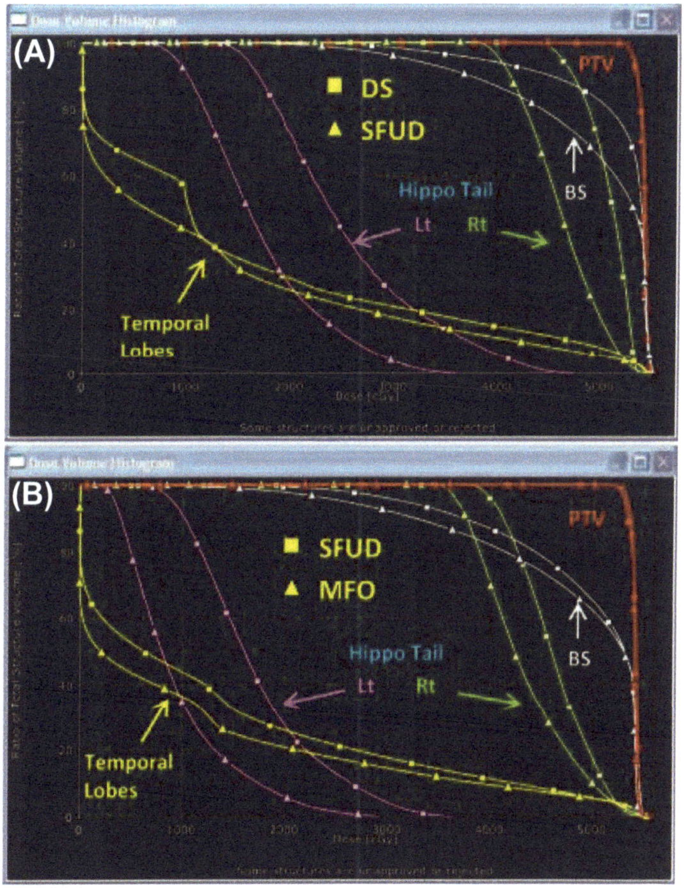

FIGURE 22.11 **A,** A dose–volume histogram (DVH) comparison between double-scatter proton therapy and intensity-modulated proton therapy (IMPT) with single-field uniform dose (SFUD) optimization and range shifters. Target coverage was achieved with both plans, but IMPT resulted in a lower dose to the organs at risk. Three fields with the same beam angles were used for both plans. **B,** A DVH comparison between SFUD and multi-field optimization (MFO). MFO further reduced the dose to the organs at risk. Range shifters were not needed for the MFO technique for this case; the sharper penumbra resulted in better sparing, especially for the left hippocampal tail. *Reprinted with permission from Yeung, D., McKenzie, C., Indelicato, D., A dosimetric comparison of intensity-modulated proton therapy optimization techniques for pediatric craniopharyngiomas: a clinical case study. Pediatric Blood and Cancer 2014; 61(1), 89–94.*

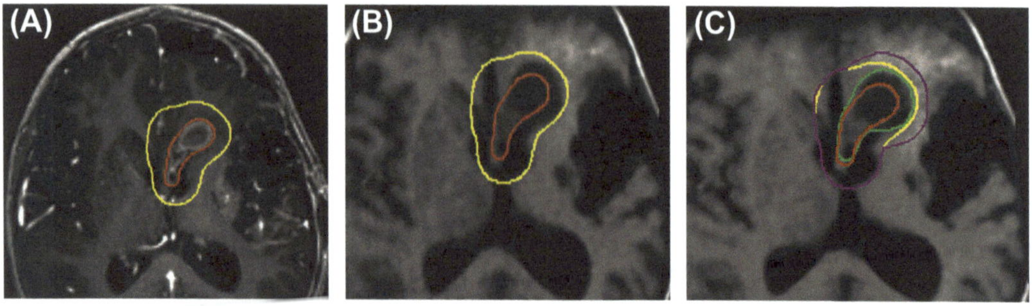

FIGURE 22.12 An image of a patient with cyst growth during radiotherapy resulting in replanning. **A,** Planning magnetic resonance images with the initial gross tumor volume (GTV) outlined in red and the initial clinical target volume (CTV) outlined in yellow. **B,** Week 1 scan. The initial GTV is outlined in red and the initial CTV is outlined in yellow. **C,** The same Week 1 MRI slice with the new GTV outlined in green and the new CTV outlined in purple. Note that the cyst now touches the initial CTV, indicating the need for replanning.

proton range uncertainties than IMPT" (Amsbaugh et al., 2012). At present, spot scanning techniques lack clinical maturity, and therefore the optimal technique remains debatable.

As with the transition from 3D conformal photon radiotherapy to IMRT, concern about marginal misses exists, since the more highly conformal dose distribution is less forgiving of the inherent uncertainty in target delineation and daily setup variations. This risk is accentuated in proton therapy, as the effect of these uncertainties on the range must also be accounted for. For this reason, a 5-mm CTV margin is being investigated with proton therapy in the prospective phase II RT2CR study. In a tumor such as craniopharyngioma, for which weekly MRI is recommended during radiotherapy due to concern for cyst expansion (Beltran et al., 2010), the fear of underdosing the target or overdosing adjacent structures is quite poignant (Figure 22.12). In one study of 17 patients treated with proton therapy who underwent imaging during radiotherapy, significant cyst growth occurred in six patients (Winkfield et al., 2009). Of the 17 patients, four (24%) required actual revision of the RT plan to accommodate cyst enlargement. Beltran et al. suggest that adaptive planning is required if a change in target volume $\geq 5\%$ develops for IMPT, $\geq 10\%$ for IMRT and $\geq 25\%$ for double-scatter proton therapy (Beltran et al., 2012). Replanning for proton therapy is more complex than for conventional radiation therapy. In double-scattered treatments, extending the CTV and PTV requires a change in the aperture and compensator, first on the planning computer and then with the actual hardware manufacture. In addition, the distal margin of one or more beams may require adjustment.

SUMMARY

Mature data from multiple institutions suggest that proton therapy is a highly effective and well-tolerated radiation therapy modality for patients with craniopharyngioma. The dosimetric advantage of proton therapy allows radiation oncologists to spare critical areas of the developing brain without compromising local control. Irradiating a craniopharyngioma that contains dynamic cystic elements presents a unique challenge to the delivery of proton therapy. Meticulous planning and frequent tumor monitoring are necessary to ensure successful treatment. Reductions in target volume should ideally be approached cautiously under prospective study. In the future, new technological developments such as IMPT may further advance the therapeutic ratio of proton therapy.

Acknowledgments

We would like to thank the Pediatric Proton Foundation and the National Association of Proton Therapy for providing the data for Figure 22.3. For assistance with editing and preparing the manuscript for publication, we would also like to thank Jessica Kirwan and the editorial staff in the Department of Radiation Oncology at the University of Florida.

References

Alapetite, C., Puget, S., Ruffier, A., Habrand, J.L., Bolle, S., Noel, G., Nauraye, C., De Marzy, L., Boddaert, N., Brisse, H., Sainte-Rose, C., Zerah, M., Boetto, S., Laffond, C., Chevignard, M., Grill, J., Doz, F., 2012. Proton therapy for craniopharyngioma in children: update of the Orsay Proton Center Experience. Neuro. Oncol. 14, i22–i25. CR-09.

Aldana, P.R., Macgregor, T.L., James, H.E., Marcus Jr., R.B., Indelicato, D.J., 2010. Titanium screws as fiducial markers for image-guided stereotactic proton irradiation in pediatric central nervous system tumors: a technical report. Pediatr. Neurosurg. 46, 227–231.

Amsbaugh, M.J., Zhu, X.R., Palmer, M., Poenisch, F., Mcaleer, M.F., Mahajan, A., Grosshans, D.R., 2012. Spot scanning proton therapy for craniopharyngioma. Practical Radiat. Oncol. 2, 314–318.

Beltran, C., Naik, M., Merchant, T.E., 2010. Dosimetric effect of target expansion and setup uncertainty during radiation therapy in pediatric craniopharyngioma. Radiother. Oncol. 97, 399–403.

Beltran, C., Roca, M., Merchant, T.E., 2012. On the benefits and risks of proton therapy in pediatric craniopharyngioma. Int. J. Radiat. Oncol. Biol. Phys. 82, e281–e287.

Bishop, A.J., Mahajan, A., Okcu, M.F., Allen, P.K., Kahalley, L.S., Mcaleer, M.F., Mcgovern, S.L., Grosshans, D.R., 2013. Proton therapy for the treatment of childhood craniopharyngiomas: cyst dynamics and initial outcomes. American Radium Society 95th Annual Meeting, P054.

Boehling, N.S., Grosshans, D.R., Bluett, J.B., Palmer, M.T., Song, X., Amos, R.A., Sahoo, N., Meyer, J.J., Mahajan, A., Woo, S.Y., 2012. Dosimetric comparison of three-dimensional conformal proton radiotherapy, intensity-modulated proton therapy, and intensity-modulated radiotherapy for treatment of pediatric craniopharyngiomas. Int. J. Radiat. Oncol. Biol. Phys. 82, 643–652.

Chang, A.L., Fitzek, M.M., Kruter, L.E., Roach, K., Thornton, A.F., 2009. Outcomes of pediatric craniopharyngioma treated with proton radiation therapy. Int. J. Radiat. Oncol. Biol. Phys. 75. S513.

Chapman, C.H., Nagesh, V., Sundgren, P.C., Buchtel, H., Chenevert, T.L., Junck, L., Lawrence, T.S., Tsien, C.I., Cao, Y., 2012. Diffusion tensor imaging of normal-appearing white matter as biomarker for radiation-induced late delayed cognitive decline. Int. J. Radiat. Oncol. Biol. Phys. 82, 2033–2040.

Chung, C.S., Yock, T.I., Nelson, K., Xu, Y., Keating, N.L., Tarbell, N.J., 2013. Incidence of second malignancies among patients treated with proton versus photon radiation. Int. J. Radiat. Oncol. Biol. Phys. 87, 46–52.

Confer, M.E., Mcnall-Knapp, R.S.K., Gross, N., 2012. Proton radiation therapy for pediatric craniopharyngiomas: initial results. Int. J. Radiat. Oncol. Biol. Phys. 84. S635.

Cushing, H., 1932. Intracranial tumors. Notes upon a series of two thousand cases with surgical mortality percentages pertaining thereto. Thomas, Springfield, IL.

Durante, M., Loeffler, J.S., 2010. Charged particles in radiation oncology. Nat. Rev. Clin. Oncol. 7, 37–43.

Farr, J.B., Mascia, A.E., Hsi, W.C., Allgower, C.E., Jesseph, F., Schreuder, A.N., Wolanski, M., Nichiporov, D.F., Anferov, V., 2008. Clinical characterization of a proton beam continuous uniform scanning system with dose layer stacking. Med. Phys. 35, 4945–4954.

Fitzek, M.M., Linggood, R.M., Adams, J., Munzenrider, J.E., 2006. Combined proton and photon irradiation for craniopharyngioma: long-term results of the early cohort of patients treated at Harvard Cyclotron Laboratory and Massachusetts General Hospital. Int. J. Radiat. Oncol. Biol. Phys. 64, 1348–1354.

Friedman, D.L., Whitton, J., Leisenring, W., Mertens, A.C., Hammond, S., Stovall, M., Donaldson, S.S., Meadows, A.T., Robison, L.L., Neglia, J.P., 2010. Subsequent neoplasms in 5-year survivors of childhood cancer: the Childhood Cancer Survivor Study. J. Natl. Cancer Inst. 102, 1083–1095.

Halperin, E.C., 2006. Particle therapy and treatment of cancer. Lancet. Oncol. 7, 676–685.

Indelicato, D.J., Rotondo, R., Flampouri, S., Kowalchik, K., Sandler, E., Aldana, P., Merchant, T.E., Mendenhall, N.P., Marcus, R.B., 2012. Proton therapy for craniopharyngioma: early clinical outcomes. Int. J. Radiat. Oncol. Biol. Phys. 84. S634.

Khong, P.L., Leung, L.H., Fung, A.S., Fong, D.Y., Qiu, D., Kwong, D.L., Ooi, G.C., Mcalonan, G., Cao, G., Chan, G.C., 2006. White matter anisotropy in post-treatment childhood cancer survivors: preliminary evidence of association with neurocognitive function. J. Clin. Oncol. 24, 884–890.

Laffond, C., Dellatolas, G., Alapetite, C., Puget, S., Grill, J., Habrand, J.L., Doz, F., Chevignard, M., 2012. Quality-of-life, mood and executive functioning after childhood craniopharyngioma treated with surgery and proton beam therapy. Brain Inj. 26, 270–281.

Laser, B.S., Merchant, T.E., Indelicato, D.J., Hua, C.H., Shulkin, B.L., Snyder, S.E., 2013. Evaluation of children with craniopharyngioma using carbon-11 methionine PET prior to proton therapy. Neuro. Oncol. 15, 506–510.

Lomax, A.J., 2008a. Intensity modulated proton therapy and its sensitivity to treatment uncertainties 1: the potential effects of calculational uncertainties. Phys. Med. Biol. 53, 1027–1042.

Lomax, A.J., 2008b. Intensity modulated proton therapy and its sensitivity to treatment uncertainties 2: the potential effects of inter-fraction and inter-field motions. Phys. Med. Biol. 53, 1043–1056.

Luu, Q.T., Loredo, L.N., Archambeau, J.O., Yonemoto, L.T., Slater, J.M., Slater, J.D., 2006. Fractionated proton radiation treatment for pediatric craniopharyngioma: preliminary report. Cancer J. 12, 155–159.

Merchant, T.E., Conklin, H.M., Onar-Thomas, A., Boop, F.A., 2013. Longitudinal models of cognitive function in children with craniopharyngioma demonstrate the effect of radiation dose. Int. J. Radiat. Oncol. Biol. Phys. 87, S38–S39.

Merchant, T.E., Hua, C.H., Shukla, H., Ying, X., Nill, S., Oelfke, U., 2008. Proton versus photon radiotherapy for common pediatric brain tumors: comparison of models of dose characteristics and their relationship to cognitive function. Pediatr. Blood Cancer 51, 110–117.

Merchant, T.E., Kiehna, E.N., Kun, L.E., Mulhern, R.K., Li, C., Xiong, X., Boop, F.A., Sanford, R.A., 2006. Phase II trial of conformal radiation therapy for pediatric patients with craniopharyngioma and correlation of surgical factors and radiation dosimetry with change in cognitive function. J. Neurosurg. 104, 94–102.

Merchant, T.E., Kiehna, E.N., Sanford, R.A., Mulhern, R.K., Thompson, S.J., Wilson, M.W., Lustig, R.H., Kun, L.E., 2002. Craniopharyngioma: the St. Jude Children's Research Hospital experience 1984–2001. Int. J. Radiat. Oncol. Biol. Phys. 53, 533–542.

Miralbell, R., Lomax, A., Cella, L., Schneider, U., 2002. Potential reduction of the incidence of radiation-induced second cancers by using proton beams in the treatment of pediatric tumors. Int. J. Radiat. Oncol. Biol. Phys. 54, 824–829.

Nagesh, V., Tsien, C.I., Chenevert, T.L., Ross, B.D., Lawrence, T.S., Junick, L., Cao, Y., 2008. Radiation-induced changes in normal-appearing white matter in patients with cerebral tumors: a diffusion tensor imaging study. Int. J. Radiat. Oncol. Biol. Phys. 70, 1002–1010.

Robertson, J.B., Williams, J.R., Schmidt, R.A., Little, J.B., Flynn, D.F., Suit, H.D., 1975. Radiobiological studies of a high-energy modulated proton beam utilizing cultured mammalian cells. Cancer 35, 1664–1677.

Suneja, G., Poorvu, P.D., Hill-Kayser, C., Lustig, R.A., 2013. Acute toxicity of proton beam radiation for pediatric central nervous system malignancies. Pediatr. Blood Cancer 60, 1431–1436.

Uh, J., Hua, C., Lam, M., Indelicato, D.J., Merchant, T.E., 2013. Assessment of structural integrity of normal brain tissues in craniopharyngioma patients after proton therapy. ISMRM 21st Annual Meeting and Exhibition, 3639.

Visser, J., Hukin, J., Sargent, M., Steinbok, P., Goddard, K., Fryer, C., 2010. Late mortality in pediatric patients with craniopharyngioma. J. NeuPlsrooncol 100, 105.

Winkfield, K.M., Linsenmeier, C., Yock, T.I., Grant, P.E., Yeap, B.Y., Butler, W.E., Tarbell, N.J., 2009. Surveillance of craniopharyngioma cyst growth in children treated with proton radiotherapy. Int. J. Radiat. Oncol. Biol. Phys. 73, 716–721.

Winkfield, K.M., Tsai, H.K., Yao, X., Larson, E., Neuberg, D., Pomeroy, S.L., Ullrich, N.J., Cohen, L.E., Kieran, M.W., Scott, R.M., Goumnerova, L.C., Marcus, K.J., 2011. Long-term clinical outcomes following treatment of childhood craniopharyngioma. Pediatr. Blood Cancer 56, 1120–1126.

Yeung, D., Mckenzie, C., Indelicato, D.J., 2014. A dosimetric comparison of intensity-modulated proton therapy optimization techniques for pediatric craniopharyngiomas: A clinical case study. Pediatr. Blood Cancer 61 (1), 89–94.

CHAPTER

23

Craniopharyngioma: Radiation Toxicities

Roshan V. Sethi, Shannon M. MacDonald

Department of Radiation Oncology, Massachusetts General Hospital, Harvard Medical School, Boston, MA, USA

"Tumor dose: 2,844 r; period of treatment forty-seven days. September 5, 1934. *Hemiparesis almost disappeared; patient now able to continue her studies on the piano."* ***RC Carpenter, GW Chamberlin, and CH Frazier, 1937***

INTRODUCTION

In the treatment of craniopharyngioma, radiotherapy (RT) represents a definitive and effective therapy that avoids the morbidity associated with extensive surgical resection. However, RT also carries the risks of toxicity, many which manifest long after treatment. This is a particular concern among patients with craniopharyngioma, as the majority of these patients will become long-term survivors. These effects, which may not be clinically observed for years after treatment, include cognitive decline, endocrine deficiency, ototoxicity, optic neuropathy, vascular complications, radiation necrosis, and second malignancy.

The prevalence of these complications in survivors of craniopharyngioma is still not well understood, due to the rarity of the tumor. Many of the studies reviewed in this chapter include patients with other types of central nervous system tumors treated with cranial RT (CRT) to a portion of the brain and in some cases the whole brain. These studies should be interpreted with caution, as the therapeutic field in craniopharyngioma is limited to the tumor and a small margin. In addition, the central location of craniopharyngiomas – which grow adjacent to the optic nerves, the circle of Willis, and the hypothalamic–pituitary axis – significantly increases the morbidity of any treatment, including surgical resection. In addition, recent technological advances in imaging and radiation oncology have improved the therapeutic ratio for radiation. However, the majority of the data regarding late effects comes from outdated radiation techniques, since long-term follow-up is required to report these complications.

Craniopharyngiomas
http://dx.doi.org/10.1016/B978-0-12-416706-3.00023-4

Although craniopharyngiomas are considered to be "benign" tumors, the complications of tumor growth, surgical resection, or CRT greatly impact the quality of life of survivors. Modern treatment aims to provide tumor control while preserving overall function. Patients with craniopharyngioma who received CRT should undergo regular follow-up care to screen for late complications of treatment.

ACUTE

Toxicities related to CRT are divided into acute, sub-acute, and late effects according to the timing of the complications. Acute effects, which are usually temporary, occur during irradiation. Sub-acute or early delayed reactions occur up to six months after the completion of CRT. Late effects occur after six months, but may take years to develop.

The most common acute reactions to CRT are nausea/vomiting, fatigue, headache, and decreased appetite. Nausea and vomiting are effectively treated with anti-emetics, particularly 5-hydroxytryptamine 3 receptor antagonists (Maranzano et al., 2010). In a series of 78 pediatric patients with low-grade glioma undergoing partial brain CRT, 69% of patients required anti-emetic therapy during treatment (Merchant et al., 2009b).

In 2002, Merchant et al. described initial cyst expansion during CRT in four of 23 patients with craniopharyngioma (Merchant et al., 2002b). Cyst expansion, which reflects inflammation from tumor death rather than disease progression, may cause headache, nausea, and a transient worsening of pre-existing neurological deficits. Symptoms from the expansion may be managed with corticosteroids. The expansion generally resolves or remains stable by the completion of CRT. In order to assure accurate delivery of CRT, treatment plans should be adjusted for cyst expansion or contraction.

The majority of acute toxicities resolve after completion of CRT, although both fatigue and decreased appetite frequently persist after treatment (see the section "Sub-Acute" below and also Figure 23.1) (Merchant et al., 2009b). Alopecia, which develops after two to three weeks of CRT and resolves in the months following treatment, may be permanent in a sub-set of patients (Lawenda et al., 2004). In 2004, Lawnenda et al. correlated follicle dose with the late-term alopecia score (Lawenda et al., 2004). Patients with moderate-to-severe alopecia received a mean follicle scalp dose of 56.1 Gy, while patients with none-to-minimal alopecia received a mean scalp dose of 31.6 Gy. At a follicle dose of 43 Gy (in 30 fractions), half of patients developed permanent alopecia. The receipt of chemotherapy, a personal history of hair loss, and several classes of medications may increase the risk of permanent alopecia (Lawenda et al., 2004).

SUB-ACUTE

The most significant sub-acute reaction after CRT is somnolence syndrome, a condition characterized by extreme fatigue, and, less commonly, signs of increased intra-cranial pressure, including headache, nausea, and vomiting (Littman et al., 1984; Mandell et al., 1989; Uzal et al., 1998). The presumed etiology is transient demyelination of cerebral white matter tracts. Symptoms typically peak after six weeks and resolve by six months (Powell et al., 2011).

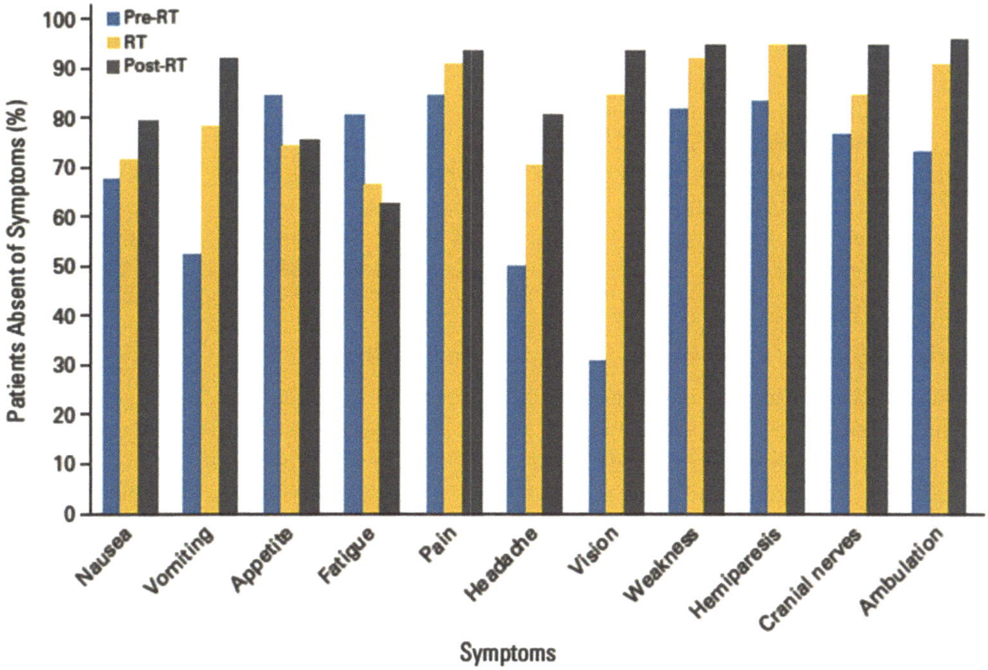

FIGURE 23.1 Presence of symptoms before, during, and after CRT for low-grade glioma. *Source: Merchant, 2009.*

The exact prevalence of the condition is not known, as symptoms are non-specific and physicians do not always evaluate patients during the period in which somnolence reaches its peak incidence. In addition, the severity of somnolence ranges widely among affected patients. In a series of 97 children treated for acute lymphocytic leukemia (ALL) who received whole-brain CRT, 58% reported some degree of somnolence in the sub-acute period (Littman et al., 1984). The risk was not related to the daily fraction size (1 Gy vs. 1.8 Gy). In 2011, Powell et al. reported that 90% of 70 patients undergoing CRT for glioblastoma multiforme reported some degree of somnolence following the completion of CRT (Powell et al., 2011). Thirty-three patients reported mild to moderate somnolence, and one patient reported severe somnolence.

Prophylactic and low-dose corticosteroids administered during or after CRT may reduce the risk of developing somnolence syndrome (Mandell et al., 1989; Uzal et al., 1998). Treatment with neuro-stimulants, such as modafinil (Provigil®) or methylphenidate (Ritalin®) may also avoid side effects associated with steroids (Butler Jr. et al., 2007).

LATE EFFECTS

Neurocognitive

Cognitive impairment in survivors of childhood primary brain tumors is related to many variables, including tumor location and extent, hydrocephalus, shunt devices, chemotherapy, and CRT dose and volume (Mulhern et al., 2004). Of these variables, CRT is likely the most significant risk factor for cognitive injury, particularly when administered to children under the age of three years (Mulhern et al., 2004).

Cognitive changes are due to failure of development rather than a decline in existing ability. In 2001, Palmer et al. studied the rate of new knowledge acquisition in 44 patients with medulloblastoma (Palmer et al., 2001). The authors found that patients who had undergone cranial RT acquired new information less rapidly than healthy age-matched peers. This finding may be due to RT-related impairment of the growth of cerebral normal-appearing white matter, which develops rapidly in very young children (Mulhern et al., 1999; Reddick et al., 2005).

Cognitive Function After Whole-Brain And Partial-Brain CRT

RT-induced cognitive decline was originally described in patients undergoing whole-brain CRT and medulloblastoma (Silber et al., 1992). The loss in full-scale intelligence quotient (FSIQ) correlated with both dose and age at the time of irradiation. In a study of 48 patients with either ALL or medulloblastoma, Silber et al. found that the follow-up FSIQ in patients who received CRT to a dose of 36 Gy was 8.2 points lower than the FSIQ of a patient who received 24 Gy, and 12.3 points lower than the FSIQ of a patient who received 18 Gy (Silber et al., 1992). These studies led to a reduction in the craniospinal dose for selected patients with medulloblastoma, and the use of chemotherapy to delay CRT (Duffner et al., 1993). Contemporary estimates of whole-brain CRT-induced cognitive decline are lower than previous series. In studies published between 2001 and 2005, estimates of the annual decline in FSIQ ranged from −1.59 points/year to −4.3 points/year (Palmer et al., 2001; Ris et al., 2001; Spiegler et al., 2004; Mulhern et al., 2005).

In contrast to patients treated with whole-brain CRT, patients treated with partial-brain CRT appear to enjoy relative stability of FSIQ (Netson et al., 2012). These findings have been attributed to the use of increasingly conformal RT techniques that significantly limit the volume of supratentorial brain receiving the highest dose (Merchant et al., 2005, 2006b). In 2009, Merchant et al. studied the cognitive outcomes in 78 patients with low-grade glioma who underwent CRT (Merchant et al., 2009a). Fifty-five patients were evaluated on at least two occasions. The estimated FSIQ at 60 months (average 95.4) was not significantly changed from baseline (98.96). Netson et al. reported similar results in a cohort of 123 patients with ependymoma (Netson et al., 2012). The estimated FSIQ did not decline significantly, with an estimated annual loss of −0.04 points/year.

While partial-brain CRT appears to preserve FSIQ, both the baseline and annual change scores are still modified significantly by age. In the Merchant series, for example, children with low-grade glioma who were 5 years old at the time of irradiation experienced an average ten-point decline in estimated FSIQ by 60 months after the administration of CRT (see Figure 23.2) (Merchant et al., 2009a). In contrast, patients with ependymoma under the age of 3 years exhibited lower baseline estimated FSIQ (89.7 vs. 98.7), but demonstrated significant improvement over time (Merchant et al., 2004). Intellectual outcomes also depend on the region of brain that receives the highest dose (Merchant et al., 2005). In a study of 86 patients with ependymoma, Merchant et al. found that estimated IQ correlated with dosimetry to the supratentorial brain (Merchant et al., 2005). Patients who received between 45 and 60 Gy to the supratentorial brain were at the greatest risk of cognitive decline.

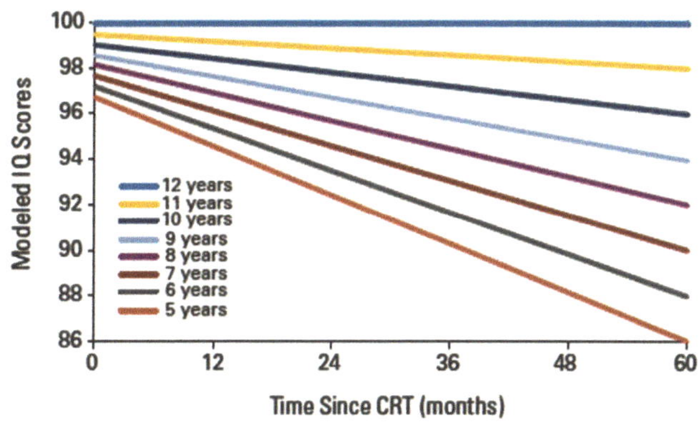

FIGURE 23.2 Cognitive decline by age in patients with low-grade glioma. *Source: Merchant, 2009.*

In addition to FSIQ, studies have investigated multiple other cognitive, behavioral, and academic domains that may be affected by CRT. In patients with low-grade glioma and ependymoma, Merchant et al. and Netson et al. observed significant declines in academic reading and spelling achievement, and the communication sub-set of adaptive behavior, though overall adaptive behavior remained intact (Conklin et al., 2008; Netson et al., 2012). In patients with ependymoma, low-grade glioma, and craniopharyngioma, verbal, and visual-auditory learning are also intact after CRT (Di Pinto et al., 2010, 2012). Inattentiveness, as measured by the Connors' Continuous Performance test, increases significantly after CRT, particularly among patients with craniopharyngioma or other diencephalic tumors (Kiehna et al., 2006).

Cognitive Function in Craniopharyngioma

Few studies have examined cognitive performance after CRT in patients with craniopharyngioma. In 2006, Merchant et al. reported the cognitive outcomes of 27 patients with craniopharyngioma at 48 months after CRT (Merchant et al., 2006a). These patients had been treated on a Phase II trial that sought to limit the clinical tumor volume margin to 1 cm around the solid and cystic complex. While patients over the age of 7.4 years at the time of CRT exhibited relative cognitive stability, patients 7.4 years or younger experienced a significant decline in estimated FSIQ (see Figure 23.3A). The risk was highly modified by other variables, including extensive surgery and pre-RT diabetes insipidus (see Figure 23.3B).

Surgical resection also impacts cognitive morbidity (Merchant et al., 2002b; Ondruch et al., 2011). In 2002, Merchant et al. studied the cognitive morbidity of different upfront treatment strategies (Merchant et al., 2002b). In this series, the authors compared 15 patients treated with surgery alone to 15 patients treated with limited surgery and irradiation. At a median cognitive follow-up of 52 months, the loss in FSIQ was 9.8 points in patients treated with upfront surgery alone (though eight received CRT at relapse) and 1.25 points in patients treated with limited surgery and irradiation. These findings suggested that the cognitive morbidity associated with maximal resection and an increased risk of recurrence outweighed the cognitive morbidity of CRT alone, though few other studies have performed a similar comparison (Cavazzuti et al., 1983).

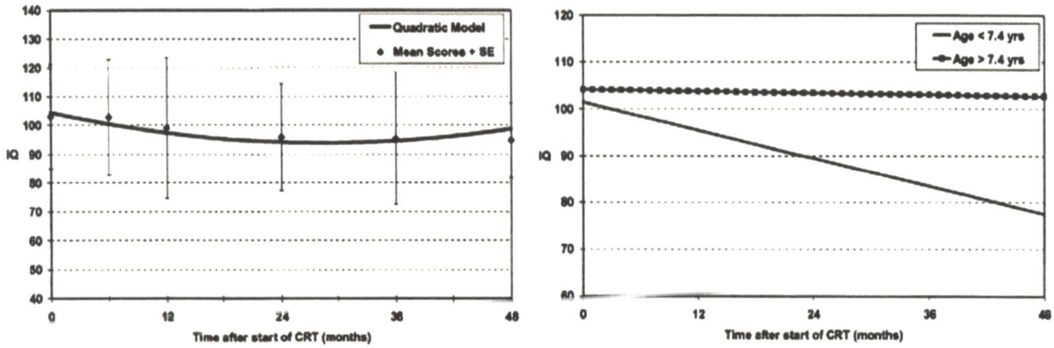

FIGURE 23.3 Cognitive decline in patients with craniopharyngioma. *Source: Merchant, 2006.*

Neuro-Endocrine

Structures at Risk

The hypothalamic–pituitary axis influences nearly every physiological function in the body, including growth, metabolism, stress response, pubertal development, and osmotic balance. The hypothalamus, a small structure located inferior to the thalamus, secretes stimulatory and inhibitory factors that regulate the action of hormones produced in the anterior pituitary: growth hormone (GH), thyroid stimulating hormone (TSH), adrenocorticotropic hormone (ACTH), luteinizing hormone (LH), follicle-stimulating hormone (FSH), and prolactin (PRL). It also synthesizes oxytocin and vasopressin (ADH), which are stored in the posterior pituitary, a neuronal projection of the hypothalamus (see Table 23.1 and Figure 23.4) (Sklar and Constine, 1995).

RT-induced injury to the hypothalamus is a widely recognized complication of CRT. It is presumed to result from direct damage to secreting parenchymal cells and the supportive vasculature (Constine et al., 1993; Sklar and Constine, 1995). Mean dose to the hypothalamus is correlated with the risk of every anterior pituitary hormone deficiency, with the exception of prolactin. The incidence of endocrinopathy increases over time, likely because of

TABLE 23.1 Hypothalamic and Pituitary Factors

Hypothalamic Factor	Effect on Pituitary Secretion	Pituitary Hormone
GH-releasing hormone Somatostatin	Stimulatory Inhibitory	Growth hormone
Dopamine	Inhibitory	Prolactin
Gonadotropin-releasing hormone	Stimulatory	Lutenizing hormone Follicle-stimulating hormone
Thyrotropin-releasing hormone	Stimulatory	Thyroid stimulating hormone
Corticotropin-releasing hormone	Stimulatory	Adrenocorticotropin

Adapted from Sklar, 1995.

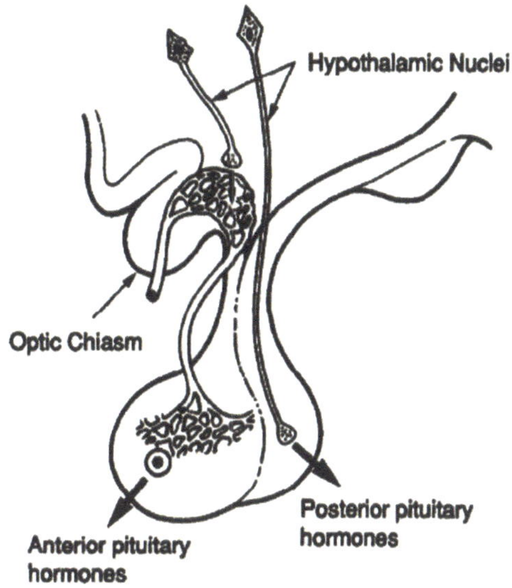

FIGURE 23.4 Hypothalamic–pituitary axis. *Source: Sklar, 1995.*

underlying progressive vascular damage. The pituitary is less radiosensitive than the hypothalamus, although pituitary damage still contributes substantially to the rate of RT-induced endocrinopathy (Constine et al., 1993; Fernandez et al., 2009). Nevertheless, most studies rely on dose to the hypothalamus, because the radiation tolerance of this organ is better understood and the dose to both structures is usually similar.

Endocrinopathy in Craniopharyngioma

The rate of pre-treatment endocrinopathy is very high in patients with craniopharyngioma, due to the suprasellar location of the tumor (Sklar, 1994a; DeVile et al., 1996). Hormonal axes are further perturbed by surgery, even when microsurgical techniques are used to avoid critical structures. The risk of post-operative endocrinopathy is related to the extent of hypothalamic tumor involvement and the extent of attempted surgical resection (Regine et al., 1993; Poretti et al., 2004; Stripp et al., 2004; Lopez-Serna et al., 2012). The estimated prevalence of any anterior or posterior pituitary endocrinopathy after surgical resection ranges from 60% to 100% in recent series (Danoff et al., 1982, 1983; Regine et al., 1993; Sklar, 1994b; Fisher et al., 1998; Habrand et al., 1999; Merchant et al., 2002b, 2006a; Karavitaki et al., 2005; Jung et al., 2009, 2010). Some deficits – including obesity related to hyperphagia and diabetes insipidus with absent thirst mechanism – are unique to the mass effect of tumor or surgical resection (Hoffman et al., 1992; Sklar, 1994b).

It is difficult to estimate the extent of the additional risk contributed by radiation therapy when used as adjuvant or salvage therapy (Danoff et al., 1982; Regine et al., 1993; Gonc et al., 2004; Karavitaki et al., 2005). Multiple studies, published as early as 1980, found that the prevalence of endocrinopathy is actually lower after limited surgery and irradiation than - after maximal resection (Thomsett et al., 1980; Weiss et al., 1989; Hetelekidis et al., 1993;

Rajan et al., 1993; Sklar, 1994a; Sughrue et al., 2011; Clark et al., 2012; Gautier et al., 2012). In 2002, Merchant et al. reported the outcomes of 30 pediatric patients with craniopharyngioma who had been treated with either upfront surgical resection only or limited surgery with irradiation (Merchant et al., 2002b). The authors found that adrenal hormone supplementation (93% vs. 67%) and ADH replacement (73% vs. 33%) were required more often by patients treated with upfront surgery alone, although over half of these patients received radiotherapy at relapse.

As a result of ongoing evolution in radiation techniques, RT is increasingly used as adjuvant treatment for craniopharyngioma. In 2013, Cohen et al. compared the outcomes of patients with craniopharyngioma treated at the Hospital for Sick Children over the last three decades (Cohen et al., 2013). Since 1975, the rate of gross total resection has decreased, while the rate of sub-total resection and adjuvant therapy (including intra-cystic chemotherapy and RT) has increased. The authors observed a corresponding decline in the prevalence of any hormonal deficiency, anterior panhypopituitarism, diabetes insipidus, and severe obesity.

Growth Hormone Deficiency

Growth hormone deficiency (GHD) is the most common and best-characterized endocrine complication of RT (Duffner et al., 1985; Lustig et al., 1985; Constine et al., 1993; Merchant et al., 2002c; Gurney et al., 2003). In children, GHD limits growth, delays bone age, alters body compositions, and worsens cognition and quality of life. In adults, GHD alters body composition and lipid profile, decreases bone mineral density, and, most significantly, depresses quality of life and overall psychological well being (Attanasio et al., 1997; Vance and Mauras, 1999; Murray et al., 2002; Maiter et al., 2006).

GHD is associated with many pre-treatment variables, including tumor location and size and hydrocephalus. Among suprasellar tumors, the prevalence of pre-CRT GHD is very high (88%) (Merchant et al., 2002c). After the delivery of high-dose RT to tumors in this location, the prevalence of GHD is near universal. In contrast, among patients with non-suprasellar primary brain tumors undergoing CRT to doses between 13 to 65 Gy, the overall prevalence of GHD is 35% (Mulder et al., 2009).

The dose–response curve of GHD has been studied in detail. In 2011, Merchant et al. performed provocative testing of GH secretion on 192 patients with primary brain tumors before and after partial-brain CRT (Merchant et al., 2002a, 2011). The risk of GHD was greater than 5% regardless of the mean dose to the hypothalamus. At a dose as low as 5 Gy, the 5-year risk of GHD was 23%. The cumulative dose associated with a 50% risk of GHD at 5 years was 16.1 Gy, which the authors recommend as the avoidance dose to the hypothalamic–pituitary axis. Higher doses to the hypothalamus shortened the time to the development of GHD; patients who received greater than 60 Gy developed GHD by 12 months, while patients who received 15–20 Gy developed GHD by 60 months (see Figure 23.5).

The most sensitive method of testing for GHD is provocative or stimulatory testing, in which the serum concentration of GH is measured after the administration of multiple possible agents, most commonly arginine plus levodopa (L-dopa). The diagnostic threshold for GHD is still controversial. The most conservative criteria require post-stimulation values less than 5–7 ng/mL (Merchant et al., 2011). Provocative testing protocols use multiple blood draws, which can be uncomfortable for children (Hua et al., 2012). As an alternative, many

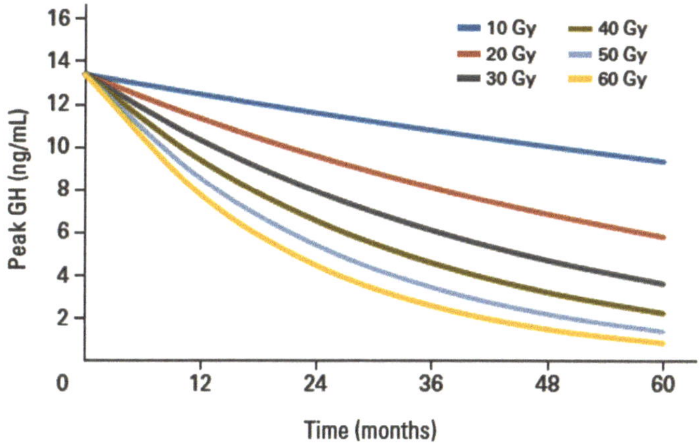

FIGURE 23.5 Risk of growth hormone (GH) deficiency correlates with mean dose to the hypothalamus. *Source: Merchant, 2011.*

centers use the serum insulin-like growth factor-1 (IGF-1) and insulin-like growth factor binding protein-3 (IGFBP-3), though these screening tests are significantly less sensitive for the detection of RT-induced GHD than provocative testing (Sklar et al., 1993; Tillmann et al., 1998; Hua et al., 2012). Both IGF-1 and IGFBP-3 are affected by age, gender, pubertal status, and obesity, which can lead to an overestimation of GHD (Sklar et al., 1993).

Early replacement with biosynthetic growth hormone analogue, sometimes administered with a gonadotropin-releasing hormone (GnRH) agonist, allows catch-up growth and normal adult height (Kanev et al., 1991; Ilveskoski et al., 1997). The therapy may be most effective in pre-pubertal children (Ogilvy-Stuart and Shalet, 1995). Most centers allow 1 year of disease control before starting treatment (Merchant et al., 2011). The theoretical risk of GH-induced tumor growth or recurrence has not been observed in multiple studies (Clayton et al., 1988; Sklar et al., 2002).

Continued replacement at the time of transition to adulthood and during adulthood may be beneficial (Abs et al., 1999; Vance and Mauras, 1999; Murray et al., 2002; Carroll et al., 2004; Koltowska-Haggstrom et al., 2010). Maiter et al. described the response to GH therapy in 1,077 adult patients with GHD and a prior history of adult-onset pituitary adenoma or craniopharyngioma (15% of the total cohort) treated by surgery and/or RT (Maiter et al., 2006). All patients were registered in the Pfizer International Metabolic Database. Among patients diagnosed with RT-induced GHD, GH therapy significantly improved body composition, lipid profile, quality of life, and bone mineral composition at 1 and 2 years.

Thyroid Hormone Deficiency

Deficiency of TSH, also known as central hypothyroidism, may be sub-clinical or cause lethargy, weight gain, and poor growth. At doses to the hypothalamic–pituitary axis between 40 and 50 Gy, central hypothyroidism may be relatively uncommon (Sklar and Constine, 1995; Schmiegelow et al., 2003; Laughton et al., 2008). At doses above 50 Gy, however, the prevalence of central hypothyroidism is similar to the prevalence of GHD

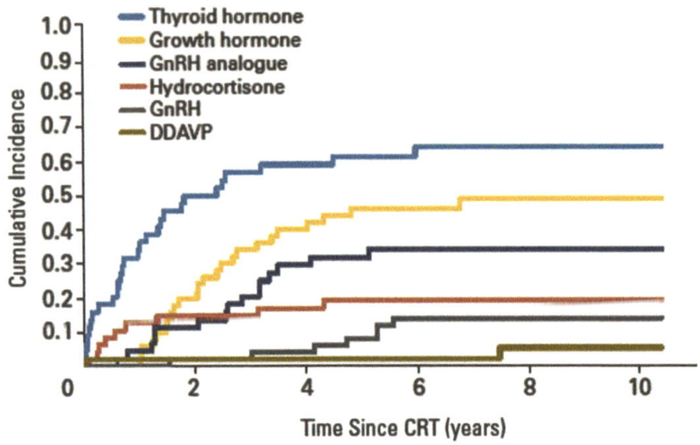

FIGURE 23.6 Cumulative incidence of hormonal replacement therapy. *Source: Merchant, 2009.*

(Constine et al., 1987, 1993). In 2009, Merchant et al. reported treatment toxicities in a cohort of 78 pediatric patients with low-grade glioma treated with 54 Gy CRT. The majority (n = 58) of tumors were located in the diencephalon. The 10-year cumulative incidence of thyroid hormone replacement (including baseline hormone replacement as a competing risk) was 64.0%. Among patients who received ≥ 40 Gy, the cumulative incidence was 69.1% (see Figure 23.6).

A substantial percentage of central hypothyroidism may be mediated by damage to the pituitary. In 1982, Samaan et al. detected central hypothyroidism in 30 of 110 patients with nasopharyngeal and paranasal sinus tumors who had received a median dose of 50 Gy to the hypothalamus and 56.18 Gy to the anterior pituitary (Samaan et al., 1982). In 21 of 30 cases, TSH failed to rise after the administration of thyroid-releasing hormone (TRH), suggesting a pituitary etiology in most cases.

Adrenocorticotropic Hormone Deficiency

ACTH deficiency (ACTHD) causes nausea/vomiting, decreased appetite, hypoglycemia, and fatigue (Sklar and Constine, 1995; Rose et al., 2005). The lack of glucocorticoid reserve is particularly dangerous during illness or surgery if the replacement therapy dose is not increased (Pemberton et al., 2005). In the Constine and Merchant series, ACTHD was the least prevalent endocrine deficiency among patients treated with CRT alone (Constine et al., 1993; Merchant et al., 2009a). The relatively low prevalence may be due to the high doses required for RT-induced ACTHD. In a retrospective review of children who received CRT for primary brain tumors and hematologic malignancies, the prevalence of ACTHD was significantly increased among patients who received doses above 24 Gy compared to patients who received less than 24 Gy (28% vs. 9%), though relatively uncommon in both dose categories (Rose et al., 2005). In Constine et al., none of the patients with ACTHD had received a dose to the hypothalamus lower than 50 Gy (Constine et al., 1993). Nevertheless, testing for ACTHD is recommended in all patients with primary brain tumors who received CRT, particularly in the presence of other hypothalamic–pituitary deficiencies (Rose et al., 2005). A morning

(08:00) serum cortisol and/or low-dose ACTH stimulation are effective screening evaluations (Rose et al., 2005).

Gonadotropin Deficiency

The effect of CRT on the pubertal axis depends on the dose to the hypothalamus, and the gender of the patient (Shalet and Brennan, 2002). At lower doses, CRT can induce precocious puberty, and, at higher doses, RT can induce deficiency of LH and FSH. In children treated with doses between 18 and 24 Gy, the mean age at menarche is earlier in females, and normal in males (Quigley et al., 1989; Didcock et al., 1995). In children treated with doses between 25 and 47.5 Gy, the average onset of puberty is early in both genders. At doses greater than 50 Gy, gonadotropin deficiency, in addition to precocious puberty, can be encountered (Rappaport et al., 1982). In the Merchant low-grade glioma series, the cumulative risk of gonadotropin-replacement treatment at 10 years was 14.1%. In contrast, the 10-year cumulative incidence of GnRH agonist use was 34.2% (some patients without precocious puberty received this treatment as an adjunct to GH replacement) (Merchant et al., 2009a).

Prolactin

The production of prolactin in the anterior pituitary is inhibited by dopamine secreted by the hypothalamus (Sklar and Constine, 1995). RT-induced damage in the hypothalamus may therefore result in hyperprolactinemia (Constine et al., 1987, 1993). Though the elevation is typically mild, and few patients are symptomatic, hyperprolactinemia has been associated with the delay of puberty in children, alteration of menstruation in women, and decreased libido in men (Rappaport et al., 1982; Samaan et al., 1982; Constine et al., 1987, 1993). In 1987, Constine et al. found that the prevalence of elevated prolactin in children and adults who underwent CRT was 14% at doses ≤ 55 Gy, 64% at doses > 55 Gy and 75% at doses > 59.5 Gy (Constine et al., 1987). Treatment is rarely required, but dopamine agonists such as bromocriptine may be used in symptomatic patients (Samaan et al., 1982; Sklar and Constine, 1995).

Significance of Endocrine Deficiencies

Due to the need for life-long replacement therapy, and the limited ability of treatment to replicate the highly choreographed actions of the hypothalamus and pituitary, endocrine deficiencies significantly affect quality of life. In addition, among survivors of craniopharyngioma, endocrine deficiency remains a leading cause of morbidity and mortality (Rajan et al., 1993; Pemberton et al., 2005; Pereira et al., 2005). In particular, diabetes insipidus with absent thirst mechanism can lead to osmotic demyelination and death (Lyen and Grant, 1982; Kang and Song, 1988; DeVile et al., 1996; Pemberton et al., 2005). Morris et al. studied the causes of death in a cohort of 643 patients with primary brain tumors treated at St. Jude's Children Research Hospital from 1995 to 2000 (Morris et al., 2007). Unlike survivors of medulloblastoma or ependymoma, survivors of craniopharyngioma and germ cell tumor were more likely to die of sepsis, cardiopulmonary collapse, and metabolic collapse than recurrent disease or second malignancy. The majority of medical deaths were attributed to hormone dysfunction, and the average age at death was 14.1 years. Early diagnosis and treatment of this class of RT- and surgery-induced toxicity are critical to the long-term survival of affected patients.

Optic Neuropathy

Craniopharyngiomas grow adjacent to the optic nerves and chiasm. As a result, even highly conformal CRT plans deliver relatively high doses of radiation to the optic apparatus. Uncommonly, CRT can damage the optic nerve, resulting in acute and permanent loss of visual acuity and/or new field deficits within 3 years of irradiation (Kline et al., 1985). The mechanism of this complication is not well understood, but may result from progressive ischemia and necrosis (Kline et al., 1985).

Habrand et al. found that the risk of optic neuropathy varied according to the volume and total dose of the treated optic nerve and/or chiasm (Habrand et al., 1989). In a retrospective review of 20 patients (15 with available neuro-ophthalmology follow-up) with upper clivus tumors treated with proton RT (for the majority of treatment) to a dose between 66.6 Gy (RBE) and 74.4 Gy (RBE) at the Harvard Cyclotron Laboratory, optic neuropathy was diagnosed in two patients. One patient received > 65 Gy (RBE) to approximately half of the optic chiasm. The second patient received > 55 Gy (RBE) to a portion on one optic nerve, but also carried a diagnosis of diabetes mellitus, which was thought by the authors to be a potential predisposing factor. From this small number of patients, the authors concluded that among patients treated to ≥ 20% of the optic apparatus the risk of optic neuropathy was 12.5% at 55 Gy (RBE) and 20% to 25% at doses of 60 Gy (RBE) to 65 Gy (RBE) at fractions between 1.8 Gy (RBE) and 2.1 Gy (RBE). The two reported cases were patients who had been treated with fractions less than 2.0 Gy (RBE) (Aristizabal et al., 1977).

The risk of neuropathy also depends on the dose per fraction. Harris et al. followed 55 adult patients with craniopharyngioma and pituitary adenomas treated with between 45 and 55 Gy. The crude prevalence of optic neuropathy was 9%. Fraction size, rather than total dose, was predictive of complications. The prevalence of optic injury was 18% (5/28) among patients treated with fraction sizes greater than 2.5 Gy, and 0% (0/27) among patients treated with fraction sizes less than 2.5 Gy. Similarly, Parsons et al. reported on 215 optic nerves in 131 patients with head and neck cancers treated with RT. None of the 106 optic nerves that had received a total dose less than 59 Gy developed an optic neuropathy. Among the optic nerves that received ≥ 60 Gy, the 15-year cumulative incidence of optic neuropathy was 11% with fraction sizes < 1.9 Gy, and 47% with fraction sizes ≥ 1.9 Gy.

Craniopharyngioma patients may be at particular risk of RT-induced optic neuropathy due to prior injury to the optic apparatus from tumor growth and surgery (Harris and Levene, 1976; Flickinger et al., 1990; van den Bergh et al., 2003). In a retrospective review of 21 children and adults with craniopharyngioma, Flickinger et al. reported an actuarial 5-year cumulative incidence of optic neuropathy of 30% if greater than a normalized total dose of 60 Gy (1.8 Gy fractions) was delivered to the optic apparatus (Flickinger et al., 1990). In studies of craniopharyngioma patients treated with less than 60 Gy, optic neuropathy is substantially less common. For example, in a large retrospective review of 173 pediatric and adult craniopharyngioma patients who underwent CRT to a median dose of 56 Gy between 1950 and 1962 and a median dose of 50 Gy between 1962 and 1986, there were no cases of optic neuropathy (Rajan et al., 1993). No patient received a fraction size greater than 2.0 Gy.

In summary, optic neuropathy is an uncommon, irreversible consequence of radiation to the optic apparatus reported at doses above 45 Gy (Harris and Levene, 1976; Habrand et al., 1989; Flickinger et al., 1990). Patients treated with a total dose greater than 60 Gy and/or fractions greater than 2 Gy are at the greatest risk of developing this complication.

Vascular

Moyamoya Syndrome and Stroke Risk

Moyamoya syndrome refers to the progressive occlusion of major cerebral vessels with compensatory collateral formation. The syndrome can result from the compressive effect of tumor, surgery, and high-dose RT to the circle of Willis (Ullrich et al., 2007). In many patients, Moyamoya is eventually complicated by ischemic events and seizures. Most patients are treated with anti-platelet therapy (Ullrich et al., 2007). A sub-set of patients with rapidly progressive or symptomatic lesions may require surgical intervention (Ullrich et al., 2007).

The estimated prevalence of Moyamoya in patients treated with CRT for primary brain tumors varies between 3.5% and 9% (Ullrich et al., 2007; Merchant et al., 2009b; Winkfield et al., 2011). In the largest published study, Ullrich et al. prospectively followed 345 children treated with CRT for primary brain tumors with serial magnetic resonance (MR) scans and neurologic exams (Ullrich et al., 2007). At a median follow-up of 54 months, Moyamoya had been diagnosed in 12 patients (3.5%). Nine of the 12 required surgery with unilateral or bilateral pial synangiosis. The risk of developing Moyamoya was increased significantly by young age at the time of RT, neurofibromatosis syndrome type 1 (NF-1), and dose to the optic chiasm (chosen as a surrogate for dose to the circle of Willis). The majority of patients with Moyamoya were treated for optic system glioma. In addition, half of affected patients carried a diagnosis of NF-1 (see Figure 23.7).

The prevalence of pre-CRT vasculopathy due to tumor growth or surgery may be relatively high. In 2009, Merchant et al. reported a cohort of 78 pediatric patients with low-grade glioma treated with CRT to a median dose of 54 Gy. Prior to RT, four patients demonstrated evidence of cerebral vasculopathy, and two patients required surgical revascularization. An additional five patients developed RT-induced Moyamoya, suggesting a similar prevalence of pre-CRT and post-CRT vasculopathy (Merchant et al., 2009b). Careful

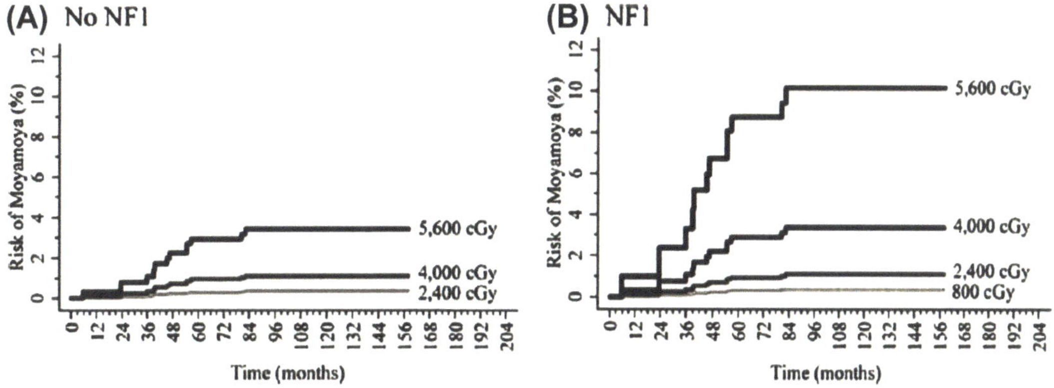

FIGURE 23.7 Risk of Moyamoya syndrome in NF-1 and non-NF1 patients. *Source: Ullrich, 2007.*

screening of patients with MR angiography prior to CRT may help to identify patients at risk of this disorder.

The prevalence of other CRT-induced vascular damage is not as well characterized as Moyamoya syndrome. In the Ullrich series, infarctions were present in 29 patients (9.6%), though ten of these strokes developed in the post-operative period. Of the 19 patients with non-surgical strokes, nine were related to Moyamoya and two were related to tumor vessel encasement. An additional ten patients developed major vessel narrowing, and three patients suffered from hemorrhagic radiation vasculopathy. As 18.8% of the patients in this series received craniospinal irradiation (CSI) for medulloblastoma, it is not clear if the prevalence of these findings would be as high among patients receiving partial brain CRT.

In 2006, Bowers et al. followed 4,828 survivors of ALL and 1,871 survivors of primary brain tumors. The 25-year cumulative incidence of patient-reported stroke was 0.84% in leukemia survivors who had received whole-brain CRT, and 0.44% in leukemia survivors who had not received CRT. Among survivors of primary brain tumors, the 25-year cumulative incidence of patient-reported stroke was 6.90% in patients who had received either partial- or whole-brain CRT, and 2.85% in patients who had not received CRT. CRT did not significantly contribute to the risk of stroke at doses below 30 Gy. In addition, in 49% of leukemia survivors with a late-occurring stroke, and in 29% of primary brain tumor survivors with a late-occurring stroke, tumor recurrence preceded the development of stroke. The risk of stroke in these patients may be related to additional treatment, or to the direct effect of the tumor.

Cavernous Hemangioma

Cavernous hemangiomas are benign vascular tumors that develop between 3 and 20 years after CRT (Lew et al., 2006; Strenger et al., 2008). Most cavernomas are asymptomatic and followed without intervention, although hemorrhage with resulting seizure or ischemia is a rare possibility (see Figure 23.8). In 2006, Lew et al. reviewed the incidence of RT-induced cavernomas in 59 patients treated with CSI for medulloblastoma to a dose of either 24 Gy or 36 Gy (Lew et al., 2006). At a mean follow-up of 7.2 years, the cumulative incidence of any lesion demonstrating susceptibility on MR was 5.6% at 3 years, 14% at 5 years, and 43% at 10 years. The relatively high prevalence of cavernomas was attributed to the increased sensitivity of the gradient-echo sequence. The majority of lesions were not clinically significant, and only one patient developed symptomatic hemorrhage requiring surgical intervention.

The incidence may be lower among patients who are not treated with whole-brain RT (Strenger et al., 2008). Strenger et al. followed 171 patients with hematological malignancies and primary brain tumors who underwent CRT (Strenger et al., 2008). The cumulative incidence at 10 and 20 years was 3.86% and 6.74%. The lesions were more common in patients younger than 10 years of age at the time of irradiation, but the risk of CRT-induced cavernoma was not related to RT dose or tumor histology.

Ototoxicity

RT may damage sensory cells in the cochlea, particularly those located in the organ of Corti. If high doses of radiation are delivered to this region, patients can suffer from

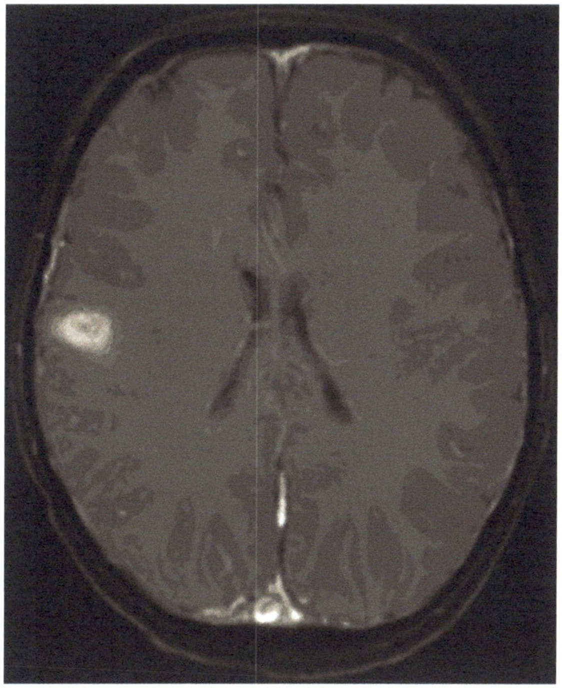

FIGURE 23.8 T1 post-contrast image of a post-RT cavernoma that has bled.

permanent sensori-neural hearing loss (SNHL) that develops between 3 and 5 years after CRT (Hua et al., 2008). The risk of this complication is increased with the addition of platinum-based chemotherapy, which is commonly used in the treatment of medulloblastoma (Bhandare et al., 2007).

The risk of RT-induced SNHL correlates with the mean dose to the cochlea. Hua et al. followed 155 ears and 78 patients with serial pure-tone audiographs and/or auditory brainstem response after the administration of CRT. None of the patients received carboplatin or cisplatin. The prevalence of high-frequency (6–8 kHz) SNHL was 0% at $\leq$ 30 Gy, 2% at 35 Gy, 4% at 40 Gy, 5% at 45 Gy, 11% at 50 Gy, 24% at 55 Gy, and 37% at 60 Gy. The incidence of intermediate- and low-frequency hearing loss was 0% at doses of 40 Gy and less. The authors concluded that the risk of permanent SNHL was minimized at doses below 35 Gy. For most craniopharyngiomas, cochlear doses below 35 Gy should be possible with modern radiation techniques.

The dose threshold for RT-induced SNHL may be higher in adult patients. In a series of 325 patients with extra-cranial head and neck tumors, Bhandare et al. found there were no cases of SNHL after doses to the cochlea less than 55 Gy (Bhandare et al., 2007). The prevalence in other dose ranges was 6.8% between 55–59.99 Gy, 13.2% between 60–64.99 Gy, and 33.8% between 65–69.99 Gy.

The overall prevalence of hearing loss is difficult to report as the severity of hearing loss varies widely; severe SNHL, for example, is uncommon at doses between 35 and 50 Gy

(Hua et al., 2008). In addition, tumor location and extent significantly influence the risk of high dose to the cochleae. In the Hua series, in which the most common diagnosis was ependymoma (n = 41), 14% of patients and 11% of cochleae suffered some extent of hearing loss (Hua et al., 2008). In the Bhandare series, a similar percentage (15%) suffered from some degree of SNHL, though many patients in this series received chemo-radiotherapy (Bhandare et al., 2007). In a series of 78 pediatric patients with low-grade glioma who were treated with CRT and/or chemotherapy, Merchant et al. reported a 10-year cumulative incidence of hearing loss of 5.7% in the right ear and 4.0% in the left ear (Merchant et al., 2009a). While a total of nine children developed hearing loss at any frequency, transient increases in hearing threshold that resolved to normal on subsequent audiology evaluation were detected in 17 children, suggesting that temporary fluctuations in testing were the most common result of RT to the cochlea.

Radiation Necrosis

Radiation necrosis is a rare complication of RT that results in permanent death of parenchymal brain tissue. The most likely etiology is RT-induced fibrinoid necrosis of vessel walls that leads to infarction. Imaging can show enhancing or non-enhancing lesions accompanied by significant edema. Most lesions develop within 6–12 months from CRT (Ruben et al., 2006). It is often difficult to distinguish radiation necrosis and/or treatment change from tumor recurrence, as both present with similar imaging findings and symptoms (Glantz et al., 1994; Giglio and Gilbert, 2003).

The risk of radiation necrosis is related to RT dose, volume, and the receipt of chemotherapy, which may sensitize normal tissue to RT damage (Marks and Wong, 1985; Ruben et al., 2006). Most cases occur in regions treated with greater than 55 Gy (Marks and Wong, 1985; Ruben et al., 2006). In 2006, Ruben et al. studied the incidence of radiation necrosis in 426 adult patients treated with CRT for glioblastoma multiforme (Ruben et al., 2006). Of the 21 patients who developed radiation necrosis, the total dose was greater than 60 Gy in 20 of 21 patients (the remaining patient was treated with 45 Gy in 20 fractions). The biological equivalent dose – a formulation of RT total dose that accounts for fraction size, the radio-sensitivity of tissue, and duration of RT – significantly increased for risk of necrosis. No patient who received a BED less than 96 Gy_2 developed radiation necrosis.

The prevalence in most series is less than 5% (Marks and Wong, 1985; Habrand et al., 1999; Merchant et al., 2002b; Ruben et al., 2006). In the Ruben series, the overall prevalence was 4.9%, though the actuarial incidence was 13.3% at 3 years (Ruben et al., 2006). In 2002, Merchant et al. reported one case of radiation necrosis after 55.8 Gy among 23 patients with craniopharyngioma treated with CRT (Merchant et al., 2002). In 1999, Habrand et al. reported one case of radiation necrosis after 55 Gy among 37 children with craniopharyngioma treated with CRT (Habrand et al., 1999).

The current standard of care is steroid therapy and/or surgical reduction. Additional experimental therapies include hyperbaric oxygen and anti-coagulation (Chuba et al., 1997). Bevacizumab, which reduces vessel proliferation and permeability, may improve imaging features, decrease the steroid requirement, and halt radiographic progression (Levin et al., 2011; Boothe et al., 2013).

Second Malignancy

The development of a second cancer due to the treatment of the first is one of the most devastating complications of radiotherapy. As demonstrated by multiple, large population studies, exposure to CRT is a dose-dependent risk for the development of meningiomas, gliomas, skin cancer, and other cancers. The risk increases at doses as low as 1 Gy (Ron et al., 1988). Second tumors may be more likely among patients irradiated at a young age, and among patients with an underlying genetic syndrome that predisposes them to multiple central nervous system (CNS) tumors, including neuro-cutaneous disorders (NF-1, NF-2, and tuberous sclerosis), Turcot's syndrome, Gorlin's syndrome, and Gardner's syndrome (Danoff et al., 1982; Neglia et al., 1991; Broniscer et al., 2004). The morbidity of this complication varies by the type of second cancer, but, after progressive or recurrent disease, secondary malignancy remains the leading cause of death among cancer survivors (Morris et al., 2007; Mertens et al., 2008; Armstrong et al., 2009). In a report on 20,483 survivors of childhood and adolescent cancers, Mertens et al. found that the cumulative mortality from second malignancy was 3.5% at 30 years (Mertens et al., 2008).

The most common tumor histology is meningioma, which develops at a median interval of 19–36 years after CRT (Sadetzki et al., 2002; Paulino et al., 2009). The interval may be shortened by higher-dose RT. Compared to spontaneous meningiomas, RT-induced meningiomas are more likely to be multiple, to recur, and to have an atypical or malignant histology (Sadetzki et al., 2002; Paulino et al., 2009). These tumors are rarely fatal, but cause significant morbidity due to the need for occasionally extensive surgery and the high rate of recurrence.

The second most common tumor histology is glioma, which occurs between 5 and 15 years after CRT. High-grade gliomas, a relative minority of second tumors, are fatal regardless of treatment (Carret et al., 2006). In contrast, the prognosis for low-grade gliomas, which may comprise up to half of all second tumors, is generally good, though these patients must also face the additional morbidity of further surgery and other treatment (Walter et al., 1998).

According to Cohen et al, the criteria for an RT-induced tumor include 1) development of the tumor within the previous RT field; 2) histology that is distinct from the primary tumor; 3) a relatively long latency period since the start of radiotherapy; and 4) the absence of any underlying genetic disorder (Cohen and Duffner, 1991).

Incidence

Among patients treated with CRT, the estimated 10-year cumulative incidence varies between 1.6% and 4.2% (Neglia et al., 1991; Packer et al., 2013), the 15-year cumulative incidence between 2.53% and 5.3% (Neglia et al., 1991; Broniscer et al., 2004) and the 20-year cumulative incidence between 1.39% (brain tumors only) and 14.8% (Walter et al., 1998; Jenkinson et al., 2004; Goshen et al., 2007; van Dijk et al., 2013). Pui et al., in a single-institution series of 597 patients with ALL treated with whole-brain CRT, found the highest reported incidence of 20.9% at 20 years. The series – which had a median follow-up of 18.9 years, longer than the majority of comparable series – detected an increase in incidence at 20 years attributed to the late onset of largely benign tumors such as meningioma.

In the case of craniopharyngioma, these estimated incidences should be viewed with caution, as most studies are based on patients treated with CSI or whole-brain CRT rather than partial-brain CRT. In addition, not all second tumors carry the same risk of morbidity and mortality. For example, non-melanoma skin cancers and thyroid neoplasms (from CSI) are frequently included in these series (van Dijk et al., 2013). In studies of patients treated for craniopharyngioma, the reported incidence of secondary malignancy is generally less than 5% (Merchant et al., 2002b, 2006a). In 2006, Morris et al. reviewed the major causes of death in 643 survivors of primary CNS tumors. Among the 57 craniopharyngioma and germ cell tumor survivors included in this series, the 10-year cumulative incidence of death from a second malignancy was 2.2% (Morris et al., 2007).

Among adults, the risk of RT-induced second malignancy may be lower than among children. Brada et al. reviewed the risk of second tumor among 335 patients treated with surgery and CRT to a median dose of 45 Gy between 1962 and 1986 (Brada et al., 1992). The cumulative risk of second tumor was 1.9% at 20 years. Four of the five tumors were benign, and meningioma was the most common histology.

CONCLUSION

CRT is associated with multiple long-term complications, including cognitive decline, endocrine deficiency, cerebral vasculopathy, second malignancy, and radiation necrosis. These complications are best characterized in patients treated with older, less conformal RT techniques and larger treatment volumes. Certain modalities, such as proton RT and stereotactic radiotherapy combined with daily image guidance, may significantly limit the dose delivered to critical brain structures (see Figure 23.9). In addition, the morbidity of maximal resection is often very extensive, and must be weighed against the effects of CRT.

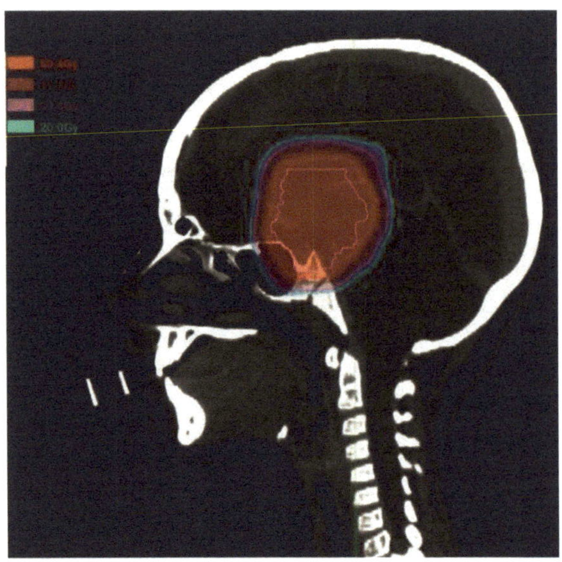

FIGURE 23.9 Proton RT plan for a patient with craniopharyngioma minimizes dose delivered to surrounding healthy brain tissue. Teal, 20 Gy (RBE); red, 50.4 Gy (RBE).

References

Abs, R., Bengtsson, B.A., Hernberg-Stahl, E., et al., 1999. GH replacement in 1034 growth hormone deficient hypopituitary adults: demographic and clinical characteristics, dosing and safety. Clin. Endocrinol. (Oxf) 50 (6), 703–713.

Aristizabal, S., Caldwell, W.L., Avila, J., 1977. The relationship of time-dose fractionation factors to complications in the treatment of pituitary tumors by irradiation. Int. J. Radiat. Oncol. Biol. Phys. 2 (7–8), 667–673.

Armstrong, G.T., Liu, Q., Yasui, Y., et al., 2009. Long-term outcomes among adult survivors of childhood central nervous system malignancies in the Childhood Cancer Survivor Study. J. Natl. Cancer. Inst. 101 (13), 946–958.

Attanasio, A.F., Lamberts, S.W., Matranga, A.M., et al., 1997. Adult growth hormone (GH)-deficient patients demonstrate heterogeneity between childhood onset and adult onset before and during human GH treatment. Adult Growth Hormone Deficiency Study Group. J. Clin. Endocrinol. Metab. 82 (1), 82–88.

Bhandare, N., Antonelli, P.J., Morris, C.G., Malayapa, R.S., Mendenhall, W.M., 2007. Ototoxicity after radiotherapy for head and neck tumors. Int. J. Radiat. Oncol. Biol. Phys. 67 (2), 469–479.

Boothe, D., Young, R., Yamada, Y., Prager, A., Chan, T., Beal, K., 2013. Bevacizumab as a treatment for radiation necrosis of brain metastases post stereotactic radiosurgery. Neuro. Oncol. 15, 1257–1263.

Brada, M., Ford, D., Ashley, S., et al., 1992. Risk of second brain tumour after conservative surgery and radiotherapy for pituitary adenoma. BMJ 304 (6838), 1343–1346.

Broniscer, A., Ke, W., Fuller, C.E., Wu, J., Gajjar, A., Kun, L.E., 2004. Second neoplasms in pediatric patients with primary central nervous system tumors: the St. Jude Children's Research Hospital experience. Cancer 100 (10), 2246–2252.

Butler Jr., J.M., Case, L.D., Atkins, J., et al., 2007. A phase III, double-blind, placebo-controlled prospective randomized clinical trial of d-threo-methylphenidate HCl in brain tumor patients receiving radiation therapy. Int. J. Radiat. Oncol. Biol. Phys. 69 (5), 1496–1501.

Carpenter, R.C., Chamberlin, G.W., Frazier, C.H., 1937. The treatment of hypophyseal stalk tumours by evacuation and irradiation. Am. J. Roent. 38, 162–167.

Carret, A.S., Tabori, U., Crooks, B., et al., 2006. Outcome of secondary high-grade glioma in children previously treated for a malignant condition: a study of the Canadian Pediatric Brain Tumour Consortium. Radiother. Oncol. 81 (1), 33–38.

Carroll, P.V., Drake, W.M., Maher, K.T., et al., 2004. Comparison of continuation or cessation of growth hormone (GH) therapy on body composition and metabolic status in adolescents with severe GH deficiency at completion of linear growth. J. Clin. Endocrinol. Metab. 89 (8), 3890–3895.

Cavazzuti, V., Fischer, E.G., Welch, K., Belli, J.A., Winston, K.R., 1983. Neurological and psychophysiological sequelae following different treatments of craniopharyngioma in children. J. Neurosurg. 59 (3), 409–417.

Chuba, P.J., Aronin, P., Bhambhani, K., et al., 1997. Hyperbaric oxygen therapy for radiation-induced brain injury in children. Cancer 80 (10), 2005–2012.

Clark, A.J., Cage, T.A., Aranda, D., Parsa, A.T., Auguste, K.I., Gupta, N., 2012. Treatment-related morbidity and the management of pediatric craniopharyngioma: a systematic review. J. Neurosurg. Pediatr. 10 (4), 293–301.

Clayton, P.E., Price, D.A., Shalet, S.M., Gattemaneni, H.R., 1988. Craniopharyngioma recurrence and growth hormone therapy. Lancet 1 (8586), 642.

Cohen, M.E., Duffner, P.K., 1991. Long-term consequences of CNS treatment for childhood cancer, Part I: Pathologic consequences and potential for oncogenesis. Pediatr. Neurol. 7 (3), 157–163.

Cohen, M., Bartels, U., Branson, H., Kulkarni, A.V., Hamilton, J., 2013. Trends in treatment and outcomes of pediatric craniopharyngioma, 1975–2011. Neuro. Oncol. 15 (6), 767–774.

Conklin, H.M., Li, C., Xiong, X., Ogg, R.J., Merchant, T.E., 2008. Predicting change in academic abilities after conformal radiation therapy for localized ependymoma. J. Clin. Oncol. 26 (24), 3965–3970.

Constine, L.S., Rubin, P., Woolf, P.D., Doane, K., Lush, C.M., 1987. Hyperprolactinemia and hypothyroidism following cytotoxic therapy for central nervous system malignancies. J. Clin. Oncol. 5 (11), 1841–1851.

Constine, L.S., Woolf, P.D., Cann, D., et al., 1993. Hypothalamic-pituitary dysfunction after radiation for brain tumors. N. Engl. J. Med. 328 (2), 87–94.

Danoff, B.F., Cowchock, F.S., Marquette, C., Mulgrew, L., Kramer, S., 1982. Assessment of the long-term effects of primary radiation therapy for brain tumors in children. Cancer 49 (8), 1580–1586.

Danoff, B.F., Cowchock, F.S., Kramer, S., 1983. Childhood craniopharyngioma: survival, local control, endocrine and neurologic function following radiotherapy. Int. J. Radiat. Oncol. Biol. Phys. 9 (2), 171–175.

DeVile, C.J., Grant, D.B., Hayward, R.D., Stanhope, R., 1996. Growth and endocrine sequelae of craniopharyngioma. Arch. Dis. Child. 75 (2), 108–114.

Di Pinto, M., Conklin, H.M., Li, C., Xiong, X., Merchant, T.E., 2010. Investigating verbal and visual auditory learning after conformal radiation therapy for childhood ependymoma. Int. J. Radiat. Oncol. Biol. Phys. 77 (4), 1002–1008.

Di Pinto, M., Conklin, H.M., Li, C., Merchant, T.E., 2012. Learning and memory following conformal radiation therapy for pediatric craniopharyngioma and low-grade glioma. Int. J. Radiat. Oncol. Biol. Phys. 84 (3), e363–e369.

Didcock, E., Davies, H.A., Didi, M., Ogilvy Stuart, A.L., Wales, J.K., Shalet, S.M., 1995. Pubertal growth in young adult survivors of childhood leukemia. J. Clin. Oncol. 13 (10), 2503–2507.

Duffner, P.K., Cohen, M.E., Voorhess, M.L., et al., 1985. Long-term effects of cranial irradiation on endocrine function in children with brain tumors. A prospective study. Cancer 56 (9), 2189–2193.

Duffner, P.K., Horowitz, M.E., Krischer, J.P., et al., 1993. Postoperative chemotherapy and delayed radiation in children less than three years of age with malignant brain tumors. N. Engl. J. Med. 328 (24), 1725–1731.

Fernandez, A., Brada, M., Zabuliene, L., Karavitaki, N., Wass, J.A., 2009. Radiation-induced hypopituitarism. Endocr. Relat. Cancer 16 (3), 733–772.

Fisher, P.G., Jenab, J., Gopldthwaite, P.T., et al., 1998. Outcomes and failure patterns in childhood craniopharyngiomas. Childs. Nerv. Syst. 14 (10), 558–563.

Flickinger, J.C., Lunsford, L.D., Singer, J., Cano, E.R., Deutsch, M., 1990. Megavoltage external beam irradiation of craniopharyngiomas: analysis of tumor control and morbidity. Int. J. Radiat. Oncol. Biol. Phys. 19 (1), 117–122.

Gautier, A., Godbout, A., Grosheny, C., et al., 2012. Markers of recurrence and long-term morbidity in craniopharyngioma: a systematic analysis of 171 patients. J. Clin. Endocrinol. Metab. 97 (4), 1258–1267.

Giglio, P., Gilbert, M.R., 2003. Cerebral radiation necrosis. Neurologist 9 (4), 180–188.

Glantz, M.J., Burger, P.C., Friedman, A.H., Radtke, R.A., Massey, E.W., Schold Jr., S.C., 1994. Treatment of radiation-induced nervous system injury with heparin and warfarin. Neurology 44 (11), 2020–2027.

Gonc, E.N., Yordam, N., Ozon, A., Alikasifoglu, A., Kandemir, N., 2004. Endocrinological outcome of different treatment options in children with craniopharyngioma: a retrospective analysis of 66 cases. Pediatr. Neurosurg. 40 (3), 112–119.

Goshen, Y., Stark, B., Kornreich, L., Michowiz, S., Feinmesser, M., Yaniv, I., 2007. High incidence of meningioma in cranial irradiated survivors of childhood acute lymphoblastic leukemia. Pediatr. Blood Cancer 49 (3), 294–297.

Gurney, J.G., Kadan-Lottick, N.S., Packer, R.J., et al., 2003. Endocrine and cardiovascular late effects among adult survivors of childhood brain tumors: Childhood Cancer Survivor Study. Cancer 97 (3), 663–673.

Habrand, I.L., Austin-Seymour, M., Birnbaum, S., et al., 1989. Neurovisual outcome following proton radiation therapy. Int. J. Radiat. Oncol. Biol. Phys. 16 (6), 1601–1606.

Habrand, J.L., Ganry, O., Couanet, D., et al., 1999. The role of radiation therapy in the management of craniopharyngioma: a 25-year experience and review of the literature. Int. J. Radiat. Oncol. Biol. Phys. 44 (2), 255–263.

Harris, J.R., Levene, M.B., 1976. Visual complications following irradiation for pituitary adenomas and craniopharyngiomas. Radiology 120 (1), 167–171.

Hetelekidis, S., Barnes, P.D., Tao, M.L., et al., 1993. 20-year experience in childhood craniopharyngioma. Int. J. Radiat. Oncol. Biol. Phys. 27 (2), 189–195.

Hoffman, H.J., De Silva, M., Humphreys, R.P., Drake, J.M., Smith, M.L., Blaser, S.I., 1992. Aggressive surgical management of craniopharyngiomas in children. J. Neurosurg. 76 (1), 47–52.

Hua, C., Bass, J.K., Khan, R., Kun, L.E., Merchant, T.E., 2008. Hearing loss after radiotherapy for pediatric brain tumors: effect of cochlear dose. Int. J. Radiat. Oncol. Biol. Phys. 72 (3), 892–899.

Hua, C., Wu, S., Chemaitilly, W., Lukose, R.C., Merchant, T.E., 2012. Predicting the probability of abnormal stimulated growth hormone response in children after radiotherapy for brain tumors. Int. J. Radiat. Oncol. Biol. Phys. 84 (4), 990–995.

Ilveskoski, I., Saarinen, U.M., Wiklund, T., et al., 1997. Growth impairment and growth hormone therapy in children treated for malignant brain tumours. Eur. J. Pediatr. 156 (10), 764–769.

Jenkinson, H.C., Hawkins, M.M., Stiller, C.A., Winter, D.L., Marsden, H.B., Stevens, M.C., 2004. Long-term population-based risks of second malignant neoplasms after childhood cancer in Britain. Br. J. Cancer 91 (11), 1905–1910.

Jung, T.Y., Jung, S., Choi, J.E., Moon, K.S., Kim, I.Y., Kang, S.S., 2009. Adult craniopharyngiomas: surgical results with a special focus on endocrinological outcomes and recurrence according to pituitary stalk preservation. J. Neurosurg. 111 (3), 572–577.

Jung, T.Y., Jung, S., Moon, K.S., Kim, I.Y., Kang, S.S., Kim, J.H., 2010. Endocrinological outcomes of pediatric craniopharyngiomas with anatomical pituitary stalk preservation: preliminary study. Pediatr. Neurosurg. 46 (3), 205–212.

Kanev, P.M., Lefebvre, J.F., Mauseth, R.S., Berger, M.S., 1991. Growth hormone deficiency following radiation therapy of primary brain tumors in children. J. Neurosurg. 74 (5), 743–748.

Kang, J.K., Song, J.U., 1988. Results of the management of craniopharyngioma in children. An endocrinological approach to the treatment. Childs. Nerv. Syst. 4 (3), 135–138.

Karavitaki, N., Brufani, C., Warner, J.T., et al., 2005. Craniopharyngiomas in children and adults: systematic analysis of 121 cases with long-term follow-up. Clin. Endocrinol. (Oxf) 62 (4), 397–409.

Kiehna, E.N., Mulhern, R.K., Li, C., Xiong, X., Merchant, T.E., 2006. Changes in attentional performance of children and young adults with localized primary brain tumors after conformal radiation therapy. J. Clin. Oncol. 24 (33), 5283–5290.

Kline, L.B., Kim, J.Y., Ceballos, R., 1985. Radiation optic neuropathy. Ophthalmology 92 (8), 1118–1126.

Koltowska-Haggstrom, M., Geffner, M.E., Jonsson, P., et al., 2010. Discontinuation of growth hormone (GH) treatment during the transition phase is an important factor determining the phenotype of young adults with non-idiopathic childhood-onset GH deficiency. J. Clin. Endocrinol. Metab. 95 (6), 2646–2654.

Laughton, S.J., Merchant, T.E., Sklar, C.A., et al., 2008. Endocrine outcomes for children with embryonal brain tumors after risk-adapted craniospinal and conformal primary-site irradiation and high-dose chemotherapy with stem-cell rescue on the SJMB-96 trial. J. Clin. Oncol. 26 (7), 1112–1118.

Lawenda, B.D., Gagne, H.M., Gierga, D.P., et al., 2004. Permanent alopecia after cranial irradiation: dose-response relationship. Int. J. Radiat. Oncol. Biol. Phys. 60 (3), 879–887.

Levin, V.A., Bidaut, L., Hou, P., et al., 2011. Randomized double-blind placebo-controlled trial of bevacizumab therapy for radiation necrosis of the central nervous system. Int. J. Radiat. Oncol. Biol. Phys. 79 (5), 1487–1495.

Lew, S.M., Morgan, J.N., Psaty, E., Lefton, D.R., Allen, J.C., Abbott, R., 2006. Cumulative incidence of radiation-induced cavernomas in long-term survivors of medulloblastoma. J. Neurosurg. 104 (Suppl. 2), 103–107.

Littman, P., Rosenstock, J., Gale, G., et al., 1984. The somnolence syndrome in leukemic children following reduced daily dose fractions of cranial radiation. Int. J. Radiat. Oncol. Biol. Phys. 10 (10), 1851–1853.

Lopez-Serna, R., Gomez-Amador, J.L., Barges-Coll, J., et al., 2012. Treatment of craniopharyngioma in adults: systematic analysis of a 25-year experience. Arch. Med. Res. 43 (5), 347–355.

Lustig, R.H., Schriock, E.A., Kaplan, S.L., Grumbach, M.M., 1985. Effect of growth hormone-releasing factor on growth hormone release in children with radiation-induced growth hormone deficiency. Pediatrics 76 (2), 274–279.

Lyen, K.R., Grant, D.B., 1982. Endocrine function, morbidity, and mortality after surgery for craniopharyngioma. Arch. Dis. Child. 57 (11), 837–841.

Maiter, D., Abs, R., Johannsson, G., et al., 2006. Baseline characteristics and response to GH replacement of hypopituitary patients previously irradiated for pituitary adenoma or craniopharyngioma: data from the Pfizer International Metabolic Database. Eur. J. Endocrinol. 155 (2), 253–260.

Mandell, L.R., Walker, R.W., Steinherz, P., Fuks, Z., 1989. Reduced incidence of the somnolence syndrome in leukemic children with steroid coverage during prophylactic cranial radiation therapy. Results of a pilot study. Cancer 63 (10), 1975–1978.

Maranzano, E., De Angelis, V., Pergolizzi, S., et al., 2010. A prospective observational trial on emesis in radiotherapy: analysis of 1020 patients recruited in 45 Italian radiation oncology centres. Radiother. Oncol. 94 (1), 36–41.

Marks, J.E., Wong, J., 1985. The risk of cerebral radionecrosis in relation to dose, time and fractionation. A follow-up study. Prog. Exp. Tumor. Res. 29, 210–218.

Merchant, T.E., Goloubeva, O., Pritchard, D.L., et al., 2002a. Radiation dose-volume effects on growth hormone secretion. Int. J. Radiat. Oncol. Biol. Phys. 52 (5), 1264–1270.

Merchant, T.E., Kiehna, E.N., Sanford, R.A., et al., 2002b. Craniopharyngioma: the St. Jude Children's Research Hospital experience 1984–2001. Int. J. Radiat. Oncol. Biol. Phys. 53 (3), 533–542.

Merchant, T.E., Williams, T., Smith, J.M., et al., 2002c. Preirradiation endocrinopathies in pediatric brain tumor patients determined by dynamic tests of endocrine function. Int. J. Radiat. Oncol. Biol. Phys. 54 (1), 45–50.

Merchant, T.E., Mulhern, R.K., Krasin, M.J., et al., 2004. Preliminary results from a phase II trial of conformal radiation therapy and evaluation of radiation-related CNS effects for pediatric patients with localized ependymoma. J. Clin. Oncol. 22 (15), 3156–3162.

Merchant, T.E., Kiehna, E.N., Li, C., Xiong, X., Mulhern, R.K., 2005. Radiation dosimetry predicts IQ after conformal radiation therapy in pediatric patients with localized ependymoma. Int. J. Radiat. Oncol. Biol. Phys. 63 (5), 1546–1554.

Merchant, T.E., Kiehna, E.N., Kun, L.E., et al., 2006a. Phase II trial of conformal radiation therapy for pediatric patients with craniopharyngioma and correlation of surgical factors and radiation dosimetry with change in cognitive function. J. Neurosurg. 104 (Suppl. 2), 94–102.

Merchant, T.E., Kiehna, E.N., Li, C., et al., 2006b. Modeling radiation dosimetry to predict cognitive outcomes in pediatric patients with CNS embryonal tumors including medulloblastoma. Int. J. Radiat. Oncol. Biol. Phys. 65 (1), 210–221.

Merchant, T.E., Conklin, H.M., Wu, S., Lustig, R.H., Xiong, X., 2009a. Late effects of conformal radiation therapy for pediatric patients with low-grade glioma: prospective evaluation of cognitive, endocrine, and hearing deficits. J. Clin. Oncol. 27 (22), 3691–3697.

Merchant, T.E., Kun, L.E., Wu, S., Xiong, X., Sanford, R.A., Boop, F.A., 2009b. Phase II trial of conformal radiation therapy for pediatric low-grade glioma. J. Clin. Oncol. 27 (22), 3598–3604.

Merchant, T.E., Rose, S.R., Bosley, C., Wu, S., Xiong, X., Lustig, R.H., 2011. Growth hormone secretion after conformal radiation therapy in pediatric patients with localized brain tumors. J. Clin. Oncol. 29 (36), 4776–4780.

Mertens, A.C., Liu, Q., Neglia, J.P., et al., 2008. Cause-specific late mortality among 5-year survivors of childhood cancer: the Childhood Cancer Survivor Study. J. Natl. Cancer. Inst. 100 (19), 1368–1379.

Morris, E.B., Gajjar, A., Okuma, J.O., et al., 2007. Survival and late mortality in long-term survivors of pediatric CNS tumors. J. Clin. Oncol. 25 (12), 1532–1538.

Mulder, R.L., Kremer, L.C., van Santen, H.M., et al., 2009. Prevalence and risk factors of radiation-induced growth hormone deficiency in childhood cancer survivors: a systematic review. Cancer. Treat. Rev. 35 (7), 616–632.

Mulhern, R.K., Reddick, W.E., Palmer, S.L., et al., 1999. Neurocognitive deficits in medulloblastoma survivors and white matter loss. Ann. Neurol. 46 (6), 834–841.

Mulhern, R.K., Merchant, T.E., Gajjar, A., Reddick, W.E., Kun, L.E., 2004. Late neurocognitive sequelae in survivors of brain tumours in childhood. Lancet. Oncol. 5 (7), 399–408.

Mulhern, R.K., Palmer, S.L., Merchant, T.E., et al., 2005. Neurocognitive consequences of risk-adapted therapy for childhood medulloblastoma. J. Clin. Oncol. 23 (24), 5511–5519.

Murray, R.D., Darzy, K.H., Gleeson, H.K., Shalet, S.M., 2002. GH-deficient survivors of childhood cancer: GH replacement during adult life. J. Clin. Endocrinol. Metab. 87 (1), 129–135.

Neglia, J.P., Meadows, A.T., Robison, L.L., et al., 1991. Second neoplasms after acute lymphoblastic leukemia in childhood. N. Engl. J. Med. 325 (19), 1330–1336.

Netson, K.L., Conklin, H.M., Wu, S., Xiong, X., Merchant, T.E., 2012. A 5-year investigation of children's adaptive functioning following conformal radiation therapy for localized ependymoma. Int. J. Radiat. Oncol. Biol. Phys. 84 (1), 217–223 e1.

Ogilvy-Stuart, A.L., Shalet, S.M., 1995. Growth and puberty after growth hormone treatment after irradiation for brain tumours. Arch. Dis. Child. 73 (2), 141–146.

Ondruch, A., Maryniak, A., Kropiwnicki, T., Roszkowski, M., Daszkiewicz, P., 2011. Cognitive and social functioning in children and adolescents after the removal of craniopharyngioma. Childs. Nerv. Syst. 27 (3), 391–397.

Packer, R.J., Zhou, T., Holmes, E., Vezina, G., Gajjar, A., 2013. Survival and secondary tumors in children with medulloblastoma receiving radiotherapy and adjuvant chemotherapy: results of Children's Oncology Group trial A9961. Neuro. Oncol. 15 (1), 97–103.

Palmer, S.L., Goloubeva, O., Reddick, W.E., et al., 2001. Patterns of intellectual development among survivors of pediatric medulloblastoma: a longitudinal analysis. J. Clin. Oncol. 19 (8), 2302–2308.

Paulino, A.C., Ahmed, I.M., Mai, W.Y., Teh, B.S., 2009. The influence of pretreatment characteristics and radiotherapy parameters on time interval to development of radiation-associated meningioma. Int. J. Radiat. Oncol. Biol. Phys. 75 (5), 1408–1414.

Pemberton, L.S., Dougal, M., Magee, B., Gattamaneni, H.R., 2005. Experience of external beam radiotherapy given adjuvantly or at relapse following surgery for craniopharyngioma. Radiother. Oncol. 77 (1), 99–104.

Pereira, A.M., Schmid, E.M., Schutte, P.J., et al., 2005. High prevalence of long-term cardiovascular, neurological and psychosocial morbidity after treatment for craniopharyngioma. Clin. Endocrinol. (Oxf) 62 (2), 197–204.

Poretti, A., Grotzer, M.A., Ribi, K., Schonle, E., Boltshauser, E., 2004. Outcome of craniopharyngioma in children: long-term complications and quality of life. Dev. Med. Child. Neurol 46 (4), 220–229.

Powell, C., Guerrero, D., Sardell, S., et al., 2011. Somnolence syndrome in patients receiving radical radiotherapy for primary brain tumours: a prospective study. Radiother. Oncol. 100 (1), 131–136.

Quigley, C., Cowell, C., Jimenez, M., et al., 1989. Normal or early development of puberty despite gonadal damage in children treated for acute lymphoblastic leukemia. N. Engl. J. Med. 321 (3), 143–151.

Rajan, B., Ashley, S., Gorman, C., et al., 1993. Craniopharyngioma—a long-term results following limited surgery and radiotherapy. Radiother. Oncol. 26 (1), 1–10.

Rappaport, R., Brauner, R., Czernichow, P., et al., 1982. Effect of hypothalamic and pituitary irradiation on pubertal development in children with cranial tumors. J. Clin. Endocrinol. Metab. 54 (6), 1164–1168.

Reddick, W.E., Glass, J.O., Palmer, S.L., et al., 2005. Atypical white matter volume development in children following craniospinal irradiation. Neuro. Oncol. 7 (1), 12–19.

Regine, W.F., Mohiuddin, M., Kramer, S., 1993. Long-term results of pediatric and adult craniopharyngiomas treated with combined surgery and radiation. Radiother. Oncol. 27 (1), 13–21.

Ris, M.D., Packer, R., Goldwein, J., Jones-Wallace, D., Boyett, J.M., 2001. Intellectual outcome after reduced-dose radiation therapy plus adjuvant chemotherapy for medulloblastoma: a Children's Cancer Group study. J. Clin. Oncol. 19 (15), 3470–3476.

Ron, E., Modan, B., Boice Jr., J.D., et al., 1988. Tumors of the brain and nervous system after radiotherapy in childhood. N. Engl. J. Med. 319 (16), 1033–1039.

Rose, S.R., Danish, R.K., Kearney, N.S., et al., 2005. ACTH deficiency in childhood cancer survivors. Pediatr. Blood Cancer 45 (6), 808–813.

Ruben, J.D., Dally, M., Bailey, M., Smith, R., McLean, C.A., Fedele, P., 2006. Cerebral radiation necrosis: incidence, outcomes, and risk factors with emphasis on radiation parameters and chemotherapy. Int. J. Radiat. Oncol. Biol. Phys. 65 (2), 499–508.

Sadetzki, S., Flint-Richter, P., Ben-Tal, T., Nass, D., 2002. Radiation-induced meningioma: a descriptive study of 253 cases. J. Neurosurg. 97 (5), 1078–1082.

Samaan, N.A., Vieto, R., Schultz, P.N., et al., 1982. Hypothalamic, pituitary and thyroid dysfunction after radiotherapy to the head and neck. Int. J. Radiat. Oncol. Biol. Phys. 8 (11), 1857–1867.

Schmiegelow, M., Feldt-Rasmussen, U., Rasmussen, A.K., Poulsen, H.S., Muller, J., 2003. A population-based study of thyroid function after radiotherapy and chemotherapy for a childhood brain tumor. J. Clin. Endocrinol. Metab. 88 (1), 136–140.

Shalet, S.M., Brennan, B.M., 2002. Puberty in children with cancer. Horm. Res. 57 (Suppl. 2), 39–42.

Silber, J.H., Radcliffe, J., Peckham, V., et al., 1992. Whole-brain irradiation and decline in intelligence: the influence of dose and age on IQ score. J. Clin. Oncol. 10 (9), 1390–1396.

Sklar, C.A., Constine, L.S., 1995. Chronic neuroendocrinological sequelae of radiation therapy. Int. J. Radiat. Oncol. Biol. Phys. 31 (5), 1113–1121.

Sklar, C., Sarafoglou, K., Whittam, E., 1993. Efficacy of insulin-like growth factor binding protein 3 in predicting the growth hormone response to provocative testing in children treated with cranial irradiation. Acta Endocrinol. (Copenh) 129 (6), 511–515.

Sklar, C.A., Mertens, A.C., Mitby, P., et al., 2002. Risk of disease recurrence and second neoplasms in survivors of childhood cancer treated with growth hormone: a report from the Childhood Cancer Survivor Study. J. Clin. Endocrinol. Metab. 87 (7), 3136–3141.

Sklar, C.A., 1994a. Craniopharyngioma: endocrine abnormalities at presentation. Pediatr. Neurosurg. 21 (Suppl. 1), 18–20.

Sklar, C.A., 1994b. Craniopharyngioma: endocrine sequelae of treatment. Pediatr. Neurosurg. 21 (Suppl. 1), 120–123.

Spiegler, B.J., Bouffet, E., Greenberg, M.L., Rutka, J.T., Mabbott, D.J., 2004. Change in neurocognitive functioning after treatment with cranial radiation in childhood. J. Clin. Oncol. 22 (4), 706–713.

Strenger, V., Sovinz, P., Lackner, H., et al., 2008. Intracerebral cavernous hemangioma after cranial irradiation in childhood. Incidence and risk factors. Strahlenther. Onkol. 184 (5), 276–280.

Stripp, D.C., Maity, A., Janss, A.J., et al., 2004. Surgery with or without radiation therapy in the management of craniopharyngiomas in children and young adults. Int. J. Radiat. Oncol. Biol. Phys. 58 (3), 714–720.

Sughrue, M.E., Yang, I., Kane, A.J., et al., 2011. Endocrinologic, neurologic, and visual morbidity after treatment for craniopharyngioma. J. Neurooncol. 101 (3), 463–476.
Thomsett, M.J., Conte, F.A., Kaplan, S.L., Grumbach, M.M., 1980. Endocrine and neurologic outcome in childhood craniopharyngioma: Review of effect of treatment in 42 patients. J. Pediatr. 97 (5), 728–735.
Tillmann, V., Shalet, S.M., Price, D.A., et al., 1998. Serum insulin-like growth factor-I, IGF binding protein-3 and IGFBP-3 protease activity after cranial irradiation. Horm. Res. 50 (2), 71–77.
Ullrich, N.J., Robertson, R., Kinnamon, D.D., et al., 2007. Moyamoya following cranial irradiation for primary brain tumors in children. Neurology 68 (12), 932–938.
Uzal, D., Ozyar, E., Hayran, M., Zorlu, F., Atahan, L., Yetkin, S., 1998. Reduced incidence of the somnolence syndrome after prophylactic cranial irradiation in children with acute lymphoblastic leukemia. Radiother. Oncol. 48 (1), 29–32.
van den Bergh, A.C., Hoving, M.A., Links, T.P., et al., 2003. Radiation optic neuropathy after external beam radiation therapy for acromegaly: report of two cases. Radiother. Oncol. 68 (2), 101–103.
van Dijk, I.W., Cardous-Ubbink, M.C., van der Pal, H.J., et al., 2013. Dose-effect relationships for adverse events after cranial radiation therapy in long-term childhood cancer survivors. Int. J. Radiat. Oncol. Biol. Phys. 85 (3), 768–775.
Vance, M.L., Mauras, N., 1999. Growth hormone therapy in adults and children. N. Engl. J. Med. 341 (16), 1206–1216.
Walter, A.W., Hancock, M.L., Pui, C.H., et al., 1998. Secondary brain tumors in children treated for acute lymphoblastic leukemia at St Jude Children's Research Hospital. J. Clin. Oncol. 16 (12), 3761–3767.
Weiss, M., Sutton, L., Marcial, V., et al., 1989. The role of radiation therapy in the management of childhood craniopharyngioma. Int. J. Radiat. Oncol. Biol. Phys. 17 (6), 1313–1321.
Winkfield, K.M., Tsai, H.K., Yao, X., et al., 2011. Long-term clinical outcomes following treatment of childhood craniopharyngioma. Pediatr. Blood Cancer 56 (7), 1120–1126.

SECTION V

INTRACAVITARY THERAPY

CHAPTER

24

Intracavitary Therapy: Radioisotopes ^{32}P, ^{90}Y, and ^{186}Re

Edward A. Monaco III, Zachary Tempel, Ajay Niranjan, L. Dade Lunsford

Center for Image Guided Neurosurgery, Department of Neurological Surgery, University of Pittsburgh Medical Center, Pittsburgh, PA, USA

"On March 4th, 1952, fifteen months after application of P^{32}, his visual fields remained improved...the future course cannot be predicted. It is probable that the cyst will eventually start to grow again but so far the treatment seems to have postponed an impending blindness." **Lars Leksell, 1949**

Management of craniopharyngiomas must include an emphasis on both long-term quality of life as well as tumor control. Where radical surgical resection is possible and safe, this remains the favored approach for select patients regardless of the composition of the tumor (i.e., solid, cystic). However, the need for maximal tumor resection must be balanced with the potential risks of surgery, including hypothalamic dysfunction, hypopituitarism, and vision loss. Often craniopharyngiomas are found to be adherent to critical structures like the optic apparatus, the hypothalamus, and the pituitary stalk. Even at experienced centers, the frequency of surgical morbidities is meaningful (Sughrue et al., 2011). When complete resection is not possible or has not occurred, other modalities must be employed, either alone, or more often in combination. For example, patients with residual tumor following partial resection are candidates for stereotactic radiosurgery (Niranjan et al., 2010).

Ninety percent of craniopharyngiomas possess cystic components, and often there is a single dominant cyst (Pollack et al., 1988; Habrand et al., 1999; Savas et al., 1999). Frequently, it is the cystic portion of the tumor that causes clinical symptoms. When cystic pathology is the predominant feature of a craniopharyngioma, intracavitary radiation is designed to treat the thin-walled cyst, leading to cessation of cyst fluid accumulation and gradual cyst shrinkage. Leksell and Lidėn first reported on the use of intracavitary therapy for cystic craniopharyngiomas with the colloidal, purely beta-emitting radioisotope phosphorus-32 (^{32}P) in 1952 (Leksell and Lidėn, 1952). Since this initial report, the technique of stereotactic intracavitary therapy for cystic craniopharyngiomas has been established as a

Craniopharyngiomas
http://dx.doi.org/10.1016/B978-0-12-416706-3.00024-6

safe and effective tool in the multimodal management often necessary to treat these challenging tumors. In this review, we will discuss the indications for intracavitary therapy for craniopharyngiomas, the technical details of the surgery, and the reported outcomes and complications of this treatment.

INDICATIONS FOR INTRACAVITARY THERAPY

To be considered for intracavitary therapy, a patient's tumor must be purely or predominantly monocystic, a situation that is present in up to two-thirds of cases (Kickingereder et al., 2012). It is indicated in patients with solitary cysts, for patients harboring recurrent cysts after previous treatments, and in patients experiencing clinical deterioration from the cystic portion of their tumors. Although intracavitary therapy is often used after other therapies have been exacted, it can be used as a primary treatment of primarily cystic tumors, especially in patients for whom open surgery may harbor high risks due to age or medical comorbidities, or where complete or aggressive surgical resection is considered particularly hazardous. In these situations, a stereotactic procedure can yield a pathologic diagnosis via polarized light microscopic examination of aspirated cyst fluid and the detection of cholesterol crystals. Because of the need to perform accurate dose calculation in order to deliver a specific dose of radiation to the cyst wall using volumes less than 1 cc of the instilled isotope, treatable cysts generally are larger than 3 cc in volume (Janicki and Seuntjens, 2003). Patients referred for intracavitary radiation after prior placement of cyst reservoir drainage devices (Ommaya type reservoirs) must be screened to make sure that the cyst wall is intact. Prior to therapeutic instillation of the radioactive isotope, the cyst integrity can be assessed using a diagnostic injection of a radionuclide (technetium-99m) into the cyst followed by serial imaging using a gamma camera. Cyst leakage excludes patients from intracavitary therapy (Kickingereder et al., 2012). Prior to surgery, all patients should undergo thorough neurological, ophthalmological, and endocrinological evaluations.

SURGICAL TECHNIQUE

The surgical technique for performing stereotactic intracavitary radiation is based on several basic principles: accurate determination of the cyst volume, selection of the radioisotope, calculation of the prescription dose, and stereotactic puncture of the cyst followed by injection and barbotage of the radioisotope.

Determination of Cyst Volume

Cyst volume estimates are performed in a number of ways, although the exact method is often not explicitly described in published reports. Our group typically utilizes the preoperative computed tomography (CT) or magnetic resonance imaging (MRI) scans to make a pre-operative estimate of the cyst volume. Using the equation for a simple ellipsoidal volume, we calculate the estimated cyst volume: $(\pi/6) \times (x, y, z)$ (Hasegawa et al., 2004). This volume is then communicated in advance of the procedure to the nuclear pharmacist who orders the radioisotope. Then, on the day of surgery, a high-resolution axial contrasted

CT is obtained after the patient has been placed in a stereotactic head frame. The images from this study are imported into the radiation therapy treatment planning software (i.e., Gamma Plan) to contour the cyst edges and determine the cyst area of each slice in square centimeters (Hasegawa et al., 2004; Barriger et al., 2011). This value is multiplied by the slice thickness, which provides the cyst volume in cubic centimeters. This approach has proven simpler and more reliable than using a prior intracystic injection of technetium-99m to perform a volume calculation.

Choice of Radioisotope

The bulk of intracavitary radiation therapy has been performed using one of three radioisotopes: phosphorus-32 (^{32}P), yttrium-90 (^{90}Y), and rhenium-186 (^{186}Rh). While both ^{32}P and ^{90}Y are pure beta (β) particle-emitting isotopes that are made in colloidal suspensions, ^{186}Re has both β and γ emission. In addition, ^{186}Re preparations are reported to be less viscous, and potentially could extravasate beyond the cyst wall. Pure β-emitting intracavitary agents are preferred because of the short penetrance of their emitted radiation, their relatively short half-lives, and their ease of handling (Julow et al., 1985; Backlund et al., 1989; Lunsford, 1989). It is generally accepted that the ideal isotope should be a pure β emitter of high energy (Blackburn et al., 1999). The efficacy of mixed-emitting isotopes is limited by the gamma emissions. When comparing the two pure β emitters, ^{32}P has a lower energy, a shorter penetrance, and a longer half-life than ^{90}Y. Theoretically, the shorter penetrance minimizes the amount of radiation exposure that critical surrounding structures receive with treatment. A longer half-life allows prolonged exposure of the cyst's epithelium to the radioactivity. These theoretical advantages favor ^{32}P, which delivers the radiation dose during five half-lives of decay, or 70 days. The penetrance of the β energy (0.9 mm) is related to the distance from the source and follows the inverse square law wherein the penetrance falls off by one over the square of the distance from the source. Therefore, most energy is delivered within the 2–3 mm that typifies a cyst wall. The ^{90}Y half-life is much shorter, and the entire effect is delivered over 3–5 days. Yttrium-90 may be more efficacious in patients who require early re-aspiration of cyst contents to reduce mass effect. Phosphorus-32 is the only radioisotope approved for intracavitary therapy in the United States, while ^{90}Y has been favored in Europe and Japan. The authors' experience is limited to the use and handling of ^{32}P. Table 24.1 summarizes the different properties of these three radioisotopes. Although ^{186}Rh has a lower beta energy and a shorter tissue range than ^{90}Y, it possesses the disadvantages of emitting a gamma component and it

TABLE 24.1 Characteristics of the Most Commonly Utilized β-Emitting Radionuclides

	^{32}P	^{90}Y	^{186}Re
Half-life (days)	14.3	2.7	3.8
Mean β-energy (MeV)	0.69	0.93	0.36
Max. β-energy (MeV)	1.71	2.28	1.08
γ-Emission	No	No	Yes
Half value depth (mm)	0.8	2.9	1
Max. tissue range (mm)	7.9	11	4.5

converts to an unstable perrhenate form in water (Voges et al., 1997). Due to these limitations, the focus of this review will be on the pure beta-emitting isotopes. The efficacy of the intracavitary technique was confirmed by *in vitro* experiments using ^{32}P in cultures of lining cells from craniopharyngiomas (Young et al., 1976). Moreover, Szeifert et al. confirmed the utility of intracavitary irradiation from pathological specimens after treatment (Szeifert et al., 1990).

Selection and Calculation of Prescription Dose

Prescription doses vary somewhat from group to group, but for ^{32}P most groups report doses ranging from 200−300 Gy delivered over the course of five half-lives (Pollack et al., 1988; Pollock et al., 1995; Hasegawa et al., 2004; Barriger et al., 2011; Kickingereder et al., 2012). Zhao et al. prescribed a dose of 400−500 Gy per injection because of concerns that previously published doses were inadequate (Zhao et al., 2010). Yttrium-90 dosing has been reported in a similar range (Van den Berge et al., 1992; Voges et al., 1997; Julow et al., 1997, 2007). Specific details regarding the calculation of prescription doses are beyond the scope of this review. In brief, at the authors' institution a nuclear pharmacist assumes this task and orders an adequate amount of a ^{32}P stock solution based on a pre-operative calculation of cyst volume and the desired dose. This solution is assayed for its radioactivity on the day of its delivery and on the day of the operation. After the precise cyst volume calculation is made intra-operatively, the volume data are given to the pharmacist who prepares the isotope and calculates the volume necessary to provide a dose of 200−250 Gy over five half-lives (Hasegawa et al., 2004). Typically the entire dose of 200 Gy is delivered from a volume of ^{32}P as small as 0.6 ml. Dose calculation has been based on nomogram tables from numerical calculations of the dose delivered to a surface element on the inner wall of a hollow sphere filled with a homogeneous mixture of radiocolloid and water and assumes a uniform distribution of the colloid in the cyst (Barriger et al., 2011). Some investigators are examining the adequacy of this dose calculation technique and have suggested alternatives that may be more accurate and lead to improved efficacy of the technique (Denis-Bacelar et al., 2013).

Surgical Procedure

The two most commonly utilized procedures to administer radioisotope are frame-based stereotactic needle insertion into the cyst(s) (Van den Berge et al., 1992; Hasegawa et al., 2004; Barriger et al., 2011; Kickingereder et al., 2012) or placement of an Ommaya reservoir into the cyst with subsequent dosing (Blackburn et al., 1999; Zhao et al., 2010). The potential advantage of an Ommaya reservoir is in the setting of a need to aspirate cyst contents frequently, or in a situation where it is felt that several radioisotope administrations will be necessary. The main disadvantage is that holes in the proximal catheter in the cyst may also lie outside the cyst in the ventricle or cistern. Injection of the isotope in such a patient raises the risk that some isotope may be outside the cyst itself.

Stereotactic needle insertion facilitates targeting of multiple cysts in the same surgical procedure. The authors use the frame-based stereotactic needle insertion technique (Pollack et al., 1988; Pollock et al., 1995; Hasegawa et al., 2004). Briefly, after the placement of a Leksell stereotactic head frame under intravenous sedation, the patient undergoes a contrasted high-resolution CT scan in a dedicated intra-operative CT scanner (Figure 24.1A). The images

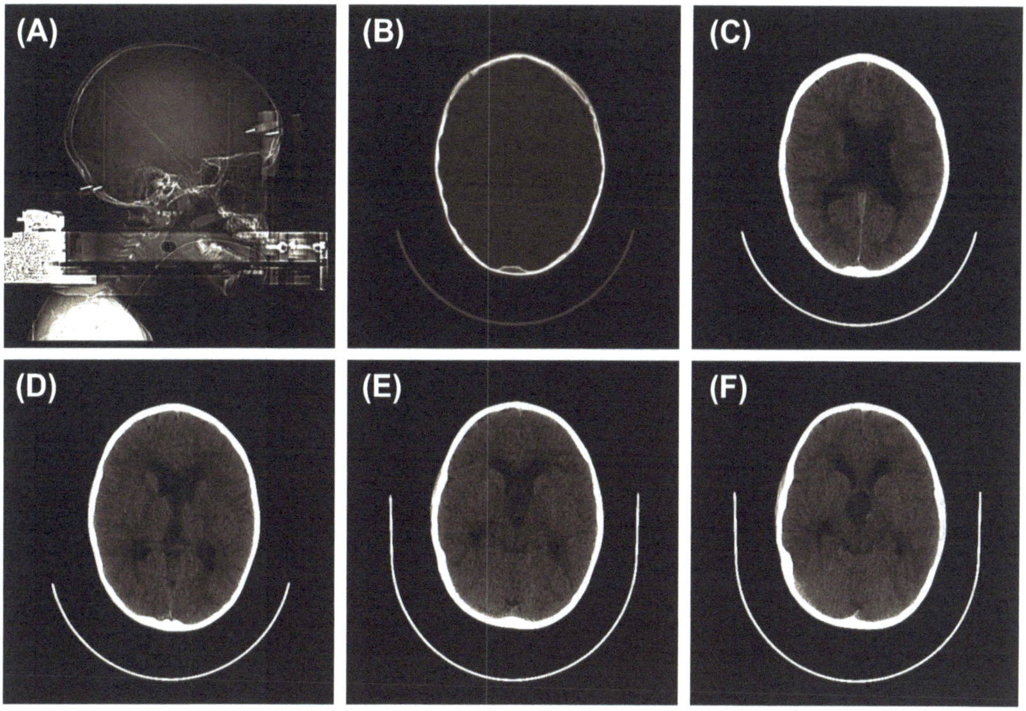

FIGURE 24.1 **A,** a sagittal scout tomogram shows a pediatric patient's head in a Leksell stereotactic head frame taken prior to high-definition CT imaging. **B–F,** select axial non-contrast CT images depicting the twist drill craniostomy and small air bubbles along the needle tract as well as in the ventral portion of the cyst.

are transferred via Ethernet to a computer workstation possessing stereotactic planning software. These images are used to calculate the cyst volume as described previously, and to select the ideal stereotactic path to the cyst. Typically, a frontal, coronal suture approach is selected. A target 7 to 10 mm inferior to the dorsal margin of the cyst is chosen to allow for cyst wall depression while performing the needle puncture. A twist drill craniostomy is performed, and a 0.9 mm outer-diameter sharp-tipped needle is passed through a 15.5 cm long 1.5 mm diameter stabilizing cannula to puncture the cyst (Figure 24.1B). After the cyst is punctured, the stylet is removed and a three-way stopcock is applied to the needle. A tuberculin syringe is used to aspirate 1 cc of cyst fluid, which is examined by a neuropathologist using polarized light microscopy to detect cholesterol crystals. Two tuberculin syringes are then attached to the three-way stopcock, one containing the calculated volume of ^{32}P colloidal suspension in a 30% glucose solution and the other containing 0.2 cc sterile saline flush. The isotope is then injected into the cyst and barbotaged three to five times, followed by an injection of a small volume of saline to restore the original cyst volume and to eject any isotope remaining from the needle into the cyst. The goal is to maintain the original cyst volume in order to provide optimum exposure of the cyst wall to the radiation by avoiding wrinkling of the cyst wall, recalling that the isotope β radiation effect is limited to 2–3 mm. After the injection is completed, all instruments are examined for residual radioactivity and the nuclear pharmacist calculates the exact dose administered to the patient. All patients undergo an immediate post-operative CT scan that often reveals a small air bubble at the anterior margin of the cyst (Figure 24.1C–F).

Although early adopters of intracavitary treatment report freehand cyst punctures, the most common variation of the procedure is the use of different stereotactic frame systems (i.e., Julow et al., 2007; Kickingereder et al., 2012). Kickingereder et al. perform additional volumetry during the procedure via the pre-therapeutic injection of technetium-99m human serum microaggregates into the cyst (Kickingereder et al., 2012). After instillation of the technetium, it is aspirated to identify any decrease in radioactivity, suggesting intracranial dispersal and cyst leakage, a contraindication to proceeding with a therapeutic injection. Very small cysts are not considered ideal targets for intracavitary therapy. A minimum cyst volume of 0.5 cc has been suggested, because of the inaccuracy of dose calculations below this volume (Kickingereder et al., 2012). The authors dilute the ^{32}P suspension with a 30% glucose solution to facilitate accurate and precise dose delivery to cysts less than 20 cc in volume (Hasegawa et al., 2004). Several groups make use of bremstrahllung localization scans at various intervals post-operatively to continue to evaluate for leakage of the radioactive cyst contents (Julow et al., 2007; Barriger et al., 2011). In the setting of neurological or visual deterioration thought to be due to mass effect from a cyst, a cyst's volume can be therapeutically reduced by aspiration, followed by administration of the radioisotope in the same surgical procedure (Kickingereder et al., 2012).

OUTCOMES AND COMPLICATIONS

The goal of intracavitary radiotherapy is to achieve cyst control while preserving visual, endocrine, and neurological functioning (Figure 24.2). There are no prospective trials in this field, and all studies in this area are limited by the fact that they represent retrospective case series and hence have the associated biases.

The results of clinical series published from 1981 to 2004 have been exhaustively reviewed by Cáceres in 2005 (Caceres, 2005). In a majority of these studies, either ^{32}P or ^{90}Yt was the primary radioisotope used for therapy. The total number of patients in each series ranged from six to 62, with the three largest including 49, 57, and 62 patients respectively (Hasegawa et al., 2004, Sturm et al., 1981, Voges et al., 1997). The follow-up period was not reported in five studies, and ranged from six to 156 months in the other 13. The percentage of patients who were progression-free from cyst growth ranged from 0% to 100% at last follow-up. For series using ^{32}P, the percentage of patients free from cyst progression ranged from 76 to 100% (Kobayashi et al., 1981; Sturm et al., 1981; Pollack et al., 1988; Pollock et al., 1995; Voges et al., 1997; Jiang et al., 2002; Schefter et al., 2002), whereas the studies using ^{90}Yt reported a range typically from 55 to 100% (Strauss et al., 1982; Musolino et al., 1985; Julow et al., 1985; Guevara et al., 1988; Sturm et al., 1981; Backlund et al., 1989; Van den Berge et al., 1992; Voges et al., 1997; Blackburn et al., 1999), with a single study reporting 0% (Netzeband et al., 1984). A minority of series involve the use of ^{186}Re, with results also ranging from 0 to 100% tumor-free progression (Sturm et al., 1981; Netzeband et al., 1984; Szilka et al., 1984; Musolino et al., 1985). Unfortunately, many early studies reported primarily on tumor response and did not expand on the ophthalmological and endocrine results. Three of the

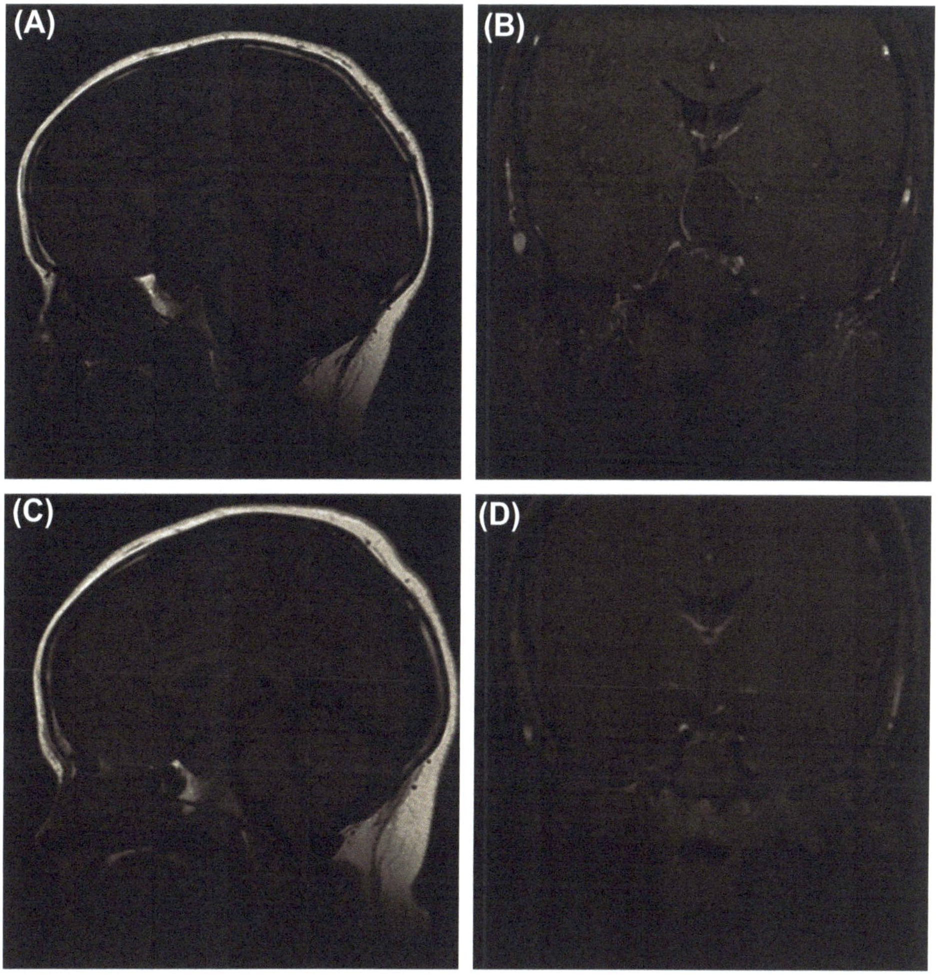

FIGURE 24.2 **A** and **B**, sagittal non-contrast and coronal post-contrast MRI images of a pediatric patient harboring a monocystic craniopharyngioma prior to ^{32}P intracavitary therapy. **C** and **D**, sagittal non-contrast and coronal post-contrast MRI images of the same patient approximately 2 years after ^{32}P intracavitary therapy with no residual cyst detectable.

larger studies are illustrative for the attention given to these three outcome measures together (Table 24.2). Voges et al. treated 66 cysts with ^{90}Yt and reported a partial or complete response in 83% of cases (Voges et al., 1997). Eight cysts were treated with ^{32}P and only one did not respond. Four cysts were treated with ^{186}Re, with two remaining stable and two increasing in size. Mean survival after intracavitary therapy in this series was 9.0 years with actuarial survival rates at 5 and 10 years of 55 and 45%, respectively. Patients with solitary cysts had improved mean and actuarial survival (mean = 12.5 years, 5- and 10-year actuarial survivals of 80 and 64%, respectively). Interestingly, in patients treated with only intracavitary therapy, survival was the longest (10-year survival of 90%). Twenty-three of the 38

TABLE 24.2 Selected Clinical Series of Intracavitary Radionuclide Therapy

	Patients	Radionuclide	Follow-up (months)	Dose (Gy)	Cyst volume (median, ml)	Cyst control	Vision stable or improved	Hormonal status stable or improved
Van den Berge et al. (1992)	31	^{90}Y	2–80	200	2–150 (range)	91%	*42%/48%	77.4%
Voges et al. (1997)	62	^{90}Y, ^{32}P, ^{186}Re	18–196.8	200	18.5	79.5%	93.5%	95.2%
Hasegawa et al. (2004)	49	^{32}P	49 (mean)	224	13	76%	77%	$71%
Julow et al. (2007)	60	^{90}Y	8–360	300	10.6	100%	94.2%	NR
Derrey et al. (2008)	42	^{186}Re	8–148	400	8	87%	91%	74%
Zhao et al. (2010)	20	^{32}P	36–336	400–500	29	100%	95%	85%
Barriger et al. (2011)	19	^{32}P	8–136	300	9	63%	81%	74%
Kickingereder et al. (2012)	53	^{32}P	3–196.7	200	6.1	88.2%	90.2%	80.4%

** 42% reported for visual acuity, 48% for visual fields.*
$of the patients who had normal pre-operative pituitary function.
NR, not reported.

patients with pre-operative visual deficits showed improvement while the remaining 15 were stable. Four patients suffered worsened vision and were all treated with ^{90}Y. In 33 patients with pre-operative endocrine dysfunction, there were no changes in status with treatment. Three patients developed worsened endocrine function following treatment. Other notable complications included: cyst leakage in 10% of interventions and one death attributed to direct radiation damage to the hypothalamus.

Van den Berge et al. treated 31 patients with primarily cystic craniopharyngiomas using intracavitary ^{90}Yt (Van den Berge et al., 1992). Twenty-six of these patients were treated primarily with intracavitary therapy and had undergone no other previous therapies. The follow-up period ranged from 2 to 80 months, and during this period, five patients died from tumor-related causes. In 22 of the 31 patients, the treated cyst either completely resolved or showed radiographic regression. In six other patients, the cyst volume remained stable, while only three patients showed increases in cyst size, for a total cyst progression-free rate of 91%. Visual fields were evaluated in 64 eyes during the study, of which 26 had normal vision pre-operatively and 38 had a partial deficit. Following intracavitary treatment, 58% of the eyes investigated developed decreased visual acuity and 52% developed worsened field cuts. All nine patients who possessed normal pre-operative endocrine function retained this during follow-up. One patient demonstrated complete resolution of endocrinopathy after intracavitary therapy. Ten patients harbored three or more insufficiencies prior to treatment, while this was true in 17 patients after treatment.

Hasegawa et al. reported the largest series using ^{32}P (Hasegawa et al., 2004). Fifty-four tumor cysts were treated with stereotactic intracavitary therapy in 49 patients, of which 51% were treated primarily and had undergone no previous therapy. Ten of these patients were known to have died from tumor-related causes. The mean follow-up period was 49 months. The overall actuarial tumor control rate was 76% at 5 years and 70% at 10 years. Patients harboring solid tumor components had little or no reduction in the solid portions of their tumors with intracavitary treatment (12%). Thirteen percent of patients developed a new cyst during follow-up. In patients treated primarily, 48% of the patients with diminished pre-operative acuity improved and 52% had improved visual fields. These numbers were similar in the adjuvant treatment group (47% and 41%, respectively). Nine patients (23%) developed visual abnormalities following intracavitary therapy: six were attributed to tumor progression, while the remaining three were attributed to an adverse effect of ^{32}P as vision deteriorated in a delayed fashion despite tumor remission. Of the 17 patients who possessed either normal pituitary function or stalk effect pre-operatively, 71% of these had preserved endocrine function. No other complications were noted in this series.

Since the review by Cáceres, there have been several meaningful reports published on this topic (Table 24.2). Julow et al. reviewed their 30-year experience treating cystic craniopharyngiomas with intracavitary ^{90}Y (Julow et al., 2007). Ninety-four cysts were treated in 66 patients using a planned 300 Gy dose, with all of the patients having previously undergone surgical excision. The mean overall survival for this patient cohort was 9.4 years during a follow-up period ranging from 8 to 360 months. At last follow-up, all 60 patients had experienced tumor shrinkage after the 73 implantation procedures. In this series, 5.8% of patients developed visual deterioration. Thirteen (13.5%) patients had improved ophthalmological status after the procedure. There were three peri-operative deaths. No data on the endocrine status of this cohort was reported.

In 2008, Derrey et al. reported on the largest ever series of patients treated with intracavitary ^{186}Re (Derrey et al., 2008). Using a calculated wall dose of 400 Gy, this group analyzed their results in a total of 39 patients over a mean follow-up period of 43 months. All but five patients (13%) demonstrated stability or cyst regression. All patients with normal vision prior to treatment maintained this through follow-up. Only one patient with a pre-existing deficit in visual acuity worsened and two patients with pre-existing field cuts worsened. In total, three patients developed worsened visual function despite evidence of tumor control on imaging. The 17 patients with normal endocrine function did not worsen during follow-up. In the patients with pre-existing hormonal dysfunction, no patient worsened and 86.5% demonstrated no change. No patients suffered other permanent morbidities from surgery and there were no mortalities directly attributed to intracavitary therapy.

Zhao et al. treated 20 pediatric patients with predominantly cystic craniopharyngiomas with intracavitary ^{32}P (Zhao et al., 2010). A total dose of 400–500 Gy was used per injection with only six of the patients undergoing a solitary procedure. Over half of this cohort had intracavitary therapy as the primary treatment (55%). Reporting on a median follow-up period of 47.7 months, Zhao et al. noted that in 90% of cysts there was a reduction in size of more than 50%. Five-year survival was 100% in the patient cohort. During follow-up, the vision of only one patient worsened. From an endocrine standpoint, growth hormone deficiency was stable, adrenocorticotropic and thyroid stimulating hormone deficiencies improved, and hyperprolactinemia worsened.

Barriger et al. retrospectively analyzed the results of intracavitary therapy with ^{32}P in 19 patients with a median follow-up of 62 months (Barriger et al., 2011). The median prescribed dose to the cyst wall was 300 Gy. Of the 19 cysts treated, 63.2% were controlled. Four of these developed new cysts, and several demonstrated growth in the solid portion of the tumor. Vision was stable or improved in 81% of the patients. Fourteen of these patients had at least some pre-operative pituitary hormone function, and this was preserved in 57.1%.

Kickingereder et al. summarized their experience most recently (Kickingereder et al., 2012). After a median follow-up of 53 months in 53 patients treated with a median of 200 Gy to the inner cyst wall by ^{32}P, 82.3% of cysts regressed completely or partially. Nearly six percent of cysts remained stable, while 11.8% increased in volume. All failures occurred within the first 12 months of treatment. New cysts formed in 27.5% of patients and the solid portion of the tumors progressed in 7.8% of patients. Visual acuity was improved or remained stable in 92.2%, whereas patients' visual fields improved or remained stable in 90.2% of the cohort. Ten patients (19.6%) in the series developed worsened endocrine function following treatment. Nearly 14% of the cohort suffered new transient neurological deficits following treatment. Two patients suffered permanent deficits, one a hemiparesis and the second a third nerve palsy. There were no treatment-related mortalities.

CONCLUSIONS

Although craniopharyngiomas are histologically benign tumors, they cause a high degree of morbidity due to the sensitive nature of the neighboring structures that are compressed or invaded. Historically, maximum resection has been considered the goal of treatment. However, even in the most experienced hands, attempted gross total resection may be associated with unacceptably high rates of morbidity and mortality. Sughrue et al. performed an extensive review of studies in which outcome data were reported on surgically managed patients (Sughrue et al., 2011). They found that gross total resection was associated with new endocrinopathy in 37% of cases. Visual loss was associated with approximately 4% of these cases. The risk of visual loss was twice as high with fractionated radiation therapy and radiosurgery alone (8.6%). Yang et al. reviewed tumor control rates with various treatment strategies (Yang et al., 2010). Tumor recurrence rates at 2 and 5 years were 12–23% after gross total resection, and 9–31% after subtotal resection combined with adjuvant external beam radiation. In our single-institution series of patients treated with gamma knife stereotactic radiosurgery, local failure rates at 1, 3, and 5 years were 9, 19, and 32%, respectively (Niranjan et al., 2010).

Craniopharyngiomas are unique tumors because they are variably composed of different proportions of cystic and solid components, with many tumors harboring a dominant cystic component (Pollack et al., 1988; Habrand et al., 1999; Savas et al., 1999). Thus, treatment for craniopharyngiomas should be tailored to the individual, and the modern goals of management include not only maximum tumor control, but also maintenance of visual, endocrine, and neurological function whenever possible. Often, patients will require multimodal therapy to accomplish these goals. Intracavitary radionuclide therapy has evolved as a minimally invasive primary or salvage strategy for predominantly cystic craniopharyngiomas. It is thought to have certain advantages over radical surgery and other forms of radiotherapy: it is minimally invasive, it well suited to cystic tumors, and the short tissue penetrance of the β-emitting radionuclides can limit toxicity to local structures. The literature on intracavitary therapy suggests that control of cystic tumors compares favorably with other treatment modalities. Moreover, the risks of new visual loss and endocrinopathy are relatively low. The choice of radionuclide is typically determined by local laws and availability, but there do not appear to be demonstrated differences in the control and complication rates with ^{32}P and ^{90}Y. The pure β emitters possess an advantage over ^{186}Re because of a lack of γ emissions, although the limited literature on ^{186}Re does not suggest dramatically higher complication rates. As with many different therapies, primary intracavitary therapy seems more efficacious and safer than salvage therapy (Van den Berge et al., 1992). As expected, it does not have a meaningful effect on the solid portions of these tumors (Julow et al., 2007; Barriger et al., 2011).

The studies on intracavitary therapy for craniopharyngiomas suffer from several important limitations. There are few or no standardized methods for the technique. Specifically, ophthalmological, endocrine, and neurological data are not always presented, and when presented, are done so variably, making comparisons between studies difficult. There is a dearth of data on validated quality-of-life measures in these studies. These measures should be formally included in the future evaluation of all treatments for craniopharyngiomas. Despite these limitations, intracavitary radionuclide therapy should be considered in a multimodality regimen for any patient harboring a predominantly cystic craniopharyngioma.

References

Backlund, E.O., Axelsson, B., Bergstrand, C.G., Eriksson, A.L., Noren, G., Ribbesjo, E., Rahn, T., Schnell, P.O., Tallstedt, L., Saaf, M., et al., 1989. Treatment of craniopharyngiomas – the stereotactic approach in a ten to twenty-three years' perspective. I. Surgical, radiological and ophthalmological aspects. Acta Neurochir. (Wien) 99, 11–19.

Barriger, R.B., Chang, A., Lo, S.S., Timmerman, R.D., Desrosiers, C., Boaz, J.C., Fakiris, A.J., 2011. Phosphorus-32 therapy for cystic craniopharyngiomas. Radiother. Oncol. 98, 207–212.

Blackburn, T.P., Doughty, D., Plowman, P.N., 1999. Stereotactic intracavitary therapy of recurrent cystic craniopharyngioma by instillation of 90 yttrium. Br. J. Neurosurg. 13, 359–365.

Caceres, A., 2005. Intracavitary therapeutic options in the management of cystic craniopharyngioma. Childs Nerv. Syst. 21, 705–718.

Denis-Bacelar, A.M., Romanchikova, M., Chittenden, S., Saran, F.H., Mandeville, H., Du, Y., Flux, G.D., 2013. Patient-specific dosimetry for intracavitary ^{32}P-chromic phosphate colloid therapy of cystic brain tumours. Eur. J. Nucl. Med. Mol. Imaging 40, 1532–1541.

Derrey, S., Blond, S., Reyns, N., Touzet, G., Carpentier, P., Gauthier, H., Dhellemmes, P., 2008. Management of cystic craniopharyngiomas with stereotactic endocavitary irradiation using colloidal 186Re: a retrospective study of 48 consecutive patients. Neurosurgery 63, 1045–1052; discussion 1052–1053.

Guevara, J.A., Bunge, H.J., Heinrich, J.J., Weller, G., Villasante, A., Chinela, A.B., 1988. Cystic craniopharyngioma treated by 90yttrium silicate colloid. Acta Neurochir. Suppl. (Wien) 42, 109–112.

Habrand, J.L., Ganry, O., Couanet, D., Rouxel, V., Levy-Piedbois, C., Pierre-Kahn, A., Kalifa, C., 1999. The role of radiation therapy in the management of craniopharyngioma: a 25-year experience and review of the literature. Int. J. Radiat. Oncol. Biol. Phys. 44, 255–263.

Hasegawa, T., Kondziolka, D., Hadjipanayis, C.G., Lunsford, L.D., 2004. Management of cystic craniopharyngiomas with phosphorus-32 intracavitary irradiation. Neurosurgery 54, 813–820; discussion 820–822.

Janicki, C., Seuntjens, J., 2003. Re-evaluation of the dose to the cyst wall in P-32 radiocolloid treatments of cystic brain tumors using the dose-point-kernel and Monte Carlo methods. Med. Phys. 30, 2475–2481.

Jiang, R., Liu, Z., Zhu, C., 2002. Preliminary exploration of the clinical effect of bleomycin on craniopharyngiomas. Stereotact. Funct. Neurosurg. 78, 84–94.

Julow, J., Lanyi, F., Hajda, M., Simkovics, M., Arany, I., Toth, S., Pasztor, E., 1985. The radiotherapy of cystic craniopharyngioma with intracystic installation of 90Y silicate colloid. Acta Neurochir. (Wien) 74, 94–99.

Julow, J., Lanyi, F., Hajda, M., Szeifert, G.T., Balint, K., Drasny, G., Pasztor, E., Fedorcsak, I., Borbely, K., Nyary, I., 1997. Treatment of cystic craniopharyngiomas with yttrium-90 colloid solution. Neurosurg. Focus. 3, e6.

Julow, J., Backlund, E.O., Lanyi, F., Hajda, M., Balint, K., Nyary, I., Szeifert, G.T., 2007. Long-term results and late complications after intracavitary yttrium-90 colloid irradiation of recurrent cystic craniopharyngiomas. Neurosurgery 61, 288–295; discussion 295–296.

Kickingereder, P., Maarouf, M., El Majdoub, F., Fuetsch, M., Lehrke, R., Wirths, J., Luyken, K., Schomaecker, K., Treuer, H., Voges, J., Sturm, V., 2012. Intracavitary brachytherapy using stereotactically applied phosphorus-32 colloid for treatment of cystic craniopharyngiomas in 53 patients. J. Neurooncol. 109, 365–374.

Kobayashi, T., Kageyama, N., Ohara, K., 1981. Internal irradiation for cystic craniopharyngioma. J. Neurosurg. 55, 896–903.

Leksell, L., 1949. A therapeutic trial with radioactive isotopes in cystic brain tumour. Acta Chir. Scan. 99, 76–78.

Leksell, L., Liden, K., 1952. A therapeutic trial with radioactive isotopes in cystic brain tumours. Radioisotope techniques. J. Med. Physiol. Appl. 4, 1–4.

Lunsford, L.D., 1989. Stereotactic treatment of craniopharyngioma: Intracavitary irradiation and radiosurgery. Cont. Neurosurg. 11, 1–6.

Musolino, A., Munari, C., Blond, S., Betti, O., Lajat, Y., Schaub, C., Askienazy, S., Chodkiewicz, J.P., 1985. [Stereotaxic treatment of expanding cysts in craniopharyngiomas by endocavitary beta-irradiation (Re-186; Au-198; Y-90)]. Neurochirurgie 31, 169–178.

Netzeband, G., Sturm, V., Georgi, P., 1984. Results of stereotactic intracavitary irradiation of cystic craniopharyngiomas. Comparison of the effects of Yttrium-90 and Rhenium-186. Acta Neurochir. (Wien) (Suppl. 33), 341–344.

Niranjan, A., Kano, H., Mathieu, D., Kondziolka, D., Flickinger, J.C., Lunsford, L.D., 2010. Radiosurgery for craniopharyngioma. Int. J. Radiat. Oncol. Biol. Phys. 78, 64–71.

Pollack, I.F., Lunsford, L.D., Slamovits, T.L., Gumerman, L.W., Levine, G., Robinson, A.G., 1988. Stereotaxic intracavitary irradiation for cystic craniopharyngiomas. J. Neurosurg. 68, 227–233.

Pollock, B.E., Lunsford, L.D., Kondziolka, D., Levine, G., Flickinger, J.C., 1995. Phosphorus-32 intracavitary irradiation of cystic craniopharyngiomas: current technique and long-term results. Int. J. Radiat. Oncol. Biol. Phys. 33, 437–446.

Savas, A., Arasil, E., Batay, F., Selcuki, M., Kanpolat, Y., 1999. Intracavitary chemotherapy of polycystic craniopharyngioma with bleomycin. Acta Neurochir. (Wien) 141, 547–548; discussion 549.

Schefter, J.K., Allen, G., Cmelak, A.J., Johnson, M., Toms, S., Duggan, D., Blevins, L.S., 2002. The utility of external beam radiation and intracystic 32P radiation in the treatment of craniopharyngiomas. J. Neurooncol. 56, 69–78.

Strauss, L., Sturm, V., Georgi, P., Schlegel, W., Ostertag, H., Clorius, J.H., Van Kaick, G., 1982. Radioisotope therapy of cystic craniopharyngomas. Int. J. Radiat. Oncol. Biol. Phys. 8, 1581–1585.

Sturm, V., Rommel, T., Strauss, L., 1981. Preliminary results of intracavitary irradiation of cystic craniopharyngiomas by means of stereotactically applied yttrium-90. In: Schiefer, W., Klinger, M., Brock, M. (Eds.), Advances in neurosurgery 9. Springer, Berlin Heidelberg New York, p. 401–404.

Sughrue, M.E., Yang, I., Kane, A.J., Fang, S., Clark, A.J., Aranda, D., Barani, I.J., Parsa, A.T., 2011. Endocrinologic, neurologic, and visual morbidity after treatment for craniopharyngioma. J. Neurooncol. 101, 463–476.

Szeifert, G.T., Julow, J., Slowik, F., Balint, K., Lanyi, F., Pasztor, E., 1990. Pathological changes in cystic craniopharyngiomas following intracavital 90yttrium treatment. Acta Neurochir. (Wien) 102, 14–18.

Szilka, G., Musolino, A., Miyahara, S., 1984. Colloidal rhenium-186 endocavitary irradiation of cystic craniopharyngiomas and active glioma cysts. Long term results, side effects and clinical dosimetry. Acta Neurochir. (Wien) (Suppl. 33), 331–339.

Van Den Berge, J.H., Blaauw, G., Breeman, W.A., Rahmy, A., Wijngaarde, R., 1992. Intracavitary brachytherapy of cystic craniopharyngiomas. J. Neurosurg. 77, 545–550.

Voges, J., Sturm, V., Lehrke, R., Treuer, H., Gauss, C., Berthold, F., 1997. Cystic craniopharyngioma: long-term results after intracavitary irradiation with stereotactically applied colloidal beta-emitting radioactive sources. Neurosurgery 40, 263–269; discussion 269–270.

Yang, I., Sughrue, M.E., Rutkowski, M.J., Kaur, R., Ivan, M.E., Aranda, D., Barani, I.J., Parsa, A.T., 2010. Craniopharyngioma: a comparison of tumor control with various treatment strategies. Neurosurg. Focus 28, E5.

Young, H.F., Fu, Y.S., Fratkin, M.J., 1976. Organ culture of craniopharyngioma and its cellular effects induced by colloidal chromic phosphate. J. Neuropathol. Exp. Neurol. 35, 404–412.

Zhao, R., Deng, J., Liang, X., Zeng, J., Chen, X., Wang, J., 2010. Treatment of cystic craniopharyngioma with phosphorus-32 intracavitary irradiation. Childs Nerv. Syst. 26, 669–674.

CHAPTER

25

Intracavitary Therapy: Intracavitary Chemotherapy

Eric Bouffet, Jennifer Adamski, Ute Bartels

Division of Haematology/Oncology, The Hospital for Sick Children, Toronto, Ontario, Canada

"The oncological characteristics of craniopharyngiomas are: 1) that in most cases the tumor is associated with a cyst; and 2) that it is an epithelial tumor." ***H Takahasi, et al., 1985***

INTRODUCTION

Craniopharyngiomas are benign non-glial intracranial neoplasms that occur both in children and in adults (Karavitaki and Wass, 2008). They are thought to arise from squamous epithelial remnants of Rathke's pouch. In the pediatric age group, they account for 4–10% of central nervous system tumors and represent the most common sellar and suprasellar tumors in this population. The WHO classification of craniopharyngiomas describes two variants. The adamantinomatous type is typically seen in the pediatric group; this variant is predominantly cystic, with or without solid components, and often shows calcifications on CT scan. Papillary craniopharyngiomas are more common in adults and are essentially solid (Rushing et al., 2007). While complete excision has traditionally been the primary goal of treatment, aggressive surgery has been associated with significant complications, including pituitary and hypothalamic damage, which has devastating consequences (De Vile et al., 1996; Honegger and Tatagiba, 2008). Over the last two decades, the management of this tumor has evolved and a number of retrospective and prospective studies have contributed to clarifying the respective role of surgery and irradiation (Merchant et al., 2013). The optimal management of predominantly or purely cystic craniopharyngiomas remains controversial. Evacuation of the cyst is a temporary measure that relieves pressure; however, early refilling of the cyst is common, and intermittent aspiration of the cystic contents generally fails to control cystic fluid secretion (Bartels et al., 2012). While some advocate for surgical decompression followed by stereotactic irradiation, a number of reports have described the potential benefit of radioisotope therapy or intracystic treatment, either using chemotherapy with bleomycin or

Craniopharyngiomas
http://dx.doi.org/10.1016/B978-0-12-416706-3.00025-8

immunotherapy with interferon-α. This chapter reviews the published experience of intracystic chemotherapy in craniopharyngiomas.

PATHOLOGICAL CONSIDERATIONS

Craniopharyngiomas are thought to arise from squamous epithelial rests in the remnant of Rathke's pouch (Rushing et al., 2007). More specifically, it is thought that they arise from rests of pharyngeal epithelium remaining from embryogenesis that subsequently forms benign neoplastic cells. Of the two recognized variants, the adamantinomatous type is typically seen in the pediatric age group and can be predominantly cystic, whereas the papillary type is more common in adults and is usually essentially solid. Histologically, the wall of craniopharyngioma cysts is lined by a stratified squamous epithelium associated with keratinization. Cyst walls can vary from very thin membranes to thick and tough structures, which may be hard to puncture because of calcium salt deposition. The consistency of the cystic fluid can vary, but it is usually thick and contains suspended cholesterol crystals. The consistency and brownish color of the fluid is typically described as "machine oil." Many children present initially with one large craniopharyngioma cyst that can be considered for intracystic therapy.

INTRACYSTIC DEVICES

Historically, radical cyst fenestration has been used as the treatment of choice for cystic craniopharyngiomas. However, early on, neurosurgeons became aware that recurrence of symptoms in craniopharyngioma patients was primarily related to the reaccumulation of cystic fluid. In the Boston experience, Katz noted that children whose tumors had a large cystic component generally did less well than those with non-cystic tumors (Katz, 1975). Cyst re-accumulation was traditionally an indication for repeat craniotomy. While the benefit of these reoperations was identified, the risk associated with radical surgery of recurrent craniopharyngioma was well recognized (Miles, 1977). Over time, various alternative treatment modalities have been advocated to alleviate or decrease the secretion of cystic fluid. The first experiences of intracystic treatment were described in the 1950s and consisted of stereotactic injections of radioactive material into the cystic cavity (Leksell et al., 1967). However, as craniopharyngioma cysts usually require repeated drainage, initiatives were taken to consider permanent intracystic devices. Fox described the use of the Ommaya reservoir in a craniopharyngioma patient in 1967 (Fox, 1967). Ten years later, Miles described four patients treated with the same technique, including one patient who experienced sustained control after one aspiration only (Miles, 1977). The main advantage of this device was that it offered the possibility of performing intermittent drainage and decompression of cystic craniopharyngiomas without the need for major craniotomy.

In 1963, Dr. Ayub Ommaya, a neurosurgeon from Pakistan invented a device that was initially designed to gain sterile access to cerebrospinal fluid and treat CNS infections (Ommaya, 1963). It consists of a small capsule to which a straight ventricular catheter is attached. The catheter tip has multiple side holes to facilitate the aspiration of cystic fluid. The capsule is made of silicone rubber with a base that can fit into a burr hole. The dome of the capsule is made of thickened silicone rubber that allows repeated (up to 200) punctures.

The catheter is also made of silicone and its length can be adjusted at the time of insertion. This Ommaya reservoir is the most commonly used device for aspirating cysts, although some teams have described intracystic treatment using the Rickham reservoir, which is metal based with a plastic cap (Rickham, 1964). Different techniques of insertion have been described, either under direct vision after a frontal or pterional craniotomy, by stereotaxy with a stereotactic frame, or using freehand placement of the catheter through a burr hole with or without ultrasound guidance (Zanon et al., 2008).

Injections of chemotherapeutic agents or isotopes into the cyst require the system (reservoir–catheter–cyst) to be a perfectly enclosed cavity. This is confirmed by a permeability test that is usually performed 2–4 weeks after the insertion of the device. Practically, a small amount of fluid (2–3 cc) is removed from the cyst and 2 cc of contrast material is introduced. The volume and concentration of contrast needed depends of the volume of the cyst. Thirty to 60 minutes after the injection, a post-contrast CT is performed that will detect areas of extravasations (Figures 25.1 and 25.2). When no extravasation is observed, the treatment can be initiated. In case of extravasation, the permeability test can be repeated 2–4 weeks later.

Leakage of the cytotoxic agent is the major risk associated with the administration of intracystic chemotherapy. Zanon and colleagues analyzed the technique of insertion of the catheter and the subsequent risk of leakage once the catheter was connected to the subcutaneous reservoir (Zanon et al., 2008). In their review of 50 cases, they reported an incidence of 16.3% of misplacement or leakage that was independent of the technique of insertion. Alternative techniques have been suggested to minimize the risk of misplacement and/or leakage (Mori et al., 2013).

However, cystic craniopharyngiomas have the propensity to grow new cysts at different locations. This represents one limitation of this technique, as each individual cyst will require the separate insertion of a device to facilitate therapy. Another potential limitation is the presence of septations in the cyst that will limit the diffusion of the medication (Korinth et al., 2001; Nicolato et al., 2004).

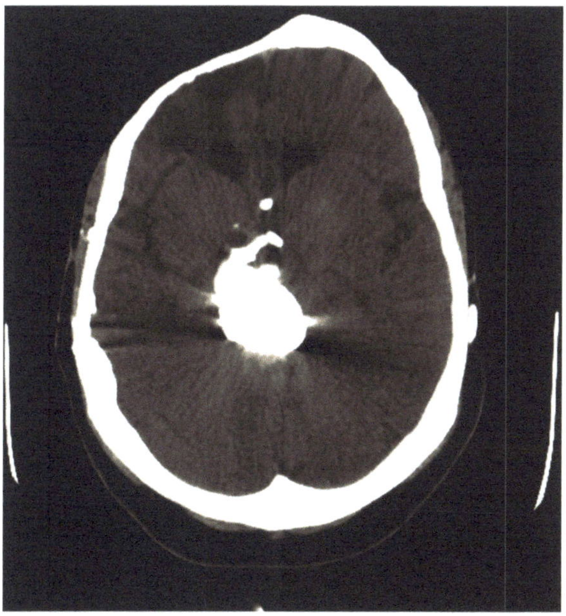

FIGURE 25.1 Permeability test showing contrast material in the cyst without evidence of leakage.

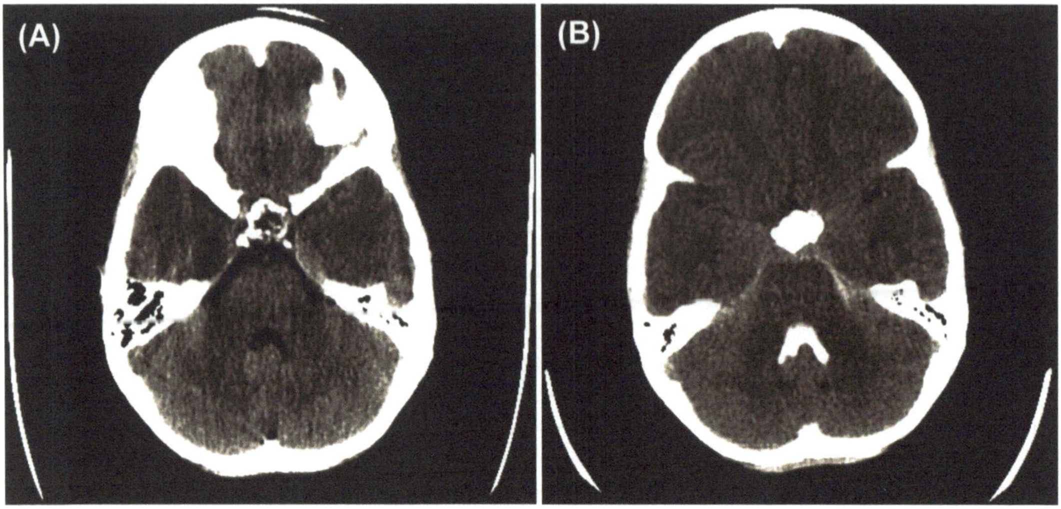

FIGURE 25.2 **Permeability test. A,** CT scan prior contrast injection. **B,** Leakage in the fourth ventricle following administration of contrast in the Ommaya reservoir.

INTRACYSTIC BLEOMYCIN

Bleomycin is a natural glycopeptide antibiotic that interferes with DNA production. This agent has shown interesting activity in the management of patients with squamous cell carcinomas (Crooke and Bradner, 1976; Smith et al., 1986). In 1985, Takayashi reported the first institutional series of seven pediatric craniopharyngioma patients treated with intracystic bleomycin (Takahashi et al., 1985). Bleomycin was injected through an Ommaya reservoir at a dose of 1–5 mg per injection administered every other day. The number of administrations was based on the level of lactate dehydrogenase (LDH) in the cyst and response to bleomycin administration. The treatment was discontinued when the cystic fluid became colorless, and the LDH activity had decreased to below 1000 units. The cumulative dose of bleomycin injected ranged from 13 to 95 mg. Four patients had essentially cystic tumors and showed a sustained response to treatment without recurrence after a follow-up of 2–7 years. The three other patients had mostly solid (one patient) or mixed solid-cystic lesions (two patients) that showed no or only transient response to bleomycin administration. Several small series have been reported since, which confirmed the activity of this technique (Broggi and Franzini, 1996; Cavalheiro et al., 1996; Mottolese et al., 2001; Jiang et al., 2002; Park et al., 2002). In a review of the literature on this topic in 2006, Hargrave collected 68 cases (Hargrave, 2006). The median age of the patients treated was 11 years (range 2–65). Treatment protocols showed variations between centers, with most following a Monday–Wednesday–Friday regimen. The amount of fluid aspirated prior to bleomycin administration varied between patients and within patients (i.e., the amount aspirated was larger during the early phase of the treatment) and averaged 5 ml. The average dose of bleomycin injected was 5 mg, ranging from 2 to 15 mg. The average length of a course of bleomycin was 4 weeks (range, 2–15 weeks) and the median dose per course was 36 mg (range,

5–150 mg). Some patients received multiple courses of bleomycin, either because of incomplete response or recurrence of the cyst (Figure 25.3).

Several authors have reported results of institutional or multicenter series of treatment with intracystic bleomycin (Table 25.1). The response rate to bleomycin reported in the different series is high, with a complete disappearance of the cysts in 43–74% of cases (Jiang et al., 2002). However, interpretation of response following such treatment with repeated aspirations is obviously difficult to interpret. The rate of sustained control is a more reliable indicator. In a collaborative review of the Canadian experience, Hukin reported a sustained benefit of over one year (median 3.6 years, range, 1.6–9.3 years) in 11 of 17 patients before another modality of therapy was required (Hukin et al., 2007). Data from the different published series are in agreement with this figure, with a total number of 48 patients with sustained control out of 87 treated patients in our literature review (Table 25.1). There is no clear correlation between the dose of bleomycin administered and response to treatment. Similarly, no schedule seems to appear more effective. However, Hukin noticed that patients who received < 9 mg/wk and 0.09 mg/mL/dose had a lower chance of significant cyst shrinkage and shorter duration of response (Hukin et al., 2007).

Although the administration of this agent is usually well tolerated, the toxicity of intracystic bleomycin has been documented throughout these experiences, including fatal consequences. The most common side effects include mild headaches, sometimes associated with nausea and/or vomiting, and transient episodes of fever during or shortly after the

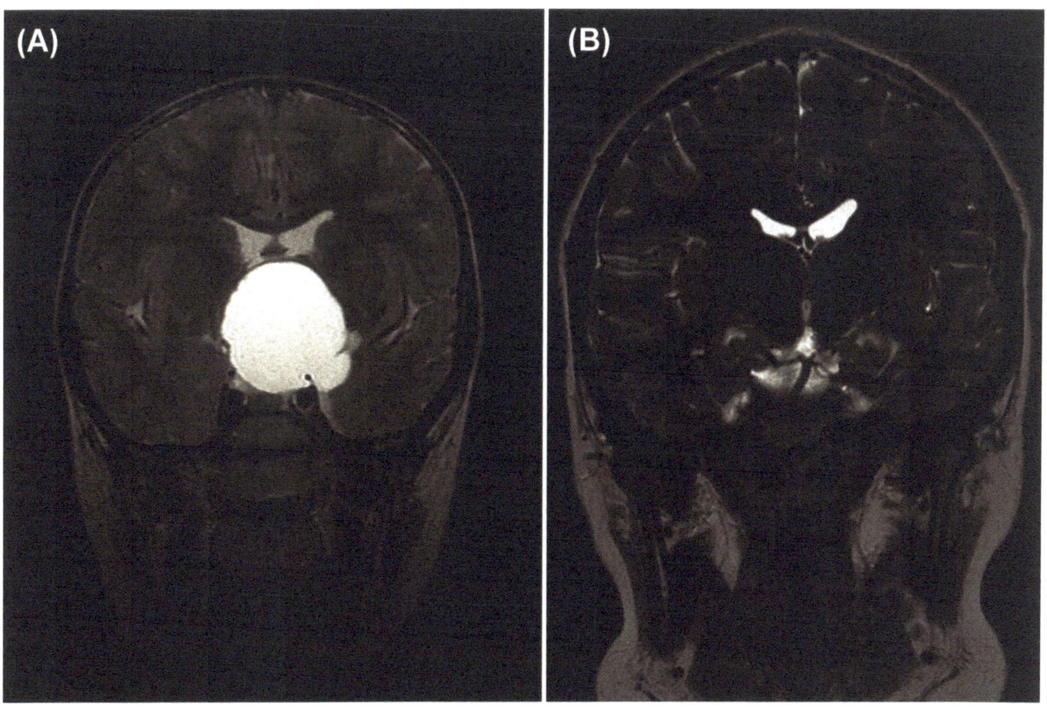

FIGURE 25.3 **Cystic craniopharyngioma. A,** Initial MRI at the time of diagnosis. **B,** Follow-up MRI scan 12 years later. The patient required two treatments with intracystic interferon. She remains endocrinologically intact.

TABLE 25.1 Summary of Published Series (> 5 Patients) of Intracystic Bleomycin

Author (reference)	Number of patients	Number of treatments (patient number)	Dose	Schedule	Total dose	Responding patients (number with CR)	Sustained response	Follow-up (median)	Complications (patient number)
Mottolese (Mottolese et al., 2001)	24	1 (23); > 1 (1)	3–5 mg	alternate days	30–150 mg	24 (7)	16	2–10 (NA)	Blindness (1) Leakage on CT (2)
Hukin* (Hukin et al., 2007)	17	1(12); > 1 (5)	2–5 mg	various	15–75 mg		11	1.6–9.3 (3.6)	Leakage with neurologic symptoms (2) Precocious puberty (1) Panhypopituitarism (1)
Takahashi (Takahashi et al., 1985)	7	1 (6); 2(1)	1–5 mg	alternate days	13–95 mg	6 (NA)	4	21–26 (NA)*	None
Takahashi (Takahashi et al., 2005)	11	1 (11)	NA	NA	NA	11 (NA)	7	3–16	None
Park (Park et al., 2002)	10	1 (9); 2 (1)	2–5 mg	2 to 7 days	NA	10	6	1–6.6 (2.8)	Cerebellar infarction (1)
Frank (Frank et al., 1995)	6	NA	NA	NA	NA	NA	0	NA	Bilateral deafness (1)
Jiang (Jiang et al., 2002)	5	1 (5)	5–15 mg	daily	14.5–120 mg	3 (0)	0	0.6–2 (NA)	None
Hader* (Hader et al., 2000)	7	1 (6); 4 (1)	2–5 mg	3 times/ week	18–115	7(0)	4	0.5–5 (NA)	Asymptomatic intracystic hemorrhage (2) Leakage complicated by panhypopituitarism (1)

** Some patients from the Hukin series may overlap with previous report from Hader; NA: not available; CR: complete response.*

injection. The incidence of these side effects varies between series from 10–70%. More severe toxicity has been described mostly in adults. Savas and coworkers reported a fatal toxicity in a 47-year-old woman who developed progressive neurological deterioration after daily administration of bleomycin for a total dose of 56 mg over 8 days (Savas et al., 2000). This patient developed progressive brainstem dysfunction and died 45 days after completion of treatment. The MRI disclosed diffuse edema at the level of the diencephalon and the brainstem. Haisa et al. reported thermal dysfunction, somnolence, memory difficulties, and personality changes in a 48-year-old patient following a course of intracystic bleomycin (Haisa et al., 1994). More recently, Lafay-Cousin and colleagues described neuroradiological findings of bleomycin leakage in three children. All patients had a permeability study that ruled out leakage prior to initiation of therapy (Lafay-Cousin et al., 2007). They underwent serial MRI scans during treatment, and FLAIR and T2 sequences revealed extensive vasogenic edema surrounding the cyst in all three patients, consistent with evidence of bleomycin leakage. Patients were asymptomatic or had mild symptoms at the time of neuroimaging. Subsequently, two patients developed clinical symptoms suggestive of hypothalamic injury. They both improved following a short course of steroids. Based on these findings, the authors recommended close clinical monitoring and radiological evaluation during treatment using MR imaging, and particularly FLAIR or T2 sequences, to detect early signs of bleomycin leakage (Figure 25.4).

Some authors have analyzed histological changes following administration of bleomycin. Takahasi et al. reported the autopsy findings of a patient who experienced tumor progression

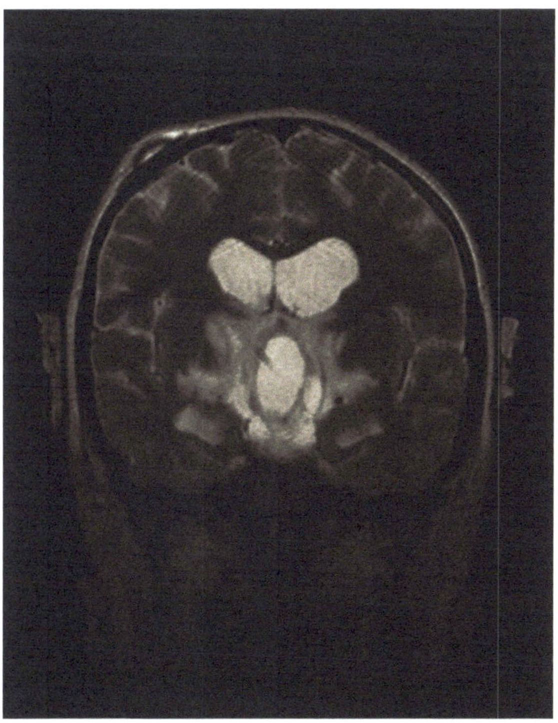

FIGURE 25.4 T2 coronal sequence in a patient treated with intracystic bleomycin, showing diffuse changes in adjacent basal ganglia and thalamus. The pretreatment permeability test did not show any leakage.

despite treatment. They did not identify any significant hemorrhagic or necrotic changes in the region where the Ommaya catheter was inserted. Hukin and coworkers described histological findings in three patients who underwent surgery after intracystic bleomycin. In all cases, there were only the usual features of normal, thin-walled vessels in the gliotic brain adjacent to the craniopharyngioma. No unusual features related to bleomycin toxicity in the tumor or its vasculature were identified on histological examination.

There has been only one small randomized trial that has compared intracystic bleomycin with intracystic ^{32}P in craniopharyngioma treatment. Jiang treated 19 patients, either with bleomycin, ^{32}P, or bleomycin followed by a single injection of ^{32}P (Jiang et al., 2002; Liu et al., 2012). This study did not demonstrate any statistical difference between the three groups in terms of response or side effects. However, two patients in the combined treatment group developed bithalamic infarction leading to death in one.

INTRACYSTIC INTERFERON ALPHA

The use of interferon in craniopharyngioma is based on the same rationale as bleomycin. Immunotherapy with interferon alpha has indeed shown evidence of activity in the treatment of squamous cell carcinoma. Jakacki conducted a phase II study of alpha interferon (IFNα) given daily by subcutaneous injection for 16 consecutive weeks (Jakacki et al., 2000). Fifteen patients were enrolled in this trial and three of the 12 evaluable patients showed radiological response, including one complete response. Interestingly, all three responders had predominantly cystic tumors.

IFNα had been used intrathecally in the management of CNS diseases, particularly subacute sclerosing panencephalitis and neoplastic meningitis (Mitchell and Crawford, 1987; Sobczyk et al., 1987; Chamberlain, 2002; Tomoda et al., 2003). Side effects are usually transient using this route, and mild to moderate in nature. Chemical arachnoiditis is common and characterized by nausea, vomiting, headache, and fever. These symptoms are easily treated with analgesics, antiemetics, and antipyretics. Chronic fatigue is the other common side effect and seems to increase with repeated intrathecal administrations. Importantly, for the purpose of intracystic administration, there are no specific concerns of neurotoxicity associated with IFNα leakage.

In 2005, Cavalheiro reported the first experience of the use of intracystic interferon alpha for patients with cystic craniopharyngiomas (Cavalheiro et al., 2005). Nine children were treated with repeated injections of 3 million units (MU) of IFNα on alternate days, to a total dose of 36 MU per course. Tumor volume was assessed prior to and immediately after completion of treatment. The treatment was repeated if there was no evidence of a significant decrease in the cyst size. Six patients received more than one course of IFNα (maximum three). In all patients, the end-of-treatment imaging study showed a significant reduction in the volume of the cyst, including a complete response in seven patients. The same author provided an update in 2010, with 60 cases treated at three different institutions (Cavalheiro et al., 2010). The number of cycles ranged from one to nine, with a median of five cycles. All patients were treated in the ambulatory setting. The pretreatment volume ranged from 3.3 to 134.5 ml and the post-treatment volume from 0.14 to 70.7 ml. With a follow-up of 44 months, 47 patients showed sustained control, defined as persistent cyst shrinkage of $> 50\%$. Thirteen patients had no or transient response and required surgery and radiotherapy. Eighteen patients developed side effects during treatment; the majority were headaches, palpebral edema, and/or fever. However, no side effect was significant enough to affect the course of administration. Interestingly, three patients previously treated with bleomycin showed sustained response to IFNα. The authors concluded that this technique allows sustained control of predominantly cystic craniopharyngiomas, offering an alternative to more aggressive surgical approaches. They emphasized the low morbidity of this treatment and, in particular, its hypothalamus-sparing potential

CONCLUSIONS AND FUTURE DIRECTIONS

Despite evidence of activity, the local treatment of cystic craniopharyngioma has not been adopted as a standard of care in many institutions. There are many reasons for this. Some physicians still advocate maximal resection. Others recommend limited surgical intervention including cyst aspiration or drainage to minimize cyst size followed by conformal radiation. Implementation of intracystic administration of radioisotopes or chemotherapeutic agents has been limited by the potential toxicity of these techniques, and in particular the risks of hypothalamic damage or visual impairment, as has been documented in several series (Caceres, 2005; Lafay-Cousin et al., 2007). The long-term efficacy of IFNα needs to be confirmed in larger collaborative studies. One of the main limitations of this technique is the natural history of craniopharyngioma. While some patients show sustained benefit from intracystic therapies, other may develop new cysts that require placement of a new Ommaya catheter (Figure 25.5). The impact of repeated intracystic treatment and multiple

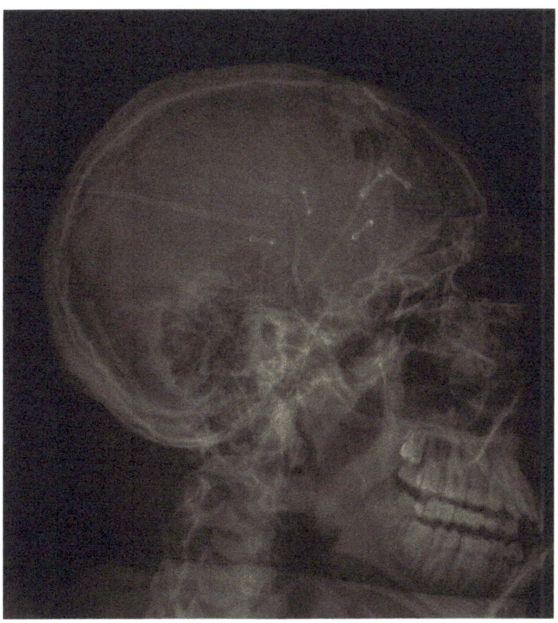

FIGURE 25.5 Skull X-ray of a patient who required multiple Ommaya insertions for intracystic therapy.

aspirations is still poorly documented. In a review of the St. Jude experience on 28 patients, Merchant et al. reported a negative association between placement of an Ommaya reservoir or repeated cyst aspirations and long-term cognitive function (Merchant et al., 2006). However, this radiation series may represent a selection of patients who failed one or several intracystic therapies, and the overriding concerns with regards to long-term cognitive outcome in this series were young age at the time of radiation and extensive surgery with two or more surgical procedures. Comparative results of the cognitive outcome of patients who were successfully treated with intracystic bleomycin or interferon are needed to clarify the impact of these interventions on cognition.

The future of intracystic therapies may come from identification of candidate genes and mutations and the development of targeted treatment. With the discovery of aberrant WNT/β-catenin pathway signaling in the pathogenesis of adamantinomatous craniopharyngioma (Campanini et al., 2010) and recurrent mutations in BRAF in papillary craniopharyngiomas (Brastianos et al., 2014), we can anticipate new treatment options for craniopharyngiomas in the near future. This may include the use of WNT or BRAF inhibitors, either systemically or injected locally in patients with predominantly cystic lesions.

References

Bartels, U., Laperriere, N., Bouffet, E., Drake, J., 2012. Intracystic therapies for cystic craniopharyngioma in childhood. Front. Endocrinol. 3, 39.

Brastianos, P.K., Taylor-Weiner, A., Manley, P.E., Jones, R.T., Dias-Santagata, D., Thorner, A.R., et al., 2014. Exome sequencing identifies BRAF mutations in papillary craniopharyngiomas. Nat. Genet. 46 (2), 161–165.

Broggi, G., Franzini, A., 1996. Bleomycin for cystic craniopharyngioma. J. Neurosurg. 84 (6), 1080–1081.

Caceres, A., 2005. Intracavitary therapeutic options in the management of cystic craniopharyngioma. Childs Nerv. Syst. 21 (8–9), 705–718.

Campanini, M.L., Colli, L.M., Paixao, B.M., Cabral, T.P., Amaral, F.C., Machado, H.R., et al., 2010. CTNNB1 gene mutations, pituitary transcription factors, and MicroRNA expression involvement in the pathogenesis of adamantinomatous craniopharyngiomas. Hormones & Cancer 1 (4), 187–196.

Cavalheiro, S., Sparapani, F.V., Franco, J.O., da Silva, M.C., Braga, F.M., 1996. Use of bleomycin in intratumoral chemotherapy for cystic craniopharyngioma. Case report. J. Neurosurg. 84 (1), 124–126.

Cavalheiro, S., Dastoli, P.A., Silva, N.S., Toledo, S., Lederman, H., da Silva, M.C., 2005. Use of interferon alpha in intratumoral chemotherapy for cystic craniopharyngioma. Child's nervous system: ChNS. J. Int. Soc. Pediatr. Neurosurg. 21 (8–9), 719–724.

Cavalheiro, S., Di Rocco, C., Valenzuela, S., Dastoli, P.A., Tamburrini, G., Massimi, L., et al., 2010. Craniopharyngiomas: intratumoral chemotherapy with interferon-alpha: a multicenter preliminary study with 60 cases. Neurosurg. Focus 28 (4), E12.

Chamberlain, M.C., 2002. A phase II trial of intra-cerebrospinal fluid alpha interferon in the treatment of neoplastic meningitis. Cancer 94 (10), 2675–2680.

Crooke, S.T., Bradner, W.T., 1976. Bleomycin, a review. J. Med. 7 (5), 333–428.

De Vile, C.J., Grant, D.B., Kendall, B.E., Neville, B.G., Stanhope, R., Watkins, K.E., et al., 1996. Management of childhood craniopharyngioma: Can the morbidity of radical surgery be predicted? J. Neurosurg. 85 (1), 73–81.

Fox, J.L., 1967. Intermittent drainage of intracranial cyst via the subcutaneous Ommaya reservoir. Technical note. J. Neurosurg. 27 (3), 272–273.

Frank, F., Fabrizi, A.P., Frank, G., Fioravanti, A., 1995. Stereotactic management of craniopharyngiomas. Stereotact. Funct. Neurosurg. 65 (1–4), 176–183.

Hader, W.J., Steinbok, P., Hukin, J., Fryer, C., 2000. Intratumoral therapy with bleomycin for cystic craniopharyngiomas in children. Pediatr. Neurosurg. 33 (4), 211–218.

Haisa, T., Ueki, K., Yoshida, S., 1994. Toxic effects of bleomycin on the hypothalamus following its administration into a cystic craniopharyngioma. Br. J. Neurosurg 8 (6), 747–750.

Hargrave, D.R., 2006. Does chemotherapy have a role in the management of craniopharyngioma? JPEM 19 (Suppl. 1), 407–412.

Honegger, J., Tatagiba, M., 2008. Craniopharyngioma surgery. Pituitary 11 (4), 361–373.

Hukin, J., Steinbok, P., Lafay-Cousin, L., Hendson, G., Strother, D., Mercier, C., et al., 2007. Intracystic bleomycin therapy for craniopharyngioma in children: The Canadian experience. Cancer 109 (10), 2124–2131.

Jakacki, R.I., Cohen, B.H., Jamison, C., Mathews, V.P., Arenson, E., Longee, D.C., et al., 2000. Phase II evaluation of interferon-alpha-2a for progressive or recurrent craniopharyngiomas. J. Neurosurg. 92 (2), 255–260.

Jiang, R., Liu, Z., Zhu, C., 2002. Preliminary exploration of the clinical effect of bleomycin on craniopharyngiomas. Stereotact. Funct. Neurosurg. 78 (2), 84–94.

Karavitaki, N., Wass, J.A., 2008. Craniopharyngiomas. Endocrinol. Metab. Clin. North Am. 37 (1), 173–193, ix–x.

Katz, E.L., 1975. Late results of radical excision of craniopharyngiomas in children. J. Neurosurg. 42 (1), 86–93.

Korinth, M.C., Weinzierl, M.R., Krings, T., Gilsbach, J.M., 2001. Occurrence and therapy of space-occupying cystic lesions after brain tumor surgery. Zentralbl. Neurochir. 62 (3), 87–92.

Lafay-Cousin, L., Bartels, U., Raybaud, C., Kulkarni, A.V., Guger, S., Huang, A., Lafay-Cousin, L., Bartels, U., Raybaud, C., Kulkarni, A.V., Guger, S., Huang, A., Bouffet, E., 2007. Neuroradiological findings of bleomycin leakage in cystic craniopharyngioma. Report of three cases. J. Neurosurg. 107 (Suppl. 4), 318–323.

Leksell, L., Backlund, E.O., Johansson, L., 1967. Treatment of craniopharyngiomas. Acta chirurgica Scandinavica. 133 (5), 345–350.

Liu, W., Fang, Y., Cai, B., Xu, J., You, C., Zhang, H., 2012. Intracystic bleomycin for cystic craniopharyngiomas in children (abridged republication of Cochrane systematic review). Neurosurgery 71 (5), 909–915.

Merchant, T.E., Kiehna, E.N., Kun, L.E., Mulhern, R.K., Li, C., Xiong, X., et al., 2006. Phase II trial of conformal radiation therapy for pediatric patients with craniopharyngioma and correlation of surgical factors and radiation dosimetry with change in cognitive function. J. Neurosurg. 104 (Suppl. 2), 94–102.

Merchant, T.E., Kun, L.E., Hua, C.H., Wu, S., Xiong, X., Sanford, R.A., et al., 2013. Disease control after reduced volume conformal and intensity modulated radiation therapy for childhood craniopharyngioma. Int. J. Radiat. Oncol. Biol. Phys. 85 (4), e187–e192.

Miles, J., 1977. Sump drainage: A palliative manoeuvre for the treatment of craniopharyngioma. J. Neurol. Neurosurg. Psychiat. 40 (2), 120–126.

Mitchell, W.G., Crawford, T.O., 1987. Intraventricular alpha 2b interferon for SSPE. Neurology 37 (12), 1884.

Mori, R., Joki, T., Nonaka, Y., Ikeuchi, S., Abe, T., 2013. Parallel insertion endoscopic technique for precise catheter placement in cystic craniopharyngiomas. J. Neurol. Surg. A. Cent. Eur. Neurosurg.

Mottolese, C., Stan, H., Hermier, M., Berlier, P., Convert, J., Frappaz, D., et al., 2001. Intracystic chemotherapy with bleomycin in the treatment of craniopharyngiomas. Childs Nerv. Syst. 17 (12), 724–730.

Nicolato, A., Foroni, R., Rosta, L., Gerosa, M., Bricolo, A., 2004. Multimodality stereotactic approach to the treatment of cystic craniopharyngiomas. Minimally invasive neurosurgery. MIN 47 (1), 32–40.

Ommaya, A.K., 1963. Subcutaneous reservoir and pump for sterile access to ventricular cerebrospinal fluid. Lancet 2 (7315), 983–984.

Park, D.H., Park, J.Y., Kim, J.H., Chung, Y.G., Lee, H.K., Lee, K.C., et al., 2002. Outcome of postoperative intratumoral bleomycin injection for cystic craniopharyngioma. J. Korean Med. Sci. 17 (2), 254–259.

Rickham, P.P., 1964. A Ventriculostomy Reservoir. Br. Med. J. 2 (5402), 173. Epub 1964/07/18.

Rushing, E.J., Giancaspero, F., Paulus, W., Burger, P.C., 2007. Craniopharyngioma. In: Cavenee, W.K. (Ed.), WHO Classification of Tumours of the Central Nervous System, fourth ed. IARC Press, Lyon, pp. 238–240.

Savas, A., Erdem, A., Tun, K., Kanpolat, Y., 2000. Fatal toxic effect of bleomycin on brain tissue after intracystic chemotherapy for a craniopharyngioma: case report. Neurosurgery 46 (1), 213–216; discussion 216–217.

Smith, R.E., Heilbrun, L.K., Bottomley, R.M., Gad-el-Mawla, N., Fletcher, W., 1986. Therapy of recurrent squamous cell carcinoma of the head and neck using combination vincristine, bleomycin, and methotrexate. A Southwest Oncology Group Study. Cancer 58 (11), 2382–2385.

Sobczyk, W., Kulczycki, J., Iwinska, B., Buksowicz, C., Pilkowska, E., 1987. [Intrathecal administration of interferon in the treatment of SSPE]. Neurol. Neurochir. Pol. 21 (6), 516–519.

Takahashi, H., Nakazawa, S., Shimura, T., 1985. Evaluation of postoperative intratumoral injection of bleomycin for craniopharyngioma in children. J. Neurosurg. 62 (1), 120–127.

Takahashi, H., Yamaguchi, F., Teramoto, A., 2005. Long-term outcome and reconsideration of intracystic chemotherapy with bleomycin for craniopharyngioma in children. Childs Nerv. Syst. 21 (8–9), 701–704.

Tomoda, A., Nomura, K., Shiraishi, S., Miike, T., Hamada, A., Hosoya, M., 2003. [Trial of intraventricular ribavirin and interferon-alpha combination therapy for subacute sclerosing panencephalitis (SSPE) in Japan]. No to hattatsu Brain Dev. 35 (4), 321–326.
Zanon, N., Cavalheiro, S., da Silva, M.C., 2008. Does the choice of surgical approach to insert an intratumoral catheter influence the results of intratumoral cystic treatment? Surg. Neurol. 70 (1), 66–69; discussion 69.

SECTION VI

MANAGEMENT OF RECURRENCE

CHAPTER

26

Management of the Recurrence of Craniopharyngiomas

Benjamin A. Rubin, Irene Kim, Jeffrey H. Wisoff

Division of Pediatric Neurosurgery, NYU Langone Medical Center, New York, NY, USA

"Almost all of our major intraoperative and postoperative problems, and all of our operative fatalities, have come with secondary and tertiary attempts to remove tumors that had again become symptomatic after a previous subtotal surgical procedure." **DD Matson and JF Crigler Jr, 1969**

INTRODUCTION

The management of recurrent craniopharyngioma is a challenging and controversial area of discussion in the field of neurosurgery. Owing to the relative rarity of craniopharyngiomas, consensus on optimal primary treatment has not been reached. Additionally, the patients who present with recurrent tumors are an even more select group, and again, treatment paradigms are not necessarily agreed upon. Overall and progression-free survival rates are similar for radical resection compared to limited resection followed by radiation therapy, for primary tumors (Hetelekidis et al., 1993; Merchant et al., 2002; Caldarelli et al., 2005; Di Rocco et al., 2006; Minniti et al., 2007; Elliott et al., 2010; Schoenfeld et al., 2012).

When recurrence does occur, it is of paramount importance that a multidisciplinary approach be taken when considering the optimal treatment strategy for the patient. A team of specialists including a neurosurgeon, endocrinologist, neuro-opthalmologist, oncologist, neuropsychologist, and radiation oncologist should all agree on a plan of treatment. Additionally, and perhaps, most importantly, the patients and their families should be assessed for their ability and willingness to tolerate whatever side effects or deficits may be suffered as a result of any given intervention. In this chapter we will discuss the patterns and rates of recurrence, the options for treatment of recurrent tumors, and the factors associated with various outcomes.

Craniopharyngiomas
http://dx.doi.org/10.1016/B978-0-12-416706-3.00026-X

RECURRENCE

The primary treatment strategy for craniopharyngioma remains controversial. The various options for curative treatment include radical resection, gross total resection (GTR), combined resection of solid tumor and intracystic therapy for mixed solid-cystic tumors, intracystic therapy for purely cystic tumors, and limited resection or subtotal resection (STR) with adjuvant radiation therapy (XRT) (Elliott et al., 2010). Most literature suggests that there are similar rates of disease control for primary tumors between patients undergoing GTR alone compared with STR with adjuvant XRT (Hetelekidis et al., 1993; Merchant et al., 2002; Caldarelli et al., 2005; Di Rocco et al., 2006; Minniti et al., 2007; Elliott et al., 2010; Schoenfeld et al., 2012). STR, cyst aspiration, or XRT alone are not optimal first-line strategies; they do not provide the same durability of disease control and recurrence occurs earlier and more frequently (Rajan et al., 1993; Wisoff, 1994; Bulow et al., 1998; Fahlbusch et al., 1999; Duff et al., 2000; Minamida et al., 2005; Gupta et al., 2006; Shi et al., 2006, 2008; Lin et al., 2008; Elliott et al., 2010; Yang et al., 2010). Median time to recurrence varies from 2–8 years depending on the initial modality of treatment (Liubinas et al., 2011). After primary treatment is completed, surveillance is performed with serial imaging. As MRI techniques and capabilities have advanced, screening sensitivity for recurrence has improved. Recurrence may be seen earlier than with previous imaging modalities (Zada et al., 2010; Liubinas et al., 2011).

While a large percentage of recurrences can be diagnosed by frequent surveillance imaging in asymptomatic patients, the majority of recurrences are symptomatic prior to imaging confirmation of recurrence. The most common presentation is visual deterioration, with both acuity and field deficits. Other symptoms of recurrence include progressive headaches, development of hydrocephalus, hormonal disturbances, and seizures (Karavitaki et al., 2005; Elliott et al., 2010; Liubinas et al., 2011).

The single factor most closely associated with recurrence appears to be the extent of resection at initial surgery (Liubinas et al., 2011). However several studies have shown lower recurrence rates when XRT is used post-operatively regardless of GTR or STR (Hoogenhout et al., 1984; Hetelekidis et al., 1993; Gupta et al., 2006). Other factors associated with increased recurrence rates appear to be larger tumors (> 5 cm), highly calcified tumors, and tumors that extend beyond the suprasellar space (Fahlbusch et al., 1999; Duff et al., 2000; Di Rocco et al., 2006; Shi et al., 2006; Liubinas et al., 2011). It is our anecdotal observation that tumors with large or calcified intrasellar components also tend to have higher recurrence rates, owing largely to the difficulty of access into this space from a transcranial approach and possible invasion of the dura of the sella turcica.

Molecular diagnostics will inevitably become an increasingly important adjunct when determining risk of recurrence. There is evidence that increased rates of expression within the tumor involving osteonectin, epithelial cell adhesion molecule (Ep-CAM), and pituitary transforming gene (PTTG-1) may increase the risk of recurrence (Tena-Suck et al., 2009; Ebrahimi et al., 2013). As the signaling pathways within these tumors become better understood, our ability to predict the future behavior of the tumor and guide therapy appropriately will also improve.

There are also increasing reports in the literature of ectopic recurrence of craniopharyngioma. While it is still considered a rare phenomenon, approximately 50 cases have been reported to date. Most were of the adamantinous histological subtype. These recurrences are thought to arise from contamination of tumor cells along the surgical tract during the primary transcranial resection, or by spreading through CSF pathways into distant locations of the subarachnoid space (Elliott et al., 2009; Kordes et al., 2011; Jakobs and Orakcioglu, 2012). In general, these ectopic lesions should be treated with curative intent, especially when found in isolation. Surgical resection can be curative with low morbidity given that these lesions, for the most part, maintain excellent arachnoidal planes. With GTR of these lesions and close surveillance, adjuvant XRT can be avoided. This may minimize late radiation-induced morbidity, especially in pediatric patients (Elliott et al., 2009).

TREATMENT

Once tumor recurrence has been identified, a decision to treat must be made. Not every patient is a candidate for treatment and, as discussed previously, patients and families must be aware of the potential for complications and development of new deficits. Options for treatment include reoperation for tumor resection, intracystic treatment with bleomycin or a beta-emitting radionuclide, fractionated radiotherapy, stereotactic radiosurgery, or some combination thereof.

Reoperation for tumor resection should be considered whenever possible, both for recurrences following GTR, and after STR and XRT. Pediatric patients in particular should almost always be considered for surgery, as should patients with predominantly solid tumor recurrence. Patients who may potentially not be candidates for reoperation include elderly patients who are relatively asymptomatic from their recurrence or patients with predominantly cystic tumor recurrence (Wisoff, 1994; Vinchon and Dhellemmes, 2008).

The possibility of reoperation is also dependent on the previous treatments for the tumor. In an initial operation for tumor resection, there is typically a natural cleavage plane between the tumor and the hypothalamus as the result of a dense gliotic reaction. This plane may be destroyed by radical resection, which can make reoperation after radical surgery extremely challenging or even impossible, and increases the potential for complications (Wisoff, 1994; Jang et al., 2009). Similarly, prior irradiation can cause significant fibrosis, which can also make surgery difficult (Vinchon and Dhellemmes, 2008; Elliott et al., 2010).

Once a decision is made to proceed with reoperation, the best surgical approach must be determined. Some favor reopening the previous craniotomy, which can be challenging due to the dissection through adhesions and scar tissue and the difficulty in determining the plane between tumor and normal neurohypophyseal structures (Stagno and Cappabianca, 2013). Others suggest that pterional craniotomy with or without removal of the supraorbital rim and zygomatic process of the frontal bone, regardless of the previous approach, may be associated with a lower incidence of secondary recurrence. This approach provides access to tumors varying from small suprasellar recurrences to very large tumors that extend from the foramen of Munro to the pontomedullary junction. In patients who have had previous resection through a different approach, this approach with a wide, clean dissection of the Sylvian fissure allows identification of normal landmarks and vasculature while avoiding adhesions and scar tissue (Yasargil et al., 1990; Wisoff, 1994). The transsphenoidal approach has typically been reserved for tumor recurrence that was limited to the sella tursica (Wisoff, 1994). However, with the advent and improvement of extended endoscopic approaches, more surgeons are favoring this approach when considering both primary resection and reoperation strategies (Cavallo et al., 2009).

Patients with predominantly cystic tumor recurrence who are not candidates for resection or who choose not to pursue aggressive surgery may be treated with intracystic or intracavitary therapies, including bleomycin or beta-emitting radionuclides. Stereotactic cyst aspiration or Ommaya reservoir placement for serial cyst aspirations can also be performed, but this is usually reserved for palliation (Wisoff, 1994).

Bleomycin is an antineoplastic agent that is commonly used in the treatment of squamous cell carcinoma, lymphoma, and testicular cancer, but has also been used in the treatment of gliomas and cystic craniopharyngiomas (Cho et al., 2012). In craniopharyngiomas, it is typically injected directly into the cyst itself via an Ommaya reservoir, and has been demonstrated to be effective in inducing cyst shrinkage (Takahashi et al., 2005; Steinbok and Hukin, 2010; Cho et al., 2012). However, its use has been debated as it has been associated with significant side effects and toxicities, most of which are thought to be secondary to leakage or diffusion. As many as 70% of patients experience mild symptoms such as low-grade fever, headache, nausea/vomiting, and fatigue, which usually occur shortly after treatment and are typically self-limiting. Delayed complications, which are less common but potentially more serious, include peritumoral edema, seizure, hypothalamic dysfunction, and vasculopathy (Vinchon and Dhellemmes, 2008; Steinbok and Hukin, 2010; Cho et al., 2012).

Beta-emitting radionuclides can also be used as intracystic treatment for cystic tumor recurrence. Sometimes referred to as intracystic or intracavitary irradiation, the most commonly used radionuclides are phosphorus-32 (^{32}P) and yttrium-90 (^{90}Y), although radioisotopes of rhenium, gold, and bismuth have also been used (Lunsford et al., 1994; Steinbok and Hukin, 2010). The volume of radionuclide to be delivered is calculated using a formula based on the volume of the cyst(s) to be treated, and this is then injected into the cyst under stereotactic guidance. The procedure is generally well tolerated by patients. Cyst shrinkage occurs gradually over a period of 3–18 months (Lunsford et al., 1994).

Another option available for the treatment of tumor recurrence is XRT, which can be used as adjunctive therapy after STR or at the time of tumor progression or recurrence (Vinchon and Dhellemmes, 2008; Jang et al., 2009). Significant consideration must be given to the potential long-term consequences of irradiation, particularly in children, given their long life expectancies. These include visual deterioration, hypothalamic–pituitary axis dysfunction, cognitive deficits, secondary radiation-induced CNS tumors, and moyamoya syndrome or other vasculopathies (Wisoff, 1994; Elliott et al., 2010).

More recently, the use of stereotactic radiosurgery (SRS) has become much more popular because it allows the delivery of a high dose of radiation to a small, stereotactically targeted field, usually in a single fraction. The steep radiation dose fall-off beyond the target limits the amount of radiation received by the surrounding normal tissues, thereby avoiding many of the complications of conventional external beam radiation therapy (Gopalan et al., 2008). Gamma knife (GK) radiosurgery is generally used in the treatment of predominantly solid tumors no more than 3 cm in diameter that are at least a few millimeters away from the optic apparatus (Kobayashi et al., 1994; Suh and Gupta, 2006). It is generally tolerated extremely well by patients; the most common morbidities are related to visual deterioration or worsening endocrine dysfunction (Niranjan et al., 2010). While the vast majority of the published literature on SRS in craniopharyngiomas is on GK, several studies also indicate that these tumors are also responsive to Cyber knife SRS (Suh and Gupta, 2006; Lee et al., 2008).

The use of these various treatment modalities is not mutually exclusive, especially given that recurrence can occur more than once. In fact, multimodal treatment is often necessary in the treatment of tumor recurrence. This again highlights the importance of the multidisciplinary approach to treatment of tumor recurrence.

OUTCOMES

Reported outcomes after treatment for tumor recurrence vary widely. Mortality rates for reoperation range from 2.2 to 42% in the literature, largely due to the wide variability in degree of surgical aggressiveness. The challenges of reoperation have been discussed previously, and GTR rates for second operations vary from 21% to 71% for transcranial approaches, and from 6% to 62% for transsphenoidal approaches. Specifically, larger tumor size and prior radiation therapy have both been identified as statistically significant risk factors for STR rather than GTR at reoperation. Regardless of the actual numbers, most studies indicate that mortality rates appear to be slightly higher and the likelihood of achieving GTR slightly lower for reoperations compared to initial operations (Elliott et al., 2010; Liubinas et al., 2011).

While multiple studies have indicated that reoperation is associated with higher morbidity rates, particularly with respect to vision, endocrine dysfunction, and overall functional outcome, some have reported that reoperations for tumor recurrence are actually better tolerated by patients than initial operations in terms of peri-operative morbidity, because endocrine disturbances have already been identified and stabilized with medical therapy (Yasargil et al., 1990; Wisoff, 1994; Fahlbusch et al., 1999; Caldarelli et al., 2005; Di Rocco et al., 2006; Vinchon and Dhellemme, 2008; Jang et al., 2009; Elliott et al., 2010; Liubinas et al., 2011). In the hands of an experienced surgeon, it has been demonstrated that reoperation for tumor recurrence is not associated with higher mortality, morbidity, or worsened overall functional outcome (Elliott et al., 2010). Second recurrences occur in 14–33% of patients after reoperation for tumor recurrence (Elliott et al., 2010; Liubinas et al., 2011).

CONCLUSION

Tumor recurrence is the most common complication after treatment of craniopharyngiomas. To date, there is no consensus on the paradigm for treatment of tumor recurrence or progression of residual tumor. Available options include reoperation for tumor resection, radiation therapy, stereotactic radiosurgery, intracystic therapy with bleomycin or a beta-emitting radionuclide, or some combination thereof. Because of the potentially significant and long-term complications associated with any and all of these treatment modalities, particularly visual deterioration and worsening endocrine dysfunction, a multidisciplinary approach is essential in the treatment of these patients. It is our opinion that reoperation should be considered whenever feasible. Although GTR rates with reoperation are slightly lower than at the time of initial operation, it can be performed safely without significantly higher risk of mortality or morbidity in the hands of the experienced surgeon.

References

Bulow, B., Attewell, R., Hagmar, L., Malmstrom, P., Nordstrom, C.H., Erfurth, E.M., 1998. Postoperative prognosis in craniopharyngioma with respect to cardiovascular mortality, survival, and tumor recurrence. J. Clin. Endocrinol. Metab. 83, 3897–3904.

Caldarelli, M., Massimi, L., Tamburrini, G., Cappa, M., Di Rocco, C., 2005. Long-term results of the surgical treatment of craniopharyngioma: the experience at the Policlinico Gemelli, Catholic University, Rome. Childs. Nerv. Syst. 21, 747–757.

Cavallo, L.M., Prevedello, D.M., Solari, D., Gardner, P.A., Esposito, F., Snyderman, C.H., Carrau, R.L., Kassam, A.B., Cappabianca, P., 2009. Extended endoscopic endonasal transsphenoidal approach for residual or recurrent craniopharyngiomas. J. Neurosurg. 111, 578–589.

Cho, W.S., Kim, S.K., Wang, K.C., Phi, J.H., Cho, B.K., 2012. Vasculopathy after intracystic bleomycin administration for a recurrent cystic craniopharyngioma: case report. J. Neurosurg. Pediatr. 9, 394–399.

Di Rocco, C., Caldarelli, M., Tamburrini, G., Massimi, L., 2006. Surgical management of craniopharyngiomas—experience with a pediatric series. J. Pediatr. Endocrinol. Metab. 19 (Suppl. 1), 355–366.

Duff, J., Meyer, F.B., Ilstrup, D.M., Laws Jr., E.R., Schleck, C.D., Scheithauer, B.W., 2000. Long-term outcomes for surgically resected craniopharyngiomas. Neurosurgery 46, 291–302; discussion 302–305.

Ebrahimi, A., Honegger, J., Schluesener, H., Schittenhelm, J., 2013. Osteonectin Expression in Surrounding Stroma of Craniopharyngiomas: Association With Recurrence Rate and Brain Infiltration. Int. J. Surg. Pathol 21, 591–598.

Elliott, R.E., Moshel, Y.A., Wisoff, J.H., 2009. Surgical treatment of ectopic recurrence of craniopharyngioma. Report of 4 cases. J. Neurosurg. Pediatr. 4, 105–112.

Elliott, R.E., Hsieh, K., Hochm, T., Belitskaya-Levy, I., Wisoff, J., Wisoff, J.H., 2010. Efficacy and safety of radical resection of primary and recurrent craniopharyngiomas in 86 children. J. Neurosurg. Pediatr. 5, 30–48.

Fahlbusch, R., Honegger, J., Paulus, W., Huk, W., Buchfelder, M., 1999. Surgical treatment of craniopharyngiomas: experience with 168 patients. J. Neurosurg. 90, 237–250.

Gopalan, R., Dassoulas, K., Rainey, J., Sherman, J.H., Sheehan, J.P., 2008. Evaluation of the role of Gamma Knife surgery in the treatment of craniopharyngiomas. Neurosurg. Focus 24, E5.

Gupta, D.K., Ojha, B.K., Sarkar, C., Mahapatra, A.K., Mehta, V.S., 2006. Recurrence in craniopharyngiomas: analysis of clinical and histological features. J. Clin. Neurosci. 13, 438–442.

Hetelekidis, S., Barnes, P.D., Tao, M.L., Fischer, E.G., Schneider, L., Scott, R.M., Tarbell, N.J., 1993. 20-year experience in childhood craniopharyngioma. Int. J. Radiat. Oncol. Biol. Phys. 27, 189–195.

Hoogenhout, J., Otten, B.J., Kazem, I., Stoelinga, G.B., Walder, A.H., 1984. Surgery and radiation therapy in the management of craniopharyngiomas. Int. J. Radiat. Oncol. Biol. Phys. 10, 2293–2297.

Jakobs, M., Orakcioglu, B., 2012. Ectopic recurrent craniopharyngioma of the frontal bone. J. Neurosurg. 117, 490–497.

Jang, W.Y., Lee, K.S., Son, B.C., Jeun, S.S., Hong, Y.K., Lee, S.W., Yang, S.H., 2009. Repeat operations in pediatric patients with recurrent craniopharyngiomas. Pediatr. Neurosurg. 45, 451–455.

Karavitaki, N., Brufani, C., Warner, J.T., Adams, C.B., Richards, P., Ansorge, O., Shine, B., Turner, H.E., Wass, J.A., 2005. Craniopharyngiomas in children and adults: systematic analysis of 121 cases with long-term follow-up. Clin. Endocrinol. (Oxf) 62, 397–409.

Kobayashi, T., Tanaka, T., Kida, Y., 1994. Stereotactic gamma radiosurgery of craniopharyngiomas. Pediatr. Neurosurg. 21 (Suppl. 1), 69–74.

Kordes, U., Flitsch, J., Hagel, C., Goebell, E., Schwarz, R., Herberhold, T., Von Bueren, A.O., Rutkowski, S., Muller, H.L., 2011. Ectopic craniopharyngioma. Klin. Padiatr. 223, 176–177.

Lee, M., Kalani, M.Y., Cheshier, S., Gibbs, I.C., Adler, J.R., Chang, S.D., 2008. Radiation therapy and CyberKnife radiosurgery in the management of craniopharyngiomas. Neurosurg. Focus 24, E4.

Lin, L.L., El Naqa, I., Leonard, J.R., Park, T.S., Hollander, A.S., Michalski, J.M., Mansur, D.B., 2008. Long-term outcome in children treated for craniopharyngioma with and without radiotherapy. J. Neurosurg. Pediatr. 1, 126–130.

Liubinas, S.V., Munshey, A.S., Kaye, A.H., 2011. Management of recurrent craniopharyngioma. J. Clin. Neurosci. 18, 451–457.

Lunsford, L.D., Pollock, B.E., Kondziolka, D.S., Levine, G., Flickinger, J.C., 1994. Stereotactic options in the management of craniopharyngioma. Pediatr. Neurosurg. 21 (Suppl. 1), 90–97.

Matson, D.D., Crigler Jr, J.F., 1969. Management of craniopharyngioma in childhood. J. Neurosurg. 30, 377–399.

Merchant, T.E., Kiehna, E.N., Sanford, R.A., Mulhern, R.K., Thompson, S.J., Wilson, M.W., Lustig, R.H., Kun, L.E., 2002. Craniopharyngioma: the St. Jude Children's Research Hospital experience 1984–2001. Int. J. Radiat. Oncol. Biol. Phys. 53, 533–542.

Minamida, Y., Mikami, T., Hashi, K., Houkin, K., 2005. Surgical management of the recurrence and regrowth of craniopharyngiomas. J. Neurosurg. 103, 224–232.

Minniti, G., Saran, F., Traish, D., Soomal, R., Sardell, S., Gonsalves, A., Ashley, S., Warrington, J., Burke, K., Mosleh-Shirazi, A., Brada, M., 2007. Fractionated stereotactic conformal radiotherapy following conservative surgery in the control of craniopharyngiomas. Radiother. Oncol. 82, 90–95.

Niranjan, A., Kano, H., Mathieu, D., Kondziolka, D., Flickinger, J.C., Lunsford, L.D., 2010. Radiosurgery for craniopharyngioma. Int. J. Radiat. Oncol. Biol. Phys. 78, 64–71.

Rajan, B., Ashley, S., Gorman, C., Jose, C.C., Horwich, A., Bloom, H.J., Marsh, H., Brada, M., 1993. Craniopharyngioma—a long-term results following limited surgery and radiotherapy. Radiother. Oncol. 26, 1–10.

Schoenfeld, A., Pekmezci, M., Barnes, M.J., Tihan, T., Gupta, N., Lamborn, K.R., Banerjee, A., Mueller, S., Chang, S., Berger, M.S., Haas-Kogan, D., 2012. The superiority of conservative resection and adjuvant radiation for craniopharyngiomas. J. Neurooncol. 108, 133–139.

Shi, X.E., Wu, B., Zhou, Z.Q., Fan, T., Zhang, Y.L., 2006. Microsurgical treatment of craniopharyngiomas: report of 284 patients. Chin. Med. J. (Engl) 119, 1653–1663.

Shi, X.E., Wu, B., Fan, T., Zhou, Z.Q., Zhang, Y.L., 2008. Craniopharyngioma: surgical experience of 309 cases in China. Clin. Neurol. Neurosurg. 110, 151–159.

Stagno, V., Cappabianca, P., 2013. Which side tips the scale for recurrent craniopharyngiomas? World. Neurosurg. 79, 647–648.

Steinbok, P., Hukin, J., 2010. Intracystic treatments for craniopharyngioma. Neurosurg. Focus 28, E13.

Suh, J.H., Gupta, N., 2006. Role of radiation therapy and radiosurgery in the management of craniopharyngiomas. Neurosurg. Clin. N. Am. 17, 143–148, vi-vii.

Takahashi, H., Yamaguchi, F., Teramoto, A., 2005. Long-term outcome and reconsideration of intracystic chemotherapy with bleomycin for craniopharyngioma in children. Childs. Nerv. Syst. 21, 701–704.

Tena-Suck, M.L., Ortiz-Plata, A., Galan, F., Sanchez, A., 2009. Expression of epithelial cell adhesion molecule and pituitary tumor transforming gene in adamantinomatous craniopharyngioma and its correlation with recurrence of the tumor. Ann. Diagn. Pathol. 13, 82–88.

Vinchon, M., Dhellemmes, P., 2008. Craniopharyngiomas in children: recurrence, reoperation and outcome. Childs. Nerv. Syst. 24, 211–217.

Wisoff, J.H., 1994. Surgical management of recurrent craniopharyngiomas. Pediatr. Neurosurg. 21 (Suppl. 1), 108–113.

Yang, I., Sughrue, M.E., Rutkowski, M.J., Kaur, R., Ivan, M.E., Aranda, D., Barani, I.J., Parsa, A.T., 2010. Craniopharyngioma: a comparison of tumor control with various treatment strategies. Neurosurg. Focus 28, E5.

Yasargil, M.G., Curcic, M., Kis, M., Siegenthaler, G., Teddy, P.J., Roth, P., 1990. Total removal of craniopharyngiomas. Approaches and long-term results in 144 patients. J. Neurosurg. 73, 3–11.

Zada, G., Lin, N., Ojerholm, E., Ramkissoon, S., Laws, E.R., 2010. Craniopharyngioma and other cystic epithelial lesions of the sellar region: a review of clinical, imaging, and histopathological relationships. Neurosurg. Focus 28, E4.

SECTION VII

SPECIAL CONSIDERATIONS

CHAPTER

27

Craniopharyngioma – Pediatric Management

Hermann L. Müller

Department of Pediatrics, Klinikum Oldenburg, Oldenburg, Germany

"Craniopharyngioma is a benign congenital tumor. What a depressing admission it is for a surgeon, therefore, to report that every single child with this condition treated in our clinic prior to 1950 is now dead." ***DD Matson, 1962***

INTRODUCTION

Craniopharyngiomas are rare embryonic malformations of the sellar and parasellar area with low histological grade (WHO I°). Despite high survival rates (87–95% in recent series), quality of life is frequently impaired in long-term survivors due to sequelae caused by the anatomical proximity of the tumor to the optic nerve and hypothalamic–pituitary axes (Karavitaki et al., 2006; Wisoff, 2008; Muller, 2008, 2010a, 2010b, 2014). Any clinically significant improvement in the prognosis of childhood craniopharyngioma patients will require the development of risk-adapted neurosurgical and radio-oncological treatment strategies in a multidisciplinary setting that provides medical as well as psychosocial support for these patients (Muller, 2004b, 2011b, 2013b). Due to the rareness of the disease, high survival rates, and adverse quality-of-life effects, recent multicenter cooperation has already led to beneficial results (Wisoff, 2008; Muller, 2010a, 2013a).

EPIDEMIOLOGY AND PATHOLOGY

Craniopharyngioma is a non-glial intracranial tumor derived from a malformation of embryonal tissue (Garre and Cama, 2007). There are controversial hypotheses on its embryonal origin: originating from ectodermal remnants of Rathke's pouch versus originating from residual embryonal epithelium of the anterior pituitary gland and of the anterior infundibulum (Garre and Cama, 2007).

Craniopharyngiomas
http://dx.doi.org/10.1016/B978-0-12-416706-3.00027-1

The incidence of craniopharyngioma is 0.5–2 cases per million persons per year, with 30–50% of all cases presenting during childhood and adolescence (Bunin et al., 1998; Nielsen et al., 2011). Craniopharyngioma represents 1.2–4% of all childhood intracranial tumors. In childhood and adolescence, its histological type is usually adamantinomatous with cyst formation (Muller-Scholden et al., 2000; Rushing et al., 2007; Larkin and Ansorge, 2013). Peak incidence of adult-onset craniopharyngioma is between the ages of 50 and 75 years, usually presenting with a squamous-papillary histological type. More than 70% of the predominantly childhood adamantinomatous type of craniopharyngioma bear a mutation of the β-catenin gene, which is not detectable in the adult papillary type of craniopharyngioma (Holsken et al., 2010). Recently, a new mouse model of adamantinomatous childhood craniopharyngioma due to an activation of Wnt signaling has been published (Gaston-Massuet et al., 2011). Further investigation into treatment responsiveness using this animal model could yield important insights and new approaches to the treatment of patients at risk for progression of residual tumor.

The German Pediatric Cancer Registry systematically documents cases of childhood craniopharyngioma (Muller et al., 2003c). Their data, from 1980 to 2007, obtained for 496 childhood craniopharyngioma patients diagnosed aged ≤ 18 years, reveals that most patients (451; 91%) were younger than 15 years of age at the time of diagnosis, with a 1:1 gender ratio and a median age at diagnosis of 8.8 years. The 1980 to 2007 (contemporary) survival rate is 97% after 3 years from diagnosis, 96% after 5 years, and 93% after 10 years. Patients who developed the disease in the 1980s had a lower survival rate than those diagnosed in the 1990s (survival at 5 years, 91% vs. 98%) (Muller et al., 2003c; Sherlock et al., 2010).

CLINICAL MANIFESTATIONS AT THE TIME OF DIAGNOSIS

The diagnosis of childhood craniopharyngioma is often made late – sometimes years after the initial appearance of symptoms (Muller et al., 2003c) – with clinical picture at time of diagnosis often dominated by non-specific manifestations of intracranial pressure (e.g., headache and nausea). Further primary manifestations are visual impairment (62–84%) and endocrine deficits (52–87%) (Figure 27.1). Endocrine deficits are frequently caused by disturbances to the hypothalamic–pituitary axes and they affect growth hormone secretion (75%), gonadotropins (40%), adrenocorticotropic hormone (ACTH) (25%), and thyroid-stimulating hormone (TSH) (25%). At the time of diagnosis, 40–87% of patients present with at least one hormonal deficit (Hoffman et al., 1992; Caldarelli et al., 2005; Muller, 2008), and other endocrine symptoms such as neurohormonal diabetes insipidus present pre-operatively in 17–27% of patients (Hoffman et al., 1992; Muller, 2008; Elliott and Wisoff, 2010). An analysis of anthropometric data obtained from routine checkups before the diagnosis of childhood craniopharyngioma in 90 children (Muller et al., 2004a) revealed that a pathologically reduced growth rate – an early manifestation of the disease – presents in patients as young as 12 months. Significant weight gain, however, which is predictive of hypothalamic obesity, tends to occur as a later manifestation, shortly before diagnosis. Recent literature has documented that the clinical combination of headache, visual impairment, decreased growth rate, and polydipsia/polyuria should arouse suspicion of childhood craniopharyngioma in the differential diagnosis (Muller, 2010a).

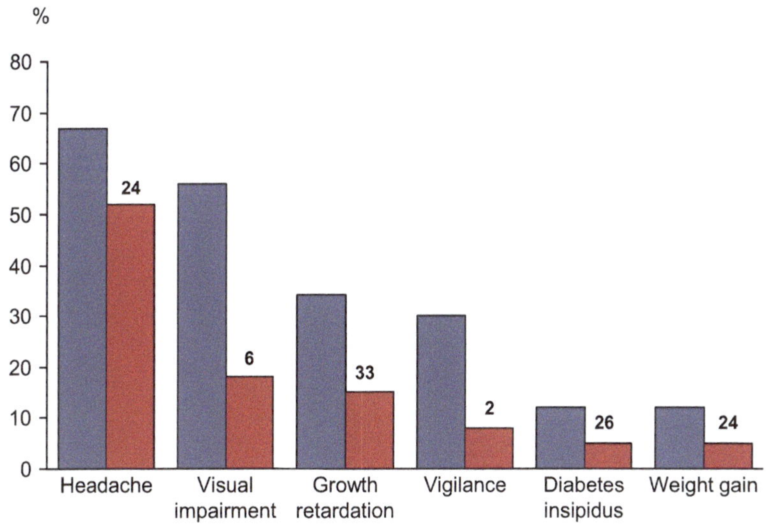

FIGURE 27.1 Manifestations before diagnosis of craniopharyngioma in children and adolescents. Frequency of occurrence of each manifestation before diagnosis (blue) and frequency of occurrence as the initial manifestation (red). The median time (months) from the appearance of each initial manifestation until diagnosis is indicated above each red column. In the overall group, the median time from the initial manifestation of disease until diagnosis was 12 months, with a range of 0.01 to 96 months. *Modified from (Muller et al., 2003c), with the kind permission of Springer.*

IMAGING STUDIES

Both computerized tomography and magnetic resonance imaging reveal that childhood craniopharyngioma is typically a cystic tumor of the intra- and/or parasellar region. The most common localization is suprasellar, with an intrasellar portion; only 20% are exclusively suprasellar and even less (5%) exclusively intrasellar (Warmuth-Metz et al., 2004; Muller, 2012b). Computerized tomography is the only way to definitively detect or exclude calcifications in craniopharyngioma tissue, which is found in approximately 90% of these tumors. The signal intensity of craniopharyngioma in magnetic resonance imaging is highly variable because it depends on the protein concentration of the cystic fluid. Solid tumor portions and cyst membranes appear isointense in T1-weighted magnetic resonance imaging, often with a mildly heterogeneous structure (Figure 27.2). The combination of solid, cystic, and calcified tumor components is an important radiological clue to the diagnosis. The differential diagnosis in imaging of sellar masses includes hypothalamic glioma and optical tract glioma, Langerhans cell histiocytosis (LCH), Rathke cleft cyst, xanthogranuloma, germinoma, epidermoid tumor, thrombosis of arachnoidal cysts, colloidal cyst of the third ventricle, pituitary adenoma, aneurysm, and rare inflammatory variations (Warmuth-Metz et al., 2004; Muller et al., 2012).

Magnetic resonance imaging before and after gadolinium application is the standard imaging for detection of childhood craniopharyngioma, further imaged by native computerized tomography to detect calcifications (Warmuth-Metz et al., 2004). After pre-operative

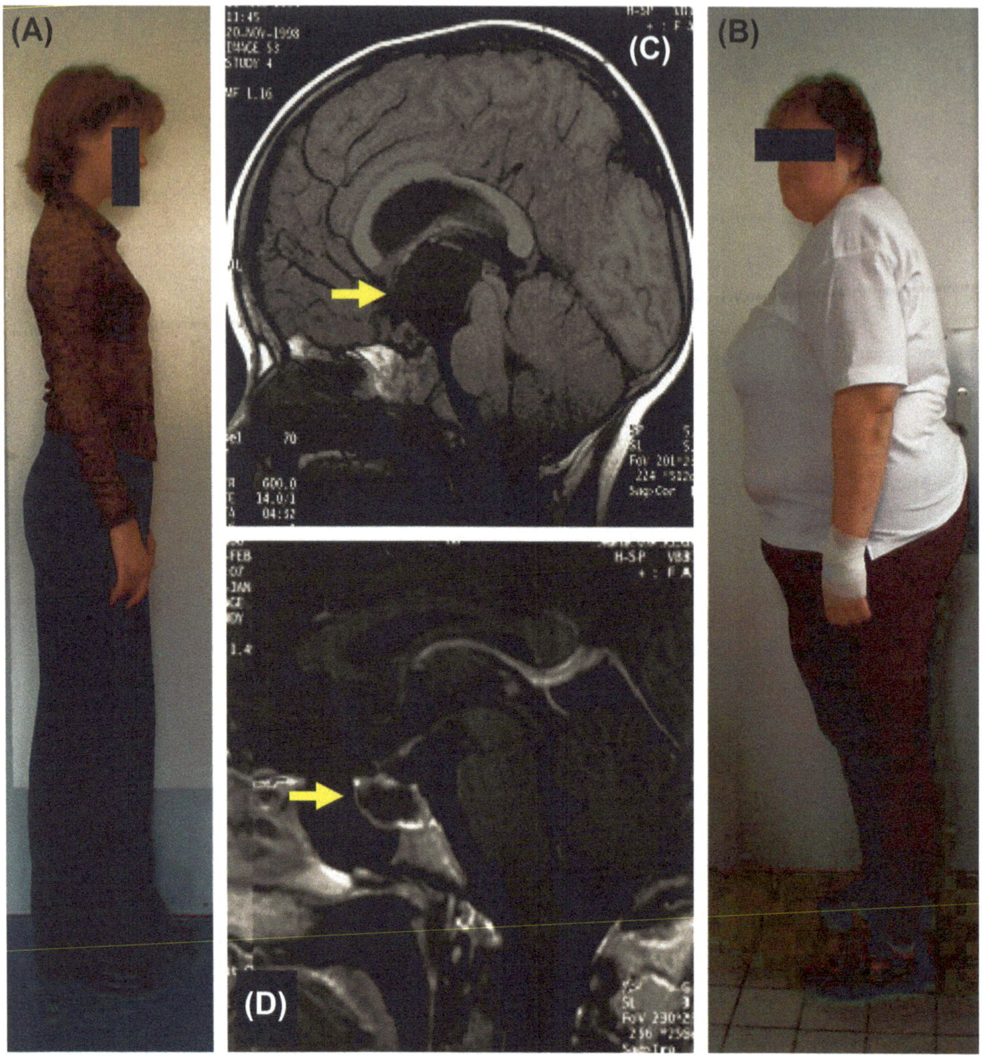

FIGURE 27.2 Degree of obesity in relation to the localization of childhood craniopharyngioma. In both patients craniopharyngioma (as indicated by arrow on magnetic resonance imaging before surgery) could be completely resected. Both patients had complete hypopituitarism after surgery requiring endocrine substitution of all hypothalamic–pituitary axes. The patient depicted in **B** developed severe obesity due to hypothalamic lesions of suprasellar parts of craniopharyngioma (**C**). The patient depicted in **A** presented with a small tumor confined to the sellar region (**D**). After complete resection she kept normal weight without any eating disorders. *Modified from (Muller et al., 2003c), with the kind permission of Springer.*

detection of calcifications, and complete resection confirmed by post-operative magnetic resonance imaging, a post-surgical native computerized tomography of the sellar/parasellar area (without contrast medium application) is recommended for definitive confirmation of complete resection (Warmuth-Metz et al., 2004).

TREATMENT STRATEGIES

Neurosurgery – Strategies and Effects

For favorably localized childhood craniopharyngioma (i.e., without involvement of hypothalamic or optical structures), the treatment of choice is an attempt at complete resection with preservation of visual and hypothalamic function (Choux and Lena, 1979; Fahlbusch et al., 1999; Flitsch et al., 2011). For unfavorably localized tumors, which are too close to or too entangled with the optic nerve and/or the hypothalamus, controversy exists over whether complete resection should still be attempted, or whether a planned, limited resection (biopsy, partial/subtotal resection) should be performed (Muller, 2010a, 2011a; Buchfelder et al., 2013). Many authors take a critical view of planned radical resection in these cases because of the risk of surgically induced deficits (mainly hypothalamic), and the high rate of recurrence in infants and small children despite apparently complete resection (Muller, 2006, 2006b). Recurrences at ectopic localizations are reported (Kordes et al., 2011). Whereas following incomplete resection the residual tumor shows progression in 71 to 90% of patients, the rate of progression after incomplete resection followed by radiotherapy is 21% (Becker et al., 1999). Elowe-Gruau and coworkers recently published the results of a single institution study at Necker, Paris, France, showing that a hypothalamus-sparing surgical strategy decreased the rate of severe long-term obesity in survivors without increasing their risk of local relapses when compared with a historical cohort treated before 2002 at the same experienced institution with a radical surgical approach (Elowe-Gruau et al., 2013).

However, the published literature to date (Hetelekidis et al., 1993; Rajan et al., 1993; Merchant et al., 2002; Karavitaki et al., 2005; Muller, 2006; Puget et al., 2006; Vinchon et al., 2009; Elliott et al., 2011; Elowe-Gruau et al., 2013) has not settled the controversy over the best treatment strategy for childhood craniopharyngioma (intended primary gross total resection versus biopsy/partial resection followed by irradiation). The therapeutic consequences of surgery and irradiation also remain a matter of debate. Above all, the effects of the chosen treatment sequence (immediate irradiation versus progression-contingent irradiation of residual tumor) on quality of life are unclear from the retrospective data published to date. A retrospective analysis cited primary therapy FSIQ (full scale IQ) losses of 9.8 points after a single complete resection compared to a loss of 1.25 points after limited resection followed by radiation therapy (Merchant et al., 2002). For a second surgical intervention carried out following a relapse, the loss was 13.1 points, statistically suggesting that radical and/or repeated surgeries seem to generate negative influences on neurocognitive function compared to limited surgical intervention plus immediate radiation treatment. However, only very limited retrospective data exist.

The German multicenter, prospective, surveillance study of children and adolescents with craniopharyngioma, KRANIOPHARYNGEOM 2000, was designed to address these issues. Newly diagnosed patients (117; 2001–2006) from Germany, Austria, and Switzerland were entered into the prospective evaluation. An analysis of 3-year, event-free survival rates (EFS) revealed frequent early events (i.e., tumor progression after incomplete resection and tumor relapse after complete resection during the 3 years following primary surgery) (Figure 27.3). In a multivariate analysis of risk factors for the observed low EFS rates, the

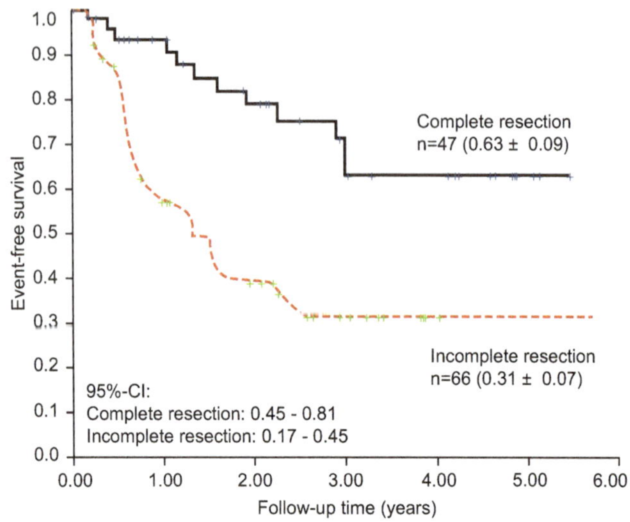

FIGURE 27.3 Kaplan-Meier analyses of event-free survival rates (EFS) depending on the extent of resection among the 117 craniopharyngioma patients recruited in the trial KRANIOPHARYNGEOM 2000. *Modified from (Muller et al., 2006b) with the kind permission of Karger.*

authors found that the risk of relapse after complete resection was 80% lower than that for incomplete resection. The risk for progression was 88% lower in irradiated patients than in patients without or before irradiation (Muller et al., 2010).

Any discussion of treatment and follow-up strategies must take into account the sequelae and quality of life experienced by childhood craniopharyngioma patients after treatment. Follow-up studies in children after complete resection of craniopharyngioma revealed that quality of life depends on the experience of the operating neurosurgeon (Sanford, 1994; Muller et al., 2011b, 2012).

Irradiation

The site and rate of progression of childhood craniopharyngioma, as well as the patient's age, are important considerations when deciding whether reoperation and/or radiotherapy should be performed. Childhood craniopharyngiomas are usually sharply bordered in the imaging. In contrast to primary brain tumors, they tend towards less infiltrative growth, permitting a small safety margin of 5 mm maximum (Kortmann, 2011; Aggarwal et al., 2013). These biological characteristics usually allow the option of using high-precision, three-dimensional conformation technology. A conventional, fractionated irradiation target (total) volume dose of 54 Gy has been established worldwide (Becker et al., 1999; Habrand et al., 2006; Merchant et al., 2006; Minniti et al., 2009; Kortmann, 2011).

Proton Beam Therapy

Fitzek and colleagues published the first series of 15 craniopharyngioma patients treated with combined proton-photon irradiation for residual or recurrent disease (Fitzek et al., 2006). Actuarial 5- and 10-year local control rates were 93% and 85%, respectively, with

10-year survival expectancy in 72% of patients. No treatment-related neurocognitive deficits were reported; functional status, academic skills, and professional abilities were unaltered after proton beam therapy. Luu and colleagues published a preliminary report on 16 patients treated with proton beam therapy (Luu et al., 2006). Local tumor control was achieved in 14 of 16 (87.5%) patients. During follow-up (12–121 months), late sequelae included newly diagnosed panhypopituitarism, a cerebrovascular accident, and an out-of-proton-field posterior fossa meningioma (59 months following proton beam therapy administered to patient who previously received photon radiotherapy). One study of proton beam therapy in craniopharyngioma assessed cyst growth during the treatment course: 24% of patients demonstrated cyst enlargement and 5% cyst reduction requiring modification of the treatment plan, while one patient required cyst drainage during treatment (Winkfield et al., 2009).

Clinical outcome data are still very limited for assessing the value of proton beam therapy compared to modern photon therapy, as the technique is available in only a few centers. However, proton beam therapy has the potential advantages of better conformation of dose to the target volume, sparing of critical structures, reduced integral dose, and lower dose of secondary neutrons, which should reduce the risk of secondary malignancies (Boehling et al., 2012; Beltran et al., 2012). Data should become available in due course with sufficient follow-up time and as more centers are able to deliver this promising therapy.

Radiosurgery

The most frequently used system for delivery of single fraction radiotherapy is gamma knife (Lee et al., 2008). Dose constraints for radiosurgery applied to the optic chiasm and brain stem were 8–9 Gy and 12–14 Gy, respectively (Mokry, 1999; Chung et al., 2000; Amendola et al., 2003; Kobayashi, 2009). In published gamma knife series, tumor control rates ranged from 67 to 94%. Complications directly attributable to gamma knife radiosurgery included visual deterioration (0–38%), endocrine morbidity (0–19%), and neurological complications (0–2%). No treatment-related mortality has been reported (Mokry, 1999; Amendola et al., 2003; Kobayashi, 2009).

Hypofractionated Stereotactic Radiotherapy – Cyber Knife

Data on the efficacy and tolerability of cyber knife in craniopharyngioma are limited (Lee et al., 2008). Tumor shrinkage was observed in seven patients and stabilized disease in three patients. No deterioration of vision or neuroendocrine function was recorded within the limited follow-up period (Lee et al., 2008).

Intracavitary β Irradiation

Stereotactic instillation of radioisotopes has been discussed as an alternative therapeutic option, mainly for monocystic craniopharyngioma recurrences. Nevertheless, this treatment method is restricted to cystic craniopharyngioma and should be considered only for post-operative recurrences and after percutaneous irradiation (Julow et al., 1989; Becker et al., 1999; Szeifert et al., 2007). A non-randomized retrospective monocentric analysis showed that patients treated with less invasive stereotactic and radiotherapeutic methods have a more favorable long-term clinical outcome than children treated with a more radical microsurgical approach (Schubert et al., 2009).

Instillation of Sclerosing Substances for Cystic Recurrent Tumors

Insertion of a catheter into a cystic craniopharyngioma may be preferable to the transient success of a cyst fenestration, since it allows repetitive drainage of the tumor cyst and the opportunity of instilling intracystic substances. Different neurosurgical techniques are employed for the placement of catheters. Even though it often relieves pressure only transiently, it is a useful therapeutic method for cystic recurrent tumors whose anatomical configuration and localization makes them difficult to resect (Cavalheiro et al., 1996; Kim et al., 2007). The instillation of sclerosing substances, such as bleomycin, in craniopharyngioma cysts using an intracystic catheter implanted by a stereotactic or open procedure, was used in such cases (Schubert et al., 2009). Severe neurotoxic side effects were observed in some cases, due to cystic leakage of bleomycin into cerebrospinal fluid (Lafay-Cousin et al., 2007). Accordingly, thorough neuroradiological imaging for exclusion of cystic leakage is warranted before instilling bleomycin.

Intracystic instillation of interferon alpha was first used by Cavalheiro and colleagues, who published the largest experience on cystic childhood craniopharyngiomas to date (Cavalheiro et al., 2005, 2010). Their most recent publication (Cavalheiro et al., 2010) included 60 children with a mean age of 11 years, who were treated at three different institutions from 2000 to 2009. Twenty-nine of the 60 patients received intracystic interferon alpha after initial surgery or bleomycin treatment had failed, and 31 were treated with interferon alpha as a first-line treatment. While in 47 children (78%) more than 50% cyst shrinkage was achieved at completion of therapy, 13 children progressed and required surgical intervention. Only one-third of the patients experienced side effects which consisted of headaches, palpebral edema, fever, chronic fatigue, or arthritis. In no patient was the associated toxicity so severe as to necessitate discontinuation of treatment. There was no mortality. These reports on the effect and tolerability of interferon alpha indicate that its intracystic instillation is a promising therapeutic option for predominantly monocystic craniopharyngiomas (Cavalheiro et al., 2010; Bartels et al., 2012).

SEQUELAE

Pituitary Deficiencies

Pituitary hormone deficiencies are common in childhood craniopharyngioma. At the time of diagnosis, 40–87% of children (Hoffman et al., 1992; Honegger et al., 1999; Caldarelli et al., 2005; Muller, 2008) present with at least one hormonal deficit and 17–27% (Hoffman et al., 1992; Muller, 2008; Elliott and Wisoff, 2010) have been reported to have diabetes insipidus neurohormonalis. The rate of post-surgical pituitary hormone deficiencies increases due to the tumor's proximity to, or even involvement in, hypothalamic–pituitary axes (Hoffman et al., 1992; De Vile et al., 1996b; Merchant et al., 2002; Muller et al., 2004a; Caldarelli et al., 2005; Elliott and Wisoff, 2010; Jung et al., 2010; Steno et al., 2011). Transient post-surgical diabetes insipidus occurs in up to 80–100% of all cases (Poretti et al., 2004; Caldarelli et al., 2005). The rate of permanent post-surgical diabetes insipidus ranges between 40–93% (Hoffman et al., 1992; De Vile et al., 1996b; Merchant et al., 2002; Poretti et al., 2004; Caldarelli et al., 2005; Ahmet et al., 2006; Elliott and Wisoff, 2010; Elliott et al., 2011; Muller et al., 2011b).

Growth hormone deficiency has been described at the time of diagnosis in 26–75% of childhood craniopharyngioma (Ahmet et al., 2006; Muller, 2008), and impaired growth may occur already years before diagnosis (Muller et al., 2004a). Growth hormone deficiency following treatment for childhood craniopharyngioma is found in about 70–92% of patients (Muller et al., 2004a, 2011b; Halac and Zimmerman, 2005; Crom et al., 2010). A positive response to growth hormone treatment is seen in most cases (Geffner et al., 2004). Normal growth in childhood craniopharyngioma patients with proven growth hormone deficiency is reported in the literature (Srinivasan et al., 2004). In fact, childhood craniopharyngioma patients with hypothalamic involvement were found to achieve normal adult height more often than those without hypothalamic involvement (Muller et al., 2004a). Even though this phenomenon of "growth without growth hormone" was described in childhood craniopharyngioma almost five decades ago (Matson, 1964), the physiology of growth in these cases is still not fully understood – although insulin and/or leptin are suspected to play a compensatory role. Both these hormones have been hypothesized to induce growth in the fetus and in obese children (Costin et al., 1976; Geffner, 1996; Phillip et al., 2002), with leptin reported to function as a bone growth factor acting directly at the level of bone growth centers, independently of growth hormone (Phillip et al., 2002). The mechanisms by which insulin stimulates growth include its known anabolic effects. At high serum levels, insulin may bind to the type 1 insulin-like growth factor (IGF) receptor and induce growth, mediated by its actions to decrease IGF-binding protein 1 levels, resulting in increased levels of free IGF-1 (Phillip et al., 2002). In support of this theory, obese childhood craniopharyngioma patients were found to present with higher height SDS at the time of diagnosis and at last follow-up with no difference in hormonal substitution, including growth hormone (Muller et al., 2001). In contrast, another study found that childhood craniopharyngioma patients who were growing despite growth hormone deficiency were not different from those requiring growth hormone substitution in terms of anthropometrical measures, body composition, and metabolic indexes, including insulin levels (Srinivasan et al., 2004).

Visual and Neurological Outcomes

Due to frequent suprasellar tumor localization, visual deficits (both visual acuity and visual fields) are relatively common in patients with childhood craniopharyngioma. Visual impairment was found as an initial clinical manifestation of childhood craniopharyngioma in more than half of affected patients (Muller, 2008), with some post-surgical improvement of vision in 41–48% of patients (Caldarelli et al., 2005; Elliott et al., 2011). Factors associated with a lack of post-surgical visual impairment include tumor localization in the pre-chiasmatic area and severe pre-surgical visual deficits (Caldarelli et al., 2005; Steno et al., 2011).

Neurological sequelae include hemiparesis, epilepsy, cranial nerve deficits, cerebrovascular disease manifestations, headaches, and learning problems (Merchant et al., 2002; Elliott and Wisoff, 2010; Crom et al., 2010). Most of these are transient and the total prevalence of long-term neurological complications is reported to be 8% (Caldarelli et al., 2005). This rate, however, rises to 36% for large-sized tumors (Elliott and Wisoff, 2010) and 30% when including both visual and neurological complications (Poretti et al., 2004).

Hypothalamic Dysfunction

Symptoms related to hypothalamic dysfunction, such as obesity, behavioral changes, disturbed circadian rhythm and sleep irregularities, daytime sleepiness, and imbalances in regulation of body temperature, thirst, heart rate, and/or blood pressure, have been found at diagnosis in 35% of childhood craniopharyngioma patients (Elliott and Wisoff, 2010). The rate of hypothalamic dysfunction dramatically increases following radical surgical treatment; in some series up to 65–80% (Poretti et al., 2004; Elliott and Wisoff, 2010). Even though pre-surgical evaluation of hypothalamic damage is difficult both clinically and radiologically (Steno et al., 2011), tumor involvement of the third ventricle or obstructive hydrocephalus are suggestive findings (Caldarelli et al., 2005). A three-level clinical grading system for hypothalamic dysfunction has been suggested based on the degree of obesity and hypothalamic tumor involvement (De Vile et al., 1996b).

Associated with high morbidity, supra-chiasmatic lesions with hypothalamic involvement are difficult to treat. Surgical removal of tumor tissue beyond the mammillary bodies (i.e., in the posterior hypothalamic area) endangers hypothalamic structures and may cause hypothalamic obesity (Muller, 2011a, 2011b). With the aid of imaging studies, several reports have indicated that the degree of obesity of affected childhood craniopharyngioma patients is positively correlated with the degree and extent of hypothalamic damage (de Vile et al., 1996a; Holmer et al., 2009, 2010; Muller et al., 2011b; Hoffmann et al., 2014a). Fjalldal et al. recently published the results of a cross-sectional study of 42 patients who were analyzed for cognitive performance and psychosocial health at a median follow-up of 20 years (1–40 years) after diagnosis of childhood craniopharyngioma. The authors observed disturbed attention and impaired processing speed in adults with childhood craniopharyngioma when compared with matched normal controls. The deficits were most pronounced in patients with hypothalamic involvement of childhood craniopharyngioma (Fjalldal et al., 2013). Taking these considerations into account, a novel classification of pre-surgical involvement and post-surgical lesions of hypothalamic structures based on magnetic resonance imaging was recently published (Flitsch et al., 2011). The classification might help to establish more risk-adapted surgical strategies (Figure 27.4) based on a grading of pre-surgical hypothalamic involvement and post-surgical hypothalamic lesions.

Obesity and Eating Disorders

Rapid weight gain and severe obesity are the most perplexing complications due to hypothalamic involvement and/or hypothalamic surgical damage of childhood craniopharyngioma. Weight gain in childhood craniopharyngioma patients often occurs years before diagnosis (Muller et al., 2004a), with 12–19% of patients reported to be obese at diagnosis (Hoffman et al., 1992; Poretti et al., 2004; Ahmet et al., 2006; Muller, 2008). Weight gain occurs despite adequate endocrine replacement of pituitary hormone deficiencies. The hypothalamic disturbance in energy management contributes to the development of severe obesity and is exacerbated by factors limiting physical activity, such as marked daytime sleepiness, disturbances of circadian rhythms, and neurological deficits (Muller et al., 2002). The degree of obesity frequently increases soon after treatment, and rapid weight gain frequently occurs during the first 6–12 months after treatment (Muller et al., 2001; Ahmet et al., 2006; Holmer et al., 2010).

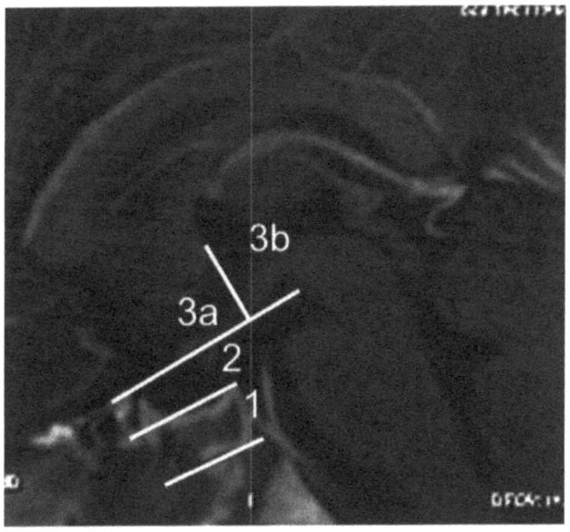

FIGURE 27.4 Sagittal magnetic resonance imaging (MRI) of the midline. Suggestion of a classification system of craniopharyngiomas by pre-operative MRI criteria. The intra- and suprasellar region can be divided into three sections. Section 1 is limited by the diaphragm sella, section 2 is below the optic chiasm and the mammillary bodies, and section 3 is above the chiasm and mammillary bodies, subdivided into an area anterior and posterior of the mammillary bodies. In this particular patient, a transsphenoidal surgery of a type 1 craniopharyngioma was performed previously. Section 1 is usually reached by the transsphenoidal route, whereas section 3A and 3B is mostly reserved for transcranial procedures. Depending on the tumor extension, section 2 can be reached by transcranial as well as transsphenoidal procedures. *Modified from (Flitsch et al., 2011), with the kind permission of Frontiers Endocrinology).*

Following treatment, the prevalence of severe obesity is higher, reaching up to 55% (Hoffman et al., 1992; Muller et al., 2001, 2003b; Poretti et al., 2004; Srinivasan et al., 2004; Ahmet et al., 2006; Lek et al., 2010; O'Gorman et al., 2010; Elliott et al., 2011). Obesity and eating disorders result in increased risks of metabolic syndrome (Srinivasan et al., 2004) and cardiovascular disease (Holmer et al., 2009), including sudden death events (Mong et al., 2008), multisystem morbidity (Pereira et al., 2005), and mortality (Scott et al., 1994; Fisher et al., 1998; Khafaga et al., 1998; Kalapurakal et al., 2003; Poretti et al., 2004; Tomita and Bowman, 2005; Habrand et al., 2006; Lin et al., 2008; Visser et al., 2010).

Although the relationship between severe obesity and hypothalamic lesions is obvious in childhood craniopharyngioma patients (Lustig et al., 2003b; Holmer et al., 2009, 2010), the mechanisms responsible for increased prevalence of cardiometabolic complications in these patients are still unclear. It is likely that in case of suprasellar extension, hypothalamic function will be compromised and will remain compromised to a certain extent when treated surgically or with irradiation. Although it is a relatively small structure of only 4 ml volume, the hypothalamic area contains several groups of nerve cell bodies forming distinct nuclei, which have highly diverse molecular, functional, and structural organization (Swaab et al., 1992). The hypothalamus plays a predominant role in keeping the internal environment stable by synchronizing biological clock mechanisms and circadian rhythms. Recent data indicate that an adequate balance of the autonomic nervous system equilibrium is crucial for metabolism. It is well known that adipose tissue is richly innervated by sympathetic nerve fibers that control lipolysis. Consequently, it appears that lipogenesis is also controlled by parasympathetic innervation of adipose tissue originating from separate sympathetic and parasympathetic neurons in the periventricular nucleus and suprachiasmatic nucleus (Kreier et al., 2002).

Such a high level of differentiation puts the suprachiasmatic nucleus in a key position to balance circadian activity of both branches of the autonomous nervous system. Considering the large proportion of childhood craniopharyngioma patients with damage to suprasellar structures, it is likely that craniopharyngiomas involving hypothalamic areas and/or the effects of treatment of these tumors damage the suprachiasmatic hypothalamic nucleus. This in turn affects the regulation of central clock mechanisms, which predisposes to alterations in metabolism. Clearly, surgical strategies to preserve hypothalamic integrity are mandatory in order to prevent sequelae such as severe obesity owing to hypothalamic lesions.

When elevated serum leptin levels relative to body mass index were found in childhood craniopharyngioma patients with a suprasellar tumor extension (Roth et al., 1998), researchers suggested that normal appetite inhibition failed to occur in these patients due to disruption of hypothalamic receptors that regulate a negative feedback loop in which leptin, formed in adipocytes, binds to hypothalamic leptin receptors. However, a study involving self-assessment by nutritional diaries revealed that hypothalamic obesity also occurs in patients with childhood craniopharyngioma, even when caloric intake is comparable to controls matched for body mass index (Harz et al., 2003).

Physical Activity and Energy Expenditure

An analysis of physical activity by accelerometric assessments showed that childhood craniopharyngioma patients had a markedly lower level of physical activity than healthy controls matched for body mass index (Harz et al., 2003). Markedly increased daytime sleepiness and disturbances of circadian rhythms have been demonstrated in patients with childhood craniopharyngioma and severe obesity (Muller et al., 2002). Daytime sleepiness and obesity in these patients were both correlated with low nocturnal and early morning melatonin concentrations in saliva. The proposed pathogenic mechanism involves impaired hypothalamic regulation of circadian melatonin secretion in patients with childhood craniopharyngioma extending to the suprasellar area. Initial experiences with oral melatonin substitution in childhood craniopharyngioma patients (6 mg melatonin per day) were promising: melatonin levels normalized and physical activity and daytime sleepiness improved significantly (Muller et al., 2006c). However, data on the long-term effect of melatonin substitution on weight development and daytime sleepiness have not yet been published.

Polysomnographic studies in patients with childhood craniopharyngioma and severe daytime sleepiness have revealed sleeping patterns typical for hypersomnia and secondary narcolepsy, i.e., frequent "sleep-onset REM phases" (SOREM) (Muller et al., 2006d; Muller, 2010c; O'Gorman et al., 2010). Medication with central stimulating agents (methylphenidate, modafinil) had a markedly beneficial effect on daytime sleepiness in these patients (Muller et al., 2006d). Secondary narcolepsy should be taken into consideration as a pathogenic factor in severely obese childhood craniopharyngioma patients. Mason et al. (2002) treated five patients with childhood craniopharyngioma and severe hypothalamic obesity (age range: 6.0–9.8 years) with the central stimulating agent, dextro-amphetamine, for the purpose of weight reduction. Dextro-amphetamine therapy stabilized patient body mass index. The patients' parents reported noticeable improvements in their child's physical activity and alertness.

A decreased metabolic rate, in terms of both resting and total energy expenditure, has been suggested to contribute to weight gain in patients with childhood craniopharyngioma. Adults and pediatric patients with childhood-onset craniopharyngioma were found to have a lower resting-energy expenditure (REE) compared to controls (Shaikh et al., 2008; Holmer et al., 2010; Kim et al., 2010) that was not explained by differences in terms of body composition. This energy intake/REE ratio was lower in those with tumors involving the third ventricle (Holmer et al., 2010). Impaired physical activity might contribute to an overall lowering of total energy expenditure (Harz et al., 2003; Shaikh et al., 2008; Holmer et al., 2009, 2010). Further factors potentially contributing to decreased physical activity are neurological and visual deficits, psychosocial difficulties, and increased daytime sleepiness.

Autonomous Nervous System

Lustig and colleagues (Lustig et al., 2003a; Lustig, 2011) hypothesized that hypothalamic disinhibition of vagal output is a cause of increased β-cell stimulation in patients with childhood craniopharyngioma, and that this disinhibition leads to hyperinsulinism and severe obesity. They therefore studied treatment with the somatostatin analog octreotide, which suppresses β-cell activity (Lustig et al., 2003a).

Several reports (Roth et al., 2007; Cohen et al., 2013) have hypothesized that decreased physical activity and severe obesity in patients with childhood craniopharyngioma could be related to impaired central sympathetic output. Roth observed reduced urine concentrations of catecholamine metabolites correlating with the degree of obesity and the level of physical activity (Roth, 2011).

Appetite Regulation

Roth and colleagues recently analyzed the gastrointestinal hormones ghrelin and peptide YY and their effect on satiety regulation in patients with childhood craniopharyngioma and hypothalamic obesity (Roth et al., 2011). Their findings support the hypothesis that reduced ghrelin secretion and impaired postprandial suppression of ghrelin in these patients leads to disturbed regulation of appetite and satiety. Peptide YY serum concentrations did not differ between normal weight, obese, and severely obese patients with childhood craniopharyngioma. A possible pathogenic role of peripheral α-melanocyte-stimulating hormone in childhood craniopharyngioma obesity has also been reported (Roth et al., 2010).

Functional magnetic resonance imaging was used in childhood craniopharyngioma patients to examine the hypothesis that hypothalamic damage due to the tumor and its treatment results in enhanced perception of food reward and/or impaired central satiety processing (Roth et al., 2012). Following the test meal, controls showed suppression of activation by food cues while childhood craniopharyngioma patients showed trends towards higher activation. The authors conclude that perception of food cues may be altered in hypothalamic obesity, especially after eating, i.e., in the satiated state. The functional magnetic resonance imaging approach is encouraging for performing future mechanistic studies of the brain response to food cues and satiety in patients with hypothalamic obesity due to childhood craniopharyngioma.

Pharmacological Treatment of Hypothalamic Obesity

Due to disturbances in energy expenditure, central sympathetic output, and appetite regulation, childhood craniopharyngioma patients with hypothalamic obesity typically develop morbid obesity that is mainly unresponsive to conventional lifestyle modifications (diet and exercise). Based on impairment of sympatho-adrenal activation and epinephrine production manifesting as a reduced hormonal response to hypoglycemia, treating this disorder with amphetamine derivates has been suggested (Schofl et al., 2002; Coutant et al., 2003). Use of dextro-amphetamine started at 10 months post-surgical intervention for craniopharyngioma and lasting for 24 months was shown to diminish continuous weight gain and stabilize body mass index (Mason et al., 2002); importantly, spontaneous physical activity increased significantly. Even shorter periods of dextro-amphetamine treatment have caused a subjective improvement in daytime sleepiness (Ismail et al., 2006). Elfers and Roth observed beneficial effects of central stimulating agents (methylphenidate) on weight development in childhood craniopharyngioma patients (Elfers and Roth, 2011).

Sibutramine is a neurotransmitter reuptake-inhibitor that reduces the reuptake of serotonin, norepinephrine, and dopamine, thereby increasing the levels of these substances in synaptic clefts and helping enhance satiety. Sibutramine has been widely used to treat obesity, leading to a weight loss of 7–10% when combined with a regulated diet. Sibutramine was tested in a randomized placebo-controlled crossover trial in patient cohorts with different obesity syndromes (Danielsson et al., 2007). While the drug was well tolerated and safe, the weight loss response in patients with hypothalamic obesity was less pronounced in comparison to other participants (such as trisomy 21 and Prader Willi syndrome). While the effect on body mass index was promising, sibutramine has been taken off the market due to adverse side effects and further clinical trials are not expected.

Childhood craniopharyngioma patients with hypothalamic obesity have a "parasympathetic predominance" of the autonomic nervous system induced by vagal activation and manifesting as daytime sleepiness, and reduced body temperature and heart rate (Lustig, 2008). Parasympathetic stimulation causes insulin secretion by way of direct activation of β cells, and it also promotes adipogenesis. As insulin is an anabolic hormone, it has been suggested as an important driver of weight gain in hypothalamic obesity. Octreotide is a somatostatin analog and thus can cause a reduction in insulin secretion. Lustig and colleagues used octreotide in a double-blind, randomized, controlled study in children with hypothalamic obesity, and demonstrated moderate reductions in weight gain (Lustig et al., 2003a). The authors showed that insulin levels during a proof-of-concept oral glucose tolerance test decreased without leading to major changes in glucose tolerance. This study was followed by a larger trial performed using octreotide LAR in 60 patients with cranial surgical interventions that led to hypothalamic obesity (http://clinicaltrials.gov/ct2/show/NCT00076362 [accessed 06/27/14]). This 6-month intervention showed no efficacy at all in changing body mass index and the open label segment of this study was terminated earlier than planned due to an increased risk of gallstone formation.

Bariatric Treatment of Hypothalamic Obesity

Initial experiences with bariatric surgery in severely obese childhood craniopharyngioma patients achieved sufficient tolerability and short-term weight reduction (Muller et al., 2007;

Inge et al., 2007; Bingham et al., 2012). An instant improvement of binge-eating behavior in patients with childhood craniopharyngioma immediately after laparoscopic adjustable gastric banding (LAGB) was observed, but failed in long-term weight reduction. Nevertheless, weight stabilization could be achieved during regular follow-up monitoring (Muller et al., 2011a).

In a systematic review and meta-analysis of the literature, Bretault et al. (2013) analyzed the 12-month outcomes after bariatric surgery for hypothalamic obesity due to craniopharyngioma treatment. At 1 year, of 18 cases with follow-up data, six had lost more than 20% of their initial weight; all had undergone either Roux Y gastric bypass (n = 3), sleeve gastrectomy, (n = 2), or biliopancreatic diversion (n = 1). All patients who had lost less than 5% of their initial weight had undergone LAGB except one Roux Y gastric bypass case. These findings indicate that Roux Y gastric bypass, sleeve gastrectomy, and biliopancreatic diversion are the most efficient bariatric procedures for weight reduction in hypothalamic obesity of childhood craniopharyngioma. However, treatment with invasive, non-reversible bariatric methods is controversial in the pediatric population because of medical, ethical, and legal considerations (Rottembourg et al., 2009; Schultes et al., 2009; Muller et al., 2011a).

Despite the availability of above-mentioned promising therapeutic approaches, it must be emphasized that at present no generally accepted (pharmacological or bariatric) therapy for hypothalamic obesity in childhood craniopharyngioma has been shown to be effective in randomized studies (Bereket et al., 2012).

Quality of Life, Neurocognitive Outcome, and Psychosocial Functioning

Quality of life in children can be affected by both the tumor itself and the treatment received. Reports assessing psychosocial and physical functioning show variable results, ranging from excellent in a majority of subjects to impaired function in almost half of patients (Hoffman et al., 1992; Van Effenterre and Boch, 2002; Muller et al., 2003a, 2005a; Poretti et al., 2004). The most common areas of difficulty include social and emotional functioning, with patients rating their psychosocial status to be lower than their physical health (Poretti et al., 2004). Other challenges include somatic complaints such as reduced mobility, pain, and self-care (Merchant et al., 2002; Poretti et al., 2004). Behavioral questionnaires indicate a high rate of psychopathological symptoms, including depression, withdrawal, and anxiety. The most frequent problems in children's everyday functioning include difficulties in learning, inability to control emotions, unsatisfactory peer relationships, and concerns regarding physical appearance and body image (Crom et al., 2010; Ondruch et al., 2011).

Factors associated with worsening quality of survival outcomes as well as neurocognitive and psychosocial functioning include younger age at diagnosis, pre-operative functional impairment, and certain tumor characteristics including larger tumor volume, hypothalamic and third ventricle involvement at presentation. Treatment strategies have also been implicated, with worse outcomes for surgery alone compared to limited surgery followed by irradiation and for multiple operations for tumor recurrence. Endocrine, neurological, and ophthalmological sequelae all adversely affect quality of life outcome (Hoffman et al., 1992; Merchant et al., 2002; Van Effenterre and Boch, 2002; Muller et al., 2003a; Poretti et al., 2004; Elliott and Wisoff, 2010; Steno et al., 2011). Hypothalamic dysfunction was found to have the most important negative impact on social functioning, physical ability, and body image (Muller et al., 2001, 2003a; Poretti et al., 2004).

Long-term neurocognitive complications following treatment for childhood craniopharyngioma include cognitive problems, particularly those affecting executive function, attention, episodic memory, and working memory (Cavazzuti et al., 1983; Riva et al., 1998; Carpentieri et al., 2001; Poretti et al., 2004; Sands et al., 2005; Kiehna et al., 2006; Crom et al., 2010; Ondruch et al., 2011). In a recent report, Özyurt and coworkers provided first evidence that hypothalamic damage impacts on neural correlates of memory retrieval in medial prefrontal cortex, indicating a less efficient use of a prefrontal area involved in executive control processes. The authors propose that the deactivation failure in the patients' anterior rostral medial prefrontal cortex is related to an increased coupling with the thalamus and reflects a reduced efficiency to flexibly adapt to task demands (Özyurt et al., 2014a, 2014b).

Furthermore, long-term survivors of childhood craniopharyngioma treated primarily with subtotal surgical resection followed by irradiation were also found to have psychological and educational deficits (Crom et al., 2010). Neurocognitive deficits include memory disturbances, slower cognitive speed, attention problems, and behavioral instability (Cavazzuti et al., 1983; Colangelo et al., 1990; Carpentieri et al., 2001; Kiehna et al., 2006; Crom et al., 2010; Ondruch et al., 2011). While intact intellectual functioning has been reported in up to 82% of patients, visual memory is impaired despite normal visual-spatial abilities (Crom et al., 2010; Ondruch et al., 2011). The acquired deficits in higher cognitive processing such as attention problems are considered precursors to poor academic achievement.

Despite over a quarter of a century of literature documenting the neurocognitive challenges encountered by individuals treated for childhood craniopharyngioma, intervention efforts have lagged. Recent case studies have examined the efficacy of cognitive rehabilitation for dysexecutive problems and behavioral lability (Metzler-Baddeley and Jones, 2010; Hammond and Hall, 2011). In a case report of a 2-month intervention using a combination of goal management therapy and naturally occurring distractions within the patients' work environment, significant improvements in cognitive tests requiring organized behavior were reported. Social, emotional, and/or behavior problems, most notably aggression, have been reported (Anderson et al., 1997; Riva et al., 1998; Poretti et al., 2004). Despite their occurrence, the assumption of the biological underpinning of the behavioral disturbance appears to have limited attempts to effectively manage it with intervention. Behavioral treatment was used for severely aggressive behaviors (Hammond and Hall, 2011); the intervention included functional behavioral analysis followed by differential reinforcement of alternative behaviors and extinction with the goal of decreasing the frequency of aggressive behavior. Aggressive behavior subsequently decreased to below 88% of baseline levels and adaptive behaviors were found to increase significantly. These results suggest that the patient's aggression was maintained by inadvertent social reinforcement. Taken together, these case studies suggest that cognitive rehabilitation approaches such as goal management therapy and functional behavioral analysis may be useful in supporting survivors of childhood craniopharyngioma adapt to and compensate for cognitive and psychosocial challenges (Cohen et al., 2011).

Survival and Late Mortality

Survival rates in patients treated for childhood craniopharyngioma are generally high (Müller et al., 2003). However, disease-related mortality can occur even many years after treatment. Data regarding survival include primarily surgically treated patients. The reported post-surgical 5-year overall survival is 88–94% (De Vile et al., 1996b; Muller et al., 2001, 2006b; Van Effenterre and Boch, 2002), and the reported 10-year overall survival is 70–92% (Hoffman et al., 1992; Van Effenterre and Boch, 2002; Poretti et al., 2004; Elliott and Wisoff, 2010; Visser et al., 2010), with a 20-year survival of 76%. Causes of late mortality include those directly related to the tumor or treatment such as progressive disease with multiple recurrences, chronic hypothalamic insufficiency, hormonal deficiencies, cerebrovascular disease, and seizures (De Vile et al., 1996b; Poretti et al., 2004; Elliott and Wisoff, 2010; Visser et al., 2010; Steno et al., 2011). Other causes have been described, including decreased mineral bone density and non-alcoholic steatohepatitis leading to liver cirrhosis in some cases (Basenau et al., 1994; Altuntas et al., 2002; Muller et al., 2003b, 2003c; Poretti et al., 2004; Caldarelli et al., 2005; Visser et al., 2010; Holmer et al., 2011). A recent review reports on substantial long-term morbidity with hypopituitarism, increased cardiovascular risk, hypothalamic damage, visual and neurological deficits, reduced bone health, and reduction in quality of life and cognitive function. The standardized overall mortality rate varies from 2.88–9.28 in cohort studies. Patients with childhood craniopharyngioma have a 3–19-fold higher cardiovascular mortality in comparison to the general population. Women with childhood craniopharyngioma have an even higher risk (Erfurth et al., 2013).

Cerebrovascular Morbidity

Radiation-induced vasculopathies are a rare consequence of radiation therapy for craniopharyngioma. In patients irradiated for childhood craniopharyngioma, Moyamoya syndrome (a radiation-induced cerebrovascular condition predisposing to stroke) has been described (Hetelekidis et al., 1993; Liu et al., 2009). A retrospective estimate was that 27% of 22 patients treated with irradiation and some combination of surgery and intracystic chemotherapy with a median radiation dose of 52.2 Gy developed some kind of vasculopathy, only half of which were symptomatic (Liu et al., 2009). No association was found between age, radiation dose, and maximum or mean dose to the internal carotid arteries with the presence of vascular abnormalities. Regine and colleagues reported a 13.7% rate of cerebrovascular events, all in irradiated cases receiving over 61 Gy (Regine and Kramer, 1992). No cerebrovascular clinical events were reported in any other series of conventionally fractionated radiotherapy for childhood craniopharyngioma, including those with large patient numbers (Rajan et al., 1993; Stripp et al., 2004; Karavitaki et al., 2005; Moon et al., 2005; Pemberton et al., 2005; Merchant et al., 2006; Combs et al., 2007).

Secondary Malignant Neoplasms

In the largest reported series no secondary malignancies were observed in 173 treated patients with a median follow-up of 12 years (Rajan et al., 1993). Overall, only four cases of secondary malignancies have been reported (Hetelekidis et al., 1993; Regine et al., 1993; Habrand et al., 1999; Winkfield et al., 2009) comprising two glioblastomas (Regine et al., 1993, Habrand et al., 1999), one glioma with unspecified grade of malignancy (Hetelekidis et al., 1993) and a posterior fossa meningioma (Winkfield et al., 2009).

ADULT-ONSET CRANIOPHARYNGIOMA

According to a recent study, there are no significant differences in neuroradiological characteristics of craniopharyngiomas between children and adults with the exception of lower rates of tumor calcification in adult patients (Mortini et al., 2011). In some studies hydrocephalus occurred less frequently in adults than in children, however other authors reported no differences in this regard (Van Effenterre and Boch, 2002; Karavitaki et al., 2005).

Age-dependent differences between childhood-onset and adult-onset craniopharyngioma are related to histological diagnosis, biological behavior, clinical manifestations, treatment options, and follow-up period (Kendall-Taylor et al., 2005; Gautier et al., 2012; Zoicas and Schofl, 2012).

Growth retardation and short stature are predominant manifestations of childhood craniopharyngioma (Muller et al., 2004a). Due to high overall survival rates and irradiation in childhood craniopharyngioma the risk of development of second malignancies should be considered in long-term follow-up.

The Kendall-Taylor et al. study compared childhood-onset craniopharyngioma patients with adult-onset craniopharyngioma patients and reported a poor state of health and quality of life in both cohorts. The majority of childhood- and adult-onset craniopharyngioma patients displayed pituitary insufficiency, with 60% suffering from diabetes insipidus. Nearly all patients were overweight or obese, reporting a poor quality of life (Kendall-Taylor et al., 2005).

QUESTIONS AND TREATMENT PERSPECTIVES

Surgical Treatment Strategies – Degree of Resection

One of the biggest challenges in treating childhood craniopharyngioma is identifying the best candidates for a radical versus conservative treatment approach. Experiential expertise in large centers has increased the likelihood of safe gross total resection, as evidenced by two reports representing historically different attitudes: the first at Necker Hospital, Paris, France (Puget et al., 2006), which is more surgically oriented; and the second in North America (Merchant et al., 2006), which is more oriented towards a conservative approach. The North American experience shows that most recent cases now receive moderate to aggressive surgery and only 42% have limited surgery before irradiation. The Necker authors (Puget et al., 2007) show in a contemporary series that 96% of their recent cases achieve complete (23%) or subtotal resection (73%), and that radiotherapy is performed in 50% of cases after subtotal resection. It appears there is a trend towards radiotherapy in centers with past predominantly surgical approaches, and towards more radical surgical treatment strategies in centers historically conservative-oriented (Puget, 2012). There are current prospective studies underway on a national and multinational level to adopt strategies tailored to risk factors for morbidity and quality of life (Muller et al., 2006a; Puget et al., 2007; Trivin et al., 2009).

Elowe-Gruau and coworkers recently reported on a single-institute treatment comparison of childhood patients with craniopharyngioma (Elowe-Gruau et al., 2013). A historical cohort of 60 children underwent extensive resection surgery between 1985 and 2002 and a prospective cohort of 65 patients underwent a hypothalamus-sparing surgical strategy between 2002 and 2010. During this second time period, the indication for hypothalamus-sparing surgery was made using an algorithm that graded pre-surgical hypothalamic tumor involvement (Puget et al., 2007). At last follow-up, patients treated by hypothalamus-sparing surgery had a significantly lower prevalence of severe obesity (BMI >3 SD score) than patients treated by extensive resection surgery (28% versus 54%, respectively). The mean number of surgical procedures was the same for both surgical groups. In the multivariate analysis, pre-operative hypothalamic involvement and hypothalamic-sparing surgery independently predicted the presence of severe obesity at last follow-up.

Controversy Over Time Point of Irradiation

In clinical practice, the timing of post-operative residual tumor irradiation is both unclear and inconsistently regarded (Sung, 1982; Regine and Kramer, 1992; Stripp et al., 2004; Moon et al., 2005; Tomita and Bowman, 2005; Muller et al., 2005b, 2006b; Trivin et al., 2009). Some favor immediate post-operative irradiation in the event of life-impairing clinical conditions, proactively preventing tumor progression (Merchant et al., 2002). On the other hand, some authors favor a wait-and-see procedure, delaying irradiation in order to reduce both its necessity and the negative consequences associated with radiation therapy. Inarguably, immediate post-operative irradiation significantly delays tumor progression (Stripp et al., 2004). However, progression-contingent irradiation has proven to be effective, as overall survival is statistically unaffected by this wait-and-see strategy (Regine and Kramer, 1992). Three recent series retrospectively compared the immediate post-operative irradiation strategy with progression-contingent deployment (Stripp et al., 2004; Moon et al., 2005; Tomita and Bowman, 2005).

No differences in overall and progression-free survival were detected between immediate irradiation and progression-contingent treatment in the series evaluated by Moon and colleagues (Moon et al., 2005). Relapse-free overall survival rates were 83% and 70% after 5 and 10 years, respectively, in the series analyzed by Tomita and colleagues (Tomita and Bowman, 2005). The corresponding numbers for patients after incomplete resection followed by immediate irradiation were 71% and 36% after 5 and 10 years, respectively. After incomplete resection without radiation therapy, the relapse-free survival rate after 5 years was merely 9%. Progression-contingent irradiation achieved similar final overall survival and progression-free survival rates of 90% and 70%, respectively, meaning progression-contingent irradiation in this series was highly effective. However, it has to be emphasized that the interpretation of these studies is difficult due to confounding factors in terms of indication for treatment, and unknown factors regarding medical staff experience and state of facilities. Regardless of concerns over quality and completeness of data, the relevant endpoint in analysis of childhood craniopharyngioma treatment should be patients' quality of life and morbidity.

KRANIOPHARYNGEOM 2007, the German prospective, childhood craniopharygioma multinational trial (Muller, 2006, 2008, 2010a, 2010b; Muller et al., 2006a, 2006b), is currently evaluating craniopharyngioma patients' prognoses (quality of life, EFS, overall survival) following defined therapeutic strategies. A stratified randomization of two treatment arms is conducted with respect to timing of post-operative irradiation (immediate radiotherapy versus radiotherapy at the time of progression) for the subgroup of patients ≥5 years of age at the time of incomplete resection. The schedule of prospective data collection and the set and definition of parameters in KRANIOPHARYNGEOM 2007 are based on a multinational European consensus (Muller et al., 2006a) (Figure 27.5).

Expertise

There are only a few studies analyzing the outcome of patients with craniopharyngioma in relation to the neurosurgeons' experience. Sanford (1994) and Boop (2007) report a marked difference in outcome according to the neurosurgeons' experience with the condition.

The degree of obesity and quality of life based on reference assessment of tumor localization and post-surgical hypothalamic lesions were analyzed in a recent report (Muller et al., 2011b) (Figure 27.6). Treatment was also analyzed regarding neurosurgical strategy and the neurosurgical center sizes based on patient load. Surgical lesions of anterior and posterior hypothalamic areas were associated with post-surgical obesity, negatively impacting quality of life in patients with posterior hypothalamic lesions. Treatment in large centers was less

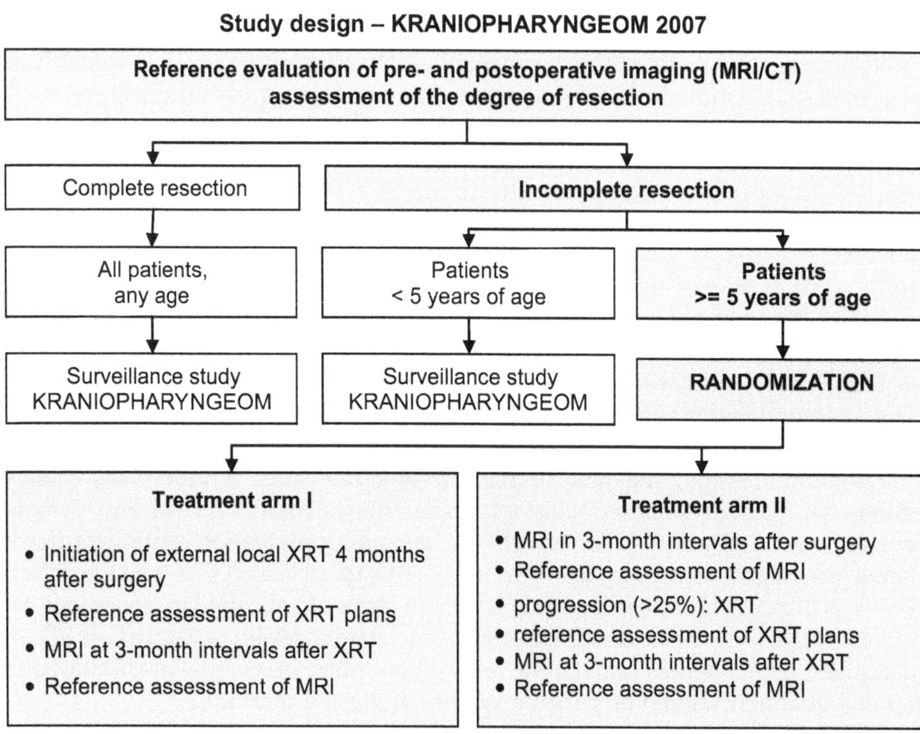

FIGURE 27.5 Study design of KRANIOPHARYNGEOM 2007 (www.kraniopharyngeom.net). *Modified from (Muller et al., 2006b), with the kind permission of Karger.*

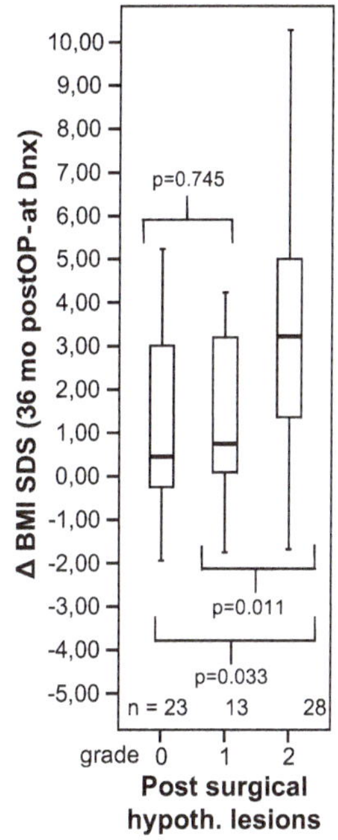

FIGURE 27.6 Changes in body mass index (BMI SDS) during first 36 months after diagnosis of 117 childhood craniopharyngioma patients recruited in KRANIOPHARYNGEOM 2000 relative to the extent of surgical hypothalamic lesions (grade 0 to 2). The horizontal line in the middle of the box depicts the median. Edges of box mark the 25th and 75th percentile. Whiskers indicate the range of values that fall within 1.5 box-lengths. *Modified from (Muller et al., 2011b), with the kind permission of Bioscientifica.*

radical, and the rates of complete resection and hypothalamic surgical lesions were lower than those of middle-sized and small centers (Muller et al., 2012; Hoffmann et al., 2014b). However, a multivariable analysis showed that pre-operative hypothalamic involvement was the only independent risk factor for severe obesity (Muller et al., 2011b).

Based on the most current literature presenting factors affecting the pathology, treatment and quality of life effects of childhood craniopharyngioma, it is advisable to have a multidisciplinary team able to discuss diagnostic and treatment strategies, adopting the most sophisticated approaches feasible based on sufficient in-house surgical, radio-oncological, and socio-psychological experience for treating patients with childhood craniopharyngioma (Muller, 2011a, 2012a 2013b).

CONCLUSIONS

Risk-adapted surgical strategies at initial diagnosis of childhood craniopharyngioma should aim at a maximal degree of resection, keenly focused on respecting the integrity of optical and hypothalamic structures to prevent severe sequelae and therein minimize consequences that could have a negative impact on patient quality of life. In case of hypothalamic involvement, hypothalamus-sparing surgical strategies are recommended in order to prevent hypothalamic damage and associated severe sequelae. Local irradiation of residual tumor is efficient in preventing tumor progression.

Because initial hypothalamic tumor involvement, especially of posterior hypothalamic structures, has an a priori effect on the clinical course (Muller et al., 2004a, 2011b), childhood craniopharyngioma should be recognized as a chronic disease requiring constant monitoring of the consequences and medical resources for treatment, in order to provide not only optimal quality of life for patients, but also to garner additional information with the intent of minimizing what at present are severe consequences of both the disease and its treatment (Muller, 2011a, 2013b).

This chapter was composed in the absence of any commercial or financial relationships that could be construed as a potential conflict of interest. The author was supported by the German Childhood Cancer Foundation, Bonn, Germany.

References

Aggarwal, A., Fersht, N., Brada, M., 2013. Radiotherapy for craniopharyngioma. Pituitary 16, 26–33.

Ahmet, A., Blaser, S., Stephens, D., Guger, S., Rutkas, J.T., Hamilton, J., 2006. Weight gain in craniopharyngioma – a model for hypothalamic obesity. J. Pediatr. Endocrinol. Metab. 19, 121–127.

Altuntas, B., Ozcakar, B., Bideci, A., Cinaz, P., 2002. Cirrhotic outcome in patients with craniopharyngioma. J. Pediatr. Endocrinol. Metab. 15, 1057–1058.

Amendola, B.E., Wolf, A., Coy, S.R., Amendola, M.A., 2003. Role of radiosurgery in craniopharyngiomas: a preliminary report. Med. Pediatr. Oncol. 41, 123–127.

Anderson, C., Wilkening, G., Filley, C., Reardon, M., Kleinschmidt-Demasters, B., 1997. Neurobehavioral outcome in pediatric craniopharyngioma. Pediatr. Neurosurg. 26, 255–260.

Bartels, U., Laperriere, N., Bouffet, E., Drake, J., 2012. Intracystic therapies for cystic craniopharyngioma in childhood. Front. Endocrinol. (Lausanne) 3, 39.

Basenau, D., Stehphani, U., Fischer, G., 1994. [Development of complete liver cirrhosis in hyperphagia-induced fatty liver]. Klin. Padiatr. 206, 62–64.

Becker, G., Kortmann, R.D., Skalej, M., Bamberg, M., 1999. The role of radiotherapy in the treatment of craniopharyngioma – indications, results, side effects. Front. Radiat. Ther. Oncol. 33, 100–113.

Beltran, C., Roca, M., Merchant, T.E., 2012. On the benefits and risks of proton therapy in pediatric craniopharyngioma. Int. J. Radiat. Oncol. Biol. Phys. 82, e281–e287.

Bereket, A., Kiess, W., Lustig, R.H., Muller, H.L., Goldstone, A.P., Weiss, R., Yavuz, Y., Hochberg, Z., 2012. Hypothalamic obesity in children. Obes. Rev. 13, 780–798.

Bingham, N.C., Rose, S.R., Inge, T.H., 2012. Bariatric surgery in hypothalamic obesity. Front. Endocrinol. (Lausanne) 3, 23.

Boehling, N.S., Grosshans, D.R., Bluett, J.B., Palmer, M.T., Song, X., Amos, R.A., Sahoo, N., Meyer, J.J., Mahajan, A., Woo, S.Y., 2012. Dosimetric comparison of three-dimensional conformal proton radiotherapy, intensity-modulated proton therapy, and intensity-modulated radiotherapy for treatment of pediatric craniopharyngiomas. Int. J. Radiat. Oncol. Biol. Phys. 82, 643–652.

Boop, F.A., 2007. Craniopharyngioma. J. Neurosurg. 106, 1–2; discussion 2.

Bretault, M., Boillot, A., Muzard, L., Poitou, C., Oppert, J.M., Barsamian, C., Gatta, B., Muller, H., Weismann, D., Rottembourg, D., Inge, T., Veyrie, N., Carette, C., Czernichow, S., 2013. Bariatric surgery following treatment for craniopharyngioma: a systematic review and individual-level data meta-analysis. J. Clin. Endocrinol. Metab. 98, 2239–2246.

Buchfelder, M., Schlaffer, S.M., Lin, F., Kleindienst, A., 2013. Surgery for craniopharyngioma. Pituitary 16, 18–25.

Bunin, G.R., Surawicz, T.S., Witman, P.A., Preston-Martin, S., Davis, F., Bruner, J.M., 1998. The descriptive epidemiology of craniopharyngioma. J. Neurosurg. 89, 547–551.

Caldarelli, M., Massimi, L., Tamburrini, G., Cappa, M., Di Rocco, C., 2005. Long-term results of the surgical treatment of craniopharyngioma: the experience at the Policlinico Gemelli Catholic University Rome. Child's. Nerv. Syst. 21, 747–757.

Carpentieri, S., Waber, D., Scott, R., Goumnerova, L., Kieran, M., Cohen, L., Kim, F., Billett, A., Tarbell, N., Pomeroy, S., 2001. Memory deficits among children with craniopharyngioma. Neurosurgery 49, 1053–1058.
Cavalheiro, S., Dastoli, P.A., Silva, N.S., Toledo, S., Lederman, H., Da Silva, M.C., 2005. Use of interferon alpha in intratumoral chemotherapy for cystic craniopharyngioma. Childs. Nerv. Syst. 21, 719–724.
Cavalheiro, S., Di Rocco, C., Valenzuela, S., Dastoli, P.A., Tamburrini, G., Massimi, L., Nicacio, J.M., Faquini, I.V., Ierardi, D.F., Silva, N.S., Pettorini, B.L., Toledo, S.R., 2010. Craniopharyngiomas: intratumoral chemotherapy with interferon-alpha: a multicenter preliminary study with 60 cases. Neurosurg. Focus 28, E12.
Cavalheiro, S., Sparapani, F.V., Franco, J.O., Da Silva, M.C., Braga, F.M., 1996. Use of bleomycin in intratumoral chemotherapy for cystic craniopharyngioma. Case report. J. Neurosurg. 84, 124–126.
Cavazzuti, V., Fischer, E., Welch, K., Belli, J., Winston, K., 1983. Neurological and psychophysiological sequelae following different treatments of craniopharyngioma in children. J. Neurosurg. 59, 409–417.
Choux, M., Lena, G., 1979. Bases of surgical management of craniopharyngioma in children [proceedings]. Acta Neurochir. Suppl. (Wien) 28, 348.
Chung, W.Y., Pan, D.H., Shiau, C.Y., Guo, W.Y., Wang, L.W., 2000. Gamma knife radiosurgery for craniopharyngiomas. J. Neurosurg. 93 (Suppl. 3), 47–56.
Cohen, M., Guger, S., Hamilton, J., 2011. Long term sequelae of pediatric craniopharyngioma – literature review and 20 years of experience. Front. Endocrinol. (Lausanne) 2, 81.
Cohen, M., Syme, C., Mccrindle, B.W., Hamilton, J., 2013. Autonomic nervous system balance in children and adolescents with craniopharyngioma and hypothalamic obesity. Eur. J. Endocrinol. 168, 845–852.
Colangelo, M., Ambrosio, A., Ambrosio, C., 1990. Neurological and behavioral sequelae following different approaches to craniopharyngioma. Long-term follow-up review and therapeutic guidelines. Child's. Nerv. Syst. 6, 379–382.
Combs, S.E., Thilmann, C., Huber, P.E., Hoess, A., Debus, J., Schulz-Ertner, D., 2007. Achievement of long-term local control in patients with craniopharyngiomas using high precision stereotactic radiotherapy. Cancer 109, 2308–2314.
Costin, G., Kogut, M.D., Phillips, L.S., Daughaday, W.H., 1976. Craniopharyngioma: the role of insulin in promoting post-operative growth. J. Clin. Endocrinol. Metab. 42, 370–379.
Coutant, R., Maurey, H., Rouleau, S., Mathieu, E., Mercier, P., Limal, J.M., Le Bouil, A., 2003. Defect in epinephrine production in children with craniopharyngioma: functional or organic origin? J. Clin. Endocrinol. Metab. 88, 5969–5975.
Crom, D., Smith, D., Xiong, Z., Onar, A., Hudson, M., Merchant, T., Morris, E., 2010. Health status in long-term survivors of pediatric craniopharyngiomas. Am. Assoc. Neurosci. Nurs. 42, 323–328.
Danielsson, P., Janson, A., Norgren, S., Marcus, C., 2007. Impact sibutramine therapy in children with hypothalamic obesity or obesity with aggravating syndromes. J. Clin. Endocrinol. Metab. 92, 4101–4106.
De Vile, C.J., Grant, D.B., Hayward, R.D., Kendall, B.E., Neville, B.G., Stanhope, R., 1996a. Obesity in childhood craniopharyngioma: relation to post-operative hypothalamic damage shown by magnetic resonance imaging. J. Clin. Endocrinol. Metab. 81, 2734–2737.
De Vile, C.J., Grant, D.B., Kendall, B.E., Neville, B.G., Stanhope, R., Watkins, K.E., Hayward, R.D., 1996b. Management of childhood craniopharyngioma: can the morbidity of radical surgery be predicted? J. Neurosurg. 85, 73–81.
Elfers, C.T., Roth, C.L., 2011. Effects of methylphenidate on weight gain and food intake in hypothalamic obesity. Front. Endocrinol. (Lausanne) 2, 78.
Elliott, R.E., Jane Jr., J.A., Wisoff, J.H., 2011. Surgical Management of craniopharyngiomas in children: Meta-analysis and comparison of transcranial and transsphenoidal approaches. Neurosurgery 69, 630–643.
Elliott, R.E., Wisoff, J.H., 2010. Surgical management of giant pediatric craniopharyngiomas. J. Neurosurg. Pediatr. 6, 403–416.
Elowe-Gruau, E., Beltrand, J., Brauner, R., Pinto, G., Samara-Boustani, D., Thalassinos, C., Busiah, K., Laborde, K., Boddaert, N., Zerah, M., Alapetite, C., Grill, J., Touraine, P., Sainte-Rose, C., Polak, M., Puget, S., 2013. Childhood craniopharyngioma: hypothalamus-sparing surgery decreases the risk of obesity. J. Clin. Endocrinol. Metab 98, 2353–3262.
Erfurth, E.M., Holmer, H., Fjalldal, S.B., 2013. Mortality and morbidity in adult craniopharyngioma. Pituitary 16, 46–55.
Fahlbusch, R., Honegger, J., Paulus, W., Huk, W., Buchfelder, M., 1999. Surgical treatment of craniopharyngiomas: experience with 168 patients. J. Neurosurg. 90, 237–250.

Fisher, P.G., Jenab, J., Gopldthwaite, P.T., Tihan, T., Wharam, M.D., Foer, D.R., Burger, P.C., 1998. Outcomes and failure patterns in childhood craniopharyngiomas. Childs. Nerv. Syst. 14, 558–563.

Fitzek, M.M., Linggood, R.M., Adams, J., Munzenrider, J.E., 2006. Combined proton and photon irradiation for craniopharyngioma: long-term results of the early cohort of patients treated at Harvard Cyclotron Laboratory and Massachusetts General Hospital. Int. J. Radiat. Oncol. Biol. Phys. 64, 1348–1354.

Fjalldal, S., Holmer, H., Rylander, L., Elfving, M., Ekman, B., Osterberg, K., Erfurth, E.M., 2013. Hypothalamic involvement predicts cognitive performance and psychosocial health in long term survivors of childhood craniopharyngioma. J. Clin. Endocrinol. Metab 98, 3253–3262.

Flitsch, J., Muller, H.L., Burkhardt, T., 2011. Surgical strategies in childhood craniopharyngioma. Front. Endocrinol. (Lausanne) 2, 96.

Garre, M.L., Cama, A., 2007. Craniopharyngioma: modern concepts in pathogenesis and treatment. Curr. Opin. Pediatr. 19, 471–479.

Gaston-Massuet, C., Andoniadou, C.L., Signore, M., Jayakody, S.A., Charolidi, N., Kyeyune, R., Vernay, B., Jacques, T.S., Taketo, M.M., Le Tissier, P., Dattani, M.T., Martinez-Barbera, J.P., 2011. Increased Wingless (Wnt) signaling in pituitary progenitor/stem cells gives rise to pituitary tumors in mice and humans. Proc. Natl. Acad. Sci. U. S. A. 108, 11482–11487.

Gautier, A., Godbout, A., Grosheny, C., Tejedor, I., Coudert, M., Courtillot, C., Jublanc, C., De Kerdanet, M., Poirier, J.Y., Riffaud, L., Sainte-Rose, C., Van Effenterre, R., Brassier, G., Bonnet, F., Touraine, P., 2012. Markers of recurrence and long-term morbidity in craniopharyngioma: a systematic analysis of 171 patients. J. Clin. Endocrinol. Metab. 97, 1258–1267.

Geffner, M., Lundberg, M., Koltowska-Haggstrom, M., Abs, R., Verhelst, J., Erfurth, E.M., Kendall-Taylor, P., Price, D.A., Jonsson, P., BakkER, B., 2004. Changes in height, weight, and body mass index in children with craniopharyngioma after three years of growth hormone therapy: analysis of KIGS (Pfizer International Growth Database). J. Clin. Endocrinol. Metab. 89, 5435–5440.

Geffner, M.E., 1996. The growth without growth hormone syndrome. Endocrinol. Metab. Clin. North. Am. 25, 649–663.

Habrand, J.L., Ganry, O., Couanet, D., Rouxel, V., Levy-Piedbois, C., Pierre-Kahn, A., Kalifa, C., 1999. The role of radiation therapy in the management of craniopharyngioma: a 25-year experience and review of the literature. Int. J. Radiat. Oncol. Biol. Phys. 44, 255–263.

Habrand, J.L., Saran, F., Alapetite, C., Noel, G., El Boustany, R., Grill, J., 2006. Radiation therapy in the management of craniopharyngioma: current concepts and future developments. J. Pediatr. Endocrinol. Metab. 19 (Suppl. 1), 389–394.

Halac, I., Zimmerman, D., 2005. Endocrine manifestations of craniopharyngioma. Childs. Nerv. Syst. 21, 640–648.

Hammond, J., Hall, S., 2011. Functional analysis and treatment of aggressive behavior following resection of a craniopharyngioma. Deve. Med. Child. Neurol. 53, 369–374.

Harz, K.J., Muller, H.L., Waldeck, E., Pudel, V., Roth, C., 2003. Obesity in patients with craniopharyngioma: assessment of food intake and movement counts indicating physical activity. J. Clin. Endocrinol. Metab. 88, 5227–5231.

Hetelekidis, S., Barnes, P.D., Tao, M.L., Fischer, E.G., Schneider, L., Scott, R.M., Tarbell, N.J., 1993. 20-year experience in childhood craniopharyngioma. Int. J. Radiat. Oncol. Biol. Phys. 27, 189–195.

Hoffman, H.J., De Silva, M., Humphreys, R.P., Drake, J.M., Smith, M.L., Blaser, S.I., 1992. Aggressive surgical management of craniopharyngiomas in children. J. Neurosurg. 76, 47–52.

Hoffmann, A., Gebhardt, U., Sterkenburg, A., Warmuth-Metz, M., Müller, H.L., 2014a. Diencephalic syndrome in childhood craniopharyngioma - Results of German multicentre studies on 485 long-term survivors of childhood craniopharyngioma. J Clin Endocrinol Metab. Jul 31:jc20141680. [Epub ahead of print].

Hoffmann, A., Warmth-Metz, M., Gebhardt, U., Pietsch, T., Pohl, F., Kortmann, R.D., Calaminus, G., Müller, H.L., 2014b. Childhood craniopharyngioma - changes of treatment strategies in the trials KRANIOPHARYNGEOM 2000/2007. Klin Padiatr. 226, 161–168.

Holmer, H., Ekman, B., Bjork, J., Nordstom, C.H., Popovic, V., Siversson, A., Erfurth, E.M., 2009. Hypothalamic involvement predicts cardiovascular risk in adults with childhood onset craniopharyngioma on long-term GH therapy. Eur. J. Endocrinol. 161, 671–679.

Holmer, H., Popovic, V., Ekman, B., Follin, C., Siversson, A.B., Erfurth, E.M., 2011. Hypothalamic involvement and insufficient sex steroid supplementation are associated with low bone mineral density in women with childhood onset craniopharyngioma. Eur. J. Endocrinol. 165, 25–31.

Holmer, H., Pozarek, G., Wirfalt, E., Popovic, V., Ekman, B., Bjork, J., Erfurth, E.M., 2010. Reduced energy expenditure and impaired feeding-related signals but not high energy intake reinforces hypothalamic obesity in adults with childhood onset craniopharyngioma. J. Clin. Endocrinol. Metab. 95, 5395–5402.

Holsken, A., Buchfelder, M., Fahlbusch, R., Blumcke, I., Buslei, R., 2010. Tumour cell migration in adamantinomatous craniopharyngiomas is promoted by activated Wnt-signalling. Acta Neuropathol. 119, 631–639.

Honegger, J., Buchfelder, M., Fahlbusch, R., 1999. Surgical treatment of craniopharyngiomas: endocrinological results. J. Neurosurg. 90, 251–257.

Inge, T.H., Pfluger, P., Zeller, M., Rose, S.R., Burget, L., Sundararajan, S., Daniels, S.R., Tschop, M.H., 2007. Gastric bypass surgery for treatment of hypothalamic obesity after craniopharyngioma therapy. Nat. Clin. Pract. Endocrinol. Metab. 3, 606–609.

Ismail, D., O'Connell, M.A., Zacharin, M.R., 2006. Dexamphetamine use for management of obesity and hypersomnolence following hypothalamic injury. J. Pediatr. Endocrinol. Metab. 19, 129–134.

Julow, J., Lanyi, F., Hajda, M., Szeifert, G., Simkovits, M., Pasztor, E., 1989. [Intracystic instillation of yttrium 90 silicate colloid in cystic craniopharyngioma]. Orv. Hetil. 130, 1367–1368, 1371–5.

Jung, T.Y., Jung, S., Moon, K.S., Kim, I.Y., Kang, S.S., Kim, J.H., 2010. Endocrinological outcomes of pediatric craniopharyngiomas with anatomical pituitary stalk preservation: preliminary study. Pediatr. Neurosurg. 46, 205–212.

Kalapurakal, J.A., Goldman, S., Hsieh, Y.C., Tomita, T., Marymont, M.H., 2003. Clinical outcome in children with craniopharyngioma treated with primary surgery and radiotherapy deferred until relapse. Med. Pediatr. Oncol. 40, 214–218.

Karavitaki, N., Brufani, C., Warner, J.T., Adams, C.B., Richards, P., Ansorge, O., Shine, B., Turner, H.E., Wass, J.A., 2005. Craniopharyngiomas in children and adults: systematic analysis of 121 cases with long-term follow-up. Clin. Endocrinol. (Oxf) 62, 397–409.

Karavitaki, N., Cudlip, S., Adams, C.B., Wass, J.A., 2006. Craniopharyngiomas. Endocr. Rev. 27, 371–397.

Kendall-Taylor, P., Jonsson, P.J., Abs, R., Erfurth, E.M., Koltowska-Haggstrom, M., Price, D.A., Verhelst, J., 2005. The clinical, metabolic and endocrine features and the quality of life in adults with childhood-onset craniopharyngioma compared with adult-onset craniopharyngioma. Eur. J. Endocrinol. 152, 557–567.

Khafaga, Y., Jenkin, D., Kanaan, I., Hassounah, M., Al Shabanah, M., Gray, A., 1998. Craniopharyngioma in children. Int. J. Radiat. Oncol. Biol. Phys. 42, 601–606.

Kiehna, E., Mulhern, R., Li, C., Xiong, X., Merchant, T., 2006. Changes in attentional performance of children and young adults iwth localized primary brain tumors after conformal radiation therapy. J. Clin. Oncol. 24, 5283–5290.

Kim, R.J., Shah, R., Tershakovec, A.M., Zemel, B.S., Sutton, L.N., Grimberg, A., Moshang, T., 2010. Energy expenditure in obesity associated with craniopharyngioma. Childs. Nerv. Syst. 26, 913–917.

Kim, S.D., Park, J.Y., Park, J., Lee, J.B., Kim, S.H., Lim, D.J., 2007. Radiological findings following postsurgical intratumoral bleomycin injection for cystic craniopharyngioma. Clin. Neurol. Neurosurg. 109, 236–241.

Kobayashi, T., 2009. Long-term results of gamma knife radiosurgery for 100 consecutive cases of craniopharyngioma and a treatment strategy. Prog. Neurol. Surg. 22, 63–76.

Kordes, U., Flitsch, J., Hagel, C., Goebell, E., Schwarz, R., Herberhold, T., Von Bueren, A.O., Rutkowski, S., Muller, H.L., 2011. Ectopic craniopharyngioma. Klin. Padiatr. 223, 176–177.

Kortmann, R.D., 2011. Different approaches in radiation therapy of craniopharyngioma. Front. Endocrinol. (Lausanne) 2, 100.

Kreier, F., Fliers, E., Voshol, P.J., Van Eden, C.G., Havekes, L.M., Kalsbeek, A., Van Heijningen, C.L., Sluiter, A.A., Mettenleiter, T.C., Romijn, J.A., Sauerwein, H.P., Buijs, R.M., 2002. Selective parasympathetic innervation of subcutaneous and intra-abdominal fat – functional implications. J. Clin. Invest. 110, 1243–1250.

Lafay-Cousin, L., Bartels, U., Raybaud, C., Kulkarni, A.V., Guger, S., Huang, A., Bouffet, E., 2007. Neuroradiological findings of bleomycin leakage in cystic craniopharyngioma. Report of three cases. J. Neurosurg. 107, 318–323.

Larkin, S.J., Ansorge, O., 2013. Pathology and pathogenesis of craniopharyngiomas. Pituitary 16, 9–17.

Lee, M., Kalani, M.Y., Cheshier, S., Gibbs, I.C., Adler, J.R., Chang, S.D., 2008. Radiation therapy and CyberKnife radiosurgery in the management of craniopharyngiomas. Neurosurg. Focus 24, E4.

Lek, N., Prentice, P., Williams, R.M., Ong, K.K., Burke, G.A., Acerini, C.L., 2010. Risk factors for obesity in childhood survivors of suprasellar brain tumours: a retrospective study. Acta Paediatr. 99, 1522–1526.

Lin, L.L., El Naqa, I., Leonard, J.R., Park, T.S., Hollander, A.S., Michalski, J.M., Mansur, D.B., 2008. Long-term outcome in children treated for craniopharyngioma with and without radiotherapy. J. Neurosurg. Pediatr. 1, 126–130.

Liu, A.K., Bagrosky, B., Fenton, L.Z., Gaspar, L.E., Handler, M.H., Mcnatt, S.A., Foreman, N.K., 2009. Vascular abnormalities in pediatric craniopharyngioma patients treated with radiation therapy. Pediatr. Blood Cancer 52, 227–230.

Lustig, R.H., 2008. Hypothalamic obesity: causes, consequences, treatment. Pediatr. Endocrinol. Rev. 6, 220–227.

Lustig, R.H., 2011. Hypothalamic obesity after craniopharyngioma: mechanisms, diagnosis, and treatment. Front. Endocrinol. (Lausanne) 2, 60.

Lustig, R.H., Hinds, P.S., Ringwald-Smith, K., Christensen, R.K., Kaste, S.C., Schreiber, R.E., Rai, S.N., Lensing, S.Y., Wu, S., Xiong, X., 2003a. Octreotide therapy of pediatric hypothalamic obesity: a double-blind, placebo-controlled trial. J. Clin. Endocrinol. Metab. 88, 2586–2592.

Lustig, R.H., Post, S.R., Srivannaboon, K., Rose, S.R., Danish, R.K., Burghen, G.A., Xiong, X., Wu, S., Merchant, T.E., 2003b. Risk factors for the development of obesity in children surviving brain tumors. J. Clin. Endocrinol. Metab. 88, 611–616.

Luu, Q.T., Loredo, L.N., Archambeau, J.O., Yonemoto, L.T., Slater, J.M., Slater, J.D., 2006. Fractionated proton radiation treatment for pediatric craniopharyngioma: preliminary report. Cancer. J. 12, 155–159.

Mason, P.W., Krawiecki, N., Meacham, L.R., 2002. The use of dextroamphetamine to treat obesity and hyperphagia in children treated for craniopharyngioma. Arch. Pediatr. Adolesc. Med. 156, 887–892.

Matson, D.D., 1964. Craniopharyngioma. Clin. Neurosurg. 10, 14.

Matson, D.D., 1962. From Clinical Neurosurgery.

Merchant, T.E., Kiehna, E.N., Kun, L.E., Mulhern, R.K., Li, C., Xiong, X., Boop, F.A., Sanford, R.A., 2006. Phase II trial of conformal radiation therapy for pediatric patients with craniopharyngioma and correlation of surgical factors and radiation dosimetry with change in cognitive function. J. Neurosurg. 104, 94–102.

Merchant, T.E., Kiehna, E.N., Sanford, R.A., Mulhern, R.K., Thompson, S.J., Wilson, M.W., Lustig, R.H., Kun, L.E., 2002. Craniopharyngioma: the St. Jude Children's Research Hospital experience 1984–2001. Int. J. Radiat. Oncol. Biol. Phys. 53, 533–542.

Metzler-Baddeley, C., Jones, R., 2010. Brief Communication: Cognitive rehabilitation of executive functioning in a case of craniopharyngioma. Appl. Neuropsychol. 17, 299–304.

Minniti, G., Esposito, V., Amichetti, M., Enrici, R.M., 2009. The role of fractionated radiotherapy and radiosurgery in the management of patients with craniopharyngioma. Neurosurg. Rev. 32, 125–132; discussion 132.

Mokry, M., 1999. Craniopharyngiomas: A six year experience with Gamma Knife radiosurgery. Stereotact. Funct. Neurosurg. 72 (Suppl. 1), 140–149.

Mong, S., Pomeroy, S.L., Cecchin, F., Juraszek, A., Alexander, M.E., 2008. Cardiac risk after craniopharyngioma therapy. Pediatr. Neurol. 38, 256–260.

Moon, S.H., Kim, I.H., Park, S.W., Kim, I., Hong, S., Park, C.I., Wang, K.C., Cho, B.K., 2005. Early adjuvant radiotherapy toward long-term survival and better quality of life for craniopharyngiomas–a study in single institute. Childs. Nerv. Syst. 21, 799–807.

Mortini, P., Losa, M., Pozzobon, G., Barzaghi, R., Riva, M., Acerno, S., Angius, D., Weber, G., Chiumello, G., Giovanelli, M., 2011. Neurosurgical treatment of craniopharyngioma in adults and children: early and long-term results in a large case series. J. Neurosurg. 114, 1350–1359.

Muller, H.L., 2006. More or less? Treatment strategies in childhood craniopharyngioma. Childs. Nerv. Syst. 22, 156–157.

Muller, H.L., 2008. Childhood craniopharyngioma. Recent advances in diagnosis, treatment and follow-up. Horm. Res. 69, 193–202.

Muller, H.L., 2010a. Childhood craniopharyngioma – current concepts in diagnosis, therapy and follow-up. Nat. Rev. Endocrinol. 6, 609–618.

Muller, H.L., 2010b. Childhood craniopharyngioma: current controversies on management in diagnostics, treatment and follow-up. Expert. Rev. Neurother. 10, 515–524.

Muller, H.L., 2010c. Increased daytime sleepiness in patients with childhood craniopharyngioma and hypothalamic tumor involvement: review of the literature and perspectives. Int. J. Endocrinol. 2010, 519607.

Muller, H.L., 2011a. Consequences of craniopharyngioma surgery in children. J. Clin. Endocrinol. Metab. 96, 1981–1991.

Muller, H.L., 2011b. Diagnostics, treatment, and follow-up in craniopharyngioma. Front. Endocrinol. (Lausanne) 2, 70.

Muller, H.L., 2012a. Childhood craniopharyngioma. Pituitary 16, 56–67.

Muller, H.L., 2012b. Craniopharyngioma – a childhood and adult disease with challenging characteristics. Front. Endocrinol. (Lausanne) 3, 80.

Muller, H.L., 2013a. Childhood craniopharyngioma. Pituitary 16, 56–67.

Muller, H.L., 2013b. Paediatrics: Surgical strategy and quality of life in craniopharyngioma. Nat. Rev. Endocrinol 9, 447–449.

Müller, H.L., 2014. Craniopharyngioma. Endocr. Rev. 35, 513–543.

Muller, H.L., Albanese, A., Calaminus, G., Hargrave, D., Garre, M.L., Gebhardt, U., Saran, F., Sorensen, N., Spoudeas, H.A., 2006a. Consensus and perspectives on treatment strategies in childhood craniopharyngioma: results of a meeting of the Craniopharyngioma Study Group (SIOP), Genova, 2004. J. Pediatr. Endocrinol. Metab. 19 (Suppl. 1), 453–454.

Muller, H.L., Bruhnken, G., Emser, A., Faldum, A., Etavard-Gorris, N., Gebhardt, U., Kolb, R., Sorensen, N., 2005a. Longitudinal study on quality of life in 102 survivors of childhood craniopharyngioma. Childs. Nerv. Syst. 21, 975–980.

Muller, H.L., Bueb, K., Bartels, U., Roth, C., Harz, K., Graf, N., Korinthenberg, R., Bettendorf, M., Kuhl, J., Gutjahr, P., Sorensen, N., Calaminus, G., 2001. Obesity after childhood craniopharyngioma – German multicenter study on pre-operative risk factors and quality of life. Klin. Padiatr. 213, 244–249.

Muller, H.L., Emser, A., Faldum, A., Bruhnken, G., Etavard-Gorris, N., Gebhardt, U., Oeverink, R., Kolb, R., Sorensen, N., 2004a. Longitudinal study on growth and body mass index before and after diagnosis of childhood craniopharyngioma. J. Clin. Endocrinol. Metab. 89, 3298–3305.

Muller, H.L., Faldum, A., Etavard-Gorris, N., Gebhardt, U., Oeverink, R., Kolb, R., Sorensen, N., 2003a. Functional capacity, obesity and hypothalamic involvement: cross-sectional study on 212 patients with childhood craniopharyngioma. Klin. Padiatr. 215, 310–314.

Muller, H.L., Gebhardt, U., Etavard-Gorris, N., Kolb, R., Warmuth-Metz, M., Sorensen, N., 2005b. Current strategies in diagnostics and endocrine treatment of patients with childhood craniopharyngioma during follow-up – recommendations in KRANIOPHARYNGEOM 2000. Onkologie 28, 150–156.

Muller, H.L., Gebhardt, U., Etavard-Gorris, N., Korenke, E., Warmuth-Metz, M., Kolb, R., Sorensen, N., Calaminus, G., 2004b. Prognosis and sequela in patients with childhood craniopharyngioma – results of HIT-ENDO and update on KRANIOPHARYNGEOM 2000. Klin. Padiatr. 216, 343–348.

Muller, H.L., Gebhardt, U., Faldum, A., Warmuth-Metz, M., Pietsch, T., Pohl, F., Calaminus, G., Sorensen, N., 2012. Xanthogranuloma, Rathke's cyst, and childhood craniopharyngioma: results of prospective multinational studies of children and adolescents with rare sellar malformations. J. Clin. Endocrinol. Metab 97, 3935–3943.

Muller, H.L., Gebhardt, U., Maroske, J., Hanisch, E., 2011a. Long-term follow-up of morbidly obese patients with childhood craniopharyngioma after laparoscopic adjustable gastric banding (LAGB). Klin. Padiatr. 223, 372–373.

Muller, H.L., Gebhardt, U., Pohl, F., Flentje, M., Emser, A., Warmuth-Metz, M., Kolb, R., Calaminus, G., Sorensen, N., 2006b. Relapse pattern after complete resection and early progression after incomplete resection of childhood craniopharyngioma. Klin. Padiatr. 218, 315–320.

Muller, H.L., Gebhardt, U., Schroder, S., Pohl, F., Kortmann, R.D., Faldum, A., Zwiener, I., Warmuth-Metz, M., Pietsch, T., Calaminus, G., Kolb, R., Wiegand, C., Sorensen, N., 2010. Analyses of treatment variables for patients with childhood craniopharyngioma–results of the multicenter prospective trial KRANIOPHARYNGEOM 2000 after three years of follow-up. Horm. Res. Paediatr. 73, 175–180.

Muller, H.L., Gebhardt, U., Teske, C., Faldum, A., Zwiener, I., Warmuth-Metz, M., Pietsch, T., Pohl, F., Sorensen, N., Calaminus, G., 2011b. Post-operative hypothalamic lesions and obesity in childhood craniopharyngioma: results of the multinational prospective trial KRANIOPHARYNGEOM 2000 after three-year follow-up. Eur. J. Endocrinol. 165, 17–24.

Muller, H.L., Gebhardt, U., Wessel, V., Schroder, S., Kolb, R., Sorensen, N., Maroske, J., Hanisch, E., 2007. First experiences with laparoscopic adjustable gastric banding (LAGB) in the treatment of patients with childhood craniopharyngioma and morbid obesity. Klin. Padiatr. 219, 323–325.

Muller, H.L., Handwerker, G., Gebhardt, U., Faldum, A., Emser, A., Kolb, R., Sorensen, N., 2006c. Melatonin treatment in obese patients with childhood craniopharyngioma and increased daytime sleepiness. Cancer. Causes. Control. 17, 583–589.

Muller, H.L., Handwerker, G., Wollny, B., Faldum, A., Sorensen, N., 2002. Melatonin secretion and increased daytime sleepiness in childhood craniopharyngioma patients. J. Clin. Endocrinol. Metab. 87, 3993–3996.

Muller, H.L., Heinrich, M., Bueb, K., Etavard-Gorris, N., Gebhardt, U., Kolb, R., Sorensen, N., 2003b. Peri-operative dexamethasone treatment in childhood craniopharyngioma – influence on short-term and long-term weight gain. Exp. Clin. Endocrinol. Diabetes 111, 330–334.

Muller, H.L., Muller-Stover, S., Gebhardt, U., Kolb, R., Sorensen, N., Handwerker, G., 2006d. Secondary narcolepsy may be a causative factor of increased daytime sleepiness in obese childhood craniopharyngioma patients. J. Pediatr. Endocrinol. Metab. 19 (Suppl. 1), 423–429.

Muller, H.L., Schneider, P., Bueb, K., Etavard-Gorris, N., Gebhardt, U., Kolb, R., Sorensen, N., 2003c. Volumetric bone mineral density in patients with childhood craniopharyngioma. Exp. Clin. Endocrinol. Diabetes 111, 168–173.

Muller-Scholden, J., Lehrnbecher, T., Muller, H.L., Bensch, J., Hengen, R.H., Sorensen, N., Stockhausen, H.B., 2000. Radical surgery in a neonate with craniopharyngioma. report of a case. Pediatr. Neurosurg. 33, 265–269.

Nielsen, E.H., Feldt-Rasmussen, U., Poulsgaard, L., Kristensen, L.O., Astrup, J., Jorgensen, J.O., Bjerre, P., Andersen, M., Andersen, C., Jorgensen, J., Lindholm, J., Laurberg, P., 2011. Incidence of craniopharyngioma in Denmark (n = 189) and estimated world incidence of craniopharyngioma in children and adults. J. Neurooncol. 104, 755–763.

O'Gorman, C.S., Simoneau-Roy, J., Pencharz, P., Macfarlane, J., Maclusky, I., Narang, I., Adeli, K., Daneman, D., Hamilton, J., 2010. Sleep-disordered breathing is increased in obese adolescents with craniopharyngioma compared with obese controls. J. Clin. Endocrinol. Metab. 95, 2211–2218.

Ondruch, A., Maryniak, A., Kropiwnicki, T., Roszkowski, M., Daszkiewicz, P., 2011. Cognitive and social functioning in children and adolescents after the removal of craniopharyngioma. Child's. Nervous. System. 27, 391–397.

Ozyurt, J., Lorenzen, A., Gebhardt, U., Warmuth-Metz, M., Müller, H.L., Thiel, C.M., 2014a. Remote effects of hypothalamic lesions in the prefrontal cortex of craniopharygioma patients. Neurobiol Learn Mem. 111, 71–80.

Ozyurt, J., Thiel, C.M., Lorenzen, A., Gebhardt, U., Calaminus, G., Warmuth-Metz, M., Müller, H.L., 2014b. Neuropsychological outcome in patients with childhood craniopharyngioma and hypothalamic involvement. J Pediatr. 164, 876–881.

Pemberton, L.S., Dougal, M., Magee, B., Gattamaneni, H.R., 2005. Experience of external beam radiotherapy given adjuvantly or at relapse following surgery for craniopharyngioma. Radiother. Oncol. 77, 99–104.

Pereira, A.M., Schmid, E.M., Schutte, P.J., Voormolen, J.H., Biermasz, N.R., Van Thiel, S.W., Corssmit, E.P., Smit, J.W., Roelfsema, F., Romijn, J.A., 2005. High prevalence of long-term cardiovascular, neurological and psychosocial morbidity after treatment for craniopharyngioma. Clin. Endocrinol. (Oxf) 62, 197–204.

Phillip, M., Moran, O., Lazar, L., 2002. Growth without growth hormone. J. Pediatr. Endocrinol. Metab. 15 (Suppl. 5), 1267–1272.

Poretti, A., Grotzer, M.A., Ribi, K., Schonle, E., Boltshauser, E., 2004. Outcome of craniopharyngioma in children: long-term complications and quality of life. Dev. Med. Child. Neurol. 46, 220–229.

Puget, S., 2012. Treatment strategies in childhood craniopharyngioma. Front. Endocrinol. (Lausanne) 3, 64.

Puget, S., Garnett, M., Wray, A., Grill, J., Habrand, J.L., Bodaert, N., Zerah, M., Bezerra, M., Renier, D., Pierre-Kahn, A., Sainte-Rose, C., 2007. Pediatric craniopharyngiomas: classification and treatment according to the degree of hypothalamic involvement. J. Neurosurg. 106, 3–12.

Puget, S., Grill, J., Habrand, J.L., Sainte-Rose, C., 2006. Multimodal treatment of craniopharyngioma: defining a risk-adapted strategy. J. Pediatr. Endocrinol. Metab. 19 (Suppl. 1), 367–370.

Rajan, B., Ashley, S., Gorman, C., Jose, C.C., Horwich, A., Bloom, H.J., Marsh, H., Brada, M., 1993. Craniopharyngioma – long-term results following limited surgery and radiotherapy. Radiother. Oncol. 26, 1–10.

Regine, W.F., Kramer, S., 1992. Pediatric craniopharyngiomas: long term results of combined treatment with surgery and radiation. Int. J. Radiat. Oncol. Biol. Phys. 24, 611–617.

Regine, W.F., Mohiuddin, M., Kramer, S., 1993. Long-term results of pediatric and adult craniopharyngiomas treated with combined surgery and radiation. Radiother. Oncol. 27, 13–21.

Riva, D., Pantaleoni, C., Devoti, M., Saletti, V., Nichelli, F., Giorgi, C., 1998. Late neuropsychological and behavioral outcome of children surgically treated for craniopharyngioma. Child's. Nerv. Syst. 14, 179–184.

Roth, C., Wilken, B., Hanefeld, F., Schroter, W., Leonhardt, U., 1998. Hyperphagia in children with craniopharyngioma is associated with hyperleptinaemia and a failure in the downregulation of appetite. Eur. J. Endocrinol. 138, 89–91.

Roth, C.L., 2011. Hypothalamic obesity in patients with craniopharyngioma: profound changes of several weight regulatory circuits. Front. Endocrinol. (Lausanne) 2, 49.

Roth, C.L., Aylward, E., Liang, O., Kleinhans, N.M., Pauley, G., Schur, E.A., 2012. Functional neuroimaging in craniopharyngioma: a useful tool to better understand hypothalamic obesity? Obes. Facts 5, 243–253.

Roth, C.L., Enriori, P.J., Gebhardt, U., Hinney, A., Muller, H.L., Hebebrand, J., Reinehr, T., Cowley, M.A., 2010. Changes of peripheral alpha-melanocyte-stimulating hormone in childhood obesity. Metabolism 59, 186–194.

Roth, C.L., Gebhardt, U., Muller, H.L., 2011. Appetite-regulating hormone changes in patients with craniopharyngioma. Obesity (Silver Spring) 19, 36–42.

Roth, C.L., Hunneman, D.H., Gebhardt, U., Stoffel-Wagner, B., Reinehr, T., Muller, H.L., 2007. Reduced sympathetic metabolites in urine of obese patients with craniopharyngioma. Pediatr. Res. 61, 496–501.

Rottembourg, D., O'Gorman, C.S., Urbach, S., Garneau, P.Y., Langer, J.C., Van Vliet, G., Hamilton, J., Huot, C., 2009. Outcome after bariatric surgery in two adolescents with hypothalamic obesity following treatment of craniopharyngioma. J. Pediatr. Endocrinol. Metab. 22, 867–872.

Rushing, E.J., Giangaspero, F., Paulus, W., Burger, P.C., 2007. Craniopharyngioma. In: Louis, D.N., Ohgaki, H., Wiestler, O.D., Webster, K.C. (Eds.), WHO Classification of Tumours of the Central Nervous System, third ed. World Health Organization Press, Geneva, Switzerland, pp. 238–240.

Sands, S., Milner, J., Goldberg, J., Mukhi, V., Moliterno, J., Maxfield, C., Wisoff, J., 2005. Quality of life and behavioral follow-up study of pediatric survivors of cranipharyngioma. J. Neurosurg. (Pediatrics) 103, 302–311.

Sanford, R.A., 1994. Craniopharyngioma: results of survey of the American Society of Pediatric Neurosurgery. Pediatr. Neurosurg. 21 (Suppl. 1), 39–43.

Schofl, C., Schleth, A., Berger, D., Terkamp, C., Von Zur Muhlen, A., Brabant, G., 2002. Sympathoadrenal counterregulation in patients with hypothalamic craniopharyngioma. J. Clin. Endocrinol. Metab. 87, 624–629.

Schubert, T., Trippel, M., Tacke, U., Van Velthoven, V., Gumpp, V., Bartelt, S., Ostertag, C., Nikkhah, G., 2009. Neurosurgical treatment strategies in childhood craniopharyngiomas: is less more? Childs. Nerv. Syst. 25, 1419–1427.

Schultes, B., Ernst, B., Schmid, F., Thurnheer, M., 2009. Distal gastric bypass surgery for the treatment of hypothalamic obesity after childhood craniopharyngioma. Eur. J. Endocrinol. 161, 201–206.

Scott, R.M., Hetelekidis, S., Barnes, P.D., Goumnerova, L., Tarbell, N.J., 1994. Surgery, radiation, and combination therapy in the treatment of childhood craniopharyngioma – a 20-year experience. Pediatr. Neurosurg. 21 (Suppl. 1), 75–81.

Shaikh, M.G., Grundy, R.G., Kirk, J.M., 2008. Reductions in basal metabolic rate and physical activity contribute to hypothalamic obesity. J. Clin. Endocrinol. Metab. 93, 2588–2593.

Sherlock, M., Ayuk, J., Tomlinson, J.W., Toogood, A.A., Aragon-Alonso, A., Sheppard, M.C., Bates, A.S., Stewart, P.M., 2010. Mortality in patients with pituitary disease. Endocr. Rev. 31, 301–342.

Srinivasan, S., Ogle, G.D., Garnett, S.P., Briody, J.N., Lee, J.W., Cowell, C.T., 2004. Features of the metabolic syndrome after childhood craniopharyngioma. J. Clin. Endocrinol. Metab. 89, 81–86.

Steno, J., Bizik, I., Steno, A., Matejcik, V., 2011. Craniopharyngiomas in children: how radical should the surgeon be? Childs. Nerv. Syst. 27, 41–54.

Stripp, D.C., Maity, A., Janss, A.J., Belasco, J.B., Tochner, Z.A., Goldwein, J.W., Moshang, T., Rorke, L.B., Phillips, P.C., Sutton, L.N., Shu, H.K., 2004. Surgery with or without radiation therapy in the management of craniopharyngiomas in children and young adults. Int. J. Radiat. Oncol. Biol. Phys. 58, 714–720.

Sung, D.I., 1982. Suprasellar tumors in children: a review of clinical manifestations and managements. Cancer 50, 1420–1425.

Swaab, D.F., Gooren, L.J., Hofman, M.A., 1992. The human hypothalamus in relation to gender and sexual orientation. Prog. Brain. Res. 93, 205–217; discussion 217–219.

Szeifert, G.T., Balint, K., Sipos, L., Sarker, M.H., Czirjak, S., Julow, J., 2007. Pathological findings in cystic craniopharyngiomas after stereotactic intracavitary irradiation with yttrium-90 isotope. Prog. Neurol. Surg. 20, 297–302.

Tomita, T., Bowman, R.M., 2005. Craniopharyngiomas in children: surgical experience at Children's Memorial Hospital. Childs. Nerv. Syst. 21, 729–746.

Trivin, C., Busiah, K., Mahlaoui, N., Recasens, C., Souberbielle, J.C., Zerah, M., Sainte-Rose, C., Brauner, R., 2009. Childhood craniopharyngioma: greater hypothalamic involvement before surgery is associated with higher homeostasis model insulin resistance index. BMC. Pediatr. 9, 24.

Van Effenterre, R., Boch, A.L., 2002. Craniopharyngioma in adults and children: a study of 122 surgical cases. J. Neurosurg. 97, 3–11.

Vinchon, M., Weill, J., Delestret, I., Dhellemmes, P., 2009. Craniopharyngioma and hypothalamic obesity in children. Childs. Nerv. Syst. 25, 347–352.

Visser, J., Hukin, J., Sargent, M., Steinbok, P., Goddard, K., Fryer, C., 2010. Late mortality in pediatric patients with craniopharyngioma. J. Neurooncol. 100, 105–111.

Warmuth-Metz, M., Gnekow, A.K., Muller, H., Solymosi, L., 2004. Differential diagnosis of suprasellar tumors in children. Klin. Padiatr. 216, 323–330.

Winkfield, K.M., Linsenmeier, C., Yock, T.I., Grant, P.E., Yeap, B.Y., Butler, W.E., Tarbell, N.J., 2009. Surveillance of craniopharyngioma cyst growth in children treated with proton radiotherapy. Int. J. Radiat. Oncol. Biol. Phys. 73, 716–721.

Wisoff, J.H., 2008. Craniopharyngioma. J. Neurosurg. Pediatr. 1, 124–125; discussion 125.

Zoicas, F., Schofl, C., 2012. Craniopharyngioma in adults. Front. Endocrinol. (Lausanne) 3, 46.

CHAPTER

28

Surgery of Craniopharyngiomas in Children

James A. Balogun, James T. Rutka

Division of Neurosurgery, the Hospital for Sick Children, The University of Toronto, Toronto, Canada

"The tumors are difficult, dangerous and at times impossible of complete extirpation." **Walter Dandy, 1945**

INTRODUCTION

The term craniopharyngioma was coined by Harvey Cushing, the father of modern neurosurgery, in 1932. He stated that "this admittedly cumbersome term has been employed for want of something more brief to include the kaleidoscopic tumors, solid and cystic, which take origin from epithelial rests ascribable to an imperfect closure of the hypophysis or craniopharyngeal duct" (Cushing, 1932). This term serves to unify the numerous terminologies that had been employed by previous workers (May et al., 2006).

Craniopharyngiomas are relatively rare, benign tumors, which tend to occur more commonly in children, comprising 10% of pediatric brain tumors diagnosed annually in the United States (Cook and Rutka, 2009). These tumors arise from remnants of the Rathke's pouch. They are mainly suprasellar in location but can occur anywhere along the track of an incompletely involuted hypophyseal-pharyngeal duct (Ohmori et al., 2007). The close proximity of these tumors to critical neurovascular structures such as the optic nerves/chiasm, hypothalamus, and vessels of the circle of Willis influence the clinical presentations of the affected children and also pose a challenge to their treatment. The untreated tumor in children can result in a syndrome of optic, pituitary, and hypothalamic dysfunction with a tendency to blindness, and affectation of growth and development. Obstructive hydrocephalus may result from the extension of the tumor into the third ventricle, causing raised intracranial pressure and ultimately death in some cases. The treatment of craniopharyngiomas remains controversial to this day. There are many opinions regarding the choice of the appropriate treatment that is curative and associated with the least morbidities. The challenge of care

Craniopharyngiomas
http://dx.doi.org/10.1016/B978-0-12-416706-3.00028-3

is further compounded by the high risk of recurrence even in radically resected tumors, or progression in residual tumors. It is a disease that continues to evoke passion and lively debate amongst clinicians.

INCIDENCE AND EPIDEMIOLOGY

Craniopharyngiomas consist of about 1–3% of intracranial tumors in children (Bunin et al., 1998; Haupt et al., 2006). There is a bimodal distribution by age, with peaks between the ages of 5 and 11 years, and 50 and 74 years. The incidence in North America is 0.13 per 100,000 per year (Bunin et al., 1998). A Danish study estimated a similar incidence of 0.14 (Nielsen et al., 2011) in children though a slightly higher incidence of 0.38 per 100,000 was observed in an Asian childhood population (Makino et al., 2010). There are suggestions that the incidence of craniopharyngiomas may be higher in Africa, but there is no conclusive evidence to corroborate this due to lack of detailed epidemiological studies (Bunin et al., 1998; Stagno et al., 2014). There is no gender predilection.

PATHOLOGY

The development of craniopharyngiomas is hinged on an understanding of the embryological formation of the hypophyseal-pharyngeal duct, which begins in the fourth week of gestation, when the neurohypophysis and buccopharyngeal membrane come into contact. The neurohypophysis arises from an outpouching at the junction of the diencephalon and mesencephalon, which forms a tubular structure as the neural tube flexes. The buccopharyngeal membrane forms an ectodermal outpouching, Rathke's pouch, that projects to the neurohypophysis. These two structures fuse at gestational age 8 weeks, forming the tubular structure that goes on to collapse into the solid anterior infundibulum.

There are two distinct histological types of craniopharyngiomas, the adamantinomatous and papillary types. A third variant, referred to as mixed or transitional and containing features of both has also been described (Miller, 1994; Ohmori et al., 2007). The adamantinomatous variant is the most common variant in children, while the papillary variant is almost exclusively a disease of adults, although a few cases have been reported in children (Adamson et al., 1990; Miller, 1994; Yoshimoto et al., 2004; Cook and Rutka, 2009; Pekmezci et al., 2010). The pathogenesis of both types is based mainly on the incomplete involution of the hypophyseal-pharyngeal duct, even though each of the types has a peculiar underlying mechanism. There are two theories that have been proposed to explain the origin of each of the histological variants. The embryogenetic theory suggests that adamantinomatous craniopharyngiomas arise from epithelial remnants of the craniopharyngeal duct or Rathke's pouch that themselves were derived from parts of the stomadeum destined to form tooth primordium, hence its similarity to dental tissue (Prabhu and Brown, 2005). The metaplastic theory attributes the more squamous papillary tumors to metaplasia of squamous epithelial cell rests that are remnants of that portion of the stomadeum that is destined to become the buccal mucosa.

The adamantinomatous craniopharyngioma which is the more common variant in childhood, on macroscopic examination, has cysts containing a turbid, yellow-brown, cholesterol-rich fluid with solid components that may contain calcific components. On microscopy it consists of clusters of organized palisading columnar cells that form whorls, sheets, and irregular shapes around loosely arranged stellate epithelial cells. It usually produces a gliotic capsule at the tumor–brain interface with accumulation of Rosenthal fibers. This is in contrast with the papillary variant, which is usually found in adults and has a low propensity for cyst formation which when present contains less turbid fluid and cholesterol. Calcification is also uncommon. The papillary craniopharyngioma has a well-differentiated squamous epithelium arranged in pseudopapillae or papillae around a vascular core (Adamson et al., 1990; Miller, 1994; Cook and Rutka, 2009).

There is no conclusive evidence to support genetic alterations in craniopharyngiomas that can serve as reliable molecular markers in craniopharyngiomas (Pettorini et al., 2010; Hussain et al., 2013). While Reinstein et al. documented nonrandom genetic alterations and possibly activation of oncogenes located in defined chromosomal regions (Rienstein et al., 2003), Yashimoto and his co-workers posit that the identified genomic alterations in adamantinomatous craniopharyngiomas do not contribute to tumorigenesis (Yoshimoto et al., 2004).

CLASSIFICATION AND CLINICAL PRESENTATION

Classification

The classification of craniopharyngiomas has been evolving over the past decades, because of its importance in predicting clinical presentation by lesion location and growth pattern, as well as the critical role in surgical planning. An initial classification by Hoffman et al. which related the lesion to the chiasm accounted for four groups:

1. Sellar craniopharyngioma confined to the sella or protruding only a short distance above the diaphragma.
2. Prechiasmatic craniopharyngioma growing forward and pushing the optic chiasm and anterior cerebral arteries superior and posterior.
3. Retrochiasmatic craniopharyngioma displacing the optic chiasm anterior and growing back into the third ventricle.
4. Giant craniopharyngioma with varying growth patterns (Hoffman, 1994).

Wang and coworkers proposed a revision of this classification using the diaphragm as a reference: subdiaphragmatic and supradiaphragmatic craniopharyngiomas with further subgrouping of the subdiaphragmatic lesions into those with or without competent diaphragma sellae (Wang et al., 2002).

The evolving use of the endoscopic approaches for the treatment of craniopharyngiomas has led to further modifying schemes. Kassam et al. proposed a classification scheme based on the infundibulum using the endoscopic approach that divides tumors according to their suprasellar extension: Type I is preinfundibular; Type II is transinfundibular (extending into the stalk); Type III is retroinfundibular, extending behind the gland and stalk, and has two subdivisions (IIIa, extending into the third ventricle; and IIIb, extending into the interpeduncular cistern); and Type IV is isolated to the third ventricle and/or optic recess (Kassam et al., 2008).

The continuous concern regarding post-operative morbidities, particularly in the pediatric age group, led to a classification based on the involvement of the hypothalamus by Puget et al.: Grade 0, no hypothalamic involvement; Grade 1, the tumor abutting or displacing the hypothalamus; and Grade 2, hypothalamic involvement (the hypothalamus is no longer identifiable) (Puget et al., 2007).

Clinical Presentation

Craniopharyngioma can present in one of several clinical syndromes on the basis of its origin and growth pattern. Children tend to present with a higher proportion of endocrine dysfunction, insidious and progressive visual loss in the younger age groups, non-specific symptoms from raised intracranial pressure, and papilloedema. This is in contradistinction to adults who more uniformly have visual symptoms (Banna, 1973; Banna et al., 1973; Carmel et al., 1982). The diagnosis is often made late, necessitating a high index of suspicion in children (Muller, 2013). The clinical presentation in children can be subdivided into five categories:

i) **Endocrine Dysfunction**: Children can present with panhypopituitarism or selective pituitary hormone deficiency, due to compression or invasion of the pituitary gland and infundibulum. They can present with growth disorders, such as short stature. Disorders of growth rate can manifest as early as 12 months of age (Kalina et al., 2009; Muller, 2013). Older children may also present with a delay in onset of puberty which, aside from hypopituitarism, may be influenced by increased levels of serum prolactin resulting in amenorrhea/galactorrhea in the female patients. Diabetes insipidus (DI) may be found in about 9–22% of patients (Sklar, 1994; Karavitaki et al., 2005; Muller, 2008). GH deficiency is particularly prevalent in children with craniopharyngiomas, sometimes found in 100% of presenting children (Sklar, 1994; Karavitaki et al., 2005; Qi et al., 2012). However it should be noted that some children may have normal growth despite a low plasma GH, a poorly understood phenomenon of "growth without GH" (Kalina et al., 2009). Older female patients may present with infertility due to increased levels of serum prolactin. Baseline measurements of all the hypothalamic–pituitary axis hormones should be obtained and response of the hypothalamic–pituitary axis to intravenously administered stimulators should be undertaken pre-operatively and followed post-operatively (DeVile et al., 1996; Hopper et al., 2006).

ii) **Visual Disturbance**: Children can present with visual complaints that include decreased visual acuity, visual field deficits (commonly bitemporal hemianopia), and optic atrophy, present in 37–70% of children (Banna et al., 1973; Kennedy and Smith, 1975; Carmel et al., 1982; Karavitaki et al., 2005). It should be noted that although ophthalmological disturbances are common in children, they are usually not the main presenting features, because children do not complain of a mild or unilateral reduction in visual acuity (Defoort-Dhellemmes et al., 2006). The chances of reversing the visual symptoms following decompression are higher in children and this may be due to a restoration of axoplasmic flow, and remyelination of the visual fibers (Stark et al., 1999).

iii) **Hypothalamic Dysfunction**: The involvement of the hypothalamus may result in a hypothalamic obesity syndrome which can occur pre-operatively, but is more often pronounced post-operatively as a surgical morbidity. The syndrome is characterized by intractable weight gain that is unresponsive to diet or exercise, and may be associated with somnolence, rage, hypogonadism, and hyperphagia. The substrates for this syndrome are thought to be the ventromedial and paraventricular nuclei of the hypothalamus (Pierre-Kahn et al., 2005; Rosenfeld et al., 2014).

iv) **Increased Intracranial Pressure (ICP)**: Symptoms of raised ICP, resulting from obstructive hydrocephalus, such as headache, nausea and vomiting, and papilloedema occur more in children than in adults (Weiner et al., 1994; Karavitaki et al., 2005). This may be due to larger tumors with or without huge cystic components (Karavitaki et al., 2005; Cook and Rutka, 2009).

v) **Disturbance in Behavior or Mentation**: The affectation of the frontal and temporal lobes indirectly by pressure effect/hydrocephalus or directly by tumor invasion may lead to altered cognition or behavior. Psychiatric symptoms may occur in about 10% of children.

Acute clinical deterioration occurs more in children than adults and may also be related to tumors with calcification (Nielsen et al., 2013). There are very few reports of the rare occurrence of spontaneous intraventricular rupture of a cystic craniopharyngioma in children (Kumar et al., 2010). This event can produce headache, fever, nuchal rigidity, and obtundation secondary to chemical meningitis with resultant acute deterioration.

STAGING

The staging of craniopharyngioma in children is a vital step that helps to define management plans for an optimum result and minimal morbidity. Staging must be thorough and set the course for the multi-disciplinary management of this disease.

Endocrine Workup

The prevalence of biochemical abnormalities in children is high, at 80–90% of patients. The importance of these abnormalities to the growth and attainment of puberty in children makes this essential to recognize (Sklar, 1994). A full panel of the hypothalamic-pituitary hormones including growth hormone (GH), insulin growth factor-1 (IGF-1), luteinizing hormone/follicle stimulating hormone (LH/FSH), adrenocorticotrophic hormone (ACTH), thyroid stimulating hormone (TSH), triiodothyronine (T3), thyroxine (T4), and prolactin should be obtained. Evaluation for DI should also be included in the workup, with a detailed history of urinary output and thirst. The serum sodium, osmolality and urine sodium, osmolality, and specific gravity should also be measured.

Neuroimaging

Although now fallen out of favor, plain radiographs of the skull as the initial modality of evaluation can reveal enlargement and/or destruction of the sella, erosion of the clinoids and the dorsum sella, as well as calcification associated with the tumor. Splayed sutures and a copper beaten appearance of the inner table of the calvarium may also suggest raised intracranial pressure from hydrocephalus (Harwood-Nash, 1994).

Computerized tomography (CT) scanning is particularly useful for demonstrating tumor calcification in almost 100% of pediatric craniopharyngiomas (Figure 28.1)

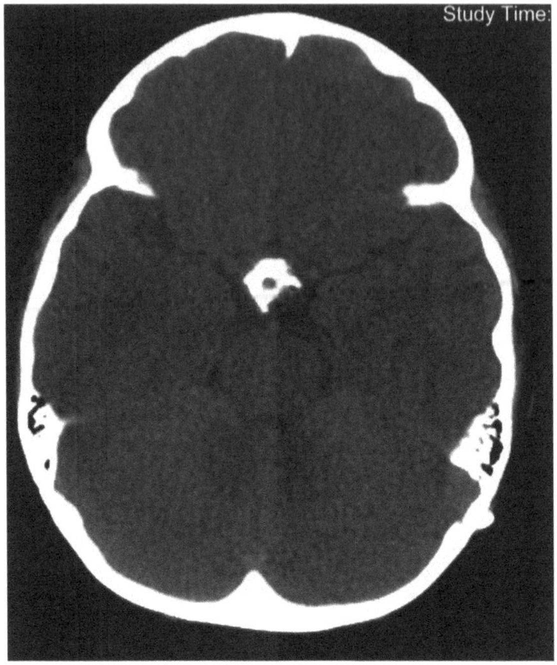

FIGURE 28.1 Axial CT of an 8-year-old male who presented with headaches, vomiting, and papilloedema. CT shows calcified suprasellar lesion.

(Harwood-Nash, 1994; Hald et al., 1995; Pekmezci et al., 2010). A contrast-enhanced CT will reveal enhancement of the solid portions and the cyst wall. Hydrocephalus can be effectively demonstrated on CT in patients presenting with acute deterioration. Coronal and sagittal reconstructions of the skull base and sella demonstrate the secondary skull bony changes better than plain radiographs. The relationship of the anterior circulation vasculature, particularly internal carotid and anterior cerebral arteries, to the tumor, is elucidated with CT angiography (Cook and Rutka, 2009).

Magnetic resonance imaging (MRI) is the imaging modality of choice. A combination of its sequences in multiple planes provides a detailed anatomy of the tumor and its relationship to the surrounding neurovascular structures, and aids in surgical planning. Gadolinium administration reveals enhancement of nodular components of the tumor and cystic walls (Figure 28.2). Cystic components are found in 97–98.9% of pediatric craniopharyngiomas (Zhang et al., 2002; Cohen et al., 2013). They are hyperintense on both T1 and T2 images, and the T2 images can also delineate the cyst wall from ventricle (Harwood-Nash, 1994; Cook and Rutka, 2009). MR angiography is also a useful tool in evaluating the relationship between the tumor and neurovasculature.

MANAGEMENT

Craniopharyngiomas present a unique challenge to management due to the diversity in clinical presentation, morphology, and location that can result in significant morbidity and mortality. This complexity therefore necessitates a multi-disciplinary approach that will

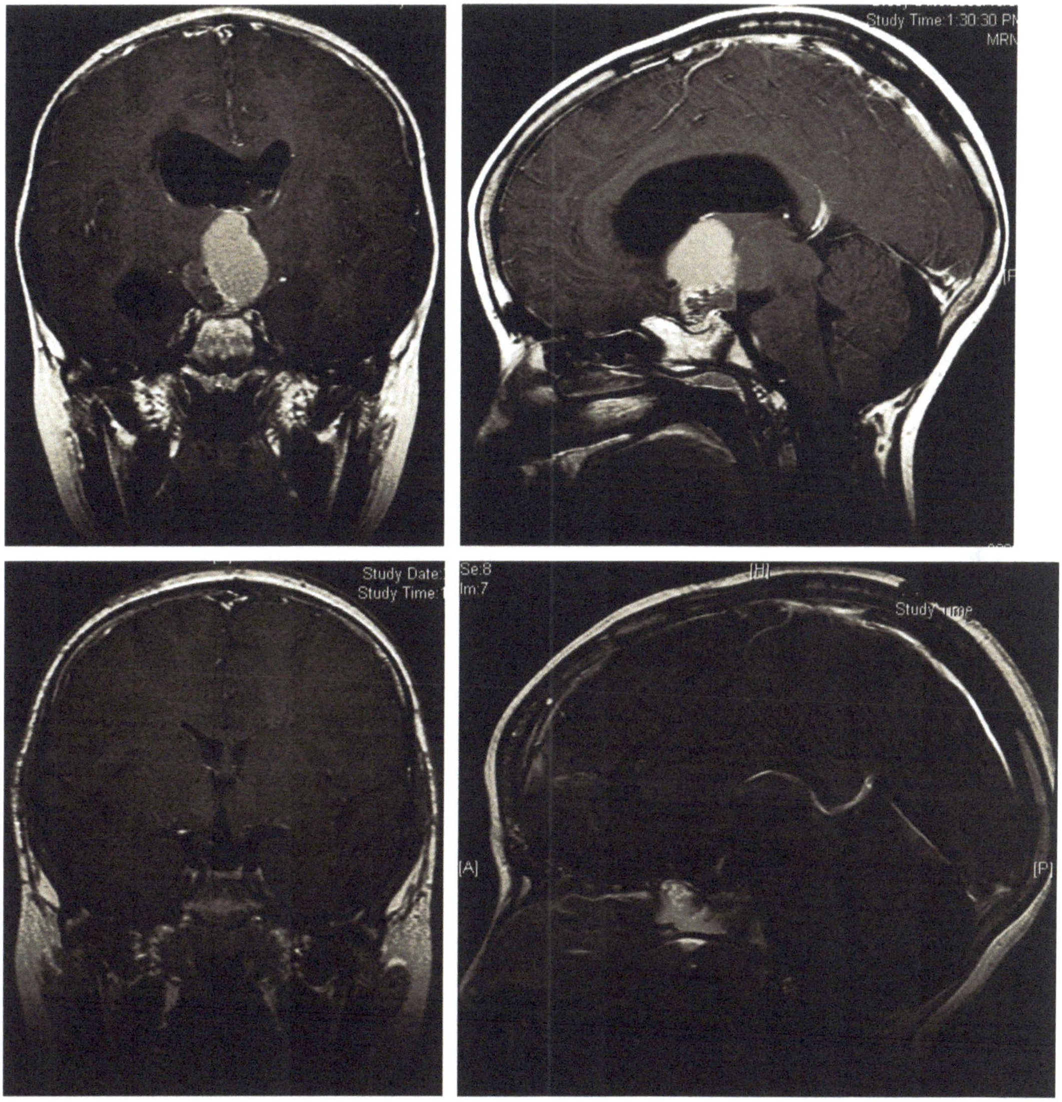

FIGURE 28.2 **A 10-year-old girl, with headaches, vomiting, and blurred vision.** Top left and right: Pre-operative coronal and sagittal MRI showing a heterogeneous lesion with solid and cystic components with a retrochiasmatic extension. The lesion fills the third ventricle and is obstructing the foramen of Monro causing hydrocephalus. Bottom left and right: Post-operative coronal and sagittal MRI showing complete resection of the lesion through a subfrontal approach.

include the neurosurgeon, neuro-ophthalmologist, neuro-endocrinologist, medical neuro-oncologist, radiation oncologist, and neuro-psychologist. Treatment should be individualized. Optimum therapy that will result in tumor control with minimal morbidity should be pursued.

Full ophthalmological assessment must be undertaken at diagnosis to document visual acuity and visual fields as well as the presence of papilloedema and optic atrophy.

Children with craniopharyngiomas should ideally have pre-operative neuropsychological testing to assess cognition and memory which can be compared to scores in the post-operative period.

The evaluation of the initial endocrinological status must be extensive and deficits corrected. ACTH deficiency, thyroid hormone deficiency, and DI have been shown to increase the intra-operative and post-operative morbidity. All patients should be assumed to be ACTH deficient and may require a stress dose of hydrocortisone. This should include patients not deficient pre-operatively, as they may develop ACTH deficiency during surgery. Additional steroid coverage is not required for patients already receiving dexamethasone for purposes such as treatment of vasogenic edema (Sklar, 1994; Halac and Zimmerman, 2005; Cook and Rutka, 2009). Hypothyroidism can manifest acutely during the early post-operative period, it is therefore important to recognize it pre-operatively and to initiate replacement therapy. When present, DI should be managed by adequate water and electrolyte balance, which may necessitate the use of synthetic vasopressin. However this abnormality is more commonly seen in the post-operative period.

Significant numbers of children present with hydrocephalus (Weiner et al., 1994; Karavitaki et al., 2005; Nielsen et al., 2013). Decompression of the ventricular pathway with resolution of the hydrocephalus is usually achieved with a gross total tumor resection or a subtotal resection directed at achieving this objective (Zuccaro, 2005). It may be necessary to place an external ventricular drain at surgery, which can be subsequently weaned in the post-operative period. Post-operative scans will direct decisions regarding the placement of a shunt. Often these patients do not require any further treatment for the hydrocephalus. The treatment of hydrocephalus will have to precede surgical intervention in patients who present *in extremis*. This is however not without some risk for deterioration in visual function due to upward herniation of the tumor under the chiasm (Tomita and McLone, 1993). The presence of pre-operative hydrocephalus has been associated with a worse prognosis (Yasargil et al., 1990; Tomita and Bowman, 2005).

NEUROSURGICAL TREATMENT

There is continuing debate over the role and the extent of surgery in the treatment of craniopharyngioma, due to the various morbidities that have been associated with surgical resection and the impact of these on the quality of life of the patients. This is particularly relevant in the pediatric age group, who are at a critical stage of growth and development. The optimum treatment will be complete microsurgical excision when safe. The availability of advanced surgical techniques and adjuncts such as neuronavigation has helped in this regard. Gross total resection (GTR) reduces the risk of tumor recurrence with the attendant challenge of repeat surgeries, and also obviates the need for early adjuvant treatment with radiotherapy (Yasargil et al., 1990; Elliott et al., 2010). It should be noted however that there have been reports of high rates of recurrence despite GTR (Tomita and Bowman, 2005). The "aggressive" surgical approach that aims for GTR may however be less than optimal in patients with large tumors and/or tumors that have infiltrated surrounding structures, who are at increased risk of significant injury and post-operative morbidities. Thus, a subtotal resection with decompression of the optic chiasm and ventricular pathway would be appropriate in this subset of patients. The advances in microsurgical and skull base techniques, coupled with surgical adjuncts such as neuronavigation and intra-operative ultrasound, as well as the availability of hormone replacement therapy, have made GTR or near-total excision of these tumors safer and associated with low rates of morbidity and mortality.

The opening of new frontiers in the care of the pediatric patient with craniopharyngioma has led to treatment with less "invasive" procedures such as tumor cyst aspiration, intracystic sclerotherapy, and intracystic radiotherapy. This is with the understanding that these procedures reduce the risk of hypothalamic injuries and endocrinological morbidities, while alleviating the symptoms of the patients. The benefit of this ongoing debate is the general acceptance that the choice of treatment should be individualized with respect to the patient's clinical presentation and the tumor morphology on neuro-imaging. We will discuss the various surgical options and approaches.

TRANSCRANIAL APPROACHES

The approach to be utilized should be predicated on the growth characteristics of the tumor, particularly in relation to the optic chiasm, as observed on CT and MRI. The approach should provide an exposure that creates the shortest distance to the lesion, adequate visualization of the lesion, control of critical neurovascular structures, and minimal brain retraction. Appropriate and realistic goals of surgery must be clearly stated and the operative approach tailored to the achievement of the goals.

The transcranial approaches to a craniopharyngioma will vary from midline anterior approaches such as a unilateral subfrontal, bifrontal (transbasal) approaches, to frontolateral approaches such as the pterional and the modified orbitozygomatic craniotomy. Some surgeons have also used the subtemporal approach and transpetrosal (Kawase) approach to extensive retrochiamatic tumors (Zada and Laws, 2010), but these are rarely utilized in the pediatric age group. There might be a need to combine a number of these approaches to facilitate safe and adequate tumor removal. Procedures may also need to be staged for large tumors.

We have a preference for the subfrontal approach in the majority of children where a transcranial approach is required, because it provides a direct trajectory to the tumor with opportunity for good visualization of the optic nerves and internal carotid arteries (Figure 28.3). The prechiasmatic extension of the tumor can be easily dissected between the optic nerves. This approach also provides a direct corridor to the lamina terminalis, allowing for the excision of the retrochiasmatic and third ventricular extensions of the tumor. This versatile approach also produces a working corridor through the opticocarotid and carotid-oculomotor cisterns. In children, the anterior fossa floor is shallow and relatively foreshortened and it may not be necessary to remove the supraorbital bar (Liu et al., 2005). The frontal sinuses are also not fully developed, thus reducing the potential for their violation and the cerebrospinal fluid (CSF) leak associated with that. The disadvantages of the approach include damage to the olfactory tract usually unilaterally and its limitation in patients with a prefixed chiasm. We often prefer the unilateral subfrontal approach, with a unilateral dural opening typically across the midline allowing for the ligation of the frontal sinus far

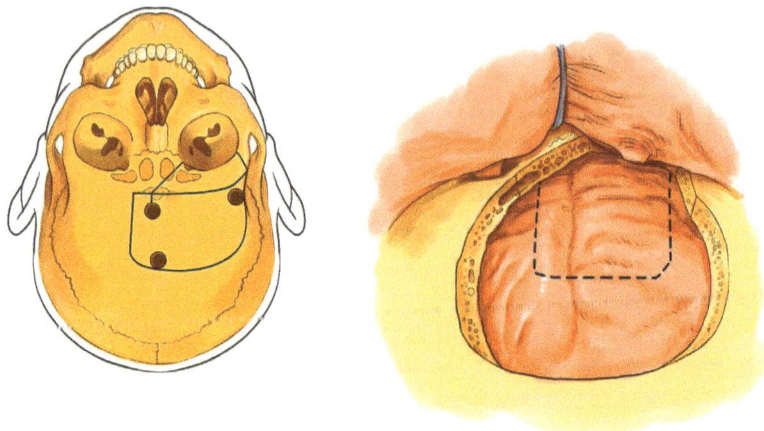

FIGURE 28.3 **Artist's depiction of a unilateral subfrontal approach.** Left: The right bone flap is carried just over the midline to the left. A unilateral orbital osteotomy is performed as depicted. The inferior and medial cut of the osteotomy is angled across the midline so as to have as much exposure at the cranial base in the midline as possible. Right: With the bone flap removed, the dural opening can be performed as indicated by the hatched line. The dura is reflected inferiorly as far as possible to reveal the anterior cranial base. The operative procedure should be conducted with as little subfrontal brain retraction as possible.

anteriorly. Microsurgical techniques are employed, after a gentle retraction of the frontal lobe, to open the interhemispheric and chiasmatic cisterns and to dissect the optic nerves and chiasm off the tumor capsule. Tumor excision is facilitated by the use of the cavitron ultrasonic aspirator (CUSA). The lamina terminalis, situated between the optic tracts, can be opened to gain access to tumors extending into the third ventricle. We acknowledge that the bifrontal transbasal approach might be preferred for large retrochiasmatic tumors, but this entails more extensive bone work. The anatomical relationship of the anterior cerebral arteries to the tumor must be well understood in the frontobasal approaches. As with many transcranial approaches, the use of neuronavigation with the frontobasal approach is frequently very helpful (Figure 28.4).

The pterional approach remains a "work horse" for craniopharyngioma surgery. It provides the shortest distance to the suprasellar region and is the preferred method in patients with a prefixed chiasm, because the tumor can be resected beneath the chiasm. The utility of this approach allows access to virtually all parts of even very large tumors (Yasargil et al., 1990). It however provides a limited view of the contralateral optico-carotid triangle and the contralateral retrocarotid space. Although it provides access into the third ventricle through the lamina terminalis, the oblique trajectory increases the risk of injury to the hypothalamus (Liu et al., 2005). This approach can be combined with a transcallosal approach for access into the third ventricle.

The modified orbitozygomatic approach has evolved over the years as an alternative approach in children. The removal of the orbital rim in this approach permits improved visualization by increasing the angle of approach and the area of exposure without significant subfrontal retraction (Miller et al., 2008; Golshani et al., 2009). The removal of the zygomatic

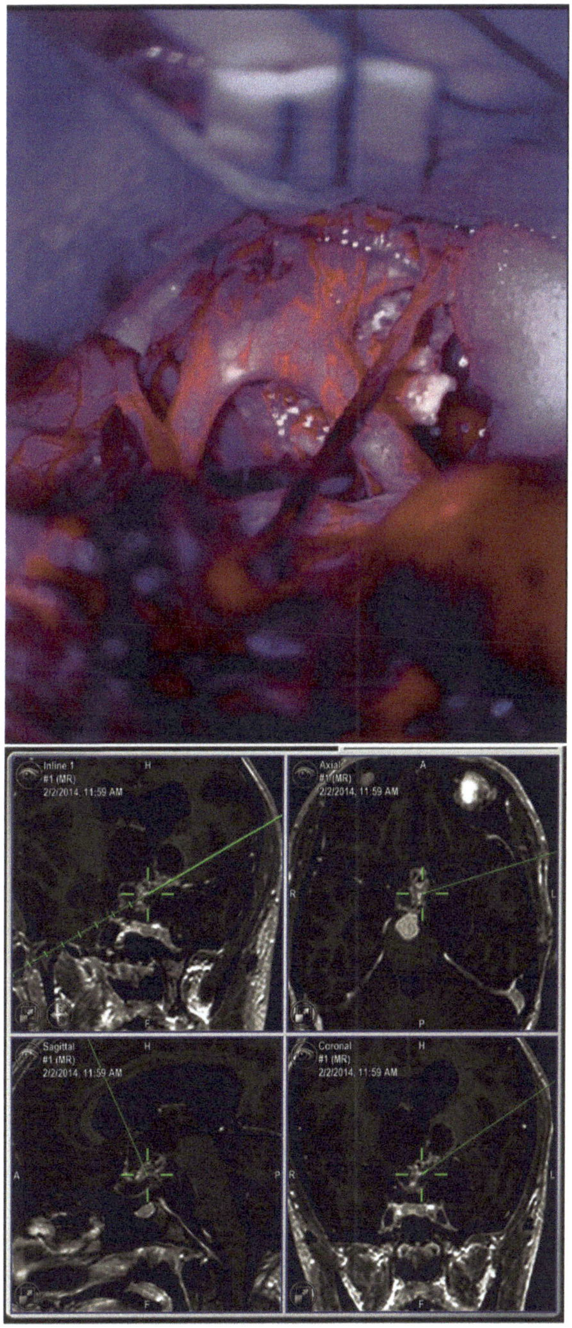

FIGURE 28.4 Left: Intra-operative use of image guidance (neuronavigation) improving safety of tumor resection. Right: Intra-operative exposure of a retrochiasmatic craniopharyngioma showing the left and right optic nerves leading to the chiasm which is stretched over the tumor. The tumor fills the chiasmatic cistern and extends to the prechiasmatic space. Calcified tumor is also appreciated lateral to the left optic nerve as shown.

arch also increases visualization by allowing for the inferior mobilization of the temporalis muscle (Liu et al., 2005). Despite the concerns for the performance of this approach in children, authors have stated that the procedure is technically simpler to perform due to thinner and more plastic bones as well as a less adherent dura. The pediatric craniofacial skeleton also appears to be exceptionally capable of excellent functional and cosmetic healing (Golshani et al., 2009).

The transcallosal or transcortical approaches provide access to tumors arising wholly in the third ventricle or with significant extension to the lateral and third ventricles. Maneuvers that can be done via the transcallosal approach include a transforaminal exposure, with an enlarged foramen of Monro, as well as the subchoroidal, transchoroidal, or interforniceal exposures. The transcallosal route does not require an enlarged lateral ventricle for access and eliminates a cortical incision, but can lead to significant injury of the fornix, anterior commissure, cortical veins, and some of the deep veins (Liu et al., 2005). These approaches can also be combined with either the subfrontal or a frontolateral approach in craniopharyngiomas with more complex morphology (Yasargil et al., 1990).

TRANSSPHENOIDAL APPROACH

Transsphenoidal resection of craniopharyngiomas is gradually becoming the neurosurgical approach of choice in the adult population, particularly in the tumors with some sellar component causing expansion of the sella. The approach and its extended modifications improve surgical access and exposure of the suprasellar and retrosellar region and the ability to achieve more extensive tumor resection. It also obviates the need for brain retraction that is required in some transcranial operations (Zada and Laws, 2010).

With technological advances, the paradigm in transsphenoidal operations is shifting from the microscopic transsphenoidal approach towards the use of the endoscopic endonasal transsphenoidal approach. This creates a ventral midline corridor to the sellar, suprasellar, and parasellar compartments that not only obviates the need for any brain retraction, but also provides a panoramic view of the tumor. This has extended the utility of the transsphenoidal approach to include purely suprasellar tumors (Kassam et al., 2008).

The challenges to the implementation of endonasal endoscopic approach in children include small working spaces, a smaller basicranium, and often in younger children the presence of a conchal sphenoid sinus that is not or is only partially pneumatized, which requires drilling with the aid of intra-operative stereotactic guidance (Chivukula et al., 2013). The tumors found in the pediatric age group also tend to be bigger than in the adult population (Koutourousiou et al., 2013). Despite these challenges, this approach is gradually becoming an alternative in the pediatric population with results that are comparable to those in adults (Figure 28.5) (Leng et al., 2012; Koutourousiou et al., 2013). The use of the nasoseptal flap has reduced post-operative CSF leak following endoscopic resection of craniopharyngiomas. Though Shah et al. suggested in their study that the pedicled nasoseptal flap may not be a viable option for reconstruction after EEA in children < 10 years of age (Shah et al., 2009), Giannoni et al. concluded that the vascularized nasoseptal flap is a feasible and reliable method of repair of dural defects in children and that age did not predict difficulty with

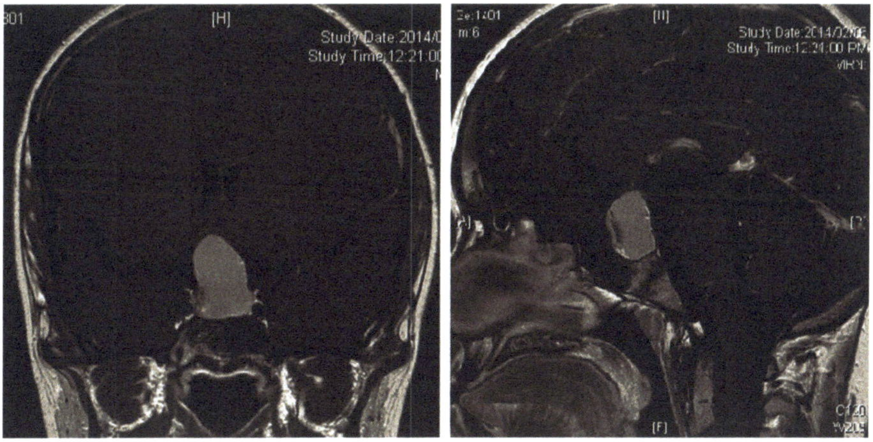

FIGURE 28.5 **A 17-year-old male with delayed puberty.** Left: Coronal MRI with contrast showing a large sellar mass with significant suprasellar extension. The tumor is infradiaphramatic with the chiasm thinned and arched over the tumor. Right: Sagittal MRI with contrast showing expanded sella, with predominantly cystic contents.The lesion was removed via a transsphenoidal approach.

flap technique, though the younger children were more challenging due to narrow spaces. The children also required operative nasal debridement (Giannoni and Whitehead, 2013).

NEUROSURGICAL TREATMENT OF CYSTIC CRANIOPHARYNGIOMAS

Wholly or predominantly cystic craniopharyngiomas can be managed through a combination of less invasive surgical options and the use of chemotherapeutic agents or radioisotopes. The evolution of these procedures is a response to the commitment to reducing morbidities associated with transcranial and transsphenoidal procedures. A high recurrence rate was reported in endoscopic fenestration with adjuvant radiotherapy (Park et al., 2011), thus making way for the placement of a ventricular catheter with a subcutaneous reservoir which permits aspiration and instillation of agents that should ideally have the ability to induce cyst shrinkage, cause adhesion of the cyst walls and remain within the cyst without leakage to the surrounding neurovascular structures (Figure 28.6). There are various options for the placement of the ventricular catheter, varying from free hand placement through a burrhole, direct placement via a transcranial approach, stereotactic (Zanon et al., 2008), and endoscopic placements (Joki et al., 2002). We have a preference for the endoscopic or the stereotactic endoscopic approach which was reported to have a low rate of complications by Hellwig et al. (1995) and can also be utilized for biopsy (Trippel and Nikkhah, 2012). The endoscopic approach also gives the surgeon the opportunity to perform a septostomy to connect the lateral ventricles and subsequently facilitates successful shunting if necessary (Bartels et al., 2012). Various agents have been used, including bleomycin, radio-isotopes such as phosphorus-32, and alpha interferon

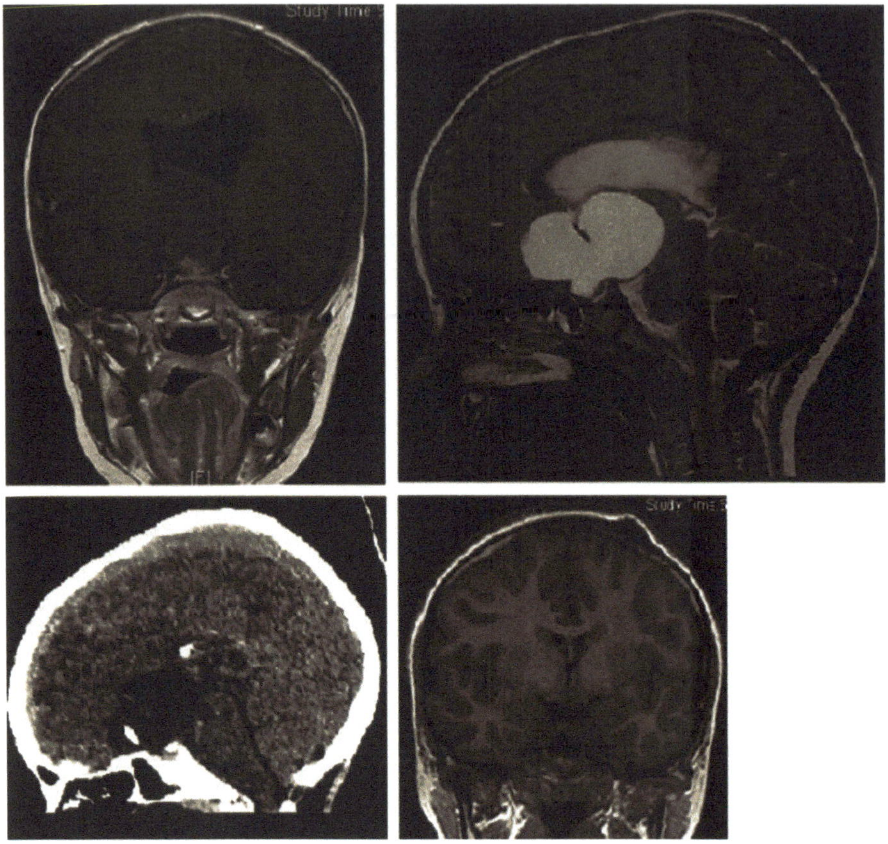

FIGURE 28.6 **A 3-year-old female with headaches, vomiting, and seizures.** Top left: Coronal T1 weighted image (T1WI) of a large mainly cystic suprasellar lesion causing obstructive hydrocephalus. Top right: Sagittal T2 weighted image (T2WI) showing the extension of the cyst into the interpenducular cistern. Bottom left: Sagittal CT showing a catheter connected to an Ommaya reservoir in place. Bottom right: A coronal T1WI post treatment with alpha interferon showing complete resolution of the cyst. The Ommaya reservoir is shown in the image.

(Steinbok and Hukin, 2010; Bartels et al., 2012; Fang et al., 2012). Alpha interferon appears to be gaining wider use due to its non-neurotoxicity (Cavalheiro et al., 2005; Steinbok and Hukin, 2010; Bartels et al., 2012). The challenges with this option of treatment include the non-treatment of the solid portion of the tumor, limitation of treatment to one cyst in a multicystic tumor, the failure of the scope/catheter to successfully penetrate the cyst wall, and volume changes during treatment which may influence the intracystic catheter tip location (Bartels et al., 2012). This approach may not only be utilized to provide treatment for wholly cystic tumors, but it is also an option for the treatment of partly cystic tumors and may potentially delay radiation therapy in the younger children. A review of our center's trend in the management of children with craniopharyngioma over three decades suggests that this approach is worth considering (Cohen et al., 2013).

ADJUVANT RADIOTHERAPY IN CHILDREN

Radiotherapy has become an important adjunct in the management of craniopharyngiomas, particularly after subtotal resection. Adjuvant radiotherapy has been associated with improved survival in the pediatric age group (Regine and Kramer, 1992; Stripp et al., 2004; Clark et al., 2012), but the effects of radiotherapy on the developing brain cannot be underscored enough. The adverse effects of radiotherapy are generally insidious, although they can occur acutely. These include acute deterioration in vision often due to rapidly enlarging cyst or hydrocephalus, new or worsening endocrine function from pituitary–hypothalamic radiation injury, impairment of neurocognitive development, vasculopathy such as moyamoya disease, as well as the development of cavernomas and secondary malignancies (Liu et al., 2009; Kiehna and Merchant, 2010; Clark et al., 2012; Dadlani et al., 2014). Radiation is preferred for children older than 5 years, but can be used in children aged 3 years and above in special circumstances (Stripp et al., 2004).

There have been various developments in the field of oncologic radiation focused on reducing the risk of radiation complications. There is a gradual shift from fractionated external beam radiation to stereotactic radiosurgery (SRS) and stereotactic radiotherapy (STR) which provide precise and focused radiation delivery. SRS also permits fractionation which has enabled these modalities to have similar or better results and outcomes (Tarbell et al., 1994; Albright et al., 2005; Kiehna and Merchant, 2010). The dose to the optic pathways is critical and should be kept as low as possible with SRS (Kobayashi et al., 1994). Treatment with proton therapy is also showing promise, with significant reduction in radiation dose (Beltran et al., 2012).

OUTCOME

The overall survival in pediatric patients with craniopharyngioma remains high irrespective of the modality of treatment (Regine and Kramer, 1992; Winkfield et al., 2011; Cohen et al., 2013). The controversy has been over the optimum treatment modality associated with the least morbidity and best long-term cure or tumor control. Advocates of radical resection of craniopharyngiomas have reported satisfactory outcomes including very low percentage of cognitive impairment (Hoffman et al., 1992; Muller-Scholden et al., 2000; Zuccaro, 2005; Elliott et al., 2010), while other reports have submitted that the neurological morbidities associated with complete resection are high and have advocated for less aggressive approaches (Bartels et al., 2012; Clark et al., 2012; Cohen et al., 2013; Ali et al., 2014). There is no doubt that complete surgical resection is the preferred mode of treatment when it is achievable with minimal morbidities. Recurrence is, however, a major concern in the treatment of this disease and remains high, with rates of 5–53% quoted even in completely resected tumors (Kim et al., 2001). The identified predictors of recurrence in children include residual tumor at surgery or post imaging (Hoffman, 1994; Stripp et al., 2004) and location of the tumor with identification of the sellar and optic chiasm as vulnerable sites (Kim et al., 2001; Qi et al., 2012).

CONCLUSION

Craniopharyngioma is a complex tumor with heterogeneous clinical and radiological characteristics that was described by Cushing as "the most baffling problem which confronts the neurosurgeon" (Cushing, 1932), evoking much debate and controversy regarding the patient's treatment. The focus of treatment in children must not be centered solely on survival as this would not be a true measure of success, but rather on the long-term quality of life of these patients. Treatment should be individualized in a multi-disciplinary setting, with clearly defined goals directed at achieving optimal outcome that encompasses cure or tumor control as well as permit a level of high functioning for these children as they grow into adulthood.

References

Adamson, T.E., Wiestler, O.D., Kleihues, P., Yasargil, M.G., 1990. Correlation of clinical and pathological features in surgically treated craniopharyngiomas. J. Neurosurg. 73 (1), 12–17.

Albright, A.L., Hadjipanayis, C.G., Lunsford, L.D., Kondziolka, D., Pollack, I.F., Adelson, P.D., 2005. Individualized treatment of pediatric craniopharyngiomas. Child's nervous system : ChNS. J. Int. Soc. Pediatr. Neurosurg. 21 (8–9), 649–654.

Ali, Z.S., Bailey, R.L., Daniels, L.B., Vakhshori, V., Lewis, D.J., Hossain, A.T., Sitterley, K.Y., Lee, J.Y., Storm, P.B., Heuer, G.G., Stein, S.C., 2014. Comparative effectiveness of treatment options for pediatric craniopharyngiomas. Journal of neurosurgery. Pediatrics 13 (2), 178–188.

Banna, M., Hoare, R.D., Stanley, P., Till, K., 1973. Craniopharyngioma in children. J. Pediatr. 83 (5), 781–785.

Banna, M., 1973. Craniopharyngioma in adults. Surg. Neurology 1 (4), 202–204.

Bartels, U., Laperriere, N., Bouffet, E., Drake, J., 2012. Intracystic therapies for cystic craniopharyngioma in childhood. Front. Endocrinol. 3, 39.

Beltran, C., Roca, M., Merchant, T.E., 2012. On the benefits and risks of proton therapy in pediatric craniopharyngioma. Int. J. Radiat. Oncol. Biol. Phys. 82 (2), e281–287.

Bunin, G.R., Surawicz, T.S., Witman, P.A., Preston-Martin, S., Davis, F., Bruner, J.M., 1998. The descriptive epidemiology of craniopharyngioma. J. Neurosurg. 89 (4), 547–551.

Carmel, P.W., Antunes, J.L., Chang, C.H., 1982. Craniopharyngiomas in children. Neurosurgery 11 (3), 382–389.

Cavalheiro, S., Dastoli, P.A., Silva, N.S., Toledo, S., Lederman, H., da Silva, M.C., 2005. Use of interferon alpha in intratumoral chemotherapy for cystic craniopharyngioma. Child's nervous system : ChNS. J. Int. Soc. Pediatr. Neurosurg. 21 (8–9), 719–724.

Chivukula, S., Koutourousiou, M., Snyderman, C.H., Fernandez-Miranda, J.C., Gardner, P.A., Tyler-Kabara, E.C., 2013. Endoscopic endonasal skull base surgery in the pediatric population. J. Neurosurg. Pediatrics 11 (3), 227–241.

Clark, A.J., Cage, T.A., Aranda, D., Parsa, A.T., Auguste, K.I., Gupta, N., 2012. Treatment-related morbidity and the management of pediatric craniopharyngioma: a systematic review. J. Neurosurg. Pediatrics 10 (4), 293–301.

Cohen, M., Bartels, U., Branson, H., Kulkarni, A.V., Hamilton, J., 2013. Trends in treatment and outcomes of pediatric craniopharyngioma, 1975–2011. Neuro. Oncol. 15 (6), 767–774.

Cook, D.J., Rutka, J.T., 2009. Craniopharyngiomas: Neurosurgical Mangement. In: Hanna, Y.E., DeMonte, F. (Eds.), Comprehensive Management of Skull Base Tumors. InformaHealthcare USA, New York, pp. 573–581.

Cushing, H., 1932. Intracranial Tumors. Notes upon Series of Two Thousand Verified Cases with Surgical Mortality Percentages Pertaining Thereto. Thomas, Springfield, IL.

Dadlani, R., Ghosal, N., Hegde, A.S., 2014. Should adjuvant radiotherapy be recommended for pediatric craniopharyngiomas? J. Korean Neurosurg. Soc. 55 (1), 54–56.

Dandy, Walter E., 1945. Surgery of the Brain. W. F. Prior Company, Inc, Hagerstown. Print, p 578.

Defoort-Dhellemmes, S., Moritz, F., Bouacha, I., Vinchon, M., 2006. Craniopharyngioma: ophthalmological aspects at diagnosis. Journal of pediatric endocrinology & metabolism. JPEM 19 (Suppl. 1), 321–324.

DeVile, C.J., Grant, D.B., Hayward, R.D., Stanhope, R., 1996. Growth and endocrine sequelae of craniopharyngioma. Arch. Dis. Child. 75 (2), 108–114.

Elliott, R.E., Hsieh, K., Hochm, T., Belitskaya-Levy, I., Wisoff, J., Wisoff, J.H., 2010. Efficacy and safety of radical resection of primary and recurrent craniopharyngiomas in 86 children. J. Neurosurg. Pediatrics 5 (1), 30–48.

Fang, Y., Cai, B.W., Zhang, H., Liu, W., Wu, B., Xu, J.G., You, C., 2012. Intracystic bleomycin for cystic craniopharyngiomas in children. Cochrane Database Syst. Rev. 4. CD008890.

Giannoni, C.M., Whitehead, W.E., 2013. Use of endoscopic vascularized nasoseptal flap in children. Otolaryngology – head and neck surgery: official journal of American Academy of Otolaryngology. Head Neck Surg. 148 (2), 344–346.

Golshani, K.J., Lalwani, K., Delashaw, J.B., Selden, N.R., 2009. Modified orbitozygomatic craniotomy for craniopharyngioma resection in children. J. Neurosurg. Pediatrics 4 (4), 345–352.

Halac, I., Zimmerman, D., 2005. Endocrine manifestations of craniopharyngioma. Childs Nerv. Syst. 21 (8–9), 640–648.

Hald, J.K., Eldevik, O.P., Skalpe, I.O., 1995. Craniopharyngioma identification by CT and MR imaging at 1.5 T. Acta Radiol. (Stockholm, Sweden : 1987) 36 (2), 142–147.

Harwood-Nash, D.C., 1994. Neuroimaging of childhood craniopharyngioma. Pediatr. Neurosurg. 21 (Suppl. 1), 2–10.

Haupt, R., Magnani, C., Pavanello, M., Caruso, S., Dama, E., Garre, M.L., 2006. Epidemiological aspects of craniopharyngioma. JPEM 19 (Suppl. 1), 289–293.

Hellwig, D., Bauer, B.L., List-Hellwig, E., 1995. Stereotactic endoscopic interventions in cystic brain lesions. Acta Neurochir. 64, 59–63. Supplement.

Hoffman, H.J., De Silva, M., Humphreys, R.P., Drake, J.M., Smith, M.L., Blaser, S.I., 1992. Aggressive surgical management of craniopharyngiomas in children. J. Neurosurg. 76 (1), 47–52.

Hoffman, H.J., 1994. Surgical management of craniopharyngioma. Pediatr. Neurosurg. 21 (Suppl. 1), 44–49.

Hopper, N., Albanese, A., Ghirardello, S., Maghnie, M., 2006. The pre-operative endocrine assessment of craniopharyngiomas. JPEM. 19 (Suppl. 1), 325–327.

Hussain, I., Eloy, J.A., Carmel, P.W., Liu, J.K., 2013. Molecular oncogenesis of craniopharyngioma: current and future strategies for the development of targeted therapies. J. Neurosurg. 119 (1), 106–112.

Joki, T., Oi, S., Babapour, B., Kaito, N., Ohashi, K., Ebara, M., Kato, M., Abe, T., 2002. Neuroendoscopic placement of Ommaya reservoir into a cystic craniopharyngioma. Childs Nerv. Syst. 18 (11), 629–633.

Kalina, M.A., Skala-Zamorowska, E., Kalina-Faska, B., Malecka-Tendera, E., Mandera, M., 2009. Practical approach to childhood craniopharyngioma: a role of an endocrinologist and a general paediatrician. Childs Nerv. Syst. 25 (9), 1053–1060.

Karavitaki, N., Brufani, C., Warner, J.T., Adams, C.B., Richards, P., Ansorge, O., Shine, B., Turner, H.E., Wass, J.A., 2005. Craniopharyngiomas in children and adults: systematic analysis of 121 cases with long-term follow-up. Clin. Endocrinol. 62 (4), 397–409.

Kassam, A.B., Gardner, P.A., Snyderman, C.H., Carrau, R.L., Mintz, A.H., Prevedello, D.M., 2008. Expanded endonasal approach, a fully endoscopic transnasal approach for the resection of midline suprasellar craniopharyngiomas: a new classification based on the infundibulum. J. Neurosurg. 108 (4), 715–728.

Kennedy, H.B., Smith, R.J., 1975. Eye signs in craniopharyngioma. Br. J. Ophthalmol. 59 (12), 689–695.

Kiehna, E.N., Merchant, T.E., 2010. Radiation therapy for pediatric craniopharyngioma. Neurosurg. Focus 28 (4), E10.

Kim, S.K., Wang, K.C., Shin, S.H., Choe, G., Chi, J.G., Cho, B.K., 2001. Radical excision of pediatric craniopharyngioma: recurrence pattern and prognostic factors. Childs Nerv. Syst. 17 (9), 531–536, discussion 537.

Kobayashi, T., Tanaka, T., Kida, Y., 1994. Stereotactic gamma radiosurgery of craniopharyngiomas. Pediatr. Neurosurg. 21 (Suppl. 1), 69–74.

Koutourousiou, M., Gardner, P.A., Fernandez-Miranda, J.C., Tyler-Kabara, E.C., Wang, E.W., Snyderman, C.H., 2013. Endoscopic endonasal surgery for craniopharyngiomas: surgical outcome in 64 patients. J. Neurosurg. 119 (5), 1194–1207.

Kumar, A., Kasliwal, M.K., Suri, A., Sharma, B.S., 2010. Spontaneous asymptomatic rupture of cystic craniopharyngioma in a child: case report and review of the literature. J. Child Neurol. 25 (12), 1555–1558.

Leng, L.Z., Greenfield, J.P., Souweidane, M.M., Anand, V.K., Schwartz, T.H., 2012. Endoscopic, endonasal resection of craniopharyngiomas: analysis of outcome including extent of resection, cerebrospinal fluid leak, return to preoperative productivity, and body mass index. Neurosurgery 70 (1), 110–123, discussion 123–124.

Liu, J.K., Cole, C.D., Kestle, J.R., Brockmeyer, D.L., Walker, M.L., 2005. Cranial base strategies for resection of craniopharyngioma in children. Neurosurg. Focus 18 (6A), E9.

Liu, A.K., Bagrosky, B., Fenton, L.Z., Gaspar, L.E., Handler, M.H., McNatt, S.A., Foreman, N.K., 2009. Vascular abnormalities in pediatric craniopharyngioma patients treated with radiation therapy. Pediatr. Blood Cancer 52 (2), 227–230.

Makino, K., Nakamura, H., Yano, S., Kuratsu, J., 2010. Population-based epidemiological study of primary intracranial tumors in childhood. Childs Nerv. Syst. 26 (8), 1029–1034.

May, J.A., Krieger, M.D., Bowen, I., Geffner, M.E., 2006. Craniopharyngioma in childhood. Adv. Pediatr. 53, 183–209.

Miller, M.L., Kaufman, B.A., Lew, S.M., 2008. Modified osteoplastic orbitozygomatic craniotomy in the pediatric population. Childs Nerv. Syst. 24 (7), 845–850.

Miller, D.C., 1994. Pathology of craniopharyngiomas: clinical import of pathological findings. Pediatr. Neurosurg. 21 (Suppl. 1), 11–17.

Muller, H.L., 2008. Childhood craniopharyngioma. Recent advances in diagnosis, treatment and follow-up. Horm. Res. 69 (4), 193–202.

Muller, H.L., 2013. Paediatrics: surgical strategy and quality of life in craniopharyngioma. Nature reviews. Endocrinology 9 (8), 447–449.

Muller, H.L., 2013. Childhood craniopharyngioma. Pituitary 16 (1), 56–67.

Muller-Scholden, J., Lehrnbecher, T., Muller, H.L., Bensch, J., Hengen, R.H., Sorensen, N., Stockhausen, H.B., 2000. Radical surgery in a neonate with craniopharyngioma. report of a case. Pediatr. Neurosurg. 33 (5), 265–269.

Nielsen, E.H., Jorgensen, J.O., Bjerre, P., Andersen, M., Andersen, C., Feldt-Rasmussen, U., Poulsgaard, L., Kristensen, L.O., Astrup, J., Jorgensen, J., Laurberg, P., 2013. Acute presentation of craniopharyngioma in children and adults in a Danish national cohort. Pituitary 16 (4), 528–535.

Nielsen, E.H., Feldt-Rasmussen, U., Poulsgaard, L., Kristensen, L.O., Astrup, J., Jorgensen, J.O., Bjerre, P., Andersen, M., Andersen, C., Jorgensen, J., Lindholm, J., Laurberg, P., 2011. Incidence of craniopharyngioma in Denmark (n = 189) and estimated world incidence of craniopharyngioma in children and adults. J. Neuro. Oncol. 104 (3), 755–763.

Ohmori, K., Collins, J., Fukushima, T., 2007. Craniopharyngiomas in children. Pediatr. Neurosurg. 43 (4), 265–278.

Park, Y.S., Chang, J.H., Park, Y.G., Kim, D.S., 2011. Recurrence rates after neuroendoscopic fenestration and Gamma Knife surgery in comparison with subtotal resection and Gamma Knife surgery for the treatment of cystic craniopharyngiomas. J. Neurosurg. 114 (5), 1360–1368.

Pekmezci, M., Louie, J., Gupta, N., Bloomer, M.M., Tihan, T., 2010. Clinicopathological characteristics of adamantinomatous and papillary craniopharyngiomas: University of California, San Francisco experience 1985–2005. Neurosurgery 67 (5), 1341–1349, discussion 1349.

Pettorini, B.L., Frassanito, P., Caldarelli, M., Tamburrini, G., Massimi, L., Di Rocco, C., 2010. Molecular pathogenesis of craniopharyngioma: switching from a surgical approach to a biological one. Neurosurg. Focus 28 (4), E1.

Pierre-Kahn, A., Recassens, C., Pinto, G., Thalassinos, C., Chokron, S., Soubervielle, J.C., Brauner, R., Zerah, M., Sainte Rose, C., 2005. Social and psycho-intellectual outcome following radical removal of craniopharyngiomas in childhood. A prospective series. Childs Nerv. Syst. 21 (8–9), 817–824.

Prabhu, V.C., Brown, H.G., 2005. The pathogenesis of craniopharyngiomas. Childs Nerv. Syst. 21 (8–9), 622–627.

Puget, S., Garnett, M., Wray, A., Grill, J., Habrand, J.L., Bodaert, N., Zerah, M., Bezerra, M., Renier, D., Pierre-Kahn, A., Sainte-Rose, C., 2007. Pediatric craniopharyngiomas: classification and treatment according to the degree of hypothalamic involvement. J. Neurosurg. 106 (Suppl. 1), 3–12.

Qi, S., Pan, J., Lu, Y., et al., 2012. The impact of the site of origin and rate of tumour growth on clinical outcome in children with craniopharyngiomas. Clin. Endocrinol. 76 (1), 103–110.

Regine, W.F., Kramer, S., 1992. Pediatric craniopharyngiomas: long term results of combined treatment with surgery and radiation. Int. J. Radiat. Oncol. Biol. Phys. 24 (4), 611–617.

Rienstein, S., Adams, E.F., Pilzer, D., Goldring, A.A., Goldman, B., Friedman, E., 2003. Comparative genomic hybridization analysis of craniopharyngiomas. J. Neurosurg. 98 (1), 162–164.

Rosenfeld, A., Arrington, D., Miller, J., Olson, M., Gieseking, A., Etzl, M., Harel, B., Schembri, A., Kaplan, A., 2014. A review of childhood and adolescent craniopharyngiomas with particular attention to hypothalamic obesity. Pediatr. Neurol. 50 (1), 4–10.

Shah, R.N., Surowitz, J.B., Patel, M.R., Huang, B.Y., Snyderman, C.H., Carrau, R.L., Kassam, A.B., Germanwala, A.V., Zanation, A.M., 2009. Endoscopic pedicled nasoseptal flap reconstruction for pediatric skull base defects. Laryngoscope 119 (6), 1067–1075.

Sklar, C.A., 1994. Craniopharyngioma: endocrine abnormalities at presentation. Pediatr. Neurosurg. 21 (Suppl. 1), 18–20.

Stagno, V., Mugamba, J., Ssenyonga, P., Kaaya, B.N., Warf, B.C., 2014. Presentation, pathology, and treatment outcome of brain tumors in 172 consecutive children at CURE Children's Hospital of Uganda. The predominance of the visible diagnosis and the uncertainties of epidemiology in sub-Saharan Africa. Childs Nerv. Syst. 30 (1), 137–146.

Stark, K.L., Kaufman, B., Lee, B.C., Primack, J., Tychsen, L., 1999. Visual recovery after a year of craniopharyngioma-related amaurosis: report of a nine-year-old child and a review of pathophysiologic mechanisms. J. AAPOS 3 (6), 366–371.

Steinbok, P., Hukin, J., 2010. Intracystic treatments for craniopharyngioma. Neurosurg. Focus 28 (4), E13.

Stripp, D.C., Maity, A., Janss, A.J., et al., 2004. Surgery with or without radiation therapy in the management of craniopharyngiomas in children and young adults. Int. J. Radiat. Oncol. Biol. Phys. 58 (3), 714–720.

Tarbell, N.J., Barnes, P., Scott, R.M., Goumnerova, L., Pomeroy, S.L., Black, P.M., Sallan, S.E., Billett, A., LaVally, B., Helmus, A., Kooy, H.M., Loeffler, J.S., 1994. Advances in radiation therapy for craniopharyngiomas. Pediatr. Neurosurg. 21 (Suppl. 1), 101–107.

Tomita, T., Bowman, R.M., 2005. Craniopharyngiomas in children: surgical experience at Children's Memorial Hospital. Childs. Nerv. Syst. 21 (8–9), 729–746.

Tomita, T., McLone, D.G., 1993. Radical resections of childhood craniopharyngiomas. Pediatr. Neurosurg. 19 (1), 6–14.

Trippel, M., Nikkhah, G., 2012. Stereotactic neurosurgical treatment options for craniopharyngioma. Front. Endocrinol. 3, 63.

Wang, K.C., Kim, S.K., Choe, G., Chi, J.G., Cho, B.K., 2002. Growth patterns of craniopharyngioma in children: role of the diaphragm sellae and its surgical implication. Surg. Neurol. 57 (1), 25–33.

Weiner, H.L., Wisoff, J.H., Rosenberg, M.E., Kupersmith, M.J., Cohen, H., Zagzag, D., Shiminski-Maher, T., Flamm, E.S., Epstein, F.J., Miller, D.C., 1994. Craniopharyngiomas: a clinicopathological analysis of factors predictive of recurrence and functional outcome. Neurosurgery 35 (6), 1001–1010, discussion 1010–1001.

Winkfield, K.M., Tsai, H.K., Yao, X., et al., 2011. Long-term clinical outcomes following treatment of childhood craniopharyngioma. Pediatr. Blood Cancer 56 (7), 1120–1126.

Yasargil, M.G., Curcic, M., Kis, M., Siegenthaler, G., Teddy, P.J., Roth, P., 1990. Total removal of craniopharyngiomas. Approaches and long-term results in 144 patients. J. Neurosurg. 73 (1), 3–11.

Yoshimoto, M., de Toledo, S.R., da Silva, N.S., Bayani, J., Bertozzi, A.P., Stavale, J.N., Cavalheiro, S., Andrade, J.A., Zielenska, M., Squire, J.A., 2004. Comparative genomic hybridization analysis of pediatric adamantinomatous craniopharyngiomas and a review of the literature. J. Neurosurg. 101 (Suppl. 1), 85–90.

Zada, G., Laws, E.R., 2010. Surgical management of craniopharyngiomas in the pediatric population. Horm. Res. Paediatr. 74 (1), 62–66.

Zanon, N., Cavalheiro, S., da Silva, M.C., 2008. Does the choice of surgical approach to insert an intratumoral catheter influence the results of intratumoral cystic treatment? Surg. Neurol. 70 (1), 66–69 discussion 69.

Zhang, Y.Q., Wang, C.C., Ma, Z.Y., 2002. Pediatric craniopharyngiomas: Clinicomorphological study of 189 cases. Pediatr. Neurosurg. 36 (2), 80–84.

Zuccaro, G., 2005. Radical resection of craniopharyngioma. Childs Nerv. Syst. 21 (8–9), 679–690.

CHAPTER

29

Pediatric Radiation

Rachel Jimenez, Shannon M. MacDonald

Radiation Oncology, Massachusetts General Hospital/Harvard Medical School, Boston, MA, USA

"The combined approach to the problem by neurosurgery and radiation therapy is likely to produce the best results." **- S Kramer, et al., 1961**

SPECIAL CONSIDERATIONS FOR CHILDREN

The diagnosis of a brain tumor is a life-changing event for any patient and their family. Although craniopharyngiomas are considered "benign" and the prospect of long-term, disease-free survival is excellent, morbidity caused by this tumor and the treatment required to control it may be devastating. When craniopharyngioma is diagnosed in a child, the risks of side effects are higher, because of the sensitivity of developing surrounding structures and the longer anticipated survival following diagnosis. Potential neurocognitive, neuroendocrine, visual, and vascular complications may need to be addressed into adulthood. Therefore, the goal of treatment should be tumor control with the best achievable quality of life. Accepted treatment modalities include surgery and radiation therapy. It is desirable to avoid or delay radiation in young children, however complete surgical resection is often difficult to achieve without substantial complications, and long-term disease control is unlikely with incomplete tumor removal. Recent technological advances should minimize some radiation-associated complications. Unfortunately, others are expected with even the most advanced radiation modalites, because craniopharyngiomas are in such close proximity to eloquent areas of the brain. Most commonly, a combination of limited surgery and radiation provides the best treatment option for children with craniopharyngioma, but each case must be considered individually.

The management of pediatric craniopharyngioma poses additional challenges because parents must make treatment choices for their child. It is a great burden to parents that they must dictate the health outcome for their child, and consequently physicians must assist parents in making these difficult treatment decisions. Management of a child with craniopharyngioma should be discussed in a multidisciplinary setting at specialty centers with pediatric neurosurgeons, pediatric oncologists, and radiation oncologists. Ultimately,

Craniopharyngiomas
http://dx.doi.org/10.1016/B978-0-12-416706-3.00029-5

determining optimal treatment for these patients is complex, depends upon both patient and tumor characteristics, and requires an experienced team of pediatric specialists to determine responsible options and to present these options clearly to parents.

MANAGEMENT OPTIONS/TREATMENT GOALS

The management of craniopharyngioma remains one of the most controversial in the field of pediatric brain tumors. Complete surgical removal of the tumor can be curative, but this may be at the expense of unacceptable morbidity (Caldarelli et al., 2005; Mottolese et al., 2005; Tomita and Bowman, 2005; Sughrue et al., 2011; Clark et al., 2012). Limited surgery and radiation is also curative, but for very young children, late radiation side effects can lead to substantial morbidity as well (Merchant et al., 2006; Liu et al., 2009). Because children with craniopharyngioma are likely to be long-term survivors, minimizing toxicity is paramount. Technical advances in both neurosurgery and radiation oncology have improved the therapeutic ratio for the treatment of this disease (Winkfield et al., 2011), but because craniopharyngioma is a rare disease, with great variety in tumor and patient characteristics, it is challenging to prove one modality superior to another. Each case must be considered individually, and reasonable management strategies may include limited surgery and radiation, complete surgical resection alone, and even subtotal resection with close surveillance. For a very young child with a small tumor that does not adhere to adjacent structures, gross total resection may be feasible and allow radiation therapy to be avoided. For large tumors with

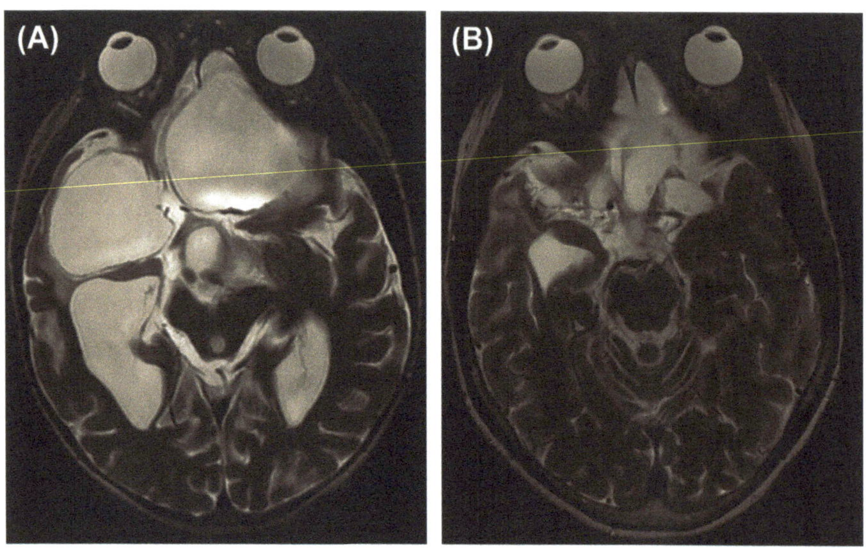

FIGURE 29.1 Axial images demonstrate a craniopharyngioma with a large cystic component in a young child before **A**, and after **B**, cyst fenestration. For this particular child the decision to fenestrate the cyst and allow time for cyst decompression and neurocognitive development prior to radiation was determined to be the best treatment course. Frequent monitoring with MRI and clinical examination were performed following cyst fenestration.

predominantly cystic components, cyst fenestration and close surveillance may allow the radiation volume to be reduced, and radiation at a young age to be avoided (Figure 29.1). However, craniopharyngiomas of adamantinomatous type, the most common type for all age groups and comprising the vast majority of craniopharyngiomas in children, are often too adherent to critical structures to allow a minimal risk resection. Therefore, for the vast majority of patients, we advocate for limited surgery followed by radiation.

IMMOBILIZATION/ANESTHESIA

Immobilization and reproducibility are critical to proper radiation delivery. Immobilization can be a challenge for young children, as they have greater difficulty staying still or cannot understand the importance of avoiding motion during treatment. In addition, some immobilization devices may be uncomfortable, as most were manufactured for adults and later adapted for use in children. For young children or those unable to tolerate treatment without sedation, anesthesia is necessary. It is crucial for pediatric radiation oncologists and nurses to have a good relationship with their anesthesia team. When patients require sedation, good teamwork enables the process to run smoothly and efficiently. Many departments prefer the use of a conscious sedative rather than full general anesthesia, which would require intubation. Propofol is often used due to its ease of administration and quick recovery in a majority of patients (McFadyen et al., 2011). Most children need only an oxygen mask, but a few will require a laryngeal mask airway (LMA) or nasal trumpet to maintain a good airway. While head positioning is optimized for radiotherapy (RT) delivery, a good airway will supersede this for children under anesthesia. Immobilization for the treatment of craniopharyngioma is usually accomplished with a molded thermoplastic mask. The mask is made before or at the time of simulation. The plastic is heated in a water bath, which allows it to become malleable. It is then placed over the child's face and secured to a board under the child's head. As it cools, it hardens and forms a mask fitting the child's face. Markers are placed on the outside of the mask to allow for laser localization to expedite the set-up process for daily treatment. Some stereotactic systems employ a more rigid frame, often with a bite block. These systems are sometimes only feasible for a single fraction treatment and usually too difficult for children to tolerate without sedation. Another method for improved localization is the use of fiducials, which are tiny metallic markers inserted into the external skull under a local anesthetic. These fiducials can be seen on X-rays taken for daily set-up and may be a good method of localization for some children (Figure 29.2).

In contrast, older children can usually tolerate treatment without sedation. Most departments have music of the patients' choice playing during the treatment, which can be very helpful for soothing anxiety or providing distraction. For some older children that become anxious or have difficulty staying still, a low dose of a medication such as Ativan can allow them to tolerate the position for the duration of treatment. Based on institutional experience, some children that cannot initially tolerate treatment do respond to coaching by nurses, child life specialists, and even other pediatric patients going through a similar treatment (Bolton, 2011). The ability to avoid anesthesia allows for maintenance of a regular meal schedule, thereby limiting impact on weight loss/gain and decreasing the amount of time spent in the radiation oncology department, permitting greater preservation of the child's routine. In addition, avoidance of

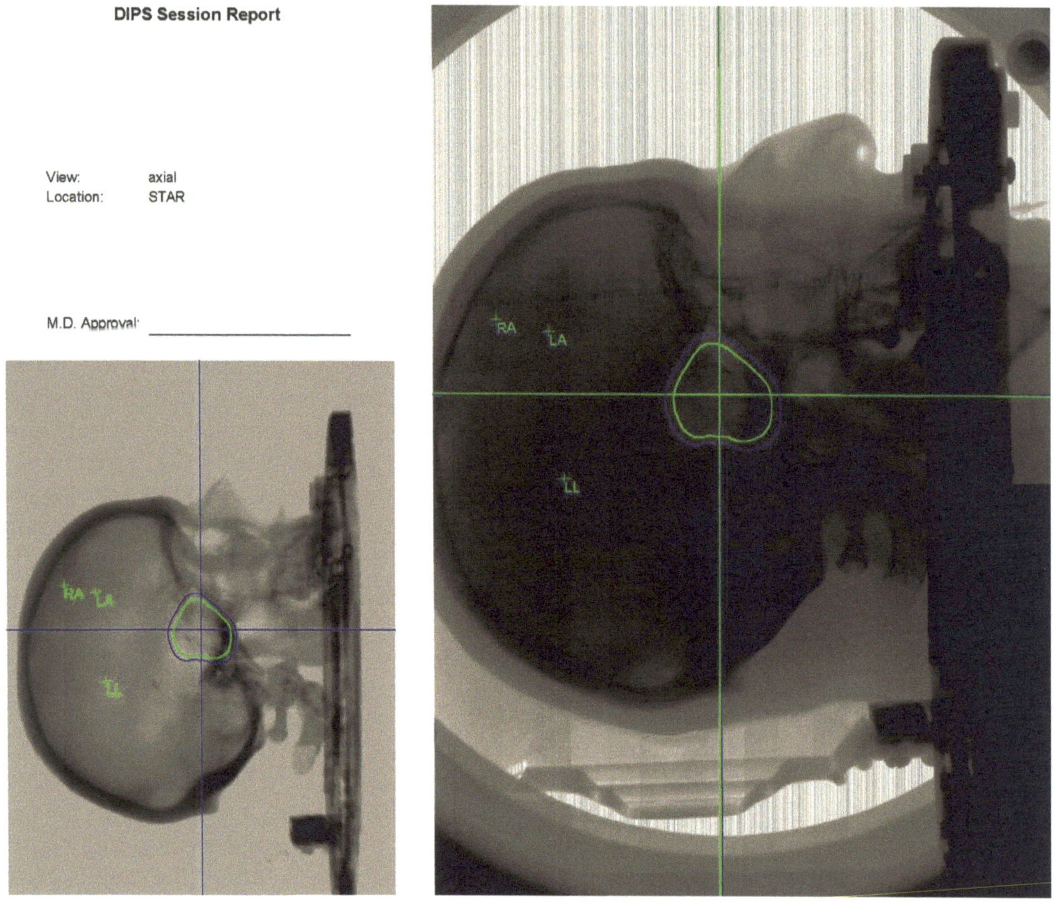

FIGURE 29.2 The figure shows a method of verifying position for radiation therapy. Diagnostic quality X-rays are performed each day prior to treatment and compared to a digitally reconstructed radiograph from the planning CT scan. Fiducial markers placed in the skull under local anesthesia allow for an efficient and accurate positioning and verification.

anesthesia limits the strain on hospital resources, including nursing and anesthesia staff, while also creating additional time on radiation treatment machines for the benefit of other patients.

RADIATION ONCOLOGY MODALITIES

3D Planning

Advances in diagnostic imaging over the past few decades have been adopted by radiation oncology, giving major improvements in radiation treatment planning. Prior to the advent of computed tomography (CT) and magnetic resonance imaging (MRI), radiation planning was performed using X-rays, referred to as 2D planning. The current use of MRI and CT now allows target volumes and avoidance structures to be defined in three dimensions, leading to markedly improved coverage of target volumes with avoidance of nearby structures. Because tumor extent is better visualized, margins for error around this volume can be made smaller, thereby giving full coverage of the tumor with improved avoidance of the surrounding normal brain and other central nervous system (CNS) structures.

More creative beam directions are also feasible. For craniopharyngiomas, most radiation oncology departments will obtain a CT scan taken while the patient is in the intended treatment position. MRI sequences of the brain are then fused to allow optimal tumor delineation using both modalities. Radiation oncologists should work closely with radiologists and neurosurgeons to define the gross tumor volume (GTV). For craniopharyngiomas, this includes any solid gross disease, cystic components of the tumor and surfaces touched directly by tumor. To account for microscopic extension, although unlikely in craniopharyngioma, most centers add a small margin (approximately 3 mm) to define a clinical tumor volume (CTV). An additional margin for set-up uncertainty and penumbra of the beam is given. This margin varies by institution and beam parameters and is often a uniform expansion referred to as a planning tumor volume (PTV).

Figure 29.3 shows an axial image with treatment volumes for a child with a craniopharygioma. For 3D treatment planning, multiple beam angles are chosen and the beam is shaped

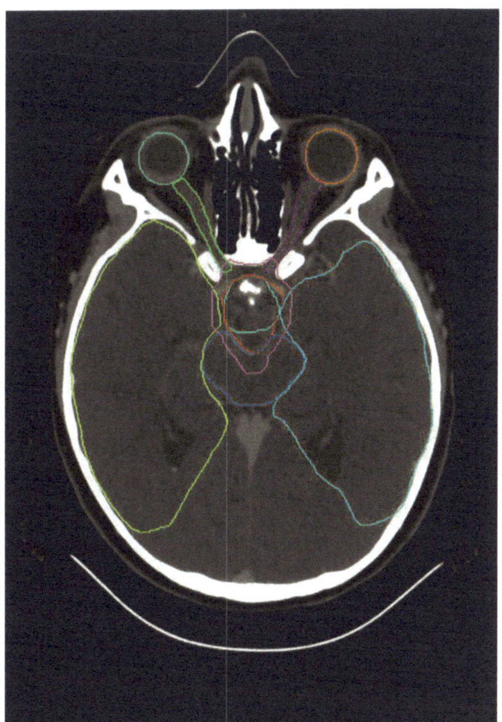

FIGURE 29.3 The figure shows an axial image with target volumes and organs at risk delineated for treatment planning. The red volume represents the tumor bed and gross tumor. The volume in magenta represents the clinical tumor volume which includes the GTV with a small margin for microscopic disease that may be present but not seen on imaging studies. Organs at risk shown include eyes, optic nerves, temporal lobes, and brainstem.

to the tumor volume using a multi-leaf collimator (MLC). This comprises a set of tungsten leaves that are moved into the path of the beam in different configurations to shape the beam to the silhouette of the tumor from the beam's eye view. This allows treatment of the target volume and blocking of the surrounding normal tissues. Typically, 4–6 beam directions are chosen to provide homogeneous coverage of the target volume and to best avoid healthy tissues.

IMRT

Intensity-modulated radiation therapy (IMRT) refers to photon radiation planning made possible by the development of sophisticated treatment planning software (Khan, 2010). For IMRT planning, the physician defines the desired dose and coverage of the target volume as well as the desired dose and volume limitations for normal healthy structures, and sets priorities for these parameters. The software program then runs multiple iterations of the treatment plan until it finds the best possible plan. This is called "inverse planning." If this plan is not satisfactory, constraints can be modified to allow for adjustments. The final plan typically consists of 5–7 beam angles and multiple "beamlets," or subfields within the defined beam angles, that are produced by MLC shaping for each of the beams. Figure 29.4 demonstrates IMRT delivery for a child with a craniopharyngioma. IMRT allows the most conformal photon plan with high-dose isodose lines "hugging" the target volume and avoiding more healthy tissues. While IMRT plans are highly conformal to the target

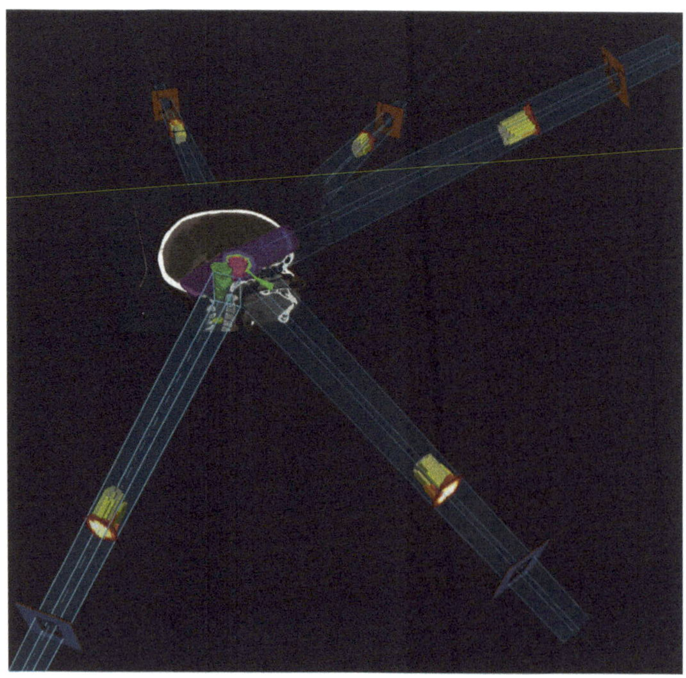

FIGURE 29.4 The figure demonstrates IMRT delivery for a child with a craniopharyngioma. Several beam angles are used that deliver several subfields of radiation to provide greater conformality of the high-dose radiation to target structures.

volume, the use of additional beam angles results in the delivery of low-dose radiation to normal tissues that would have otherwise been avoided.

SRS/SRT

The term stereotactic radiation, in part borrowed from neurosurgical localization systems, refers to high-precision radiation therapy using a 3D coordinate system. Stereotactic radiosurgery (SRS) refers to the delivery of a single treatment while stereotactic radiation therapy (SRT) refers to fractionated, or multiple treatments (Corn et al., 1997). Historically, stereotactic treatments were used only for small lesions in the brain, and the vast majority of stereotactic treatments are still reserved for CNS lesions. The idea behind these treatments is to use several beams of radiation to deliver a relatively high dose to the tumor while delivering a low dose to the surrounding normal brain. For brain tumors, these treatments are almost always delivered with a rigid frame immobilization. For children, it may not be possible to tolerate this kind of frame without sedation. For SRS, the entire process is lengthy. The treatment consists of rigid frame placement, imaging of the target volume, radiation planning and finally, radiation delivery. This can take several hours. A child is unlikely to be able to tolerate this procedure without anesthesia, and therefore demands on the anesthesia team are great. In addition, for craniopharyngioma, little data exist to support the use of SRS in children, and due to the close proximity of the optic structures, SRS is often not ideal (Adler et al., 2006). SRT, with a less rigid frame and faster delivery, can provide an effective treatment for small craniopharyngiomas (Luu et al., 2006).

Proton Radiation

Proton radiation is a form of particle radiation that allows complete sparing of tissue beyond the target volume for a given beam (MacDonald et al., 2006). Protons enter tissue and deliver a small and relatively constant dose until reaching an established distance, called the end of range, where the majority of the dose is delivered before sharply dropping off. Protons are also capable of delivering maximal dose at any depth up to 32 centimeters from the treatment machine (Smith et al., 2009). Due to these physical properties, the benefit of proton therapy is great for small, deep-seated brain tumors such as craniopharyngiomas. Proton radiation can be delivered using three-dimensional conformal proton radiation (3DCPT), also referred to as double-scattered proton technique. For this treatment, individual proton beams of the required energies are stacked to create a modulated beam or spread out Bragg peak (SOBP). This beam is passed through a brass aperture to shape the beam to the outline of the tumor, and a Lucite compensator allows the beam to conform to the distal edge of the tumor (Figures 29.5 and 29.6). Protons can also be delivered using a scanning technique. For this treatment, individual proton beams are scanned across the tumor in the required location and depth (Trofimov and Bortfeld, 2003). This type of treatment does not require a brass aperture or Lucite compensator and allows better shaping of the beam proximally with less scatter radiation. Up until 2006, only three proton centers existed in the United States. At present, 12 centers exist and many others are in the construction or planning phases despite the high capital costs involved in building a center (MacDonald et al., 2006; Loeffler and Durante,

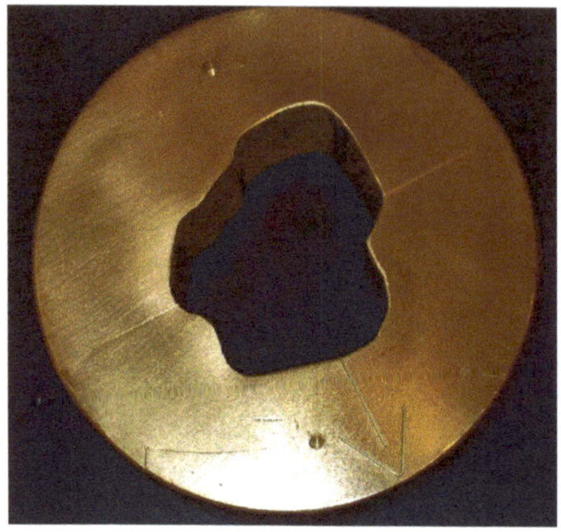

FIGURE 29.5 The figure shows a brass aperture used to block radiation from surrounding tissue and allow radiation through to treat tumor.

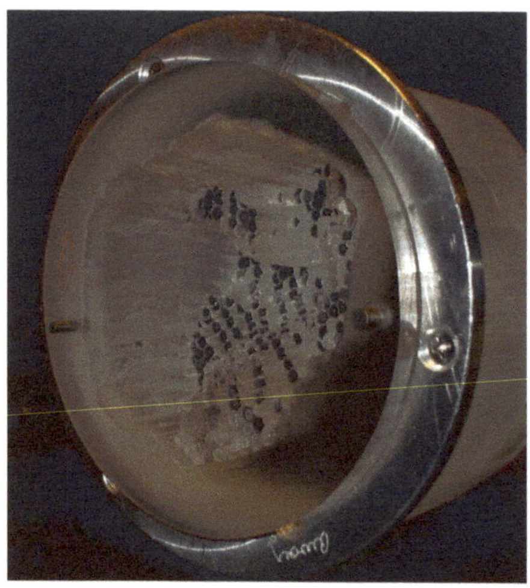

FIGURE 29.6 The figure shows a Lucite compensator used for proton delivery. The range-compensator will shift the dose distribution along the beam direction by the thickness traversed. Lucite compensator is designed to be thicker in areas requiring more shallow dose delivery and thinner in areas where the beam must penetrate more deeply to provide coverage.

2013). Pediatric brain tumors are considered one of the best indications for this type of treatment given the importance of sparing developing tissue from radiation. Although it is more costly than photon radiation, proton beam radiation for childhood brain tumors and other pediatric malignancies may prove cost-effective because it prevents costly, lifelong, medical problems (Brodin et al., 2012; Mailhot Vega et al., 2013).

Intracavitary Radiation

Intracavitary radiation is a treatment option for the cystic component of craniopharyngiomas. A pediatric neurosurgeon and radiation oncologist administer this treatment jointly. Beta-emitting particles (P32 or Y90) are administered by stereotactic cannulation of the cyst, or via an Ommaya reservoir if placement allows (Zhao et al., 2010). Cysts are often drained at the time of intracavitary treatment and a colloid suspension containing the radioactive particles is administered. The goal is to administer a dose of approximately 200 to 250 cGy evenly to the cyst wall. Cyst regression does not occur immediately and the results may take months to appreciate. Intracavitary radiation is an effective treatment, with durable response being seen in the majority of patients (Hasegawa et al., 2004). This treatment cannot be used for the solid portion of craniopharyngiomas, as the penetrance is limited to the thin cyst wall.

Image Guidance/Verification of Cyst Size

It is of paramount importance to confirm that radiation is being delivered as planned. The development of image guidance for radiation treatment has added greatly to our ability to confirm radiation delivery just prior to treatment. After aligning patients in the correct position using lasers that align to tattoos, fiducials, or marks on the immobilization mask, verification with imaging is now standard for most modern treatments. This can be performed with diagnostic quality X-rays or with cone beam CT (CBCT) while the patient is in treatment position on the treatment table. For highly precise treatments with small margins for error (less than 3 mm), daily imaging is vital. For craniopharyngioma, CBCT is more desirable because it may allow for information regarding cyst changes, in addition to verification of patient positioning. It is well known that cystic changes, more often growth of the cyst, may occur during radiation therapy (Rajan et al., 1997; Winkfield et al., 2009; Beltran et al., 2010). Since the cystic portion of the tumor is also targeted in treatment, it is crucial to make appropriate adjustments in the radiation plan to assure the cyst is covered adequately. Changes in cysts can also lead to changes in the position of the rest of the target, and can therefore impact radiation dose to normal structures as well. We recommend obtaining a CT or T2-weighted MRI approximately weekly for cystic tumors. If the initial MRI does not show change, subsequent MRIs during treatment are less likely to show change and the interval of scans may be extended. HASTE MRI, a fast MRI sequence, can be performed without gadolinium administration and without additional radiation dose, but CT scans are a more cost-effective alternative (Figure 29.7).

CLINICAL TREATMENT AND OUTCOMES

Most children are treated with fractionated external beam radiation using doses of 5040–5400 cGy at daily fractions of 180 cGy. Some series have used higher doses of radiation, but due to optical structure tolerance and lack of evidence that a greater dose provides improved tumor control, higher doses are not generally recommended (Iannalfi et al., 2013). External beam treatment options include conformal radiation, SRT, IMRT, and proton

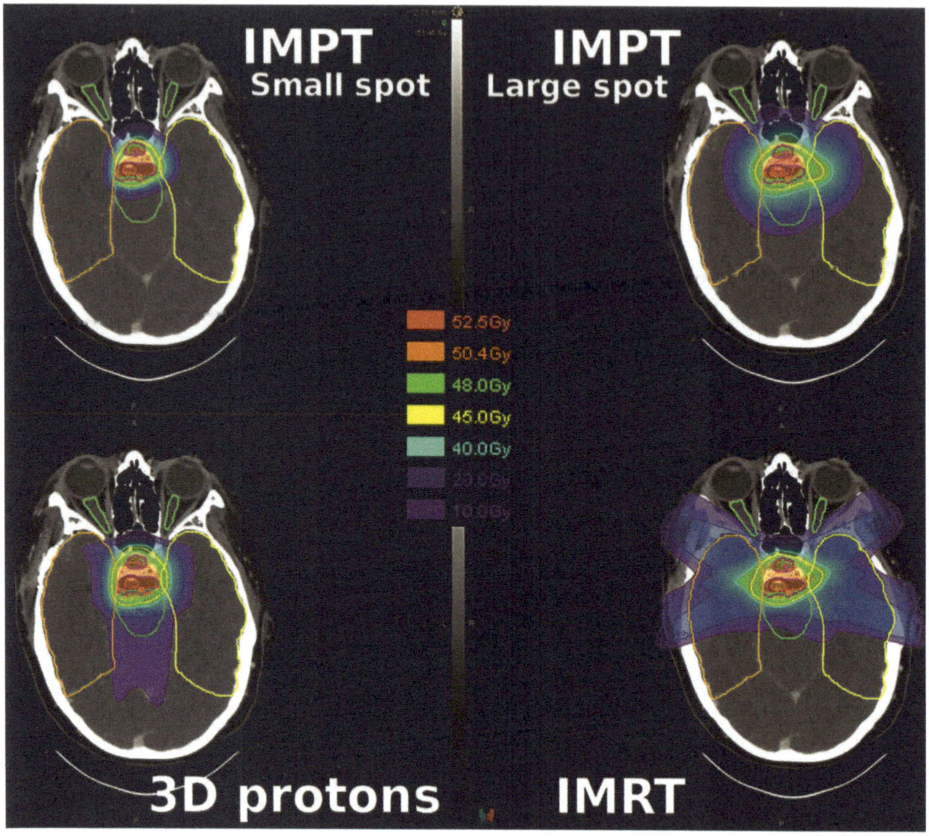

FIGURE 29.7 The figure shows comparison plans for proton (3D and IMPT (intensity-modulated proton therapy)) and photon (IMRT (intensity-modulated photon therapy)) modalities. While all modalities demonstrate excellent conformity to the target volume, proton modalities decrease low/moderate doses or integral radiation dose compared to IMRT. IMPT, especially with smaller spot sizes, decreases this unnecessary dose further.

radiation, but radiation side effects must be carefully considered. Effects may not be clinically observed for years after treatment and include, but are not limited to, neurocognitive decline, endocrine deficiency, vascular complications and second malignancy (Merchant et al., 2006; Liu et al., 2009; Kiehna and Merchant, 2010). Please refer to Chapter 22 for a detailed discussion of the side effects of radiation.

Limited surgery and radiation were first shown to be an effective treatment for craniopharygioma by investigators and physicians at the Royal Marsden Hospital in 1961 (Kramer et al., 1961). They initially reported favorable outcomes in a very small cohort of children and later for a larger cohort of patients who were mainly children (Kramer et al., 1961; Danoff et al., 1983). Many other studies followed which confirmed the excellent disease outcomes with this treatment. Publications from this era provide us with the best long-term follow-up data; however, most radiation was delivered using X-rays for treatment planning and many of these children were treated prior to the era of CT or MRI. Still, outcomes show disease control and survival on the order of 72–90% (Hoogenhout et al., 1984; Hetelekidis et al., 1993; Pemberton et al., 2005; Clark et al., 2013). Experience with 3D conformal radiation is also excellent with most modern series, suggesting disease control rates between 80–100% (Stripp et al., 2004; Jalali et al., 2005; Merchant et al., 2006; Kiehna and Merchant, 2010). Although less data on outcomes for IMRT are available, published studies also report favorable outcomes (Merchant et al., 2013). Data for proton therapy are even more scarce, but Winkfield et al. reported 100% local control for 24 patients at a median follow-up of 40.5 months (Winkfield et al., 2009).

CONCLUSIONS

Radiation therapy provides an effective treatment option for children with craniopharygioma. The risks and benefits of more aggressive surgery should be weighed against those of treating with limited surgery followed by radiation. Each individual case should be reviewed in a multidisciplinary conference to determine the best approach. Technical advances in radiation treatment including image guidance, conformal radiation, IMRT, stereotactic treatment, and proton therapy allow tumors to be targeted, giving better avoidance of healthy tissues that may be damaged by radiation. These advances, along with neurosurgical advances, should allow improved disease control with less late morbidity.

References

Adler Jr., J.R., Gibbs, I.C., Puataweepong, P., Chang, V.S.D., 2006. Visual field preservation after multisession cyberknife radiosurgery for perioptic lesions. Neurosurgery 59, 244–254.

Beltran, C., Naik, M., Merchant, T.E., 2010. Dosimetric effect of target expansion and setup uncertainty during radiation therapy in pediatric craniopharyngioma. Radiother. Oncol. 97 (3), 399–403.

Bolton, R., 2011. Show me how: peer mentoring among children receiving radiation therapy. Abstract. Sept. 8–10, 2011, Association of Pediatric Hematology Oncology Nurses. Anaheim, CA.

Brodin, N.P., Vogelius, I.R., Maraldo, M.V., et al., 2012. Life years lost – comparing potentially fatal late complications after radiotherapy for pediatric medulloblastoma on a common scale. Cancer 118 (21), 5432–5440.

Caldarelli, M., Massimi, L., Tamburrini, G., Cappa, M., Di Rocco, C., 2005. Long-term results of the surgical treatment of craniopharyngioma: the experience at the Policlinico Gemelli, Catholic University, Rome. Childs Nerv. Syst. 21 (8–9), 747–757.

Clark, A.J., Cage, T.A., Aranda, D., Parsa, A.T., Auguste, K.I., Gupta, N., 2012. Treatment-related morbidity and the management of pediatric craniopharyngioma: a systematic review. J. Neurosurg. Pediatr. 10 (4), 293–301.

Clark, A.J., Cage, T.A., Aranda, D., et al., 2013. A systematic review of the results of surgery and radiotherapy on tumor control for pediatric craniopharyngioma. Childs Nerv. Syst. 29 (2), 231–238.

Corn, B.W., Curran Jr., W.J., Shrieve, D.C., Loeffler, J.S., 1997. Stereotactic radiosurgery and radiotherapy: new developments and new directions. Semin Oncol. 24 (6), 707–714.

Danoff, B.F., Cowchock, F.S., Kramer, S., 1983. Childhood craniopharyngioma: survival, local control, endocrine, and neurologic function following radiotherapy. Int. J. Radiat. Oncol. Biol. Phys. 9 (2), 171–175.

Hasegawa, T., Kondziolka, D., Hadjipanayis, C.G., Lunsford, L.D., 2004. Management of cystic craniopharyngiomas with phosphorus-32 intracavitary irradiation. Neurosurgery 54 (4), 813–820.

Hetelekidis, S., Barnes, P.D., Tao, M.L., et al., 1993. 20-year experience in childhood craniopharyngioma. Int. J. Radiat. Oncol. Biol. Phys. 27 (2), 189–195.

Hoogenhout, J., Otten, B.J., Kazem, I., Stoelinga, G.B., Walder, A.H., 1984. Surgery and radiation therapy in the management of craniopharyngiomas. Int. J. Radiat. Oncol. Biol. Phys. 10 (12), 2293–2297.

Iannalfi, A., Fragkandrea, I., Brock, J., Saran, F., 2013. Radiotherapy in craniopharyngiomas. Clin Oncol (R Coll Radiol) 25 (11), 654–667.

Jalali, R., Budrukkar, A., Sarin, R., Sharma, D.S., 2005. High precision conformal radiotherapy employing conservative margins in childhood benign and low-grade brain tumours. Radiother. Oncol. 74 (1), 37–44.

Khan, F.K., 2010. The physics of radiation therapy, 4th. ed. Lippincott, Williams, and Wilkins, Baltimore, MD.

Kiehna, E.N., Merchant, T.E., 2010. Radiation therapy for pediatric craniopharyngioma. Neurosurg. Focus 28 (4), E10.

Kramer, S., McKissock, W., Concannon, J.P., 1961. Craniopharyngiomas. Treatment by combined surgery and radiation therapy. J. Neurosurg. 18, 217–226.

Liu, A.K., Bagrosky, B., Fenton, L.Z., et al., 2009. Vascular abnormalities in pediatric craniopharyngioma patients treated with radiation therapy. Pediatr. Blood Cancer 52 (2), 227–230.

Loeffler, J.S., Durante, M., 2013. Charged particle therapy – optimization, challenges and future directions. Nat. Rev. Clin. Oncol. 10 (7), 411–424.

Luu, Q.T., Loredo, L.N., Archambeau, J.O., Yonemoto, L.T., Slater, J.M., Slater, J.D., 2006. Fractionated proton radiation treatment for pediatric craniopharyngioma: preliminary report. Cancer J. 12 (2), 155–159.

MacDonald, S.M., Delaney, T.F., Loeffler, J.S., 2006. Proton beam radiation therapy. Cancer Invest. 23 (2), 199–208.

Mailhot Vega, R.B., Kim, J., Bussiere, M., et al., 2013. Cost effectiveness of proton therapy compared with photon therapy in the management of pediatric medulloblastoma. Cancer epub ahead of print.

McFadyen, J.G., Pelly, N., Orr, R.J., 2011. Sedation and anesthesia for the pediatric patient undergoing radiation therapy. Curr. Opin. Anaesthesiol. 24 (4), 433–438.

Merchant, T.E., Kiehna, E.N., Kun, L.E., et al., 2006. Phase II trial of conformal radiation therapy for pediatric patients with craniopharyngioma and correlation of surgical factors and radiation dosimetry with change in cognitive function. J. Neurosurg. 104 (Suppl. 2), 94–102.

Merchant, T.E., Kun, L.E., Hua, C.H., et al., 2013. Disease control after reduced volume conformal and intensity modulated radiation therapy for childhood craniopharyngioma. Int. J. Radiat. Oncol. Biol. Phys. 85 (4), e187–e192.

Mottolese, C., Szathmari, A., Berlier, P., Hermier, M., 2005. Craniopharyngioma: our experience in Lyon. Childs Nerv. Syst. 21 (8–9), 790–798.

Pemberton, L.S., Dougal, M., Magee, B., Gattamaneni, H.R., 2005. Experience of external beam radiotherapy given adjuvantly or at relapse following surgery for craniopharyngioma. Radiother. Oncol. 77 (1), 99–104.

Rajan, B., Ashley, S., Thomas, D.G., Marsh, H., Britton, J., Brada, M., 1997. Craniopharyngioma: improving outcome by early recognition and treatment of acute complications. Int. J. Radiat. Oncol. Biol. Phys. 37 (3), 517–521.

Smith, A., Gillin, M., Bues, M., et al., 2009. The M. D. Anderson proton therapy system. Med. Phys. 36 (9), 4068–4083.

Stripp, D.C., Maity, A., Janss, A.J., et al., 2004. Surgery with or without radiation therapy in the management of craniopharyngiomas in children and young adults. Int. J. Radiat. Oncol. Biol. Phys. 58 (3), 714–720.

Sughrue, M.E., Yang, I., Kane, A.K., et al., 2011. Endocrinologic, neurologic, and visual morbidity after treatment for craniopharyngioma. J. Neurooncol. 101 (3), 463–476.

Tomita, T., Bowman, R.M., 2005. Craniopharyngiomas in children: surgical experience at Children's Memorial Hospital. Childs Nerv. Syst. 21 (8–9), 729–746.

Trofimov, A., Bortfeld, T., 2003. Optimization of beam parameters and treatment planning for intensity modulated proton therapy. Technol. Cancer Res. Treat. 2 (5), 437–444.

Winkfield, K.M., Linsenmeier, C., Yock, T.I., et al., 2009. Surveillance of craniopharyngioma cyst growth in children treated with proton radiotherapy. Int. J. Radiat. Oncol. Biol. Phys. 73 (3), 716–721.

Winkfield, K.M., Tsai, H.K., Yao, X., et al., 2011. Long-term clinical outcomes following treatment of childhood craniopharyngioma. Pediatr. Blood Cancer 56 (7), 1120.

Zhao, R., Deng, J., Liang, X., Zeng, J., Chen, X., Wang, J., 2010. Treatment of cystic craniopharyngioma with phosphorus-32 intracavitary irradiation. Childs Nerv. Syst. 26 (5), 669–674.

CHAPTER

30

Management of Giant Craniopharyngiomas

Tyler J. Kenning, Matthew A. Adamo*, James J. Evans*[†]

[*]Department of Neurosurgery, Albany Medical Center, Albany, NY, USA; [†]Department of Neurological Surgery, Thomas Jefferson University Hospital, Philadelphia, PA, USA

"Some tumors of this type are attached to such a wide expanse of the base of the brain that enucleation is impossible." **Walter Dandy, 1945**

Although there is some disagreement in the literature as to what dimensions exactly characterize a "giant craniopharyngioma," tumors greater than 4–5 cm may represent up to 14–20% of these lesions and pose a significant clinical challenge (Weiner et al., 1994; Fahlbusch et al., 1999; Karavitaki et al., 2006). Their excessive size results in decreased overall survival (Elliott et al., 2010), increased mortality (Yasargil et al., 1990), increased neurological and hypothalamic morbidity (Yasargil et al., 1990; DeVile et al., 1996; Ersahin et al., 2005), decreased extent of resection and local disease control (Gordy et al., 1949; Kramer et al., 1968; Trippi et al., 1969; Kahn et al., 1973; Djordjević et al., 1979; Guidetti and Fraioli, 1979; Rougerie, 1979; Shapiro et al., 1979; Wen et al., 1989; DeVile et al., 1996; Fahlbusch and Hoffman, 1999; Mortini et al., 2011), and higher rates of recurrence (Wen et al., 1989; Hetelekidis et al., 1993; DeVile et al., 1996; Ersahin et al., 2005; Thompson et al., 2005; Gupta et al., 2006). It is well documented that giant craniopharyngiomas may have significantly higher rates of morbidity and mortality compared to tumors of smaller size and often require more surgical or adjuvant interventions. Therefore, giant craniopharyngiomas require several additional considerations, compared to tumors of a smaller size, to limit potential complications.

Radical resection while limiting operative morbidity is the primary therapy of choice, because it is associated with the best outcome in terms of overall and recurrence-free survival (Karavitaki et al., 2006; Mortini et al., 2011, 2013). It has been demonstrated that the greatest limitations to gross total resection of craniopharyngiomas are the size and the location of the mass. With increasing size, tumors can extend into multiple intracranial compartments, often needing more than one surgical approach and requiring multimodal management with post-operative adjuvant treatments, such as stereotactic radiation and intra-tumor therapies (see Chapters

Craniopharyngiomas
http://dx.doi.org/10.1016/B978-0-12-416706-3.00030-1

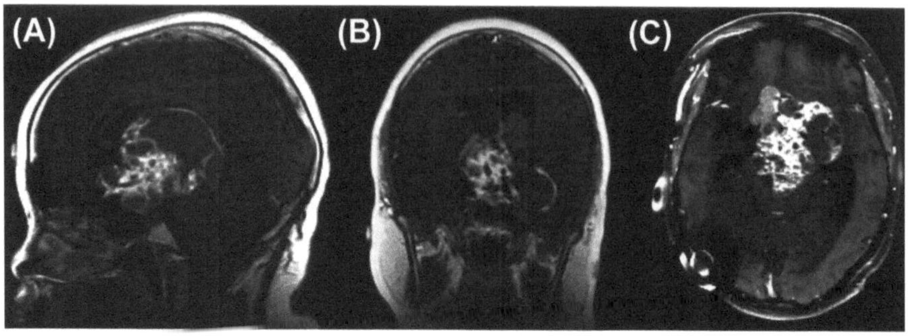

FIGURE 30.1 **A,** Sagittal, **B,** coronal, and **C,** axial contrast-enhanced T1WI MRI of a 17-year-old male with solid and cystic giant craniopharyngioma.

20–22, 24 and 25). Most (95%) craniopharyngiomas originate in the suprasellar cistern and a few (5–6%) are located purely within the sella. Giant craniopharyngiomas, on the other hand, most often extend into the anterior (72%), middle (52%), and posterior (16%) cranial fossae (Elliott et al., 2010), and often involve two or more of these intracranial compartments (Figure 30.1).

As large tumors extend into the surrounding cisternal spaces and even the ventricular system, compression, distortion, and encasement of critical neurovascular structures further complicates treatment. It can become increasingly difficult to distinguish the vascular supply to the optic apparatus, brainstem, and brain parenchyma from those branches supplying the tumor mass. This identification of vasculature is often challenging in craniopharyngiomas of even small or moderate size (Mortini et al., 2011, 2013). Tumor adherence to major vascular branches is often cited as the cause for subtotal resections (Choux and Genitori, 1991) and may also present a major source of morbidity. Ventricular obstruction can result in hydrocephalus in a significant number of patients on presentation (Elliott et al., 2010). Finally, paramount in the treatment of all craniopharyngiomas is the tumor's relationship to the hypothalamus and the effect the treatment may have on alteration of hypothalamic function or memory.

PRE-OPERATIVE CONSIDERATIONS

Prior to surgical treatment of a suspected craniopharyngioma, further evaluation is required pre-operatively. This work-up is similar to any lesion located in the suprasellar space and is discussed more thoroughly in other chapters of this text (Chapters 3, 5, and 6). Due to their excessive size, however, giant craniopharyngiomas require some special pre-operative considerations.

An ophthalmologic work-up should include an assessment of visual acuity, visual field perimetry, and optic fundoscopy. Pre-operative visual field deficits exist in 46–93% of patients (Fahlbusch and Hoffman, 2008; Elliott et al., 2010). A comprehensive endocrinological evaluation is also required, including a thorough history and physical examination as well as biochemical evaluation. Close attention should be given to both anterior and posterior pituitary gland dysfunction, especially in pediatric patients. A stimulation test of the pituitary–adrenal axis as well as an insulin-induced hypoglycemia test of the somatotrophic and corticotrophic axes may provide pre-operative information that will assist in medical management in the peri- and post-operative periods. Assessment for diabetes insipidus is also important, as it may be present in varying degrees in up to 30% of patients pre-operatively and in 70% after surgical resection (Fahlbusch and Hoffman, 2008; Elliott et al., 2010).

Prior to any surgical intervention, careful radiographic evaluation of the tumor and its relation to the adjacent neurovascular structures must be conducted. Often this can be delineated with a thin cut T2 and contrasted T1 MRI, but either computer tomography (CT) or catheter angiography may be required to best visualize the vascular anatomy, especially as structures become greatly distorted in the setting of giant tumors. MRI should also be used to detect the presence of hydrocephalus and cerebral edema, as both should be addressed pre- or intra-operatively. A CT scan should also be considered to better detect calcifications within the tumor.

SURGICAL CONSIDERATIONS

Patients who are elderly or those with significant clinical or neuropsychological deterioration that is not correctable with medical management are likely not suitable candidates for radical surgical resection, and are best treated with palliative measures aimed at symptomatic relief. Giant craniopharyngiomas with a large or predominantly cystic component may be treated with cyst aspiration, as described below, either as the primary treatment for palliation of symptoms or as the initial treatment to help a patient improve neurologically prior to a more aggressive surgical procedure for tumor resection. Those patients with a significant amount of peritumoral edema, especially within the hypothalamus, should be treated with pre-operative corticosteroids. Symptomatic hydrocephalus should be addressed with either external ventricular drainage or ventriculoperitoneal shunting.

Typically, giant craniopharyngiomas exhibit significant cystic components (Figure 30.2). There is some disagreement as to whether treatment of these cysts is helpful prior to any attempts at definitive tumor resection. Fahlbusch and Hoffman routinely perform stereotactic cyst aspiration initially, believing that it results in retraction of the tumor capsule and less significant adhesions to adjacent structures (Fahlbusch and Hoffman, 2008). In their opinion, this ultimately makes the subsequent tumor dissection easier and safer. Other groups, however, favor maintaining the cystic portion of the tumor, citing the expanded, natural corridors created by the larger tumor that aid visualization and dissection (Elliott et al., 2010). For patients with acute deterioration from mass effects or hydrocephalus due to ventricular obstruction, however, emergent decompression of any cystic tumor components via placement of an external ventricular drain or stereotactic aspiration may be required prior to definitive surgical resection.

Many surgical approaches have been described for resecting giant craniopharyngiomas, including bilateral subfrontal (Al-Mefty et al., 1985; Ammirati, 1990; Fahlbusch and Hoffman, 2008), frontobasal interhemispheric (Shirane et al., 2002), pterional with or without orbital and zygomatic osteotomies (Zuccaro, 2005), and transventricular and transpetrosal approaches (Al-Mefty et al., 2008). Reasons cited for a chosen approach include the shortest route to the pathology, access to basilar cisterns for cerebrospinal fluid drainage, limiting obstruction from critical neurovascular structures, early visualization and protection of the optic chiasm or carotid arteries, and minimizing brain retraction. Although extended endonasal endoscopic approaches have become increasingly popular in the treatment of

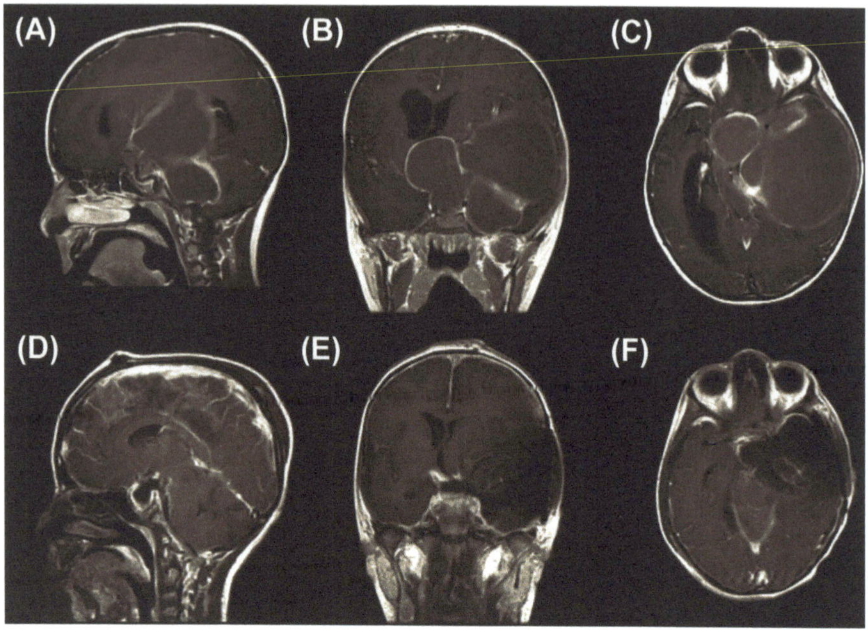

FIGURE 30.2 **A,** Sagittal, **B,** coronal, and **C,** axial contrast-enhanced T1WI MRI of an 8-year-old female with a largely cystic giant craniopharyngioma. Immediate post-operative **D,** sagittal, **E,** coronal, and **F,** axial contrast-enhanced T1WI MRI after resection through a left pterional craniotomy with some residual enhancement in the right suprasellar cistern.

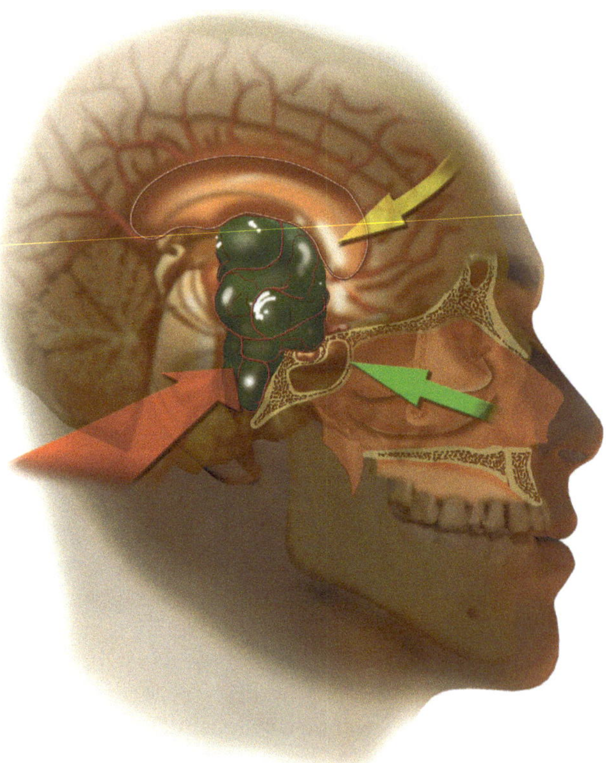

FIGURE 30.3 Sagittal illustration of a giant craniopharyngioma with significant extension down the clivus into the posterior fossa that may be best treated with a transpetrosal approach (red arrow). Additional potential approaches include endonasal (green arrow) and interhemispheric (yellow arrow).

craniopharyngiomas, many authors caution against their sole use in giant tumors with significant lateral extension. However, the utilization of an endoscope can aid a transcranial approach by permitting a greater intra-operative field of view. Staged surgical procedures with variable combinations of these approaches may be required to obtain maximal tumor resection (Figures 30.3–30.6). Some centers have advocated combined simultaneous surgical approaches as well, however most advocate staging the procedures to reduce the surgical time, blood loss, and morbidity associated with prolonged operations.

For residual or recurrent giant craniopharyngiomas, multiple treatment modalities are often required. As mentioned above, a second surgical approach in a staged procedure may be required based on post-operative imaging or planned prospectively. Serial aspiration of persistent cystic components with or without adjuvant radiotherapy has been reported as a means of controlling the tumor size and limiting morbidity (Gutin et al., 1980; Backlund, 1989; Spaziante et al., 1989). The technique and efficacy of both of these strategies is discussed elsewhere in this book. Radiotherapy for large tumors, however, may significantly increase the risk to adjacent cranial nerves and brain tissue due to the large target volumes and dosages required (Regine and Kramer, 1992; Blonigen et al., 2010; Eaton et al., 2013). Additionally, the possibility of the

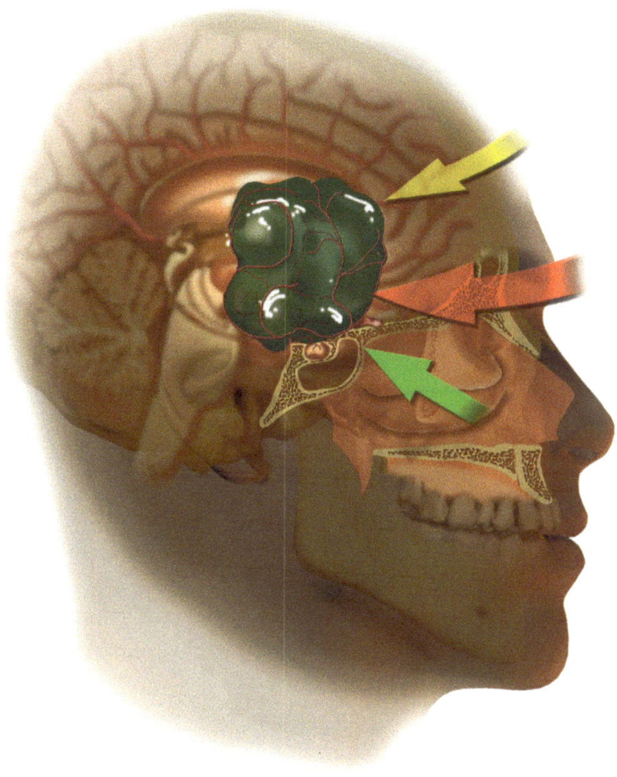

FIGURE 30.4 Sagittal illustration of a giant craniopharyngioma with extension into the anterior cranial fossa that may be best treated with a subfrontal transbasal approach (red arrow). Additional potential approaches include endonasal (green arrow) and interhemispheric (yellow arrow).

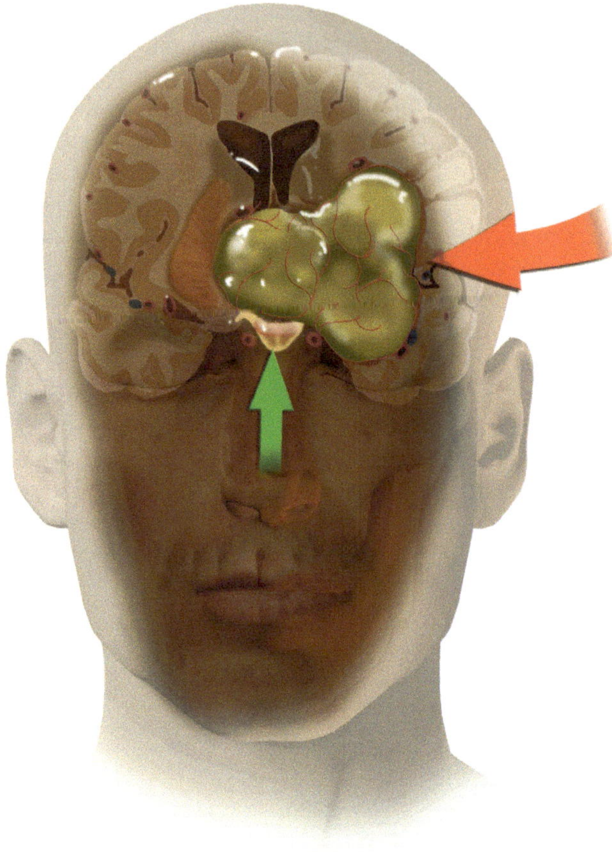

FIGURE 30.5 Coronal illustration of a giant craniopharyngioma with extension into the middle fossa that may be best treated with a transsylvian/pterional approach (red arrow). Additional potential approaches include endonasal (green arrow).

enlargement of cystic tumor components during a course of radiation treatment is widely recognized, and its occurrence in up to 28% of patients requires reimaging and potential modification of the treatment plan, with or without cyst drainage, prior to its completion (Minniti et al., 2007). Intracystic administration of either radioisotopes or chemotherapeutic agents may also be useful. Ultimately, treatment of recurrent or residual giant tumors carries greater risk than the initial presentation, with increased rates of complications, mortality, and a lower rate of effective disease control (Elliott et al., 2010).

SURGICAL OUTCOMES

Few studies are dedicated to reviewing the outcomes of giant craniopharyngiomas alone (Table 30.1). Instead, most reviews of craniopharyngioma results include these tumors within

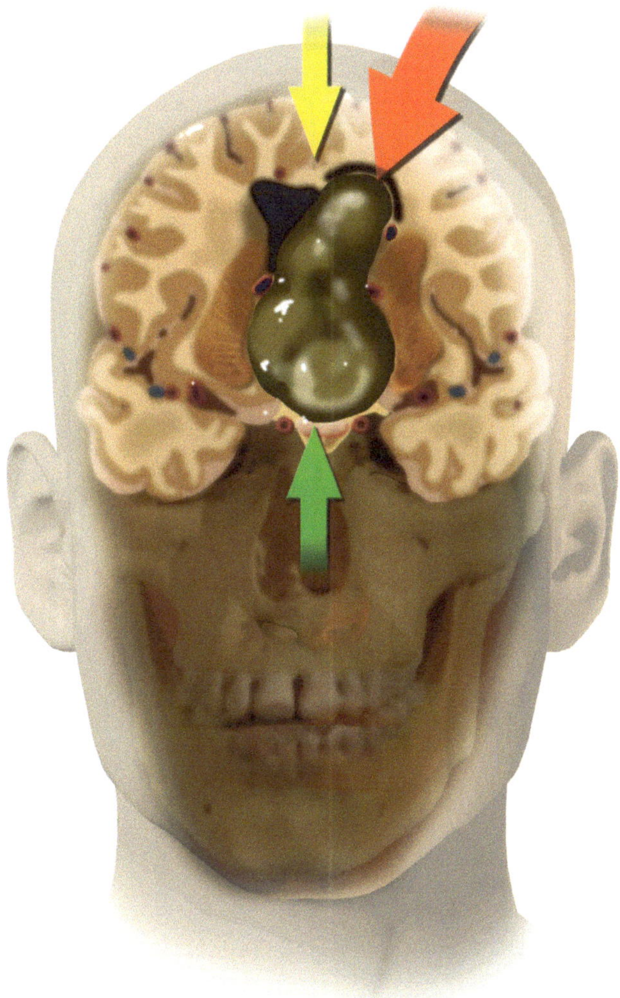

FIGURE 30.6 Coronal illustration of a giant craniopharyngioma with extension through the third ventricle and into the lateral ventricle that may be best treated with a transcortical transventricular approach (red arrow). Additional potential approaches include endonasal (green arrow) and interhemispheric (yellow arrow).

a larger series, making it difficult to extrapolate data specific to this subset. Despite this, most publications cite the potentially increased risk for peri-operative morbidity and mortality, lower rates of gross total resection, and high recurrence rates in the treatment of giant craniopharyngiomas. The most significant determinant of post-operative outcome is frequently the patient's pre-operative status, which can be profoundly affected with large cystic and solid tumors. The results of small, retrospective studies do demonstrate, however, that even giant craniopharyngiomas can be successfully managed, and even completely resected.

TABLE 30.1 Summary of Case Series Reporting On the Results of Giant Craniopharyngioma Resection

	No. patients	Mean age	Mean follow-up	Mean tumor size	% GTR	Operative mortality	Series mortality	Recurrence rate	New postop endocrinopathies	New visual deficits	New neurologic deficits	Permanent neurologic deficit
Al-Mefty et al., 1985	10	Pediatrics		> 5 cm	80	0%	20%	0%	100% DI	0	0	0
Yasargil et al., 1990	8					87.50%						
De Vile et al., 1996	25	Pediatrics		> 3.5 cm								
Fahlbusch et al., 1999	20				0							
Van Effenterre et al., 2002	13			"giant"	46							
Ersahin et al., 2005	33	Pediatrics		> 4 cm		15%						
Gupta et al., 2005	44			> 4 cm				58%				
Falhbusch and Hoffman, 2008	16	41.1 years	25.6 mos	4.8 cm	62.5	0%	0%	13%	50% DI	13%	6%	
Elliott et al., 2010	26	10.5 years	8.9 years	5.9 ± 1 cm	77	0%	31%	16% of GTR	63.2% DI	42%	65%	38%

CONCLUSION

Craniopharyngiomas pose a significant clinical challenge, which is even greater with giant tumors, since they can involve multiple intracranial compartments. Ventricular obstruction can result in hydrocephalus and adherence to the intracranial vasculature, cranial nerves, and brainstem can make surgical resection from one approach difficult. A staged surgical resection may be required. The treatment modalities used for these larger tumors are the same as for smaller craniopharyngiomas, but occasionally multimodal treatment will be required.

Acknowledgment

We would like to thank Paul Schiffmacher, BFA, Department of Medical Media Services, Thomas Jefferson University Hospital for contributing the illustrations for this chapter.

References

Al-Mefty, O., Ayoubi, S., Kadri, P.A., 2008. The petrosal approach for the resection of retrochiasmatic craniopharyngiomas. Neurosurgery 62 (5 Suppl. 2), ONS331–ONS336.

Al-Mefty, O., Hassounah, M., Weaver, P., Sakati, N., Jinkins, J.R., Fox, J.L., 1985. Microsurgery for giant craniopharyngiomas in children. Neurosurgery 17, 585–595.

Ammirati, M., Samii, M., Sephernia, A., 1990. Surgery of large retrochiasmatic craniopharyngiomas in children. Childs Nerv. Syst. 6, 13–17.

Backlund, E.O., 1989. Colloidal radioisotopes as part of a multi-modality treatment of craniopharyngiomas. J. Neurosurg. Sci. 33, 95–97.

Blonigen, B.J., Steinmetz, R.D., Levin, L., Lamba, M.A., Warnick, R.E., Breneman, J.C., 2010. Irradiated volume as a predictor of brain radionecrosis after linear accelerator stereotactic radiosurgery. Int. J. Radiat. Oncol. Biol. Phys. 77, 996–1001.

Choux, M.L.G., Genitori, L., 1991. Craniopharyngioma in children. 41st annual congress of the French Society of Neurosurgery. Neuro-Chirurgie 37 (Suppl. 1), 1–174.

Dandy, Walter E., 1945. Surgery of the Brain. W. F. Prior Company, Inc, Hagerstown. Print, p 578.

De Vile, C.J., Grant, D.B., Kendall, B.E., Neville, B.G., Stanhope, R., Watkins, K.E., Hayward, R.D., 1996. Management of childhood craniopharyngioma: can the morbidity of radical surgery be predicted? J. Neurosurg. 85, 73–81.

Djordjević, M., Djordjević, Z., Janićijević, M., Nestorović, B., Stefanović, B., Ivkov, M., 1979. Surgical treatment of craniopharyngiomas in children. Acta Neurochir. Suppl. (Wien) 28, 344–347.

Eaton, B.R., Gebhardt, B., Prabhu, R., Shu, H.K., Curran, Jr., W.J., Crocker, I., 2013. Hypofractionated radiosurgery for intact or resected brain metastases: defining the optimal dose and fractionation. Radiat. Oncol. 8, 135–201.

Elliott, R.E., Hsieh, K., Hochm, T., Belitskaya-Levy, I., Wisoff, J., Wisoff, J.H., 2010. Efficacy and safety of radical resection of primary and recurrent craniopharyngiomas in 86 children. Clinical article. J. Neurosurg. Pediatr. 5, 30–48.

Ersahin, Y., Yurtseven, T., Ozgiray, E., Mutluer, S., 2005. Craniopharyngiomas in children: Turkey experience. Childs. Nerv. Syst. 21, 766–772.

Fahlbusch, R., Hoffman, B.M., 2008. Surgical management of giant craniopharyngiomas. Acta Neurochir. 150, 1213–1226.

Fahlbusch, R., Honegger, J., Paulus, W., Huk, W., Buchfelder, M., 1999. Surgical treatment of craniopharyngiomas: experience with 168 patients. J. Neurosurg. 90, 237–250.

Gordy, P.D., Peet, M.M., Kahn, E.A., 1949. The surgery of the craniopharyngiomas. J. Neurosurg. 6, 503–517.

Guidetti, B., Fraioli, B., 1979. Craniopharyngiomas. Results of surgical treatment. Acta Neurochir. Suppl. (Wien) 28, 349–351.

Gupta, D.K., Ojha, B.K., Sarkar, C., Mahapatra, A.K., Mehta, V.S., 2006. Recurrence in craniopharyngiomas: analysis of clinical and histological features. J. Clin. Neurosci. 13, 438–442.

Gutin, P.H., Klemme, W.M., Lagger, R.L., Mackay, A.R., Pitts, L.H., Hosobuchi, Y., 1980. Management of the unresectable cystic craniopharyngioma by aspiration through an ommaya reservoir drainage system. J. Neurosurg. 52, 36–40.

Hetelekidis, S., Barnes, P.D., Tao, M.L., Fischer, E.G., Schneider, L., Scott, R.M., et al., 1993. 20-year experience in childhood craniopharyngioma. Int. J. Radiat. Oncol. Biol. Phys. 27, 189–195.

Kahn, E.A., Gosch, H.H., Seeger, J.F., Hicks, S.P., 1973. Forty-five years experience with the craniopharyngiomas. Surg. Neurol. 1, 5–12.

Karavitaki, N., Cudlip, S., Adams, C.B., Wass, J.A., 2006. Craniopharyngiomas Endocr. Rev. 27, 371–397.

Kramer, S., Southard, M., Mansfield, C.M., 1968. Radiotherapy in the management of craniopharyngiomas: further experiences and late results. Am. J. Roentgenol. Radium. Ther. Nucl. Med. 103, 44–52.

Minniti, G., Saran, F., Traish, D., Soomal, R., Sardell, S., Gonsalves, A., et al., 2007. Fractionated stereotactic conformal radiotherapy following conservative surgery in the control of craniopharyngiomas. Radiother. Oncol. 82, 90–95.

Mortini, P., Losa, M., Pozzobon, G., et al., 2011. Neurosurgical treatment of craniopharyngioma in adults and children: early and long-term results in a large case series. J. Neurosurg. 114, 1350–1359.

Mortini, P., Losa, M., Gagliardi, F., 2013. Radical removal of craniopharyngiomas. In: Hayat, M.A. (Ed.), Tumors of the central nervous system. Springer, Netherlands, pp. 249–267.

Regine, W.F., Kramer, S., 1992. Pediatric craniopharyngiomas: long-term results of combined treatment with surgery and radiation. Int. J. Radiat. Oncol. Biol. Phys. 24, 611–617.

Rougerie, J., 1979. What can be expected from the surgical treatment of craniopharyngiomas in children. Report of 92 cases. Childs Brain 5, 433–449.

Shapiro, K., Till, K., Grant, D.N., 1979. Craniopharyngiomas in childhood. A rational approach to treatment. J. Neurosurg. 50, 617–623.

Shirane, R., Ching-Chan, S., Kusaka, Y., Jokura, H., Yoshimoto, T., 2002. Surgical outcomes in 31 patients with craniopharyngiomas extending outside the suprasellar cistern: an evaluation of the frontobasal interhemispheric approach. J. Neurosurg. 96, 704–712.

Spaziante, R., De Divitiis, E., Irace, C., Cappabianca, P., Caputi, F., 1989. Management of primary or recurring grossly cystic craniopharyngiomas by means of draining systems. Topic review and 6 case reports. Acta Neurochir (Wien) 97, 95–106.

Thompson, D., Phipps, K., Hayward, R., 2005. Craniopharyngioma in childhood: our evidence-based approach to management. Childs Nerv. Syst. 21, 660–668.

Trippi, A.C., Garner, J.T., Kassabian, J.T., Shelden, C.H., 1969. A new approach to inoperable craniopharyngiomas. Am. J. Surg. 118, 307–310.

Van Effenterre, R., Boch, A.L., 2002. Craniopharyngioma in adults and children: a study of 122 surgical cases. J. Neurosurg. 97, 3–11.

Weiner, H.L., Wisoff, J.H., Rosenberg, M.E., et al., 1994. Craniopharyngiomas: a clinicopathological analysis of factors predictive of recurrence and functional outcome. Neurosurgery 35, 1001–1010 [discussion 1010–1011].

Wen, B.C., Hussey, D.H., Staples, J., Hitchon, P.W., Jani, S.K., Vigliotti, A.P., et al., 1989. A comparison of the roles of surgery and radiation therapy in the management of craniopharyngiomas. Int. J. Radiat. Oncol. Biol. Phys. 16, 17–24.

Yasargil, M.G., Curcic, M., Kis, M., Siegenthaler, G., Teddy, P.J., Roth, P., 1990. Total removal of craniopharyngiomas. Approaches and longterm results in 144 patients. J. Neurosurg. 73, 3–11.

Zuccaro, G., 2005. Radical resection of craniopharyngioma. Childs. Nerv. Syst. 21, 679–690.

CHAPTER

31

Ectopic Occurrence of Craniopharyngiomas

*Rafael Uribe**, *Henry Brem*†, *George Jallo*†

*Pontificia Universidad Javeriana, Bogotá, Colombia;

†Johns Hopkins School of Medicine, Baltimore, MD, USA

"To one who has had a large experience in dealing on the operating table with tumors in this location, the difficulties attending any attempt at radical removal at once suggest themselves." ***RC Carpenter, GW Chamberlin, and CH Frazier, 1937***

INTRODUCTION

Craniopharyngiomas are considered some of the most challenging central nervous system tumors to treat. Although histologically benign (WHO grade I), their anatomical relationship to important neuro-endocrine structures as well as critical cerebrospinal fluid (CSF) pathways makes them difficult to resect. There has been considerable controversy regarding the optimal treatment strategy for these tumors. Although gross total resection is associated with a longer progression-free survival, the morbidity and mortality associated with a more aggressive approach are potentially higher. Advances in medical management and focused forms of radiation, such as gamma knife, have allowed patients to live longer without the increased risks of radical resection.

Traditionally confined to the sellar or suprasellar space, craniopharyngiomas occasionally present in ectopic locations which can make their diagnosis and recognition more difficult until final histopathological confirmation is obtained. Ectopic craniopharyngiomas can occur primarily or through seeding after surgical removal of sellar lesions.

EPIDEMIOLOGY

Craniopharyngiomas are rare tumors. They constitute approximately 1 to 5% of all intracranial tumors (Rushing et al., 2007). They have a bimodal distribution of age at presentation, being more frequent in children (aged 5 to 14) and older adults (aged 65

Craniopharyngiomas
http://dx.doi.org/10.1016/B978-0-12-416706-3.00031-3

to 74). Their approximate incidence is 1.3 cases per million person years (Bunin et al., 1998). There is apparently no gender or racial difference in the incidence of craniopharyngiomas.

CLINICAL PRESENTATION

The anatomical proximity of craniopharyngiomas to several key anatomical structures makes the clinical presentation varied and complex. Patients may complain of headaches which may be attributable to increased intracranial pressure secondary to the presence of hydrocephalus. Compression of the optic apparatus at the level of the optic chiasm will lead to bitemporal hemianopia, and, with longstanding duration of symptoms, decreased visual acuity secondary to papilledema, and optic nerve atrophy. Displacement and compression of the pituitary stalk or gland can lead to a myriad of symptoms derived from several endocrinological disturbances.

Hypocortisolism might produce a set of vague symptoms characterized by an overall sense of fatigue and decreased energy. Hypothyroidism may lead to slowing of higher-order mental processing, weight gain, constipation, and depression. By displacing the pituitary stalk with a secondary decrease in dopamine secretion (stalk effect), prolactin levels are up-regulated, leading to decreased libido in men and menstrual cycle abnormalities, such as dysmenorrhea or amenorrhea, in women. Inhibition of growth hormone secretion might lead to restricted development in children. Lastly, compression of the posterior lobe of the pituitary might lead to alterations in secretion of vasopressin, which can produce symptoms of diabetes insipidus: increased urine output and dehydration with secondary hypernatremia. When craniopharyngiomas extend rostrally, they may compress the hypothalamus, leading to disturbances such as hyperphagia or increased somnolence. Some of these tumors might grow considerably, compressing the medial aspect of the temporal lobes, in turn leading to short-term memory disturbances.

The diagnosis of craniopharyngiomas might be delayed in children when compared to adults, since the most common presenting symptom is headache, which can be hard to evaluate especially in very young patients. Hormonal disturbances will affect the secretion of growth hormone most commonly in children (75%) followed by gonadotropins (40%), ACTH (25%), and TSH (25%). Diabetes insipidus (DI) is present pre-operatively in approximately 17% of patients (Müller, 2013).

DIAGNOSIS

In patients with suspected intracranial pathology, computed tomography (CT) or magnetic resonance imaging (MRI) is routinely performed. Craniopharyngiomas have a characteristic iso- or hypo-dense appearance on CT. They can be multicystic heterogeneously enhancing masses with calcification. This last phenomenon is more frequent in the adamantinomatous variant of the tumor. MRI denotes an iso- or hypo-intense and slightly hyperintense image on T1 and T2 weighted images, respectively. Typically these tumors enhance heterogeneously with gadolinium injection. The cystic component of these tumors often has higher signal intensity than CSF, denoting the presence of proteinaceous material inside the cysts.

PATHOLOGY

Craniopharyngiomas can be classified into three main subgroups according to their histological components. Adamantinomatous craniopharyngiomas are more frequent in children, while the papillary subtype is almost exclusively present in older adults. The former can be distinguished from the latter by the presence of calcification and a usually more cystic appearance on imaging. Adamantinomatous craniopharyngiomas are characterized histologically by the presence of squamous epithelium surrounded by columnar epithelium in a palisaded pattern. The cystic cavities are lined by flattened epithelium. The areas surrounding the tumor are marked by reactive gliosis. The papillary subtype is characterized by the presence of a well-maturated squamous epithelium which lacks surface maturation. This subtype often lacks calcification, and on occasion can have ciliated epithelium and goblet cells (Rushing et al., 2007)

EMBRYOLOGY

The pituitary is composed of two distinct lobes: anterior and posterior. During embryonic stages of development, an intermediate lobe sits between the other two, but disappears during fetal development in humans. The posterior lobe of the pituitary, also called neurohypophysis, is an evagination of the diencephalon. The anterior lobe, on the other hand, is a derivative of Rathke's pouch, an evagination of the primitive stomodeum which will develop later into the mouth (Dubois and Elamraoui, 1995). There are two main theories which have tried to explain the pathogenesis of craniopharyngiomas. An embryogenetic theory posits that craniopharyngiomas are derived from neoplastic transformation of epithelial cell remnants from the craniopharyngeal duct and Rathke's pouch. A second theory considers craniopharyngiomas to be derived from metaplastic transformation of differentiated squamous epithelium, which is part of the anterior lobe of the pituitary (Larkin and Ansorge, 2012). An argument in favor of the embryogenetic theory is the fact that there is a spectrum of disease associated with the development of Rathke's pouch in which a persistent craniopharyngeal canal (Abele, 2013) can be associated with different pathological entities, amongst them craniopharyngioma.

ECTOPIC CRANIOPHARYNGIOMAS

The most common location for these tumors is in the sellar/suprasellar space because of its spatial relationship with the pituitary and hypothalamus above and the nose and mouth below. Nevertheless, craniopharyngiomas can appear in different locations. In 2002, the senior author (HB) published a case report detailing a 73-year-old patient who had presented 8 years before, complaining of headache, dizziness, and loss of short-term memory. MRI revealed the presence of a craniopharyngioma mainly localized to the third ventricle. The patient underwent frontal craniotomy and the tumor was removed via an interhemispheric/transcallosal route. Three years after surgical removal, a small (3.0 mm), frontal, parasagittal enhancing nodule was noted next to the previous craniotomy site. The patient was followed conservatively for 8 years. Continued growth of the lesion was documented during the follow-up period, until surgery was performed on this new tumor. Intra-operatively, an extra axial lesion was documented which was found to be a craniopharyngioma with the same histological appearance as the one initially resected 8 years earlier (Liu et al., 2002). Similarly in 2011, Kordes et al. reported a 7-year-old patient who underwent a right pterional craniotomy for the removal of a craniopharyngioma. Fifteen months later, the patient was noted to have a second lesion adjacent to the site of the previous craniotomy. The lesion proved to be an adamantinomatous craniopharyngioma like the one that had been previously removed (Kordes et al., 2011). Other case reports have documented similar seeding of tumor cells distant from the original tumor site along the surgical path (Ragoowansi and Piepgras, 1991; Lee et al., 1999; Novegno et al., 2002; Ishii et al., 2004; Kawaguchi et al., 2005; Jeong et al., 2006; Yamada et al., 2006; Bikmaz, 2009; Elliott, 2009; Romani et al., 2010; Blank, 2011; Elfving et al., 2011; Jakobs and Orakcioglu, 2012). It is clear from these reports that craniopharyngioma cells have the ability to remain viable after excision, and that if implanted along the surgical tract can potentially create a second lesion (see Table 31.1).

Other authors have reported the occurrence of primary craniopharyngiomas located outside of the sellar/suprasellar region. In 2001, Jallo et al. documented a case of an 8-year-old patient who presented symptoms of headache and decreased visual acuity that had been going on for one and a half years. On exam, he was noted to have no light perception in the right eye as well as marked optic atrophy ipsilaterally. Work-up revealed on CT and MRI the presence of a large lesion within the ethmoid sinus with significant bone erosion and compression of the right optic nerve. Surgery was performed through a bifrontal transbasal approach; no evidence of sellar compromise was found and the lesion was found to be completely extradural; pathology revealed craniopharyngioma (Deutsch et al., 2001). Similarly, Bozbuga et al. reported a primary cerebellopontine angle craniopharyngioma in a 34-year-old patient with Gardner syndrome (Bozbuga et al., 2011). Likewise, Kim et al. reported a primary CP angle craniopharyngioma in a patient with suspected Gardner syndrome (Kim et al., 2014). It is unknown whether there is an association between these pathologies. Other reports have shown the presence of primary craniopharyngiomas in other locations, such as the corpus callosum (Sangiovanni et al., 1997), fourth ventricle (Shah et al., 2007), pineal gland (Usanov and Hatomkin, 1999), clivus (Kawamata et al., 2002), and the sphenoid sinus (Nourbakhsh et al., 2010) (see Table 31.2).

Although craniopharyngiomas might be seeded along a surgical tract or may appear primarily in ectopic locations, a third subset of these tumors may arise secondarily after surgical removal of a primary lesion in a distant site that harbors no relationship to the initial surgical approach. Gupta et al. reported the case of a 73-year-old man who had undergone a right pterional craniotomy for the removal of a suprasellar mass, later found to be an adamantinomatous craniopharyngioma. Seven years later, the patient presented with new-onset partial seizures. Two different lesions adjacent to the dura located on the left posterior frontal and parietooccipital lobes were documented. Surgery was performed, once again revealing adamantinomatous craniopharyngioma for both tumors (Gupta et al., 1999). In addition, Ito et al. reported a case of a 65-year-old man who had undergone prior resection of a sellar craniopharyngioma through a sub-frontal approach. Three years later, the patient was found to have a right temporal lesion that was not related to the original surgical approach (Ito et al., 2001). These last two cases raise the question of a probable metastatic potential of craniopharyngioma. Nevertheless, since there are very few cases reported and they both had prior surgical interventions, the dissemination was more likely be related to surgical manipulation. Although these cases cannot be called true metastases, they do show that craniopharyngioma cells can be viable in distant locations after possibly spreading through CSF pathways.

TABLE 31.1 Ectopic Recurrence of Craniopharyngioma after Removal of a Primary Lesion

Series	Year	Age	Gender	Primary location	Initial surgical approach	Time to recurrence	Ectopic recurrence location	Radiation therapy
Ragoowansi et al.	1991	47	M	Sellar	Right frontotemporal	1 year	Right Sylvian	No
Malik et al.	1992	28	M	Suprasellar	Right frontal	21 years	Right frontal convexity	Yes
Lee et al.	1999	31	M	Sellar	Right pterional	2 years	Right mesial temporal	Yes
Gupta et al.	1999	73	M	Sellar	Right frontal	7 years	Left frontal and parietooccipital	Yes
Ito et al.	2001	65	M	Sellar	Bifrontal	3 years	Right temporal	No
Lee et al.	2001	26	M	Sellar/suprasellar	Trans lamina terminalis	19 months	Lumbar spine	Yes (spine)
Liu et al.	2002	73	W	Third Ventricle	Interhemispheric/transcallosal	8 years	Right frontal parasaggital	No
Novegno et al.	2002	6	M	Sellar	Left pterional	3 years	Left frontal convexity	NR
Elmaci et al.	2002	62	F	Sellar	Right pterional	2 years	Left temporoparietal	No
Ishii et al.	2004	2	M	Suprasellar	Bifrontal	2 months	Frontal subdural	No
Kawaguchi et al.	2005	50	W	Sellar	Bifrontal	2 years	Left frontal	NR
De Macedo Bianco et al.	2006	27	W	Sellar	Left frontotemporal	1.5 years	Left temporal	No
Jeong et al.	2006	8	W	Suprasellar	Bifrontal	4 years	Right frontal	No
Yamada et al.	2006	27	W	Sellar	Right orbitozygomatic (OZ)	5	Left frontal	Yes
Novak et al.	2008	67	M	Suprasellar	Right minimally invasive (MI) Retrosigmoid	8 years	Right cerebellopontine angle (CPA)	NR
Bikmaz et al.	2009	52	W	Suprasellar	Not reported (NR)	15 years	Prepontine	NR
		41	M	Suprasellar	NR	9 years	Right frontal	NR
		24	M	Suprasellar	NR	12 years	Right CPA	Yes

(*Continued*)

TABLE 31.1 Ectopic Recurrence of Craniopharyngioma after Removal of a Primary Lesion—cont'd

Series	Year	Age	Gender	Primary location	Initial surgical approach	Time to recurrence	Ectopic recurrence location	Radiation therapy
Elliott et al.	2009	3	W	Retrochiasmatic	Right pterional	10 years	Right prepontine	NR
		2	M	Retrochiasmatic	Right pterional	21 months	Left CPA	NR
		3	W	Suprasellar	Right pterional	20 months	Right Sylvian + right optic	NR
		6	M	Suprasellar	NR	1 month	Left subfrontal	No
Frangou et al.	2009	10	M	Sellar	Bifrontal	6 months	Right temporal and parietal	NR
Romani et al.	2010	22	W	Suprasellar	Transcallosal	4 years	Right frontal medial	No
Wang et al.	2010	3	M	Suprasellar	Right pterional	2 years	Right frontal	Yes
Schmalisch et al.	2010	13	M	Suprasellar	Right pterional	2 years	Right Sylvian	No
		27	W	Sellar	Right pterional + transsphenoidal	4 years	Right frontal	No
		42	M	Sellar	Right frontotemporal	10 years	Right parietal	No
De Blank et al.	2011	27	F	Sellar	Right pterional	22 years	Left CPA	Yes
Kordes et al.	2011	7	M	Sellar	Transphenoidal/right Pterional	15 months	Right pterional	Yes
Elfving et al.	2011	15	F	Sellar	Right subfrontal	9 years	Right supraorbital	Yes
Jakobs et al.	2012	72	F	Suprasellar	Bifrontal	3 years	Right supraorbital	Yes
Goncalves et al.	2013	49	M	Sellar/suprasellar	Right pterional	5 years	Right frontal subgaleal	No

NR: Not reported.

TABLE 31.2 Primary Ectopic Craniopharyngiomas

Series	Year	Age	Gender	Location	Surgical Approach	Radiation Therapy
Altinors et al.	1984	14	M	Right cerebellopontine angle (CPA)	Right suboccipital	NR
Bashir et al.	1996	23	M	Left CPA/4th ventricle	Left suboccipital	NR
Sangiovanni et al.	1997	61	W	Corpus callosum	Interhemispheric	NR
Jian et al.	1998	7	M	Ethmoid sinus	Transnasal	No
Usanov et al.	1999	8	M	Pineal	Supracerebellar/infratentorial	NR
Jallo et al.	2001	8	M	Ethmoid/sphenoid sinus	Subfrontal/transbasal	Yes
Fujimoto et al.	2002	8	M	Maxillary/ethmoid	Transnasal	Yes
Kawamata et al.	2002	44	W	Clivus	Transnasal	No
Shah et al.	2006	12	W	Fourth ventricle	Suboccipital	No
Banczerowski et al.	2007	29	M	Temporal extradural	Right temporal	NR
Powers et al.	2007	12	F	Left CPA	Left retrosigmoid	Yes
Arndt et al.	2008	16	W	Clivus/ethmoid/sphenoid sinus	Mid-face degloving	NR
Yan et al.	2009	54	F	Right CPA	Right retrosigmoid	NR
Lee et al.	2009	55	M	Petroclival	Left far-lateral	Yes
Nourbakhsh et al.	2010	25	W	Sphenoid	Transphenoidal	NR
Bozbuga et al.	2011	34	M	Left CPA	Left suboccipital	NR
Singh et al.	2012	14	F	Left CPA	Left retrosigmoid	NR
Yu et al.*	2012	18	M	Infrasellar	Extradural anterior fossa approach	Yes
		30	M		Extradural anterior fossa approach	Yes
		21	F		Stereotactic	No
		7	M		Frontal base stereotactic	No
		48	M		Extradural anterior fossa approach	Yes
		52	M		Stereotactic	No
		33	F		None – Clinical observation	No

(Continued)

TABLE 31.2 Primary Ectopic Craniopharyngiomas—cont'd

Series	Year	Age	Gender	Location	Surgical Approach	Radiation Therapy
		15	F		Transnasal	No
		24	M		Stereotactic	No
		16	F		Stereotactic	Yes
		15	F		Transnasal	No
Khalatbari et al.	2012	40	M	Left CPA	Retrosigmoid	NR
		22	M	Left CPA	Retrosigmoid	NR
		28	M	Right CPA	Retrosigmoid	NR
Kundu et al.	2014	55	M	Ethmoid/sphenoid sinus	Mid-face degloving	Yes
Kim et al.	2014	31	M	Left CPA	Suboccipital	No

* *Although all the patients presented in that series had an infrasellar component, some had extensive compromise (sellar/suprasellar) which makes it difficult to discern the original primary location of the lesion.*
NR: Not reported.

CONCLUSIONS

Although rarely occurring, craniopharyngiomas can appear in ectopic locations. Direct seeding along the surgical tract is the most commonly cited reason, although primary ectopic craniopharyngiomas occur. If the mechanism by which these lesions appear is related to the pathogenesis of "usual" craniopharyngiomas, it may imply that a faulty signaling pathway during embryogenesis could result in the appearance of epithelial cells in locations other than the expected path of the craniopharyngeal duct.

On the other hand, the presence of distant secondary lesions with no anatomical relationship to the surgical approach for the treatment of a primary sellar craniopharyngioma probably relates to a different biological mechanism through which some viable cells could exhibit metastatic potential through leptomeningeal seeding. It is difficult to know whether these cases exhibit worse long-term outcomes because of their rare nature.

References

Abele, T., A, Salzman, K.L., Harnsberger, H.R., Glastonbury, C.M., 2013. Craniopharyngeal canal and its spectrum of pathology. AJNR. Am. J. Neuroradiol., 1–6.

Bikmaz, K., a, Guerrero, C., Dammers, R., Krisht, A.F., Husain, M.M., 2009. Ectopic recurrence of craniopharyngiomas: case report. Neurosurgery 64 (2), E382–E383.

Blank, P., de, Minturn, J., 2011. A rare case of ectopic recurrence of a craniopharyngioma diagnosed 17 years after initial presentation. J. Pediatr. Hematol. Oncol. 33 (5), 392–397.

Bozbuga, M., Turan Suslu, H., Hicdonmez, T., Bayindir, C., 2011. Primary cerebellopontine angle craniopharyngioma in a patient with Gardner syndrome. J. Clin. Neurosci. 18 (2), 300–301.

Bunin, G., Surawicz, T., Witman, P., Preston-Martin, S., Davis, F., Bruner, J., 1998. The descriptive epidemiology of craniopharyngioma. J. Neurosurg. 89, 547–551.

Carpenter, R.C., Chamberlin, G.W., Frazier, C.H., 1937. The treatment of hypophyseal stalk tumours by evacuation and irradiation. Am J. Roent. 38, 162–167.

Deutsch, H., Kothbauer, K., Persky, M., Epstein, F.J., Jallo, G.I., 2001. Infrasellar craniopharyngiomas: case report and review of the literature. Skull Base Off. J. North Am. Skull Base Soc. 11 (2), 121–128.

Dubois, P.M., Elamraoui, A., 1995. Embryology of the pituitary gland. Trend. Endocrinol. Metab. 6 (1), 1–7.

Elfving, M., Lundgren, J., Englund, E., Strömblad, L.-G., Erfurth, E.-M., 2011. Ectopic recurrence of a craniopharyngioma in a 15-year-old girl 9 years after surgery and conventional radiotherapy: case report. Childs Nerv. Syst. 27 (5), 845–851.

Elliott, R.E., Moshel, Y. a, Wisoff, J.H., 2009. Surgical treatment of ectopic recurrence of craniopharyngioma. Report of 4 cases. J. Neurosurg. Pediatr. 4 (2), 105–112.

Gupta, K., Kuhn, M., Shevlin, D., Wacaser, L., 1999. Metastatic craniopharyngioma. Am. J. Neuroradiol. 20 (June/July), 1059–1060.

Ishii, K., Sugita, K., Kobayashi, H., Kamida, T., Fujiki, M., Izumi, T., Mori, T., 2004. Intracranial ectopic recurrence of craniopharyngioma after Ommaya reservoir implantation. Pediatr. Neurosurg. 40 (5), 230–233.

Ito, M., Jamshidi, J., Yamanaka, K., 2001. Does craniopharyngioma metastasize? Case report and review of the literature. Neurosurgery 48 (4), 933–936.

Jakobs, M., Orakcioglu, B., 2012. Ectopic recurrent craniopharyngioma of the frontal bone. J. Neurosurg. 117 (3), 490–497.

Jeong, I.-H., Lee, J.-K., Moon, K.-S., Joo, S.P., Kwak, H.J., Kim, T.S., Kim, J.H., Kim, S.H., 2006. Ectopic recurrence of craniopharyngioma: a case report and review of the literature. J. Neurooncol. 79 (2), 191–195.

Kawaguchi, T., Fujimura, M., Shirane, R., Shoji, T., Watanabe, M., Tominaga, T., 2005. Ectopic recurrence of craniopharyngioma. J. Clin. Neurosci. 12 (3), 307–309.

Kawamata, T., Kubo, O., Kamikawa, S., Hori, T., 2002. Ectopic clival craniopharyngioma. Acta Neurochir. (Wien) 144 (11), 1221–1224.

Kim, M.S., Kim, Y.S., Lee, H.K., Lee, G.J., Choi, C.Y., Lee, C.H., 2014. Primary intracranial ectopic craniopharyngioma in a patient with probable Gardner's syndrome. J. Neurosurg. 120 (2), 337–341.

Kordes, U., Flitsch, J., Hagel, C., 2011. Ectopic craniopharyngioma. Klin Pädiatrie 223 (3), 176–177.

Larkin, S., Ansorge, O., 2013. Pathology and pathogenesis of craniopharyngiomas. Pituitary 16, 9–17 (August 2012).

Lee, J.H., Kim, C.Y., Kim, D.G., Jung, H.W., 1999. Post-operative ectopic seeding of craniopharyngioma. Case illustration. J. Neurosurg. 90 (4), 796.

Liu, J.M., Garonzik, I.M., Eberhart, C.G., Sampath, P., Brem, H., 2002. Ectopic recurrence of craniopharyngioma after an interhemispheric transcallosal approach: case report. Neurosurgery 50 (3), 639–644.

Müller, H.L., 2013. Childhood craniopharyngioma. Pituitary 16 (1), 56–67.

Nourbakhsh, A., Brown, B., Vannemreddy, P., Lian, T., Nanda, A., Guthikonda, B., 2010. Extracranial infrasellar ectopic craniopharyngioma: a case report and review of the literature. Skull Base Off. J. North Am. Skull Base Soc. 20 (6), 475–480.

Novegno, F., Di Rocco, F., Colosimo Jr., C., Lauriola, L., Caldarelli, M., 2002. Ectopic recurrences of craniopharyngioma. Childs Nerv. Syst. 18 (9–10), 468–473.

Ragoowansi, A.T., Piepgras, D.G., 1991. Post-operative ectopic craniopharyngioma. Case report. J. Neurosurg. 74 (4), 653–655.

Romani, R., Niemelä, M., Celik, O., Isarakul, P., Paetau, A., Hernesniemi, J., 2010. Ectopic recurrence of craniopharyngioma along the surgical route: case report and literature review. Acta Neurochir. (Wien) 152 (2), 297–302.

Rushing, E.J., Giangaspero, F., Paulus, W., Burger, P.C., 2007. Craniopharyngioma. In: Louis, D.N., Ohgaki, H., Wiestler, O.D., Cavenee, W.K. (Eds.), The 2007 WHO classification of tumours of the central nervous system. International Agency for Research on Cancer (IARC), Lyon, France, pp. 238–240.

Sangiovanni, G., Tancioni, F., Tartara, F., 1997. Ectopic craniopharyngioma: presentation of a case arising from the corpus callosum. Acta Neurochir. (Wien) 139 (4), 379–380.

Shah, G.B., Bhaduri, A.S., Misra, B.K., 2007. Ectopic craniopharyngioma of the fourth ventricle: case report. Surg. Neurol. 68 (1), 96–98.

Usanov, E.I., Hatomkin, D.M., Nikulina, T., a, Gorban, N. a., 1999. Craniopharyngioma of the pineal region. Childs Nerv. Syst. 15 (1), 4–7.

Yamada, Y., Haraoka, J., Akimoto, J., 2006. Ectopic recurrence of craniopharyngioma. Neurol. Med. Chir. (Tokyo) 46 (12), 598–600.

CHAPTER

32

Malignant Transformation of Craniopharyngioma

Jiang Qian, Guilian Niu, David Jones

Department of Pathology and Laboratory Medicine/Affiliated Pathology Services, Albany Medical College/Center Hospital, Albany, NY, USA

"At some point or another they seem to become a part of the brain, and they are therefore probably malignant tumors in this sense." ***CH Frazier and BJ Alpers, 1931***

INTRODUCTION

Craniopharyngioma is a rare, non-glial, primary, intracranial neoplasm of the central nervous system (CNS), with an estimated incidence of 0.13–0.18 per 100,000 population with no apparent gender differences (Bunin et al., 1998; Ostrom et al., 2013). It accounts for 0.8– 5% of all intracranial neoplasms (Burger et al., 2002; Ostrom et al., 2013), and ~30% of tumors in the sellar region (Lu and Xu, 1988; Ironside et al., 2002). Craniopharyngioma can present at any age, even in the prenatal and neonatal periods (Bailey et al., 1990; Müller-Scholden et al., 2000; Joó et al., 2009), but a bimodal distribution for age at presentation is observed, with peak ages of 5–14 years and then 50–74 years (Bunin et al., 1998). It appears to have a higher representation in the pediatric population, accounting for 10% of all pediatric brain tumors, and about 55–90% of all sellar and parasellar lesions in children (Schoenberg et al., 1976; Jagannathan et al., 2007; Delman, 2009; Schroeder and Vezina, 2011). Nearly half of craniopharyngiomas occur during childhood and adolescence (Bunin et al., 1998; Nielsen et al., 2011; Ostrom et al., 2013).

Craniopharyngiomas are thought to be derived from the remnants of Rathke's pouch or primitive craniopharyngeal duct, a related ectoderm anlage (Bigner et al., 1998), and typically originate in the region of the infundibulum, presumably from the squamoid epithelial rests known to occur there (Susman, 1932; Luse and Kernohan, 1955; Prabhu and Brown, 2005; Karavitaki et al., 2006. For further details, refer to Chapter 3 "Embryology, Pathology and Molecular Aspects").

Craniopharyngiomas are classified into adamantinomatous and papillary subtypes (Louis et al., 2007). Most are pure forms, but occasional cases are mixed, and contain both types in various proportions (Weiner et al., 1994; Crotty et al., 1995; Eldevik et al., 1996; Okada et al., 2012).

Craniopharyngiomas
http://dx.doi.org/10.1016/B978-0-12-416706-3.00032-5

These two subtypes not only exhibit distinct histopathological features, but also differ clinically in the presentation age, tumor location, and imaging characteristics (Adamson et al., 1990; Weiner et al., 1994; Crotty et al., 1995; Sartoretti-Schefer et al., 1997; Larkin and Ansorage, 2013).

The more common subtype, adamantinomatous craniopharyngioma (ACP), accounts for 60% to 80% of craniopharyngiomas (Adamson et al., 1990; Crotty et al., 1995), and is usually seen in pediatric and adolescent patients. ACP bears morphological and molecular similarities to ameloblastoma of the jaw and even more so to keratinizing and calcifying odontogenic tumor/cyst (Bernstein and Buchino, 1983; Badger and Gardner, 1997; Paulus et al., 1997; Li and Yu, 2003; Sekine et al., 2004; Lee and Kim, 2013). Grossly, ACPs are firm, calcified solid masses that are often cystic. Histopathologically (Figure 32.1), ACPs consist of anastamosing cords or trabecullae of squamoid epithelium. The central portion of the epithelium forms the so-called stellate reticulum due to its loose texture and cellular discohesion, while the periphery consists of basaloid cells forming fence-like palisades. The epithelium surrounds a stroma that is hypocellular, fibromyxoid, and often forms cystic spaces filled with amorphous cellular debris, or turbid, dark brown "machine oil" that is formed from desquamated squamous epithelium and comprised mainly of keratin and cholesterol. A characteristic finding, virtually pathognomonic although not always present, is "wet keratin", which is a nodular collection of degenerated "ghost" epithelial cells without nuclei. In addition, calcifications as well as cholesterol-rich xanthogranulomas may be present, the latter occurring as a host reaction following tissue disintegration. Variable inflammatory response can occur within or around the tumor, and dense piloid gliosis and Rosenthal fibers may be quite prominent in the adjacent brain tissue when brain invasion takes place, causing diagnostic confusion with pilocytic astrocytoma (Ironside et al., 2002; Louis et al., 2007).

The less common type is papillary craniopharyngioma (PCP), which almost exclusively occurs in adults (Adamson et al., 1990; Crotty et al., 1995; Weiner et al., 1994). As its name indicates, PCP consists of variable-sized papillary projections (Figure 32.2) with a stratified non-keratinizing squamous epithelium which encloses a loose, fibrovascular core, vaguely resembling squamous papilloma that commonly occurs in the upper aerodigestive system. Wet keratin, "ghost" cells, and calcifications are not features of PCP. PCP is more likely in solid

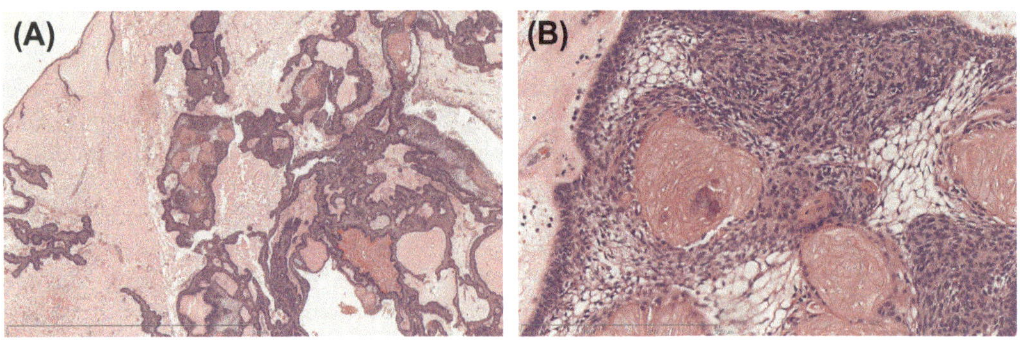

FIGURE 32.1 Photomicrographs of adamantinomatous craniopharyngioma (ACP). **A,** Low-power view of ACP revealing ribbons and lobules of epithelial cells intermixed with fluid-containing cystic spaces. **B,** High-power view of ACP revealing a stratified epithelium with palisading peripheral cells and loose "stellate reticulated" central cells. Several small collections of "wet keratin" are present showing anucleated "ghost" squamous cells with basophic calcifications. Magnifications: A at 2.5x and B at 20x objective lens.

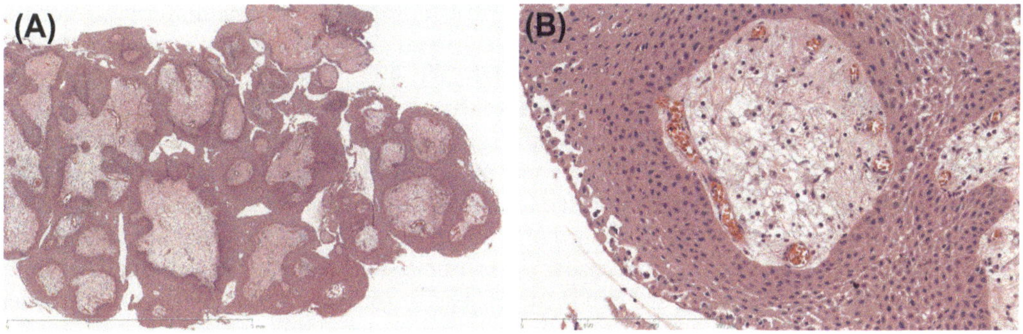

FIGURE 32.2 **Photomicrographs of papillary craniopharyngioma (PCP). A,** Low-power view of PCP, which is composed of variable-sized papillary projections formed from squamous epithelium enclosing a central loose fibrovascular core. **B,** High-power view of PCP showing non-keratinizing squamous epithelium with fibrovascular core. Magnifications: A at 2.5x and B at 20x objective lens.

form compared with ACP, and cyst formation is less common. When cysts do form, their contents tend to contain yellow clear material, rather than the "machine oil" so typical of ACP.

MALIGNANT CHANGES IN CRANIOPHARYNGIOMA

Craniopharyngioma is a histologically benign neoplasm, assigned WHO grade I (Louis et al., 2007). It can be locally aggressive and recurs quite commonly despite its benign histopathological appearance. Recurrences are reported to be about 20% to 40%, and as high as nearly 60% (Sorva and Heiskanen, 1986; Szeifert et al., 1993; Karavitaki et al., 2006; Elliott et al., 2011; Jo et al., 2012). This is at least partially due to their often infiltrative growth into critical parasellar structures (cranial nerves, intracranial vasculature, the osseous cranial base, and even into brain and the ventricular system), especially for the adamantinomatous type. As a result, complete surgical removal is often difficult, if not impossible. Thus, post-surgery radiation therapy is often needed for local disease control. The best survival is achieved in patients receiving wide tumor resection, and this group has a 5-year survival rate of over 90% (Humphreys et al., 1979; Richmond et al., 1980), and post-surgery radiation improves long-term survival further, achieving a 10-year survival rate of over 75%, even in partial or subtotal resections, comparable to that of total resection without radiation (Richmond et al., 1980; Manaka et al., 1985; Scott et al., 1994; Lin et al., 2008; Jo et al., 2012). (For further details regarding radiation therapy for craniopharyngiomas, refer to Section IV "Radiotherapy"). Most recurrences of craniopharyngioma take place in or around the original surgical site, and the recurrent tumor retains its original benign histopathology.

Although local aggressiveness and recurrences are well-recognized clinical behavior in otherwise benign-appearing craniopharyngiomas, frank histological malignancy in craniopharyngioma is only rarely documented.

Malignant craniopharyngioma, or malignant transformation of craniopharyngioma, is not well defined, and in fact is not formally listed in the latest 2007 version of the WHO tumor classification (Louis et al., 2007). However, several histopathological parameters that are usually considered typical for any malignancy are also applied to define malignancy for this tumor (Boongird et al., 2009; Stricker et al., 2010; Gao et al., 2011), including anaplastic cellular appearances, increased mitotic or proliferative activity, vascular invasion, infiltrative destruction of basement membrane, and coagulative tumor necrosis. Rare cases of craniopharyngiomas with distant recurrences that are designated as "metastatic" have been reported in the literature (Ito et al., 2001; Elmaci et al., 2002), but it is debatable whether this equates to malignancy as the term is applied to the majority of non-CNS neoplasms, for which metastasis is taken as an unequivocal sign of malignancy (Stricker and Kumar, 2010). Alternative terms are thus given to such cases as "ectopic or distant recurrent craniopharyngioma" to avoid the malignant meaning implied in metastasis. For further detailed information, interested readers are referred to Chapter 30, and this chapter will confine the discussion on malignancy in craniopharyngioma to either a craniopharyngioma that shows frank malignant histological features (malignant craniopharyngioma), or a known craniopharyngioma that has transformed into a different type of malignancy during recurrence (malignant transformation of craniopharyngioma). For the purpose of this discussion, these two descriptions, as well as the term "malignant progression" will be used interchangeably.

Malignancy in craniopharyngioma has only been reported in a small number of cases, mostly as single case reports or small series. Akachi et al. in 1987 reported in the Japanese literature the first such case of a 7-year-old girl with classical ACP diagnosed at the initial surgery, which recurred as poorly differentiated squamous cell carcinoma following surgery and radiation. In 1988, Nelson et al. described the case of a young female whose apparently benign initial craniopharyngioma underwent malignant transformation to, again, a poorly differentiated squamous cell carcinoma after 35 years of multiple recurrences and radiation therapy. Such cases are so rare that in several large series, no single case of craniopharyngioma with malignant features is reported (Crotty et al., 1995; Duff et al., 2000; Tavangar et al., 2004; Chakrabarti et al., 2005; Karavitaki et al., 2005; Pekmezci et al., 2010); and in the nearly 30 years which have passed since these early reports, only 20 cases have been documented in the literature. The major features of these cases are summarized in Table 32.1, and data analysis is given in Table 32.2.

In addition to these well-documented cases, a few other cases have been mentioned in the literature as malignant craniopharyngiomas. In 1935, Zeitlin described three cases of ACP, one of which (case 2) was diagnosed as ACP (adamantinoma was the term used then) with malignant transformation involving the sphenoid bone, infundibulum, and middle ear. However, its origin was unclear, and the nasopharynx, rather than the sellar region, might have been the primary site. Furthermore, histopathological malignancy or anaplasia was not clearly established, and therefore, it could very well represent a classical ACP with local aggressive behavior. Salyer and Carter (1973) reported a well-differentiated squamous cell carcinoma arising from an intra-sellar cyst, which could represent malignant transformation of a craniopharyngioma, although the pathological features of craniopharyngioma were not unequivocally demonstrated. There are three additional cases of malignant craniopharyngioma mentioned in reports by Akachi et al. (1987) and Suzuki et al. (1989), but details are unavailable. In an editorial comment on the relationship between Rathke cleft cyst and craniopharyngioma, Wolfe and Heros (2010) gave a brief description of a male patient who died at age 40 of squamous cell carcinoma that was transformed from a typical

TABLE 32.1 Case Summary of Craniopharyngiomas with Malignant Progression (MP) in Humans

Authors (year)[a]	Sex and age at presentation (years)	Age at MP (years)	Recurrences (n)	Treatments prior to diagnosis of MP[b]	Symptoms/ signs at MP[c]	Imaging at MP[c]	Pathology[b] including further stains (p53, beta-catenin, Ki-67, et al)	Follow-up[d]
PRIMARY CASES, DEVELOPED DE NOVO								
Yue and Da (2006)	M(17)	17 (de novo)	0	1: Rxn	Headache, vision loss	3.1 cm sellar/ suprasellar mass	ACP with MP to SCC	NA
Rodriguez et al. (2007)	M(31)	31 (de novo)	1	1: right frontal subtotal Rxn (70%) 2: gross total Rxn	1: headaches, vision problems, bitemporal hemianopsia 2: Pseudo-bulbar palsy, left hemiparesis	1: CT- 4 cm suprasellar enhancing mass 2: MRI- 3.5 cm suprasellar enhancing mass	1,2: Malignant neoplasm with odontogenic features (? malignant ACP) beta-catenin: positive p53: 82% p16: 55% Mib-1: 15%	2: gross total Rxn for recurrent MP DOD 3 mo after MP
Boongird et al. (2009)	F(46)	46 (de novo)	0	Partial Rxn followed by transcallosal residual tumor Rxn and blood removal	Impaired vision, bi-frontal headache	MRI: 4.7 cm suprasellar mass	Malignant ACP Ki-67: 44.3% p53: 98%	DOD 7 post-operative wk due to rapid growth and intra-ventricular bleed
Nishioka et al. (2009)	F(56)	56 (de novo)	1	1: gross total Rxn 2: stereotactic radiotherapy planned at time of report	18 mo history of progressive severe headache	MRI/CT: suprasellar mass	Carcinoma with odontogenic features (? malignant ACP) beta-catenin: focal membranous Ki-67/Mib-1: 15% Amelogenins: positive EM: undifferentiated epithelial cells with few tonofilaments	Recurrence 14 mo after Rxn

(Continued)

TABLE 32.1 Case Summary of Craniopharyngiomas with Malignant Progression (MP) in Humans—cont'd

Authors (year)[a]	Sex and age at presentation (years)	Age at MP (years)	Recurrences (n)	Treatments prior to diagnosis of MP[b]	Symptoms/ signs at MP[c]	Imaging at MP[c]	Pathology[b] including further stains (p53, beta-catenin, Ki-67, et al)	Follow-up[d]
Lauriola et al. (2011)	F(66)	66 (*de novo*)	0	Partial Rxn + fRT (50 Gy)	Sudden loss of right vision and deficit of left vision	MRI: Sellar/ suprasellar mass	Malignant ACP Ki-67: > 50% p53: > 50%	DOD 15 mo after MP
SECONDARY CASES, DEVELOPED IN RECURRENCE								
Akachi et al. (1987)	F(7)	10	2	1: subtotal Rxn + RT (30 Gy) 2: subtotal Rxn	Decreased left vision, right temporal anopsia, headache, nausea, vomiting	Suprasellar tumor with obstruction of the foramen of Monro	1: ACP 2,3: ACP with poorly differentiated SCC	Following Rxn 2, RT (36 Gy) 3: Debulking DOD at home 8 mo after MP (3)
Nelson et al. (1988)	F(14)	49	4	1–5: subtotal Rxn Cobalt fRT (60.6 Gy) after third Rxn	Right CN nerve palsy, left hemiparesis, and altered mental status	Heterogeneous suprasellar tumor with destruction of skull base	3: cystic CP 4: ACP 5: ACP with malignant and focal squamous features	Patient died 11 wks after last Rxn and MP due to upper GI bleeding and pneumonia (35)
Suzuki et al. (1989)	M(3)	11	3	1: left frontal subtotal Rxn + local bleomycin 2: Rxn + local bleomycin + RT (40 Gy) 3: subtotal Rxn, followed by RT (30 Gy) 4: NA (death)	4: clinical recurrence with rapid growth of mass involving orbit, nasal, and oral cavity	NA	1,2,3: ACP 4 (Autopsy): ACP with SCC	DOD 2 mo after clinical recurrence and MP diagnosed at autopsy (8)

Suzuki et al. (1989)	M(9)	14	6	1: subtotal Rxn + RT (50 Gy) 2–7: Rxn	Altered mental status	NA	1,2,3: ACP 6,7: ACP with SCC with brain invasion	DOD ~3 mo after MP (5)
Virik et al. (1999)	M(24)	34	2	1: subtotal Rxn 2: partial Rxn + adjuvant RT (55Gy) 3: 25% debulking + CTX (CCNU, procarbazine) + local RT	Left homonymous hemianopia, loss of visual acuity and diplopia	CT: 13mm mass retro-optic chiasm	1,2: ACP 3: ACP with MP to undifferentiated carcinoma	CTX (carboplatin and etoposide) + palliative RT DOD 10 mo after MP (~11)
Kristopaitis et al. (2000)	F(27)	42	7	1: transsphenoidal Rxn, followed by multiple cranial, facial and endoscopic Rxn, fRT (52 Gy) after second Rxn, Iodine 125 implants, stereotactic radiosurgery	Temporal lobe Seizures, right blindness, left visual defect	MRI: large mass involving the nasopharynx and skull base	early specimens: ACP 8: ACP with moderately differentiated SCC p53: 75% focally in SCC; < 10% in ACP	CTX (paclitaxel, carboplatin) after MP with partial response, but continuous tumor growth at 6 mo after MP. Alive with disease 5 yr after MP
Plowman et al. (2004)	F(6.5)	21	2	VPS + fRT (50 Gy) 1: subtotal Rxn 2: Rxn followed by stereotactic fRT (16 Gy) 3: Rxn	Left visual loss progressing to blindness	MRI: suprasellar cystic and solid mass extending to third ventricle	1,2: ACP 3: malignant ACP, brisk mitosis Ki-67: > 50% p53 in normal and tumor, CGH + FISH: multiple chromosomal abnormalities	3: CTX (cisplatin, etoposide), partial response, but relapsed 6 mo later followed by death (~15)
Sakai et al. (2004)	M(3 yr 8 mo)	17.5	11	1: subtotal Rxn 2: transsphenoid Rxn 3: needle cyst drainage + RT (20 mCi) 4–12: subtotal Rxn RT (60 Gy) at 5 Rxn	NA	NA	7: Malignant CP NA for other Rxn	DOD ~2 yr after MP (~17)

(*Continued*)

TABLE 32.1 Case Summary of Craniopharyngiomas with Malignant Progression (MP) in Humans—cont'd

Authors (year)[a]	Sex and age at presentation (years)	Age at MP (years)	Recurrences (n)	Treatments prior to diagnosis of MP[b]	Symptoms/ signs at MP[c]	Imaging at MP[c]	Pathology[b] including further stains (p53, beta-catenin, Ki-67, et al)	Follow-up[d]
Rodriguez et al. (2007)	F(58)	63	2	1: Rxn + RT 2: right gross total Rxn 3: right near total Rxn	Confusion, memory and behavior disturbances	2: MRI- 2 cm suprasellar mass extending to 3rd ventricle 3: CT- 2 cm 3rd ventricular mass	1: ACP 3: Malignant ACP Mib-1: up to 55% VEGF: 22% MVD: 4 X higher than ACP beta-catenin: present in both ACP and malignancy p53: 81% p16: 96%	DOD 3.5 mo after MP (5)
Rodriguez et al. (2007)	M(14)	23	3	1: Rxn 2: Rxn followed by external beam (50 Gy) 3: subtotal Rxn, followed by 32^P instillation into cyst 4: partial Rxn	Right ptosis and left arm weakness	CT: rapid growth of residual tumor	1,2,3: ACP 4: ACP with malignant myoepithelioma beta-catenin: positive in malignant part p53: 91% p16: 26% Mib-1: 16%	Died suddenly at home about 6 mo after MP (9)
Aquilina et al. (2010)	M(4)	12	4	1: near total Rxn + fRT (55.8 Gy) 2: near total Rxn 3: debulking + fRT (50.4 Gy) 4: partial Rxn 5 : subtotal Rxn	Left vision loss	MRI: recurrent tumor	1: ACP − focal PCP 5: ACP with SCC Ki-67: > 70% p53: > 95%	CMT (carboplatin + cetuximab) DOD 6 mo after MP (~8)
Aquilina et al. (2010)	F(6)	13	1	1: Subtotal Rxn + RT (54 Gy) 2: biopsy followed by subtotal Rxn	Severe progressive headache and neck pain	MRI: residual suprasellar mass and clival abnormal signal	1: ACP 2: ACP with SCC Ki-67: > 50% p53: > 95%	Rapid tumor progression, given CTX (paclitaxel and carboplatin) + RT (54 Gy), tumor stabilized 6 mo after MP

Ishida et al. (2010)	M(6)	11	3	1: subtotal Rxn 2: subtotal Rxn + RT (18 Gy) 3: intracystic CMT (bleomycin) 4: partial (50%) Rxn + CMT (cyclophosphamide, cisplatin, etoposide)	Sudden left vision loss and rapid right vision disturbance	MRI: recurrent suprasellar tumor, extending to bilateral CPA	1,2: ACP 3: no pathology 4: malignant ACP Ki-67: 27%; p53: 73%;	Alive with tumor stabilized 10 mo after MP
Ujifuku et al. (2010)	M(32)	42	3	1: Rxn + radiosurgery (11–22 Gy) 2: biopsy + fRT (50 Gy) 3: partial Rxn 4: debulking	Decreased left vision	MRI: tumor regrowth	1: no tissue 2: c/w ACP 3,4: SCC from ACP	Died due to massive SAH ~6 wk after last surgery, ~2.5 mo after MP (10)
Gao et al. (2011)	F(37)	41	2	1: subtotal Rxn 2: subtotal Rxn 3: Rxn	Headache, impaired right vision, bitemporal hemianopsia	Recurrent intra-sellar ring-enhancing mass	1: major PCP, minor ACP 2: low-grade malignant ACP 3: malignant ACP	Died 3.5 mo after 2nd Rxn due to physical deterioration and lung infection, ~1 yr after MP (5)

ACP: adamantinomatous craniopharyngioma; CGH: comparative genomic hybridization; CN: cranial nerve; CP: craniopharyngioma; CPA: cerebellopontine angle; CTX: chemotherapy; DOD: died of disease; FISH: fluorescence *in situ* hybridization; Ki-67/Mib-1: proliferation markers; MP: malignant progression; MVD: microvessel density; NA: not applicable or not available/described; PCP: papillary craniopharyngioma; RT and fRT: radiation therapy and fractionated radiation therapy; Rxn: resection; SAH: subarachnoid hemorrhage; SCC: squamous cell carcinoma; VEGF: vascular endothelial growth factor; VPS: ventriculoperitoneal shunting.

[a] *Name of the first author, and year of publication.*

[b] *Initial surgery is designated "1", and subsequent ones as "2, 3, etc".*

[c] *Clinical and imaging findings immediately prior to malignant progression.*

[d] *"wk","mo", and "yr" indicate week, month, year respectively, after malignant progression. The number in parenthesis indicates years from initial surgery to the time of death.*

Adapted and expanded from Rodriguez et al. (with permission from © 2007 Lippincott Williams & Wilkins, Inc. Published by Lippincott Williams & Wilkins, Inc).

TABLE 32.2 Data Analysis of Craniopharyngiomas with Malignant Progression (MP) in Humans

Total cases	20	
M:F ratio	10:10	
Age (years) at presentation[a]	All 20 cases 23.4±20.1 (3 – 66; 15.5)	
No of recurrences[a]	All 20 cases 2.8±2.7 (0 – 11; 2)	
	15 secondary cases 3.7±2.6 (1 – 11; 3)	5 *de novo* cases 3 cases: no recurrence 2 cases: 1 recurrence each
Years from presentation to MP[a]	15 secondary cases 10.2±7.8 (3 – 35; 8)	5 *de novo* cases NA
Months from MP to death[a]	15 of 20 cases (excluding five alive/NA cases) 7.0±6.1 (1.7 – 24; 6)	

MP: malignant progression; NA: not applicable or not available/described.
[a]*Expressed as: mean± SD (range; and median).*

craniopharyngioma resected 30 years earlier, followed by several recurrences and radiation therapy. In addition to these human cases, there are three animal tumors reported in veterinary literature: an albino rat with a spontaneously occurring, metastatic malignant craniopharyngioma (Pace et al., 1997), and two feline malignant craniopharyngiomas (Nagata et al., 2005).

CLINICAL FEATURES

Of these 20 malignant cases, five are *de novo* malignant tumors, while the remainder are secondary, malignantly transformed tumors from a previously benign craniopharyngioma following treatment and recurrences. There is no gender difference, and males and females are equally affected (ten males and ten females). The average age at presentation is 23 years, but there is a wide age range – from 3 to 66 years. The majority of these, however, have occurred in children and young adults (15 cases younger than 35 years of age). Excluding five *de novo* cases, it took on average 10 years from the presentation to malignant progression, ranging from 3 to 35 years, with the majority (9/15 cases) within 9 years, usually after multiple recurrences (~4 recurrences on average, as many as 11 reported by Sakai et al., 2004).

Because of its rarity, information is limited regarding the clinical, including imaging, features of malignant craniopharyngiomas. Among the reported cases, the most common symptoms and signs at or immediately preceding malignancy were headaches, visual disturbances, increased intracranial pressure, and focal neurological deficits such as hemiparesis, cranial nerve palsy, and unilateral ptosis. Imaging studies usually identified enlarging, recurrent tumors with variable contrast enhancement. Most of these resided in or around the sellar area, but some tumors extended further into surrounding structures such as the cerebellopontine angle (Ishida et al., 2010), the clivus (Aquilina et al., 2010), and the third ventricle (Plowman et al., 2004; Rodriguez et al., 2007). The case reported by Kristopaitis et al. (2000) was unusual in that temporal lobe seizures were the presenting symptoms, and the imaging study revealed extension of the tumor into nasopharynx and skull base. One older adult among the three cases reported by Rodriguez et al. (2007) presented with increased confusion, memory and behavior abnormalities, and MRI revealed a suprasellar mass extending into the third ventricle. One case reported by Ujifuku et al. (2010) developed moyamoya syndrome following recurrence and radiation prior to malignant craniopharyngioma, thought to be caused by radiation-induced vascular sclerosis and fibrous scarring, a well-known complication of therapeutic radiation (Cheng et al., 2004). From a diagnostic point of view, clinical and imaging findings, which may raise the concern for unfavorable clinical behavior, are unfortunately not specific enough to allow for prediction of malignant transformation, and definitive diagnosis of malignancy requires pathological confirmation.

PATHOLOGY

On pathological examination, two histological forms of malignancy account for the majority of these cases: malignant craniopharyngioma and craniopharyngioma with malignant transformation. Strictly defined, a malignant craniopharyngioma is the term given to a tumor which displays classical features of craniopharyngioma as described above, but has developed unequivocal histological changes characteristic of malignancy, such as nuclear crowding, hyperchromasia and pleomorphism, easily detected mitotic figures or increased proliferative activity as reflected by elevated Ki-67/Mib-1 labeling, and/or coagulative tumor necrosis (Figure 32.3 and Table 32.1). On the other hand, craniopharyngioma with malignant transformation is the diagnosis applied to tumors in which within the background of histologically benign craniopharyngioma, a different malignant neoplasm has evolved, most commonly squamous cell carcinoma (Figure 32.4). These two diagnostic terms are applied here to reflect distinct histological features, recognizing that when broadly defined, malignant transformation could represent both conditions, and as such these two diagnoses have sometimes been interchangeably used in literature.

Of the 20 cases, seven were malignant ACPs, while eight were ACPs with squamous cell carcinoma (SCC), which occurred either following a previous ACP as in recurrent cases, or concurrently in one *de novo* case (Yue and Da, 2006) where ACP and SCC co-existed. One interesting case was reported by Nelson et al. (1988), which exhibited features of both malignant ACP and foci of SCC. The remaining four ACP cases developed even rarer tumor types, including undifferentiated carcinoma (Virik et al., 1999), carcinoma with myoepitheliomatous features (Rodriguez et al., 2007), odontogenic ghost cell carcinoma (Rodriguez et al., 2007; Nishioka et al., 2009), and malignant ameloblastoma (Gao et al., 2011). Because of the overlapping histopathology and common origin of ameloblastoma, odontogenic ghost cell tumor, and craniopharyngioma as discussed above, it may be argued that malignant ameloblastoma (Gao et al., 2011) and odontogenic ghost cell carcinoma (Rodriguez et al., 2007; Nishioka et al., 2009) could be alternatively designated as malignant craniopharyngioma. When considered separately, of the five *de novo* cases, two developed malignant ACP, while one

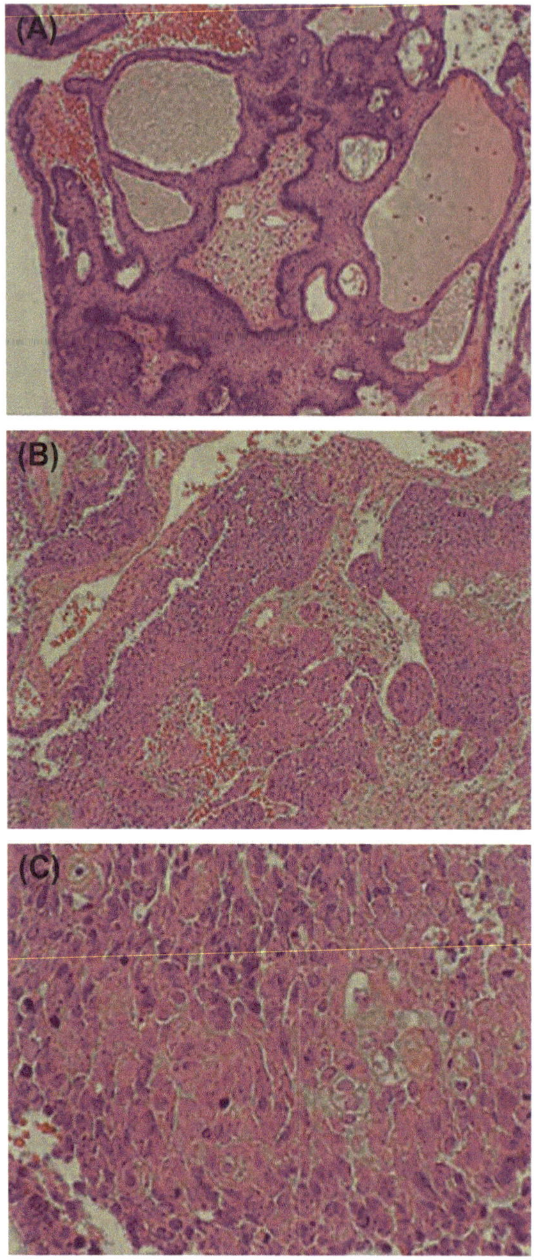

FIGURE 32.3 **Photomicrographs of malignant craniopharyngioma developed in recurrence. A,** Low-power photo of the first resection shows cysts, palisading epithelium, and stellate reticulum characteristic of adamantinomatous craniopharyngioma. **B,** The recurrent tumor exhibits an infiltrating pattern with multiple nests. **C,** High-power photo demonstrates markedly increased mitotic activity and keratin pearl formation. *(From Figure 2 in Rodriguez et al. 2007 with permission from © 2007 Lippincott Williams & Wilkins, Inc. Published by Lippincott Williams & Wilkins, Inc.)*

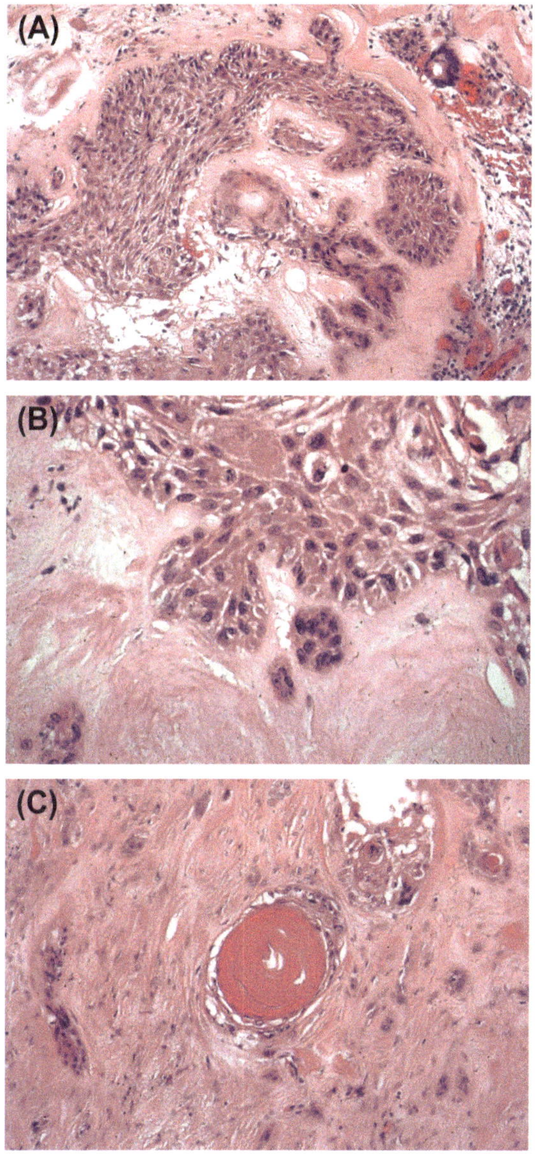

FIGURE 32.4 Photomicrographs of a case of intracranial, ventricular squamous cell carcinoma in a 56-year-old woman, demonstrating infiltrative growth (**A**), cytological atypia (**B**), and well-formed keratin pearl (**C**). It may be derived from transformed craniopharyngioma, although its relationship to sellar region could not be convincingly established. Magnifications: **A** at 10x, **B** at 100x and **C** at 40x objective lens. *(Courtesy of Dr. Arnulf Koeppen, VA Hospital, Albany, New York.)*

case was an ACP transformed into SCC; and among the 15 secondary tumors, five were malignant ACP, and seven were ACPs with transformation to SCC.

When SCC develops as transformation from ACP, the histopathology is indistinguishable from any SCC unassociated with craniopharyngioma, be it from skin, upper respiratory tract, or external genitalia. These cases displayed histological malignant changes of varying degrees with evidence of squamous differentiation typically in the form of keratinization (Figure 32.4).

These cases are so rare that any generalized conclusion may prove premature, but one cannot but notice that essentially all these cases are ACP, except for two cases with mixed histological types: one reported by Aquilina et al. which contained a minor PCP component, and the other case by Gao et al. in which a major PCP component was present initially, but it was the ACP component that underwent malignant transformation after recurrences, while the PCP component disappeared after malignant transformation. This was thought to be due to the less infiltrative growth of PCP compared with ACP, which allowed the latter to persist after surgery especially in subtotal resections (Gao et al., 2011). Like its adamantinomatous counterpart, PCP may recur and even rarely spread distantly (Elmaci et al., 2002), but malignant progression has never been reported to have developed from pure PCPs. It is unclear whether this is due to overrepresentation of ACP, or, considering the Wnt/beta-catenin pathway implicated in ACP (see below), this may actually reflect the fundamental molecular differences between these two subtypes.

MANAGEMENT AND OUTCOME

Information regarding the management of these malignant tumors is limited to a few cases. In addition to debulking (Akachi et al., 1987), these patients were treated with salvage or palliative radiation (Akachi et al., 1987; Virik et al., 1999; Aquilina et al., 2010) and several chemotherapy regimens usually combining either cisplatin or carboplatin with another agent chosen from etoposide, paclitaxel, or cetuximab (Virik et al., 1999; Kristopaitis et al., 2000; Aquilina et al., 2010). These additional treatments, however, did not appear to provide substantial benefits. As summarized in Table 32.2, most patients succumbed to the tumor relatively shortly after malignant diagnosis except for rare cases. In 15 cases with fatal outcome (12 secondary and three *de novo* cases), the time from initial presentation to death ranged from 7 weeks (Boongird et al., 2009) to 35 years (Nelson et al., 1988), with an average of 8.8 years. This reflects the wide range of the time interval from presentation to malignant progression (Table 32.2). However, it is clear that once malignancy developed, fatal outcome ensued quickly for most cases: on average, the survival time was 7 months, and for almost half of these (seven cases), it was less than 5 months, the shortest survival being 7 weeks (Boongird et al., 2009). This grave outcome is comparable to that for high-grade astrocytomas (WHO grade III and IV tumors), which have developed from radiation-treated low-grade gliomas (Dirks et al., 1994). One rare exception is the case reported by Kristopaitis et al., which showed the longest survival of 5 years after malignant progression at the time of the report publication. An interesting phenomenon is that fatal outcome appears to be related to local progression rather than distant metastasis, possibly related to time intervals that are too short for metastasis to take place.

PATHOGENESIS OF MALIGNANCY IN CRANIOPHARYNGIOMAS

Radiation

The mechanisms for malignant progression in craniopharyngioma are currently unknown. Also the reason that malignant transformation seems to target ACP remains an open question. One common finding among these rare cases stands out, that except for *de novo* cases and the case from Gao et al., tumors in all other cases have been treated at least once with radiotherapy prior to malignant transformation, at variable time intervals following initial surgery, thus suggesting a connection between radiation and malignant progression in craniopharyngiomas (Akachi et al., 1987; Nelson et al., 1988; Kristopaitis et al., 2000; Aquilina et al., 2010; Ishida et al., 2010). This is not surprising, since exposure to ionizing radiation as occurs in therapeutic radiation and atomic explosion survivors has been well established to be associated with the development of brain tumors (Modan et al., 1974; Preston et al., 2002; reviewed in Braganza et al., 2012; Michaud and Bachelor, 2014). In a large cohort study of more than 11,000 children treated with radiation for tinea capitis, Modan et al. demonstrated an increased risk for brain tumors, with higher relative risk (RR) for benign nerve sheath tumors and meningiomas (33.1 and 9.5 respectively) and a lower, but still increased over the general population, RR for malignant gliomas (2.6). It has also been reported that radiation treatment for primary intracranial tumors is associated with the development of secondary tumors within the radiation field or with the malignant transformation of benign tumors (Kohn and fry, 1984; Habrand et al., 1999; Kranzinger et al., 2001; Caldarelli et al., 2005). Meningiomas represent the best example of secondary intracranial neoplasms following radiation therapy for malignant gliomas, medulloblastomas, and other, including non-neoplastic, conditions (Strojan et al., 2000; Sadetzki et al., 2002; Al-Mefty et al., 2004; Bondy et al., 2008; Braganza et al., 2012; Godlewski et al., 2012). Examples of malignancy that have developed from benign intracranial tumors following radiation include vestibular schwannomas (Shin et al., 2002; Akamatsu et al., 2010; Yanamadala et al., 2013) and ganglioglioma (Rumana and Valadka, 1998; Tarnaris et al., 2006). Furthermore, from 55 pediatric low-grade gliomas located in the optic chiasmatic-hypothalamic-thalamic region treated with external radiation, six cases developed high-grade astrocytomas (four anaplastic astrocytomas and two glioblastomas) either at the original surgery site or within the radiation field (Dirks et al., 1994).

Treating craniopharyngiomas with radiation has also been reported to be associated with later development of both benign meningiomas and malignant gliomas (Sogg et al., 1978; Ushio et al., 1978; Maat-Schieman et al., 1985; Habrand et al., 1999; Rittinger et al., 2003; Al-Mefty et al., 2004; Caldarelli et al., 2005; Menon et al., 2007). Similarly, in a study of 123 craniopharyngiomas followed for a median of 8.9 years, three secondary CNS tumors were found, including two meningiomas occurring 24 and 27 years post-radiation, and one glioblastoma 6 years after radiation (Lo et al., 2014). Further evidence has come from the study of radiation-treated pituitary adenomas, which is relevant to craniopharyngiomas because of the similar radiation fields used. In a large cohort study of 426 pituitary adenomas treated with radiotherapy with follow-up for 5749 person-years (Minniti et al., 2005), 11 secondary brain tumors were found (five meningiomas, four high-grade astrocytomas, one meningeal sarcoma, and one primitive neuroectodermal tumor).

It is, therefore, plausible to make the same connection between malignant changes in craniopharyngiomas and therapeutic radiation, analogous to development of malignant or high-grade tumors from irradiation of benign or low-grade tumors. However, arguments still exist (Aquilina et al., 2010; Gao et al., 2011) that the vast majority of craniopharyngiomas treated with radiation to prevent recurrences do not result in secondary tumors or malignant progression; and for those *de novo* cases of malignant craniopharyngiomas, and the case from Gao et al., no prior radiation therapy was ever given. Furthermore, in one case (Akachi et al., 1987), the period of time from radiotherapy to malignant progression appears to be too short to support this argument. As pointed out by Aquilina et al., it remains to be established that malignant transformation of craniopharyngiomas is causally related to radiation therapy, because malignant transformation could represent the natural history for some tumors that are usually considered "benign" (Kubo et al., 2005).

Wnt/Beta-Catenin

The oncoprotein beta-catenin is an integral downstream component of the Wnt/beta-catenin signaling pathway. This pathway plays important physiological roles during embryogenesis, and in homeostasis of adult life, and its deregulation is implicated in human diseases including tumorigenesis (reviewed in van Es et al., 2003; MacDonald et al., 2009; Clevers and Nusse, 2012). Mutations of the beta-catenin gene *CTNNB1* lead to the beta-catenin protein being stabilized by evading ubiquitin-mediated proteasomal degradation, causing its accumulation in the nucleus and cytoplasm, and resulting in the activation of the Wnt pathway. Regulatory phosphorylation sites in the beta-catenin gene are frequently mutated in some tumors including colorectal cancer and melanoma, and activation of the pathway is identified in these tumors (Peifer and Polakis, 2000; van Es et al., 2003).

Recent studies of beta-catenin have shed light on the role of the Wnt/beta-catenin pathway in the tumorigenesis of craniopharyngiomas (reviewed in Larkin and Ansorge, 2013; Hussain et al., 2013). It has been demonstrated that more than 70% of ACPs had a mutation in the beta-catenin gene, which was not detected in PCPs (Sekine et al., 2002; Buslei et al., 2005). Furthermore, among cystic lesions in the sellar region (51 craniopharyngiomas and 30 Rathke cleft cysts) studied by Hofmann et al. (2006), nuclear beta-catenin was only detected in craniopharyngiomas (38 of 42 ACPs and none of nine PCPs). Further proof was provided in a mouse model (Gaston-Massuet et al., 2011; Andoniadou et al., 2012) that craniopharyngiomas arise from activation of beta-catenin in pituitary progenitors during embryogenesis.

The expression of beta-catenin was studied in only a few cases of craniopharyngiomas with malignant changes (Rodriguez et al., 2007; Nishioka et al., 2009). Nuclear beta-catenin was detected in all three cases of Rodriguez (one *de novo* and two secondary tumors), and interestingly, for two secondary tumors (cases 2 and 3), case 2 showed nuclear (as well as cytoplasmic) stain in both original benign tumor and the recurrent/malignant tumor, while in case 3, the nuclear stain was only observed in the malignant tumor, but not in the previous benign one.

These results support the hypothesis that the Wnt/beta-catenin pathway may play a role in the development of craniopharyngiomas, especially the ACP subtypes. However, it remains unclear whether this pathway is involved in the malignant progression of craniopharyngiomas. It is intriguing to speculate that interaction of radiation with the Wnt/beta-catenin signaling pathway may be the underlying mechanism for the malignant progression observed in these tumors. In animal models (King and Lampe, 2005), increased beta-catenin protein levels were demonstrated in liver and lung cancers that were induced by radiation, suggesting that a dysregulated beta-catenin system may interact with radiation in causing malignancy. Theoretically, it is possible that aberrant beta-catenin regulation may provide a fertile soil from which malignancy evolves from a benign craniopharyngioma due to a second hit by radiation.

p53

p53, a well-known tumor suppressor gene located on chromosome 17p13.1, and a principal mediator of growth arrest, maintenance of genomic stability, senescence, and apoptosis, is the most common target for genetic alterations in many human neoplasms (Soussi 2005; Vousden and Lane, 2007; Kandoth et al., 2013; Muller and Vousden, 2014). Variable expression of p53 protein by immunohistochemistry has been reported in craniopharyngiomas, from a low number (Lefranc et al., 2003; Momota et al., 2003) to a high number of cases (Tena-Suck et al., 2006). In ten cases of malignant craniopharyngiomas stained for p53 protein (Table 32.1), elevated expression was found in the malignant element in nine cases (three *de novo* and six secondary tumors). In one case (Plowman et al., 2004), p53 protein was found in both the initial benign tumor and the recurrent malignant tumor, but quantification was not provided. These findings raise the possibility that p53 mutations may play a role in the malignant progression of craniopharyngiomas. Confirmatory mutational analysis, however, is needed from further molecular studies. Since radiation has been shown to induce p53 mutations (De Benedetti et al., 1996; Fogelfeld et al., 1996; Brat et al., 1999; Shin et al., 2002; Henson et al., 2005; Pinto et al., 2011), it is conceivable that malignant progression in craniopharyngiomas associated with radiation may be mediated via p53 mutations.

There have been studies analyzing the tumor-stromal interactions, adhesion molecules, and growth factors in craniopharyngiomas (Hölsken et al., 2010; Qi et al., 2012; reviewed in Hussain et al., 2013). The results suggest that these factors may be involved in the tumorigenesis as well as local aggressive growth of craniopharyngiomas, but their role in malignant transformation of craniopharyngioma is not clear.

Given that squamous epithelium is the main component of craniopharyngioma, another squamous lesion may offer insights with regard to malignant progression. It is well known that uterine cervical squamous epithelium can transform from precancerous low-grade dysplasia to high-grade dysplasia/carcinoma *in situ*, to frankly invasive carcinoma, and high-risk subtypes of human papilloma virus (HPV) play a pivotal role in the process (Yugawa and Kiyono, 2009; Jaisamrarn et al., 2013; Wheeler, 2013). This dysplasia – carcinoma sequence has not been unequivocally demonstrated in craniopharyngioma with malignant transformation, suggesting intrinsic differences may exist between these two types of lesions; nonetheless, it is tempting to test the possibility that HPV may have a role in the malignant transformation of craniopharyngiomas.

CONCLUSION

Frankly malignant craniopharyngiomas are extremely rare, and prognosis is unfavorable for the vast majority of such cases. Malignant transformation of craniopharyngiomas cannot be reliably predicted; and regular follow-up with multi-disciplinary care will provide the best management. Currently, the underlying mechanisms remain to be deciphered, although an association with radiation has been suggested. One hurdle in studying this condition lies in the rarity of such cases; therefore, a multi-center coordinated approach is needed.

Acknowledgment

We greatly appreciate Dr. Dion Middleton and Mrs. Middleton for their help with the interpretation of articles written in Japanese.

References

Adamson, T.E., Wiestler, O.D., Kleihues, P., Yaşagil, M.G., 1990. Correlation of clinical and pathological features in surgically treated craniopharyngiomas. J. Neurosurg. 73 (1), 12–17.

Akachi, K., Takahashi, H., Ishijima, B., et al., 1987. Malignant changes in a craniopharyngioma. Article in Japanese No Shinkei Geka 15 (8), 843–848.

Akamatsu, Y., Murakami, K., Watanabe, M., Jokura, H., Tominaga, T., 2010. Malignant peripheral nerve sheath tumor arising from benign vestibular schwannoma treated by gamma knife radiosurgery after two previous surgeries: a case report with surgical and pathological observations. World Neurosurg. 73 (6), 751–754.

Al-Mefty O, Topsakal, C., Pravdenkova, S., Sawyer, J.R., Harrison, M.J., 2004. Radiation-induced meningiomas: clinical, pathological, cytokinetic, and cytogenetic characteristics. J. Neurosurg. 100 (6), 1002–1013.

Andoniadou, C.L., Gaston-Massuet, C., Reddy, R., Schneider, R.P., Blasco, M.A., Le Tissier, P., Jacques, T.S., Pevny, L.H., Dattani, M.T., Martinez-Barbera, J.P., 2012. Identification of novel pathways involved in the pathogenesis of human adamantinomatous craniopharyngioma. Acta Neuropathol. 124 (2), 259–271.

Aquilina, K., Merchant, T.E., Rodriguez-Galindo, C., Ellison, D.W., Sanford, R.A., Boop, F.A., 2010. Malignant transformation of irradiated craniopharyngioma in children: report of two cases. J. Neurosurg. Pediatr. 5 (2), 155–161.

Badger, K.V., Gardner, D.G., 1997. The relationship of adamantinomatous craniopharyngioma to ghost cell ameloblastoma of the jaws: a histopathologic and immunohistochemical study. J. Oral. Pathol. Med. 26, 349–355.

Bailey, W., Freidenberg, G.R., James, H.E., Hesselink, J.R., Jones, K.L., 1990. Prenatal diagnosis of a craniopharyngioma using ultrasonography and magnetic resonance imaging. Prenat. Diagn. 10, 623–629.

Bernstein, M.L., Buchino, J.J., 1983. The histologic similarity between craniopharyngioma and odontogenic lesions: a reappraisal. Oral. Surg. Oral. Med. Oral. Pathol. 56, 502–511.

Bigner, D.D., McLendon, R.E., Bruner, J.M., 1998. Russell and Rubinstein's Pathology of Tumors of the Nervous System, sixth ed, vol. 2. Oxford University Press, Inc. 629–640.

Bondy, M.L., Scheurer, M.E., Malmer, B., Barnholtz-Sloan, J.S., Davis, F.G., Il'yasova, D., Kruchko, C., McCarthy, B.J., Rajaraman, P., Schwartzbaum, J.A., Sadetzki, S., Schlehofer, B., Tihan, T., Wiemels, J.L., Wrensch, M., Buffler, P.A., 2008. Brain tumor epidemiology: Consensus from the Brain Tumor Epidemiology Consortium. Cancer 113 (Suppl. 7), 1953–1968.

Boongird, A., Laothamatas, J., Larbcharoensub, N., Phudhichareonrat, S., 2009. Malignant craniopharyngioma; case report and review of the literature. Neuropathology 29 (5), 591–596.

Braganza, M.Z., Kitahara, C.M., Berrington de González, A., Inskip, P.D., Johnson, K.J., Rajaraman, P., 2012. Ionizing radiation and the risk of brain and central nervous system tumors: a systematic review. Neuro. Oncol. 14 (11), 1316–1324.

Brat, D.J., James, C.D., Jedlicka, A.E., Connolly, D.C., Chang, E., Castellani, R.J., Schmid, M., Schiller, M, Carson, D.A., Burger, P.C., 1999. Molecular genetic alterations in radiation-induced astrocytomas. Am. J. Pathol. 154 (5), 1431–1438.

Bunin, G.R., Surawicz, T.S., Witman, P.A., Preston-Martin, S., Davis, F., Bruner, J.M., 1998. The descriptive epidemiology of craniopharyngioma. J. Neurosurg. 89, 547–551.

Burger, P.C., Scheithauer, B.W., Vogel, F.S., 2002. Surgical pathology of the nervous system and its coverings, Fourth. Ed. Churchill Livingstone. pp. 475–483.

Buslei, R., Nolde, M., Hofmann, B., et al., 2005. Common mutations of beta-catenin in adamantinomatous craniopharyngiomas but not in other tumours originating from the sellar region. Acta Neuropathol. 109 (6), 589–597. Epub 2005 May 13.

Caldarelli, M., Massimi, L., Tamburrini, G., Cappa, M., Di Rocco, C., 2005. Long-term results of the surgical treatment of craniopharyngioma: the experience at the Policlinico Gemelli, Catholic University, Rome. Childs Nerv. Syst. 21, 747–757.

Chakrabarti, I., Amar, A.P., Couldwell, W., Weiss, M.H., 2005. Long-term neurological, visual, and endocrine outcomes following transnasal resection of craniopharyngioma. J. Neurosurg. 102, 650–657.

Cheng, S.W., Ting, A.C., Ho, P., Wu, L.L., 2004. Accelerated progression of carotid stenosis in patients with previous external neck irradiation. J. Vasc. Surg. 39 (2), 409–415.

Clevers, H., Nusse, R., 2012. Wnt/β-catenin signaling and disease. Cell 149 (6), 1192–1205.

Crotty, T.B., Scheithauer, B.W., Young, J.R.W.F., et al., 1995. Papillary craniopharyngioma: a clinicopathological study of 48 cases. J. Neurosurg. 83, 206–214.

De Benedetti, V.M., Travis, L.B., Welsh, J.A., et al., 1996. p53 mutations in lung cancer following radiation therapy for Hodgkin's disease. Cancer Epidemiol. Biomarkers Prev. 5 (2), 93–98.

Delman, B.N., 2009. Imaging of pediatric pituitary abnormalities. Endocrinol. Metab. Clin. North Am. 38 (4), 673–698.

Dirks, P.B., Jay, V., Becker, L.E., et al., 1994. Development of anaplastic changes in low-grade astrocytomas of childhood. Neurosurgery 34 (1), 68–78.

Duff, J.M., Meyer, F.B., Ilstrup, D.M., Laws Jr, E.R., Schleck, C.D., Scheithauer, B.W., 2000. Long-term Outcomes for Surgically Resected Craniopharyngiomas. Neurosurgery 46 (2), 291–302.

Eldevik, O.P., Blaivas, M., Gabrielsen, T.O., Hald, J.K., Chandler, W.F., 1996. Craniopharyngioma: radiologic and histologic findings and recurrence. AJNR Am. J. Neuroradiol. 17 (8), 1427–1439.

Elmaci, L., Kurtkaya-Yapicier, O., Ekinci, G., et al., 2002. Metastatic papillary craniopharyngioma: case study and study of tumor angiogenesis. Neurooncology 4, 23–28.

Elliott, R.E., Jane, J.R.J.A., Wisoff, J.H., 2011. Surgical management of craniopharyngiomas in children: Meta-analysis and comparison of transcranial and transsphenoidal approaches. Neurosurgery 69, 630–643.

Fogelfeld, L., Bauer, T.K., Schneider, A.B., Swartz, J.E., Zitman, R., 1996. p53 gene mutations in radiation-induced thyroid cancer. J. Clin. Endocrinol. Metab. 81 (8), 3039–3044.

Frazier, C.H., Alpers, B.J., 1931. Adamantinoma of the craniopharyngeal duct. Arch. Neuro. Pysch. 26, 905–965.

Gao, S., Shi, X., Wang, Y., Qian, H., Liu, C., 2011. Malignant transformation of craniopharyngioma: case report and review of the literature. J. Neurooncol. 103 (3), 719–725.

Gaston-Massuet, C., Andoniadou, C.L., Signore, M., et al., 2011. Increased wingless (Wnt) signaling in pituitary progenitor/stem cells gives rise to pituitary tumors in mice and humans. Proc. Natl. Acad. Sci. USA. 108 (28), 11482–11487.

Godlewski, B., Drummond, K.J., Kaye, A.H., 2012. Radiation-induced meningiomas after high-dose cranial irradiation. J. Clin. Neurosci. 19 (12), 1627–1635.

Habrand, J.L., Ganry, O., Couanet, D., et al., 1999. The role of radiation therapy in the management of craniopharyngioma: a 25-year experience and review of the literature. Int. J. Radiat. Oncol. Biol. Phys. 44, 255–263.

Henson, J.W., Hobbs, W., Chakravarti, A., Louis, D.N., 2005. Alterations in p53, p21, and MIB-1 labeling index in primary human astrocytomas following radiation therapy. J. Neurooncol. 74 (2), 151–154.

Hofmann, B.M., Kreutzer, J., Saeger, W., et al., 2006. Nuclear beta-catenin accumulation as reliable marker for the differentiation between cystic craniopharyngiomas and Rathke cleft cysts: a clinico-pathologic approach. Am. J. Surg. Pathol. 30 (12), 1595–1603.

Hölsken, A., Buchfelder, M., Fahlbusch, R., Blumcke, I., Buslei, R., 2010. Tumour cell migration in adamantinomatous craniopharyngiomas is promoted by activated Wnt-signalling. Acta Neuropathol. 119 (5), 631–639.

Humphreys, R.P., Hoffman, H.J., Hendrick, E.B., 1979. A long-term postoperative follow-up in craniopharyngioma. Childs Brain 5 (6), 530–539.

Hussain, I., Eloy, J.A., Carmel, P.W., Liu, J.K., 2013. Molecular oncogenesis of craniopharyngioma: current and future strategies for the development of targeted therapies. A review. J. Neurosurg. 119, 106–112.

Ironside, J.W., Moss, T.H., Louis, D.N., Lowe, J.S., Weller, R.O., 2002. Diagnostic Pathology of Nervous System Tumours. Churchill Livingstone, 510–517.

Ishida, M., Hotta, M., Tsukamura, A., et al., 2010. Malignant transformation in craniopharyngioma after radiation therapy: a case report and review of the literature. Clin. Neuropathol. 29 (1), 2–8.

Ito, M., Jamshidi, J., Yamanaka, K., 2001. Does Craniopharyngioma metastasize? Case report and review of the literature. Neurosurgery 48, 933–936.

Jagannathan, J., Kanter, A.S., Sheehan, J.P., Jane Jr., J.A., Laws Jr., E.R., 2007. Benign brain tumors: sellar/parasellar tumors. Neurol. Clin. 25 (4), 1231–1249, xi.

Jaisamrarn, U., Castellsagué, X., Garland, S.M., et al., 2013. HPV PATRICIA Study Group. Natural history of progression of HPV infection to cervical lesion or clearance: analysis of the control arm of the large, randomised PATRICIA study. e79260 PLoS One 8 (11).

Jo, K.W., Shin, H.J., Kong, D.S., Seol, H.-J., Nam, D.-H., Lee, J.I., 2012. Treatment outcomes of pediatric craniopharyngioma: a 15-year retrospective review of 35 cases. J. Korean Neurosurg. Soc. 52, 37–41.

Joó, J.G., Rigó Jr, J., Sápi, Z., Timár, B., 2009. Foetal craniopharyngioma diagnosed by prenatal ultrasonography and confirmed by histopathological examination. Prenat. Diagn. 29 (2), 160–163.

Kandoth, C., McLellan, M.D., Vandin, F., et al., 2013. Mutational landscape and significance across 12 major cancer types. Nature 502 (7471), 333–339.

Karavitaki, N., Brufani, C., Warner, J.T., et al., 2005. Craniopharyngiomas in children and adults: systematic analysis of 121 cases with long-term follow-up. Clin. Endocrinol. 62, 397–409.

Karavitaki, N., Cudlip, S., Adams, C.B.T., Wass, J.A.H., 2006. Craniopharyngiomas. Endocr. Rev. 27 (4), 371–397.

King, T.J., Lampe, P.D., 2005. Altered tumor biology and tumorigenesis in irradiated and chemical carcinogen-treated single and combined connexin32/p27Kip1-deficient mice. Cell Commun. Adhes. 12 (5–6), 293–305.

Kohn, H.I., Fry, R.J., 1984. Radiation carcinogenesis. N. Engl. J. Med. 310, 504–511.

Kranzinger, M., Jones, N., Rittinger, O., Pilz, P., Piotrowski, W.P., Manzl, M., et al., 2001. Malignant glioma as a secondary malignant neoplasm after radiation therapy for craniopharyngioma: report of a case and review of reported cases. Onkologie 24, 66–72.

Kristopaitis, T., Thomas, C., Petruzzelli, G.J., Lee, J.M., 2000. Malignant craniopharyngioma. Arch. Pathol. Lab. Med. 124, 1356–1360.

Kubo, O., Chernov, M., Izawa, M., et al., 2005. Malignant progression of benign brain tumors after gamma knife radiosurgery: is it really caused by irradiation? Minim. Invasive Neurosurg. 48, 334–339.

Larkin, S.J., Ansorge, O., 2013. Pathology and pathogenesis of craniopharyngiomas. Pituitary 16 (1), 9–17.

Lauriola, L., Doglietto, F., Novello, M., et al., 2011. De novo malignant craniopharyngioma: case report and literature Review. J. Neurooncol. 103, 381–386.

Lee, S.K., Kim, Y.S., 2013. Current concepts and occurrence of epithelial odontogenic tumors: I. Ameloblastoma and adenomatoid odontogenic tumor. Korean J. Pathol. 47 (3), 191–202.

Lefranc, F., Chevalier, C., Vinchon, M., et al., 2003. Characterization of the levels of expression of retinoic acid receptors, galectin-3, macrophage migration inhibiting factor, and p53 in 51 adamantinomatous craniopharyngiomas. J. Neurosurg. 98 (1), 145–153.

Li, T.J., Yu, S.F., 2003. Clinicopathologic spectrum of the so-called calcifying odontogenic cysts: a study of 21 intraosseous cases with reconsideration of the terminology and classification. Am. J. Surg. Pathol. 27 (3), 372–384.

Lin, L.L., El Naqa, I., Leonard, J.R., et al., 2008. Long-term outcome in children treated for craniopharyngioma with and without radiotherapy. J. Neurosurg. Pediatr. 1 (2), 126–130.

Lo, A.C., Howard, A.F., Nichol, A., et al., 2014. Long-term outcomes and complications in patients with craniopharyngioma: The British Columbia cancer agency experience. Int. J. Radiat. Oncol. Biol. Phys. 88 (5), 1011–1018.

Louis, D.N., Ohgaki, H., Wiestler, O.D., et al., 2007. The 2007 WHO Classification of Tumours of the Central Nervous System. Acta Neuropathol. 114, 97–109.

Lu, D.H., Xu, Q.Z., 1988. Pathological analysis of 1458 cases of tumor in the sella turcica region. Article in Chinese Zhonghua Zhong Liu Za Zhi 10 (3), 205–208.

Luse, S.A., Kernohan, J.W., 1955. Squamous-cell nests of the pituitary gland. Cancer 8 (3), 623–628.

Maat-Schieman, M.L., Bots, G.T., Thomeer, R.T., Vielvoye, G.J., 1985. Malignant astrocytoma following radiotherapy for craniopharyngioma. Br. J. Radiol. 58, 480–482.

MacDonald, B.T., Tamai, K., He, X., 2009. Wnt/beta-catenin signaling: components, mechanisms, and diseases. Dev. Cell 17 (1), 9–26.

Manaka, S., Teramoto, A., Takakura, K., 1985. The efficacy of radiotherapy for craniopharyngioma. J. Neurosurg. 62 (5), 648–656.

Menon, G., Nair, S., Rajesh, B.J., Rao, B.R., Radhakrishnan, V.V., 2007. Malignant astrocytoma following radiotherapy for craniopharyngioma. J. Cancer. Res. Ther. 3, 50–52.

Michaud, D., Batchelor, T., 2014. Risk factors for brain tumors. UpToDate. updated July, 2013.

Minniti, G., Traish, D., Ashley, S., Gonsalves, A., Brada, M., 2005. Risk of second brain tumor after conservative surgery and radiotherapy for pituitary adenoma: update after an additional 10 years. J. Clin. Endocrinol. Metab. 90 (2), 800–804.

Modan, B., Mart, H., Baidatz, D., Steinitz, R., Levin, S.G., 1974. Lancet 303 (7852), 277–279.

Momota, H., Ichimiya, S., Ikeda, T., et al., 2003. Immunohistochemical analysis of the p53 family members in human craniopharyngiomas. Brain Tumor Pathol. 20, 73–77.

Muller, P.A., Vousden, K.H., 2014. Mutant p53 in cancer: new functions and therapeutic opportunities. Cancer Cell 25 (3), 304–317.

Müller-Scholden, J., Lehrnbecher, T., Müller, H.L., et al., 2000. Radical surgery in a neonate with craniopharyngioma. report of a case. Pediatr. Neurosurg. 33 (5), 265–269.

Nagata, T., Nakayama, H., Uchida, K., et al., 2005. Two cases of feline malignant craniopharyngioma. Vet. Pathol. 42, 663–665.

Nelson, G.A., Bastian, F.O., Schlitt, M., White, R.L., 1988. Malignant transformation in craniopharyngioma. Neurosurgery 22 (2), 427–429.

Nielsen, E.H., Feldt-Rasmussen, U., Poulsgaard, L., et al., 2011. Incidence of craniopharyngioma in Denmark (n = 189) and estimated world incidence of craniopharyngioma in children and adults. J. Neurooncol. 104 (3), 755–763.

Nishioka, H., Shibuya, M., Izawa, H., Ikeda, Y., 2009. Primary suprasellar malignant tumor with odontogenic features: case report. Neurosurgery 65 (2), E380–E382.

Okada, T., Fujitsu, K., Ichikawa, T., et al., 2012. Coexistence of adamantinomatous and squamous-papillary type craniopharyngioma: Case report and discussion of etiology and pathology. Neuropathology 32, 171–173.

Ostrom, Q.T., Gittleman, H., Farah, P., et al., 2013. CBTRUS statistical report: Primary brain and central nervous system tumors diagnosed in the United States in 2006–2010. Neuro.Oncol. 15, ii1–ii56.

Pace, V., Heider, K., Persohn, E., Schaetti, P., 1997. Spontaneous malignant craniopharyngioma in an albino rat. Vet. Pathol. 34 (2), 146–149.

Paulus, W., Stöckel, C., Krauss, J., et al., 1997. Odontogenic classification of craniopharyngiomas: a clinicopathological study of 54 cases. Histopathology 30, 172–176.

Peifer, M., Polakis, P., 2000. Wnt signaling in oncogenesis and embryogenesis – a look outside the nucleus. Science 287 (5458), 1606–1609.

Pekmezci, M., Louie, J., Gupta, N., Bloomer, M.M., Tihan, T., 2010. Clinicopathological characteristics of adamantinomatous and papillary craniopharyngiomas: University of California, San Francisco experience 1985–2005. Neurosurgery 67, 1341–1349.

Pinto, E.M., Siqueira, S.A., Cukier, P., Fragoso, M.C., Lin, C.J., de Mendonca, B.B., 2011. Possible role of a radiation-induced p53 mutation in a Nelson's syndrome patient with a fatal outcome. Pituitary 14 (4), 400–404.

Plowman, P.N., Besser, G.M., Shipley, J., Summersgill, B., 2004. J. Geddes J, Afshar F. Dramatic response of malignant craniopharyngioma to cis-platin-based chemotherapy. Should craniopharyngioma be considered as a suprasellar 'germ cell' tumour? Br. J. Neurosurg. 18 (5), 500–505.

Prabhu, V.C., Brown, H.G., 2005. The pathogenesis of craniopharyngiomas. Childs Nerv. Syst. 21, 622–627.

Preston, D.L., Ron, E., Yonehara, S., et al., 2002. Tumors of the nervous system and pituitary gland associated with atomic bomb radiation exposure. J. Natl. Cancer. Inst. 20, 1555–1563.

Qi, S.T., Zhou, J., Pan, J., Zhang, C., Silky, C., Yan, X.R., 2012. Epithelial-mesenchymal transition and clinicopathological correlation in craniopharyngioma. Histopathology 61 (4), 711–725.

Richmond, I.L., Wara, W.M., Wilson, C.B., 1980. Role of radiation therapy in the management of craniopharyngiomas in children. Neurosurgery 6 (5), 513–517.

Rittinger, O., Kranzinger, M., Jones, R., Jones, N., 2003. Malignant astrocytoma arising 10 years after combined treatment of craniopharyngioma. J. Pediatr. Endocrinol. Metab. 16 (1), 97–101.

Rodriguez, F.J., Scheithauer, B.W., Tsunoda, S., Kovacs, K., Vidal, S., Piepgras, D.G., 2007. The spectrum of malignancy in craniopharyngioma. Am. J. Surg. Pathol. 31 (7), 1020–1028.

Rumana, C.S., Valadka, A.B., 1998. Radiation therapy and malignant degeneration of benign supratentorial gangliogliomas. Neurosurgery 42 (5), 1038–1043.

Sadetzki, S., Flint-Richter, P., Ben-Tal, T., Nass, D., 2002. Radiation-induced meningioma: a descriptive study of 253 cases. J. Neurosurg. 97 (5), 1078–1082.

Sakai, K., Tanaka, Y., Hongo, K., Tada, T., Shigeta, H., Kobayashi, S., 2004. Treatment of craniopharyngiomas in children. Article in Japanese No Shinkei Geka 32 (4), 345–353.

Salyer, D., Carter, D., 1973. Squamous carcinoma arising in the pituitary gland. Cancer 31, 713–718.

Sartoretti-Schefer, S., Wichmann, W., Aguzzi, A., Valavanis, A., 1997. MR differentiation of adamantinous and squamous-papillary craniopharyngiomas. Am. J. Neuroradiol. 18 (1), 77–87.

Schoenberg, B.S., Schoenberg, D.G., Christine, B.W., Gomez, M.R., 1976. The epidemiology of primary intracranial neoplasms of childhood. A population study. Mayo. Clin. Proc. 51, 51–56.

Schroeder, J.W., Vezina, L.G., 2011. Pediatric sellar and suprasellar lesions. Pediatr. Radiol. 41 (3), 287–298.

Scott, R.M., Hetelekidis, S., Barnes, P.D., Goumnerova, L., Tarbell, N.J., 1994. Surgery, radiation, and combination therapy in the treatment of childhood craniopharyngioma – a 20-year experience. Pediatr. Neurosurg. 21 (Suppl. 1), 75–81.

Sekine, S., Shibata, T., Kokubu, A., et al., 2002. Craniopharyngiomas of adamantinomatous type harbor beta-catenin gene mutations. Am. J. Pathol. 161 (6), 1997–2001.

Sekine, S., Takata, T., Shibata, T., et al., 2004. Expression of enamel proteins and LEF1 in adamantinomatous craniopharyngioma: evidence for its odontogenic epithelial differentiation. Histopathology 45 (6), 573–579.

Shin, M., Ueki, K., kuritha, H., Kirino, T., 2002. Malignant transformation of a vestibular schwannoma after gamma knife radiosurgery. Lancet 360 (9329), 309–310.

Sogg, R.L., Donaldson, S.S., Yorke, C.H., 1978. Malignant astrocytoma following radiotherapy of a craniopharyngioma. Case report. J. Neurosurg. 48, 622–627.

Sorva, R., Heiskanen, O., 1986. Craniopharyngioma in Finland. A study of 123 cases. Acta Neurochir. (Wien) 81 (3–4), 85–89.

Soussi, T., Lozano, G., 2005. p53 mutation heterogeneity in cancer. Biochem. Biophys. Res. Commun. 331 (3), 834–842.

Stricker, T.P., Kumar, V., 2010. Neoplasia. In: Kumar, V., Abbas, A.K., Fausto, N., Aster, J.C. (Eds.), Robbins and Cotran Pathologic Basis of Disease, Eighth. Ed. Saunders/Elsevier, pp. 259–330. Chapter 7.

Strojan, P., Popović, M., Jereb, B., 2000. Secondary intracranial meningiomas after high-dose cranial irradiation: report of five cases and review of the literature. Int. J. Radiat. Oncol. Biol. Phys. 48 (1), 65–73.

Susman, W., 1932. Embryonic epithelial rests in the pituitary. Br. J. Surg. 19, 571–576.

Suzuki, F., Konuma, I., Matsumoto, M., Aoki, M., Hayakawa, I., 1989. Craniopharyngioma with malignant transformation–a report of two cases. Article in Japanese Gan No Rinsho 35 (6), 723–728.

Szeifert, G.T., Sipos, L., Horváth, M., et al., 1993. Pathological characteristics of surgically removed craniopharyngiomas: analysis of 131 cases. Acta Neurochir. (Wien) 124 (2–4), 139–143.

Tamaris, A., O'Brien, C., Redfern, R.M., 2006. Ganglioglioma with anaplastic recurrence of the neuronal element following radiotherapy. Clin. Neurol. Neurosurg. 108 (8), 761–767.

Tavangar, S.M., Larijani, B., Mahta, A., Hosseini, S.M.A., Mehrazine, M., Bandarian, F., 2004. Craniopharyngioma: A clinicopathological study of 141 cases. Endocr. Pathol. 15 (4), 339–344.

Tena-Suck, M.L., Salinas-Lara, C., Arce-Arellano, R.I., 2006. Clinico-pathological and immunohistochemical characteristics associated to recurrence/regrowth of craniopharyngiomas. Clin. Neurol. Neurosurg. 108 (7), 661–669.

Ujifuku, K., Matsuo, T., Takeshita, T., et al., 2010. Malignant transformation of craniopharyngioma associated with moyamoya syndrome. Neurol. Med. Chir. (Tokyo) 50 (7), 599–603.

Ushio, Y., Arita, N., Yoshimine, T., Nagatani, M., Mogami, H., 1978. Glioblastoma after radiotherapy for craniopharyngioma: case report. Neurosurgery 21, 33–38.

van Es, J.H., Barker, N., Clevers, H., 2003. You Wnt some, you lose some: oncogenes in the Wnt signaling pathway. Curr. Opin. Genet. Dev. 13 (1), 28–33.

Virik, K., Turner, J., Garrick, R., Sheehy, J.P., 1999. Malignant transformation of craniopharyngioma. J. Clin. Neurosci. 6 (6), 527–530.

Vousden, K.H., Lane, D.P., 2007. p53 in health and disease. Nat. Rev. Mol. Cell Biol. 8, 275–283.

Weiner, H.L., Wisoff, J.H., Rosenberg, M.E., et al., 1994. Craniopharyngiomas: A clinicopathological analysis of factors predictive of recurrence and functional outcome. Neurosurgery 35 (6), 1001–1011.

Wheeler, C.M., 2013. The natural history of cervical human papillomavirus infections and cervical cancer: gaps in knowledge and future horizons. Obstet. Gynecol. Clin. North Am. 40 (2), 165–176.

Wolfe, S.Q., Heros, R.C., 2010. A Rathke cleft cyst to craniopharyngioma: is there a spectrum? J. Neurosurg. 112 (6), 1322–1323, discussion 1323.
Yanamadala, V., Williamson, R.W., Fusco, D.J., Eschbacher, J., Weisskopf, P., Porter, R.W., 2013. Malignant transformation of a vestibular schwannoma after gamma knife radiosurgery. World Neurosurg. 79 (3–4), 593.e-18.
Yue, Y., Da, J.P., 2006. Malignant transformation of craniopharyngioma: a case report. Article in Chinese Zhonghua Bing Li Xue Za Zhi 35 (7), 439.
Yugawa, T., Kiyono, T., 2009. Molecular mechanisms of cervical carcinogenesis by high-risk human papillomaviruses: novel functions of E6 and E7 oncoproteins. Rev. Med. Virol. 19 (2), 97–113.
Zeitlin, H., 1935. Adamantinomas of the hypophyseal stalk and sphenoid bone. Am. J. Cancer 23, 729–740.

SECTION VIII

CONTROVERSIES

CHAPTER

33

Incomplete Resection of Craniopharyngiomas

Philip V. Theodosopoulos

Department of Neurological Surgery, University of California San Francisco, San Francisco, CA, USA

"We recognize that any attempt at radical removal of the lesion is essentially attended with risk and may well be fatal in its outcome. Such is true of any radical operation which has as its objective the removal of any portion of the wall of the third ventricle or of any radical steps in this location." **RC Carpenter, GW Chamberlin, and CH Frazier, 1937**

Craniopharyngiomas vary significantly not only in their clinical and radiographic presentation, but also in their anatomical extent and patterns of growth. The majority of them are centered around the suprasellar space as they arise from the pituitary stalk. Yet, the major component of the tumor may reside in an expanded sella, the third ventricle or laterally in the middle fossa. The relationship to the optic chiasm is the main determinant of surgical accessibility and optimal approach corridor. Their invasiveness into adjacent structures, primarily the third ventricular wall, is often the limitation for surgical resection. Large invasive lesions are difficult to resect completely. At times, even smaller lesions do not allow for a gross total resection (GTR) without the sacrifice of the pituitary stalk and the resultant endocrinological abnormalities that ensue.

Surgical approaches to craniopharyngiomas therefore need to be tailored to allow the optimal visualization of the majority of the tumor. The bifrontal, subfrontal, pterional, transventricular, supraorbital, transsphenoidal and, more recently, expanded transsphenoidal approaches have all been described in surgical series of craniopharyngiomas. Each has specific limitations of visualization. Anterior and anterolateral approaches are limited by the optic chiasm, which is frequently displaced in a prefixed location by the tumor. As a result, significant tumor dissection posterior to the chiasm is limited. Transventricular approaches are usually suitable for lesions purely in the third ventricle and are limited in their lateral reach secondary to ventricular anatomy. Transsphenoidal approaches are limited because of the narrow corridor, long reach and lack of optimal instrumentation and vascular control.

Craniopharyngiomas
http://dx.doi.org/10.1016/B978-0-12-416706-3.00033-7

The most recent addition to the transcranial surgical corridors is the supraorbital approach with or without an orbital osteotomy (Kabil and Shahinian, 2005). It allows similar exposure to a larger craniotomy with less soft tissue dissection and provides good cosmetic results. In our experience, this approach can be safely used to fenestrate the optic canal for optic nerve mobilization as well as allowing access to third ventricular lesions through the lamina terminalis, much like the pterional approach can. We believe that for almost all lesions other than those that have a significant middle fossa component, the supraorbital approach may in time replace more extensive anterolateral approaches.

Given the limitations of all surgical approaches and the frequent complex extent of the lesions, surgical treatment often results in subtotal tumor resection (STR). As these tumors tend to recur, they can pose a difficult clinical problem. Multimodal treatment, with adjuvant radiation therapy as well as focal chemotherapy agents, is often necessary and in fact likely the optimal treatment.

As the primary treatment for craniopharyngiomas has remained surgical resection, there is plenty of literature on the post-operative rates of recurrence. A compilation of most large surgical series gives a rough average of 58% of achievement of GTR, a number that is generally optimistic in our experience (Hoogenhout et al., 1984; Hoffman, 1985; Baskin and Wilson, 1986; Fischer et al., 1990; Hoffman et al., 1992; Mark et al., 1995; Caldarelli et al., 1998, 2005; Fisher et al., 1998; Khafaga et al., 1998; Fahlbusch et al., 1999; Duff et al., 2000; Bin-Abbas et al., 2001; Kim et al., 2001; Van Effenterre and Boch, 2002; Albright et al., 2005; Chakrabarti et al., 2005; Lena et al., 2005; Mottolese et al., 2005; Sosa et al., 2005; Di Rocco et al., 2006; Lin et al., 2008). Although it comes as no surprise that the rates of local tumor control are low following STR, tumor control rates following reported GTR are similarly unimpressive, ranging between 43 and 94% (Fischer et al., 1990; Hoffman et al., 1992; Fahlbusch et al., 1999; Albright et al., 2005; Caldarelli et al., 2005; Lena et al., 2005; Dhellemmes and Vinchon, 2006; Di Rocco et al., 2006; Lin et al., 2008). Reasons for this may be multiple. The definition of GTR may vary between studies, as does the modality used to confirm radiographic extent of resection. Some argue that a GTR must include resection of the pituitary stalk while others disagree. Inadequate visualization limited by the surgical approach may disallow clear identification of small remnants in areas hidden from direct view. In our experience with expanded transsphenoidal approaches where visualization is oftentimes optimal, small areas of tumor capsule densely adherent to the undersurface of the optic chiasm or third ventricular wall often are not visible on post-operative MRI scan and could easily be missed by inspection through an anterolateral approach that is relatively blind to these anatomical locations. Additionally, as these tumors tend to be invasive, it could be that cells remain behind even after all visible tumor is resected.

Expanded transsphenoidal approaches offer a novel alternative to the traditional transcranial approaches to craniopharyngiomas (Konig et al., 1986; Norris et al., 1998; Abe and Ludecke, 1999; Im et al., 2003; Laws Jr. et al., 2003; Couldwell et al., 2004; Locatelli et al., 2004; Maira et al., 2004; Frank et al., 2006; Rudnick and DiNardo, 2006; Lunsford et al., 2007; Gardner et al., 2008a, 2008b; Kassam et al., 2008; Cavallo et al., 2009; Shah et al., 2009). Removal of the tuberculum sellae and division of the circular sinus and diaphragma sellae allows a panoramic view of the suprasellar cistern, the usual epicenter of most craniopharyngiomas. Given the trajectory, it also provides visualization along the entire axis of growth and extension of most lesions, allowing direct inspection of the interface between the tumor and both the undersurface of the chiasm and the floor of the third ventricle. No other surgical corridor provides such direct visualization. The limitations of the expanded transsphenoidal approach include suboptimal available instrumentation that still hampers micro-dissection, particularly around vascular structures, as well as lateral exposure that is bounded by the optic nerve and intracranial carotid arteries (ICAs). Additionally, reconstruction of the cranial base remains challenging although the evolution of local mucosal flaps, particularly the nasoseptal flap, have decreased the rates of cerebrospinal fluid (CSF) leak from 30% to 3–5% (Zanation et al., 2009; Eloy et al., 2012). It still remains to be seen whether collective experience will allow for further refinement of the expanded transsphenoidal approach and its universal acceptance. Nonetheless, given its technical difficulty, it likely will remain a viable surgical treatment option only in the hands of experienced endoscopic teams.

Post-operative surgical morbidity, particularly when GTR of the tumor is attempted, remains a significant consideration. Post-operative visual dysfunction ranges between 5.8 and 19% and endocrinological dysfunction ranges between 50–100%. Unlike most other brain tumors, an important consideration in the surgical treatment of craniopharyngiomas is peri-operative mortality, which ranges between 1.1 and 10% in the early post-operative phase, even with contemporary surgical techniques (Hoogenhout et al., 1984; Baskin and Wilson, 1986; Fischer et al., 1990; Symon et al., 1991; Hoffman et al., 1992; Mark et al., 1995; Fisher et al., 1998; Fahlbusch et al., 1999; Duff et al., 2000; Van Effenterre and Boch, 2002; Kalapurakal et al., 2003; Albright et al., 2005; Caldarelli et al., 2005; Chakrabarti et al., 2005; Mottolese et al., 2005; Lena et al., 2005; Dhellemmes and Vinchon, 2006; Di Rocco et al., 2006). This is undoubtedly the result of the anatomical location of these lesions and their infiltrative relationship with the hypothalamus and its vascular supply. Mortality is often not catastrophic in its cause but rather the result of severe hypothalamic dysfunction. Evidence also exists regarding improved peri-operative outcomes with decreased extent of resection (Lichter et al., 1977; Ivkov et al., 1979; Colangelo et al., 1990; Honegger et al., 1999; Merchant et al., 2002; Fraioli et al., 2006).

Cystic areas of the tumor, frequently found in craniopharyngiomas, can also pose a special difficulty in the ability to maximize extent of resection. Although, in general, fenestration of the cyst wall is achievable surgically, complete resection of the cyst wall rarely is, as adhesions to the optic apparatus, third ventricle as well as ICA and posterior communicating perforators limit its safe resectability.

Short of the purely sellar or small suprasellar lesions, the majority of craniopharyngiomas pose a significant difficulty in complete surgical resection. As a result, radiation therapy is often utilized (Onoyama et al., 1977; Thompson et al., 1978; Richmond et al., 1980; Flickinger et al., 1989, 1990; Gurkaynak et al., 1994; Moon et al., 2005; Pemberton et al., 2005; Fitzek et al., 2006; Minniti et al., 2007). The majority of studies in the literature report on fractionated radiation therapy post-operatively or at recurrence. Local control rates of these generally complex lesions range between 80 and 100%, with follow-up times of up to 12 years post-treatment (Lichter et al., 1977; Calvo et al., 1983; Hoogenhout et al., 1984; Wara et al., 1994; Varlotto et al., 2002; Combs et al., 2007). Morbidity is in general limited; no visual dysfunction is observed when doses of less than 60 Gy are used. Interestingly, when compared with patients who underwent GTR alone, patients after GTR that was followed by fractionated radiotherapy, particularly in the early post-operative period had improved local tumor control rates and decreased morbidity.

Stereotactic radiosurgery has also been used in the treatment of craniopharyngiomas following surgical resection as well as at recurrence. Local control rates range between 80 and 90% at 5 years. Median marginal doses vary between 9 and 16 Gy and are associated with 58–80% response rates (Kobayashi et al., 1994, 2005; Kim et al., 1999; Mokry, 1999; Plowman et al., 1999; Chiou et al., 2001; Pollock et al., 2002; Ulfarsson et al., 2002; Amendola et al., 2003; Jackson et al., 2003; Kondziolka et al., 2003; Adler Jr. et al., 2006). Morbidity, although low, is somewhat higher than the rates generally associated with fractionated radiation therapy, with visual dysfunction in 6.1% of patients (Kobayashi et al., 2005).

The cystic nature of many craniopharyngiomas makes them amenable to stereotactic aspiration followed by instillation of radioactive material. Several beta-emitting isotopes have been used, including phosphorus 32, yttrium 90, and rhenium 186 (Pan et al., 1990; Van den Berge et al., 1992; Lunsford et al., 1994; Lange et al., 1995; Pollock et al., 1995; Voges et al., 1997; Schefter et al., 2002; Hasegawa et al., 2004; Hechtman et al., 2005; Julow et al., 2007; Derrey et al., 2008). These colloid preparations can deliver high radiation doses of 100–200 Gy to the cyst wall and the few surrounding millimeters, effectively treating the tumor capsule and sparing the surrounding neural structures. When used as a primary treatment or at recurrence, cyst aspiration followed by intracavitary radiation therapy is associated with local control rates of 70–96% (Lunsford et al., 1994; Hasegawa et al., 2004; Derrey et al., 2008).

Finally, cyst aspiration followed by instillation of bleomycin has also been used in limited studies, particularly in children, in an effort to minimize or potentially postpone the need for radiation therapy. Although most studies are small, the reported response rates range between 57 and 100% (Hader et al., 2000; Mottolese et al., 2001; Park et al., 2002; Takahashi et al., 2005; Hukin et al., 2007; Kim et al., 2007).

In putting all the available literature together, a few conclusions with respect to craniopharyngioma treatment are worth noting. GTR is often not possible and even when attempted is often associated with higher than expected rates of tumor progression and recurrence. Morbidity can be significant with extensive resections, and there is associated peri-operative mortality. Frequent post-operative endocrinological dysfunction can be difficult for the patients and may be permanent. STR is associated with decreased morbidity but requires further treatment in order to achieve the goal of tumor control. Adjuvant radiation therapy seems to confer an advantage both in tumor control and tumor progression, and probably should be recommended to all adult patients other than very simple cystic lesions that can be confirmed to be a GTR. The literature would seem to indicate that choosing between attempting a GTR with resection of the pituitary stalk and an STR followed by post-operative radiation therapy, the least invasive surgical option confers better functional outcomes and similar tumor control rates. Minimally invasive approaches, such as supraorbital or expanded transsphenoidal, may prove to be the optimal approaches to many such lesions, minimizing the surgical morbidity and optimizing visualization.

References

Abe, T., Ludecke, D.K., 1999. Transnasal surgery for infradiaphragmatic craniopharyngiomas in pediatric patients. Neurosurgery 44 (5), 957–964; discussion 964–966.

Adler Jr., J.R., et al., 2006. Visual field preservation after multisession cyberknife radiosurgery for perioptic lesions. Neurosurgery 59 (2), 244–254; discussion 254.

Albright, A.L., et al., 2005. Individualized treatment of pediatric craniopharyngiomas. Childs Nerv. Syst. 21 (8–9), 649–654.

Amendola, B.E., et al., 2003. Role of radiosurgery in craniopharyngiomas: a preliminary report. Med. Pediatr. Oncol. 41 (2), 123–127.

Baskin, D.S., Wilson, C.B., 1986. Surgical management of craniopharyngiomas. A review of 74 cases. J. Neurosurg. 65 (1), 22–27.

Bin-Abbas, B., et al., 2001. Endocrine sequelae of childhood craniopharyngioma. J. Pediatr. Endocrinol. Metab. 14 (7), 869–874.

Caldarelli, M., et al., 1998. Management of recurrent craniopharyngioma. Acta Neurochir. (Wien) 140 (5), 447–454.

Caldarelli, M., et al., 2005. Long-term results of the surgical treatment of craniopharyngioma: the experience at the Policlinico Gemelli, Catholic University, Rome. Childs Nerv. Syst. 21 (8–9), 747–757.

Calvo, F.A., et al., 1983. Radiation therapy in craniopharyngiomas. Int. J. Radiat. Oncol. Biol. Phys. 9 (4), 493–496.

Carpenter, R.C., Chamberlin, G.W., Frazier, C.H., 1937. The treatment of hypophyseal stalk tumours by evacuation and irradiation. Am. J. Roent. 38, 162–167.

Cavallo, L.M., et al., 2009. Extended endoscopic endonasal transsphenoidal approach for residual or recurrent craniopharyngiomas. J. Neurosurg. 111 (3), 578–589.

Chakrabarti, I., et al., 2005. Long-term neurological, visual, and endocrine outcomes following transnasal resection of craniopharyngioma. J. Neurosurg. 102 (4), 650–657.

Chiou, S.M., et al., 2001. Stereotactic radiosurgery of residual or recurrent craniopharyngioma, after surgery, with or without radiation therapy. Neuro. Oncol. 3 (3), 159–166.

Colangelo, M., Ambrosio, A., Ambrosio, C., 1990. Neurological and behavioral sequelae following different approaches to craniopharyngioma. Long-term follow-up review and therapeutic guidelines. Childs Nerv. Syst. 6 (7), 379–382.

Combs, S.E., et al., 2007. Achievement of long-term local control in patients with craniopharyngiomas using high precision stereotactic radiotherapy. Cancer 109 (11), 2308–2314.

Couldwell, W.T., et al., 2004. Variations on the standard transsphenoidal approach to the sellar region, with emphasis on the extended approaches and parasellar approaches: surgical experience in 105 cases. Neurosurgery 55 (3), 539–547; discussion 547–550.

Derrey, S., et al., 2008. Management of cystic craniopharyngiomas with stereotactic endocavitary irradiation using colloidal 186Re: a retrospective study of 48 consecutive patients. Neurosurgery 63 (6), 1045–1052 discussion 1052–3.

Dhellemmes, P., Vinchon, M., 2006. Radical resection for craniopharyngiomas in children: surgical technique and clinical results. J. Pediatr. Endocrinol. Metab. 19 (Suppl. 1), 329–335.

Di Rocco, C., et al., 2006. Surgical management of craniopharyngiomas–experience with a pediatric series. J. Pediatr. Endocrinol. Metab. 19 (Suppl. 1), 355–366.

Duff, J., et al., 2000. Long-term outcomes for surgically resected craniopharyngiomas. Neurosurgery 46 (2), 291–302; discussion 302–305.

Eloy, J.A., et al., 2012. Nasoseptal flap repair after endoscopic transsellar versus expanded endonasal approaches: is there an increased risk of postoperative cerebrospinal fluid leak? Laryngoscope 122 (6), 1219–1225.

Fahlbusch, R., et al., 1999. Surgical treatment of craniopharyngiomas: experience with 168 patients. J. Neurosurg. 90 (2), 237–250.

Fischer, E.G., et al., 1990. Craniopharyngiomas in children. Long-term effects of conservative surgical procedures combined with radiation therapy. J. Neurosurg. 73 (4), 534–540.

Fisher, P.G., et al., 1998. Outcomes and failure patterns in childhood craniopharyngiomas. Childs Nerv. Syst. 14 (10), 558–563.

Fitzek, M.M., et al., 2006. Combined proton and photon irradiation for craniopharyngioma: long-term results of the early cohort of patients treated at Harvard Cyclotron Laboratory and Massachusetts General Hospital. Int. J. Radiat. Oncol. Biol. Phys. 64 (5), 1348–1354.

Flickinger, J.C., et al., 1990. Megavoltage external beam irradiation of craniopharyngiomas: analysis of tumor control and morbidity. Int. J. Radiat. Oncol. Biol. Phys. 19 (1), 117–122.

Flickinger, J.C., Deutsch, M., Lunsford, L.D., 1989. Repeat megavoltage irradiation of pituitary and suprasellar tumors. Int. J. Radiat. Oncol. Biol. Phys. 17 (1), 171–175.

Fraioli, M.F., et al., 2006. "Conservative" surgical approach and early postoperative radiotherapy in a patient with a huge cystic craniopharyngioma. Childs Nerv. Syst. 22 (2), 151–155; discussion 158–163.
Frank, G., et al., 2006. The endoscopic extended transsphenoidal approach for craniopharyngiomas. Neurosurgery 59 (1 Suppl. 1), ONS75–ONS83; discussion ONS75–ONS83.
Gardner, P.A., et al., 2008a. Outcomes following endoscopic, expanded endonasal resection of suprasellar craniopharyngiomas: a case series. J. Neurosurg. 109 (1), 6–16.
Gardner, P.A., et al., 2008b. The evolution of the endonasal approach for craniopharyngiomas. J. Neurosurg. 108 (5), 1043–1047.
Gurkaynak, M., et al., 1994. Results of radiotherapy in craniopharyngiomas analysed by the linear quadratic model. Acta Oncol. 33 (8), 941–943.
Hader, W.J., et al., 2000. Intratumoral therapy with bleomycin for cystic craniopharyngiomas in children. Pediatr. Neurosurg. 33 (4), 211–218.
Hasegawa, T., et al., 2004. Management of cystic craniopharyngiomas with phosphorus-32 intracavitary irradiation. Neurosurgery 54 (4), 813–820; discussion 820–822.
Hechtman, C.D., et al., 2005. Dose distribution outside of a sphere of P-32 chromic phosphorous colloid. Int. J. Radiat. Oncol. Biol. Phys. 63 (3), 961–968.
Hoffman, H.J., et al., 1992. Aggressive surgical management of craniopharyngiomas in children. J. Neurosurg. 76 (1), 47–52.
Hoffman, H.J., 1985. Craniopharyngiomas. Can. J. Neurol. Sci. 12 (4), 348–352.
Honegger, J., Buchfelder, M., Fahlbusch, R., 1999. Surgical treatment of craniopharyngiomas: endocrinological results. J. Neurosurg. 90 (2), 251–257.
Hoogenhout, J., et al., 1984. Surgery and radiation therapy in the management of craniopharyngiomas. Int. J. Radiat. Oncol. Biol. Phys. 10 (12), 2293–2297.
Hukin, J., et al., 2007. Intracystic bleomycin therapy for craniopharyngioma in children: the Canadian experience. Cancer 109 (10), 2124–2131.
Im, S.H., et al., 2003. Transsphenoidal microsurgery for pediatric craniopharyngioma: special considerations regarding indications and method. Pediatr. Neurosurg. 39 (2), 97–103.
Ivkov, M., et al., 1979. Surgical treatment of craniopharyngiomas in adults. Acta Neurochir. Suppl. (Wien) 28 (2), 352–356.
Jackson, A.S., et al., 2003. Stereotactic radiosurgery. XVII: Recurrent intrasellar craniopharyngioma. Br. J. Neurosurg. 17 (2), 138–143.
Julow, J., et al., 2007. Long-term results and late complications after intracavitary yttrium-90 colloid irradiation of recurrent cystic craniopharyngiomas. Neurosurgery 61 (2), 288–295; discussion 295–296.
Kabil, M.S., Shahinian, H.K., 2005. Application of the supraorbital endoscopic approach to tumors of the anterior cranial base. J. Craniofac. Surg. 16 (6), 1070–1074; discussion 1075.
Kalapurakal, J.A., et al., 2003. Clinical outcome in children with craniopharyngioma treated with primary surgery and radiotherapy deferred until relapse. Med. Pediatr. Oncol. 40 (4), 214–218.
Kassam, A.B., et al., 2008. Endoscopic endonasal pituitary transposition for a transdorsum sellae approach to the interpeduncular cistern. Neurosurgery 62 (3 Suppl. 1), 57–72; discussion 72–74.
Kassam, A.B., et al., 2008. Expanded endonasal approach, a fully endoscopic transnasal approach for the resection of midline suprasellar craniopharyngiomas: a new classification based on the infundibulum. J. Neurosurg. 108 (4), 715–728.
Khafaga, Y., et al., 1998. Craniopharyngioma in children. Int. J. Radiat. Oncol. Biol. Phys. 42 (3), 601–606.
Kim, S.K., et al., 2001. Radical excision of pediatric craniopharyngioma: recurrence pattern and prognostic factors. Childs Nerv. Syst. 17 (9), 531–536; discussion 537.
Kim, S.D., et al., 2007. Radiological findings following postsurgical intratumoral bleomycin injection for cystic craniopharyngioma. Clin. Neurol. Neurosurg. 109 (3), 236–241.
Kim, M.S., Lee, S.I., Sim, S.H., 1999. Brain tumors with cysts treated with Gamma Knife radiosurgery: is microsurgery indicated? Stereotact. Funct. Neurosurg. 72 (Suppl. 1), 38–44.
Kobayashi, T., et al., 2005. Long-term results of gamma knife surgery for the treatment of craniopharyngioma in 98 consecutive cases. J. Neurosurg. 103 (Suppl. 6), 482–488.
Kobayashi, T., Tanaka, T., Kida, Y., 1994. Stereotactic gamma radiosurgery of craniopharyngiomas. Pediatr. Neurosurg. 21 (Suppl. 1), 69–74.

Kondziolka, D., et al., 2003. Long-term results after radiosurgery for benign intracranial tumors. Neurosurgery 53 (4), 815–821; discussion 821–822.

Konig, A., Ludecke, D.K., Herrmann, H.D., 1986. Transnasal surgery in the treatment of craniopharyngiomas. Acta Neurochir. (Wien) 83 (1–2), 1–7.

Lange, M., et al., 1995. Intracavitary treatment of intrasellar cystic craniopharyngeomas with 90-Yttrium by trans-sphenoidal approach–a technical note. Acta Neurochir. (Wien) 135 (3–4), 206–209.

Laws Jr., E.R., Morris, A.M., Maartens, N., 2003. Gliadel for pituitary adenomas and craniopharyngiomas. Neurosurgery 53 (2), 255–269; discussion 259–260.

Lena, G., et al., 2005. Craniopharyngioma in children: Marseille experience. Childs Nerv. Syst. 21 (8–9), 778–784.

Lichter, A.S., et al., 1977. The treatment of craniopharyngiomas. Int. J. Radiat. Oncol. Biol. Phys. 2 (7–8), 675–683.

Lin, L.L., et al., 2008. Long-term outcome in children treated for craniopharyngioma with and without radiotherapy. J. Neurosurg. Pediatr. 1 (2), 126–130.

Locatelli, D., et al., 2004. Endoscopic approach for the treatment of relapses in cystic craniopharyngiomas. Childs Nerv. Syst. 20 (11–12), 863–867.

Lunsford, L.D., et al., 1994. Stereotactic options in the management of craniopharyngioma. Pediatr. Neurosurg. 21 (Suppl. 1), 90–97.

Lunsford, L.D., et al., 2007. Radiosurgery for miscellaneous skull base tumors. Prog. Neurol. Surg. 20, 192–205.

Maira, G., et al., 2004. The role of transsphenoidal surgery in the treatment of craniopharyngiomas. J. Neurosurg. 100 (3), 445–451.

Mark, R.J., et al., 1995. Craniopharyngioma: treatment in the CT and MR imaging era. Radiology 197 (1), 195–198.

Merchant, T.E., et al., 2002. Craniopharyngioma: the St. Jude Children's Research Hospital experience 1984–2001. Int. J. Radiat. Oncol. Biol. Phys. 53 (3), 533–542.

Minniti, G., et al., 2007. Fractionated stereotactic conformal radiotherapy following conservative surgery in the control of craniopharyngiomas. Radiother. Oncol. 82 (1), 90–95.

Mokry, M., 1999. Craniopharyngiomas: A six year experience with Gamma Knife radiosurgery. Stereotact. Funct. Neurosurg. 72 (Suppl. 1), 140–149.

Moon, S.H., et al., 2005. Early adjuvant radiotherapy toward long-term survival and better quality of life for craniopharyngiomas–a study in single institute. Childs Nerv. Syst. 21 (8–9), 799–807.

Mottolese, C., et al., 2001. Intracystic chemotherapy with bleomycin in the treatment of craniopharyngiomas. Childs Nerv. Syst. 17 (12), 724–730.

Mottolese, C., et al., 2005. Craniopharyngiomas: our experience in Lyon. Childs Nerv. Syst. 21 (8–9), 790–798.

Norris, J.S., Pavaresh, M., Afshar, F., 1998. Primary transsphenoidal microsurgery in the treatment of craniopharyngiomas. Br. J. Neurosurg. 12 (4), 305–312.

Onoyama, Y., et al., 1977. Radiation therapy of craniopharyngioma. Radiology 125 (3), 799–803.

Pan, D.H., et al., 1990. Stereotactic internal irradiation for cystic craniopharyngiomas: a 6-year experience. Stereotact. Funct. Neurosurg, 525–530, 54–55.

Park, D.H., et al., 2002. Outcome of postoperative intratumoral bleomycin injection for cystic craniopharyngioma. J. Korean Med. Sci. 17 (2), 254–259.

Pemberton, L.S., et al., 2005. Experience of external beam radiotherapy given adjuvantly or at relapse following surgery for craniopharyngioma. Radiother. Oncol. 77 (1), 99–104.

Plowman, P.N., et al., 1999. Stereotactic radiosurgery. IX. Craniopharyngioma: durable complete imaging responses and indications for treatment. Br. J. Neurosurg. 13 (4), 352–358.

Pollock, B.E., et al., 1995. Phosphorus-32 intracavitary irradiation of cystic craniopharyngiomas: current technique and long-term results. Int. J. Radiat. Oncol. Biol. Phys. 33 (2), 437–446.

Pollock, B.E., Natt, N., Schomberg, P.J., 2002. Stereotactic management of craniopharyngiomas. Stereotact. Funct. Neurosurg. 79 (1), 25–32.

Richmond, I.L., Wara, W.M., Wilson, C.B., 1980. Role of radiation therapy in the management of craniopharyngiomas in children. Neurosurgery 6 (5), 513–517.

Rudnick, E.F., DiNardo, L.J., 2006. Image-guided endoscopic endonasal resection of a recurrent craniopharyngioma. Am. J. Otolaryngol. 27 (4), 266–267.

Schefter, J.K., et al., 2002. The utility of external beam radiation and intracystic 32P radiation in the treatment of craniopharyngiomas. J. Neurooncol. 56 (1), 69–78.

Shah, R.N., et al., 2009. Endoscopic pedicled nasoseptal flap reconstruction for pediatric skull base defects. Laryngoscope 119 (6), 1067–1075.

Sosa, I.J., Krieger, M.D., McComb, J.G., 2005. Craniopharyngiomas of childhood: the CHLA experience. Childs Nerv. Syst. 21 (8–9), 785–789.

Symon, L., Pell, M.F., Habib, A.H., 1991. Radical excision of craniopharyngioma by the temporal route: a review of 50 patients. Br. J. Neurosurg. 5 (6), 539–549.

Takahashi, H., Yamaguchi, F., Teramoto, A., 2005. Long-term outcome and reconsideration of intracystic chemotherapy with bleomycin for craniopharyngioma in children. Childs Nerv. Syst. 21 (8–9), 701–704.

Thompson, I.L., et al., 1978. Craniopharyngioma: the role of radiation therapy. Int. J. Radiat. Oncol. Biol. Phys. 4 (11–12), 1059–1063.

Ulfarsson, E., et al., 2002. Gamma knife radiosurgery for craniopharyngiomas: long-term results in the first Swedish patients. J. Neurosurg. 97 (Suppl. 5), 613–622.

Van den Berge, J.H., et al., 1992. Intracavitary brachytherapy of cystic craniopharyngiomas. J. Neurosurg. 77 (4), 545–550.

Van Effenterre, R., Boch, A.L., 2002. Craniopharyngioma in adults and children: a study of 122 surgical cases. J. Neurosurg. 97 (1), 3–11.

Varlotto, J.M., et al., 2002. External beam irradiation of craniopharyngiomas: long-term analysis of tumor control and morbidity. Int. J. Radiat. Oncol. Biol. Phys. 54 (2), 492–499.

Voges, J., et al., 1997. Cystic craniopharyngioma: long-term results after intracavitary irradiation with stereotactically applied colloidal beta-emitting radioactive sources. Neurosurgery 40 (2), 263–269; discussion 269–270.

Wara, W.M., Sneed, P.K., Larson, D.A., 1994. The role of radiation therapy in the treatment of craniopharyngioma. Pediatr. Neurosurg. 21 (Suppl. 1), 98–100.

Zanation, A.M., et al., 2009. Nasoseptal flap reconstruction of high flow intraoperative cerebral spinal fluid leaks during endoscopic skull base surgery. Am. J. Rhinol. Allergy 23 (5), 518–521.

CHAPTER

34

Complete Resection of Craniopharyngiomas

Gautam U. Mehta[*,†], *John Jane, Jr.*[†], *Edward H. Oldfield*[*,†]

[*]Surgical Neurology Branch, National Institutes of Neurological Disorders and Stroke, National Institutes of Health, Bethesda, MD, USA; [†]Department of Neurosurgery, University of Virginia Health Sciences Center, University of Virginia, Charlottesville, VA, USA

"Merely to nibble at a tumor, as is so frequently done, is only meddling and making it difficult or impossible for a next operation which must inevitably follow." **Walter Dandy, 1945**

The neurosurgeon, trying his utmost to effect complete removal of a craniopharyngioma by employing meticulous microtechniques to separate normal from pathological structures, often reaches a point in dissection where to proceed further or to retreat could, in the long term, be equally damaging to the patient. **M. Gazi Yasargil, 1990 (Yasargil et al., 1990)**

Craniopharyngiomas have long been considered among the most challenging neurosurgical lesions. Despite benign histology, their relation to critical structures, including the optic apparatus, pituitary stalk, hypothalamus, and circle of Willis, occasionally makes the operative morbidity of achieving surgical cure unacceptable. In fact, surgical mortality in the initial era of craniopharyngioma surgery was 15 to 41% (Cushing, 1932; Grant, 1948; Gordy et al., 1949). Even when limited resection was planned, local recurrence greatly limited long-term survival (Ingraham and Scott, 1946; Grant, 1948).

In 1952, Franc Ingraham and Donald Matson reported the peri-operative use of synthetic adrenocorticotropic hormone (ACTH) and cortisone for craniopharyngioma surgery (Ingraham et al., 1952). This significantly reduced operative mortality, particularly when radical resection was performed (Tytus et al., 1955; Matson and Crigler, 1960). Other advances such as improved understanding of the hypothalamic–pituitary axis, the use of the operative microscope, and the reintroduction of the transsphenoidal approach led to further reductions in operative morbidity (Matson and Crigler, 1969; Hardy, 1971; Laws, 1980; Yasargil et al., 1990). Despite these advances, that total resection should be the goal for all lesions remains controversial. Even in modern series, perceived total

Craniopharyngiomas
http://dx.doi.org/10.1016/B978-0-12-416706-3.00034-9

resection is frequently subject to recurrence and operative morbidity remains high, particularly for tumors involving the hypothalamus in children (Bartlett, 1971; Yasargil et al., 1990; Symon et al., 1991; Hoffman et al., 1992; Duff et al., 2000; Elliott et al., 2010; Jane et al., 2010b). Given these findings, most surgeons no longer favor attempted complete resection of tumors that involve the hypothalamus (Yasargil et al., 1990; Muller, 2011; Gautier et al., 2012; Elowe-Gruau et al., 2013). Controversy remains regarding complete resection of tumors that do not involve the hypothalamus.

EFFECT OF EXTENT OF RESECTION ON RECURRENCE AND SURVIVAL

Before his introduction of peri-operative steroids, Ingraham recognized that a conservative resection or cyst aspiration could delay the natural history of these lesions, but found that the majority of patients had early recurrence and died within 18 months (Cushing, 1932; Ingraham and Scott, 1946; Grant, 1948; Gordy et al., 1949). With the use of corticosteroids, Matson achieved complete resection in 46 of 57 patients in whom he intended radical excision (Ingraham and Scott, 1946; Grant, 1948; Matson and Crigler, 1969). He reported good outcome in 40 patients despite five operative mortalities. From the 1950s to the mid-1990s, the treatment of choice at most centers was radical resection (Ingraham et al., 1952; Yasargil et al., 1990; Symon et al., 1991; Fahlbusch et al., 1999).

Although radiotherapy for craniopharyngioma was first described in the 1930s, during the 1960s and 1970s some groups began to report that the results of intended subtotal resection plus radiotherapy compared favorably to those of radical resection (Tytus et al., 1955; Matson and Crigler, 1960; Kramer et al., 1961; Hoff and Patterson, 1972). In 1977, Lichter and colleagues reported improved tumor control in patients who received surgery and radiation (80%) compared with patients who had surgery alone (53%) (Lichter et al., 1977). Subsequent reports reinforced these findings (Bartlett, 1971; Richmond et al., 1980; Fischer et al., 1985; Regine and Kramer, 1992; Jane et al., 2010a). However, these results were confronted by reports from experienced surgeons demonstrating good results (no impairment) in 67–79% of patients who underwent radical resection alone (Yasargil et al., 1990; Fahlbusch et al., 1999). Such discordant outcomes led to controversy regarding the optimal management of these lesions.

More recent surgical series have variably followed radical and conservative treatment paradigms (Table 34.1). Reporting has been inconsistent among surgical series. Many large studies do not include survival analyses (recurrence-free survival or overall survival) and/or do not differentiate outcomes for patients who underwent complete or limited resection (Duff et al., 2000; Van Effenterre and Boch, 2002; Caldarelli et al., 2005; Chakrabarti et al., 2005; Zuccaro, 2005; Zhang et al., 2008; Elliott et al., 2010; Hofmann et al., 2012; Elowe-Gruau et al., 2013). Furthermore, studies supporting limited resection and radiotherapy (Fischer et al., 1985; Schoenfeld et al., 2012) consistently report worse outcomes with complete resection than studies supporting complete resection (Yasargil et al., 1990; Gautier et al., 2012; Hofmann et al., 2012) (Table 34.1). Nonetheless, the majority of studies demonstrate that radical resection leads to increased freedom from recurrence and better overall survival (Table 34.1, Figure 34.1).

Few prospective studies on surgical outcomes exist for craniopharyngioma. One study, KRANIOPHARYNGEOM 2000, a multi-center prospective observational trial, analyzed the results of surgical treatment in a cohort of children with craniopharyngioma (Muller et al.,

TABLE 34.1 Progression-free Survival (PFS) in Surgical Series for Craniopharyngioma Since 2000[a]

Authors	Year	Age	N	PFS with complete resection (n)	PFS with incomplete resection and radiotherapy (n)	PFS with incomplete resection (n)
Gautier et al.[b]	2012	Pediatric/Adult	171	80% at 5 years (98)		41% at 5 years (73)[c]
Schoenfeld et al.[d]	2012	Pediatric/Adult	122	75% at 2 years (33)	73% at 2 years (48)	36% at 2 years (41)
Müller et al.[e,f]	2011	Pediatric	117	64% at 3 years (47)		31% at 3 years (64)[g]
Mortini et al.[h]	2011	Pediatric/Adult	112	86% at 5 years (78)		46% at 5 years (31)[i]
Tomita et al.[j]	2005	Pediatric	54	83% at 5 years (33)	71% at 5 years (8)	9% at 5 years (13)

[a]*Studies with greater than 50 patients and survival analyses.*
[b]*Gautier, A. et al., 2012. Markers of Recurrence and Long Term Morbidity in Craniopharyngioma: A Systematic Analysis of 171 Patients. Journal of Clinical Endocrinology & Metabolism, 97(4), pp. 1258–1267.*
[c]*Includes 30 patients who received radiotherapy.*
[d]*Schoenfeld, A. et al., 2012. The superiority of conservative resection and adjuvant radiation for craniopharyngiomas. Journal of Neuro-Oncology, 108(1), pp. 133–139.*
[e]*Müller, H.L. et al., 2010. Analyses of Treatment Variables for Patients with Childhood Craniopharyngioma – Results of the Multi-center Prospective Trial KRANIOPHARYNGEOM 2000 after Three Years of Follow-Up. Hormone Research in Paediatrics, 73(3), pp. 175–180.*
[f]*Prospective study.*
[g]*Includes 28 patients who received radiotherapy.*
[h]*Mortini, P. et al., 2011. Neurosurgical treatment of craniopharyngioma in adults and children: early and long term results in a large case series. Journal of Neurosurgery, pp. 1–10.*
[i]*Includes eight patients who received radiotherapy.*
[j]*Tomita, T. & Bowman, R.M., 2005. Craniopharyngiomas in children: surgical experience at Children's Memorial Hospital. Child's nervous system: ChNS: official journal of the International Society for Pediatric Neurosurgery, 21(8–9), pp. 729–746.*

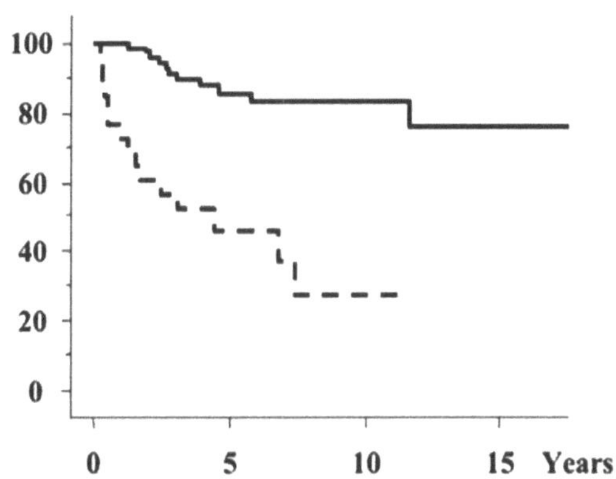

FIGURE 34.1 Recurrence-free survival in 112 patients with craniopharyngioma based on the absence (solid line) or presence (dashed line) of residual tumor on post-operative imaging. *Adapted from Mortini, P. et al., 2011. Neurosurgical treatment of craniopharyngioma in adults and children: early and long term results in a large case series. Journal of Neurosurgery, pp. 1–10.*

2010, 2011). One hundred and seventeen patients were treated at small (23 patients), medium (60 patients), and large (34 patients) centers. Although no randomization of treatment was specified, resection that spared the optic apparatus and hypothalamic structures was recommended. The study found that 3-year event-free survival was significantly improved

($P < 0.001$) in patients with complete resection (63%) compared with incomplete resection (31%). However, only 28 of 64 patients with incomplete resection received post-operative radiation. Patients who received radiation had significantly improved survival ($P < 0.001$), although the results of complete resection were not compared with those of incomplete resection and radiation. Additionally, the relationship between extent of resection and survival as it related to tumor grade was not analyzed.

LIMITATIONS OF COMPARING SURGICAL APPROACHES FOR CRANIOPHARYNGIOMAS

The results of different surgical approaches for craniopharyngioma have not been directly compared. Transcranial approaches have been most commonly used, although the transsphenoidal approach, largely re-introduced by Hardy, and popularized by Laws, Weiss, and Falhbusch, has been used since the 1970s for craniopharyngiomas originating in the sella and lying below the diaphragm sella (Hardy, 1971; Laws, 1980; Fahlbusch et al., 1999; Chakrabarti et al., 2005). A meta-analysis of surgical series for craniopharyngioma showed that the patient populations treated with the two approaches are likely different, with transcranial approaches favored for tumors arising above the diaphragm sella and the transsphenoidal preferred for tumors originating in the sella (Elliott et al., 2011). More recently, with the introduction of the extended transsphenoidal approach for craniopharyngiomas arising in the suprasellar space and in the face of a normal size sella in 2000, extended transsphenoidal approaches with the operating microscope and the endoscope have been examined, although the series are too small and the follow-up too brief for conclusions to be reached as yet (Kouri et al., 2000; Leng et al., 2012).

To date, most surgical series have reported only the results of surgery for children or have combined the results of surgery for children and adults (Matson and Crigler, 1969; Yasargil et al., 1976; Fischer et al., 1985; Fahlbusch et al., 1999; Tomita and Bowman, 2005; Elliott et al., 2010; Müller et al., 2010; Gautier et al., 2012; Elowe-Gruau et al., 2013). Relatively few data are available on the results of surgery for adults alone (Russell and Pennybacker, 1961; Jane et al., 2010a). As the biology and histological subtype of craniopharyngiomas vary with age, it is important to differentiate surgical outcomes between children and adults (Jane and Laws, 2006; Louis and Ohgaki, 2007). Only one recent retrospective study separates the results for children and adults (Gautier et al., 2012). In that report, recurrence-free survival was similar for patients 10–18 years old (n=34) and patients older than 18 years (n=106), but was substantially reduced in patients less than 10 years old at presentation (n=28).

EFFECT OF EXTENT OF RESECTION ON SECONDARY OUTCOMES AND MORBIDITY

Visual Outcomes

As many as 60–96% of patients with craniopharyngioma present with visual deficits (Chakrabarti et al., 2005; Defoort-Dhellemmes et al., 2006; Clark et al., 2012). Defoort and colleagues analyzed visual outcomes in children who underwent surgery for craniopharyngioma (Defoort-Dhellemmes et al., 2006). Improvement in visual symptoms was greater after complete resection (66%) than with limited resection. The report of the outcomes of a series of patients operated on by Weiss revealed that visual outcomes were more often improved when using the transsphenoidal approach (87%) than when transcranial approaches were used (61%) (Chakrabarti et al., 2005).

Endocrine Outcomes

Endocrine dysfunction occurs commonly with craniopharyngioma and is frequently caused by, or made worse by, surgery. Honegger and colleagues found that the rate of diabetes insipidus (DI) increased greatly with radical resection, from 16.1% pre-operatively to 59.4% post-operatively (Honegger et al., 1999). Anterior pituitary dysfunction was common at presentation and worsened after surgery, but to a lesser extent. A systematic review by Clark and colleagues demonstrated that complete resection led to a significantly greater (P=0.02) risk of post-operative DI than limited resection with radiotherapy (Clark et al., 2012). The rate of post-operative panhypopituitarism was increased in the limited resection with radiotherapy group, although this result was not statistically significant (P=0.08).

Post-Operative Obesity

A primary endpoint of the prospective KRANIOPHARYNGEOM 2000 study in children was the effect of hypothalamic lesions on post-operative obesity (Muller et al., 2011). The study demonstrated that post-operative obesity in children was related to tumor location. Patients with lesions involving the posterior hypothalamus had increased body-mass index (BMI) 3 years after surgery. This increase was significantly worse than the subgroup of patients without tumors involving the posterior hypothalamus (P=0.03). The study did not specify the effect of complete resection on post-operative obesity. Clark and colleagues in a retrospective series found the incidence of post-operative obesity to be similar in children who underwent complete resection compared to those who underwent limited resection plus radiotherapy (6% and 4%, respectively) (Clark et al., 2012).

Neuropsychologic Outcomes

Since surgery and radiotherapy are thought to have negative neurocognitive effects on developing children, Merchant and colleagues compared the effects of aggressive resection and limited resection with adjuvant radiotherapy on intelligence quotient (IQ) (Merchant et al., 2002). Over 14 years, 30 children were analyzed with 15 patients in each group. In the resection only group, gross total resection was achieved in eight patients, however nine recurrences were observed. In the limited resection plus radiotherapy group, only two recurrences were observed. Using full-scale IQ, they found that patients who underwent complete resection lost an average of 9.8 points, compared with 1.25 points after limited resection and radiation. Although the relative location of the tumors was not specified, the authors concluded that neurocognitive impairment from complete resection is worse than the effects of radiation in children. However, the outcome in adults is likely different based on a prospective study by Honegger and colleagues (Honegger et al., 1998). In the latter study, neuropsychological outcome was detailed in 13 adults who underwent radical resection. Transcranial approaches were used for ten patients and complete resection was achieved in eight patients. Mean IQ was unchanged by surgery.

Quality of Life Outcomes

Several authors have attempted to summarize the outcome of surgery using quality of life questionnaires. Sands and colleagues analyzed the outcomes of surgery using a pediatric quality of life questionnaire (Sands et al., 2005). Overall, patients who underwent surgery had a slightly lower than average quality of life. The study found that patients with retrochiasmatic tumors and those who had recurrence or needed additional surgery had worse quality of life. Quality of life was also assessed in KRANIOPHARYNGEOM 2000. This prospective study confirmed that surgery for posteriorly located tumors, specifically tumors that involved the hypothalamus, was associated with significantly worse results on a pediatric quality of life questionnaire (Muller et al., 2011).

EXTENT OF RESECTION FOR TUMORS INVOLVING THE HYPOTHALAMUS

As resection of tumors that involve the hypothalamus results in worse endocrine, neuropsychologic, and quality of life outcomes, Puget and colleagues at Hôpital Necker-Enfants Malades devised a grading scale to guide resection based on hypothalamic involvement noted on pre-operative imaging (Figure 34.2) (Puget et al., 2007). Grade 0 tumors do not involve the hypothalamus, grade 1 tumors abut or displace the hypothalamus, and grade 2 tumors involve or invade the hypothalamus. Using this classification, they devised a treatment protocol for childhood craniopharyngioma that they term hypothalamus-sparing surgery. Radical resection was recommended for grade 0 and grade 1 tumors, and grade 2 tumors should undergo subtotal resection with sparing of hypothalamic components. Post-operative radiation was used based on completeness of resection and patient age. A similar treatment paradigm has been suggested by Müller and the KRANIOPHARYNGEOM 2000 investigators as well as the Children's Cancer Leukaemia Group (Muller et al., 2011; Mallucci et al., 2012).

The surgeons at Hôpital Necker-Enfants Malades enacted this protocol recently as part of a pediatric prospective observational study (Elowe-Gruau et al., 2013). The prospective cohort underwent hypothalamus-sparing surgery as described above and was compared with a retrospective cohort treated with radical resection over the previous 18 years. They found that BMI z-scores were significantly higher in the radical resection group as early as 6 months after surgery and through last follow-up. Hypocortisolism, hypogonadism, and DI also occurred more frequently in the radical resection group. The study used the rate of surgical intervention as a surrogate for local recurrence and noted 1.45 surgeries per patient in the radical resection group compared to 1.52 surgeries per patient in the prospective cohort, although it must be acknowledged that, due to the timing of their cohorts, mean follow-up was longer in the radical resection group (103 months vs. 33 months). The timing of additional surgery was not specified and no survival analyses were performed. Furthermore, results in the different groups by tumor grade were not specified.

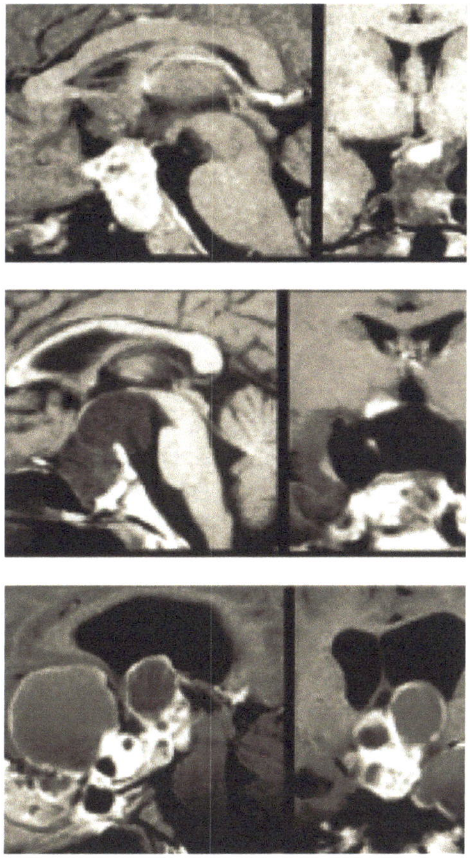

FIGURE 34.2 Pre-operative imaging classification of craniopharyngioma based on hypothalamic involvement. Grade 0 tumors do not involve the hypothalamus (top), grade 1 tumors abut the hypothalamus (middle), and grade 2 tumors invade the hypothalamus (bottom). *Adapted from Puget, S., et al., 2007. Pediatric craniopharyngiomas: classification and treatment according to the degree of hypothalamic involvement.* Journal of Neurosurgery. Pediatrics *106(1), pp. 3–12, with permission.*

Prospective data from KRANIOPHARYNGEOM 2000 also confirmed worse post-operative obesity and quality of life with resection lesions involving the hypothalamus (Muller et al., 2011). Neither study was designed to determine the effect of hypothalamus-sparing surgery on recurrence and survival. Regardless, the clear morbidity of aggressive surgery on lesions involving the hypothalamus argues for a conservative approach in this subgroup.

EXTENT OF RESECTION FOR TUMORS NOT INVOLVING THE HYPOTHALAMUS

Few data exist regarding the utility of aggressive versus conservative resection of tumors that do not involve the hypothalamus, although some groups advocate limited resection for all lesions (Schoenfeld et al., 2012). Prospective data from KRANIOPHARYNGEOM 2000 have demonstrated that complete resection results in improved freedom from recurrence and prior retrospective studies show higher rates of recurrence with residual tumor (Table 34.1, Figure 34.1) (Mortini et al., 2011; Muller, 2011). Concurrently, KRANIOPHARYNGEOM 2000 has shown the major determinant of morbidity associated with craniopharyngioma resection to be hypothalamic involvement (Muller et al., 2011). Given the limited surgical morbidity of lesions that do not involve the hypothalamus and the likelihood of increased freedom from recurrence and survival with complete resection, complete resection should be sought in adults and in children without hypothalamic involvement.

CONCLUSIONS

Level I, and arguably level II, data regarding the use of radical versus conservative surgical paradigms for craniopharyngioma do not exist. Furthermore, inconsistent reporting and surgical outcomes make it difficult to extract aggregate or definitive conclusions from even modern prospective trials. Regardless, when surgical outcomes at centers of excellence are analyzed, achieved or intended complete resection results in improved progression-free survival and has an acceptable risk profile in adults and in children without involvement of the hypothalamus (Yasargil et al., 1990; Tomita and Bowman, 2005; Gautier et al., 2012; Hofmann et al., 2012). The sole exception supported by recent prospective data is tumors in children that invade the hypothalamus (Elowe-Gruau et al., 2013). In this instance, risks of hypothalamic obesity, endocrine disturbance, and worsened quality of life outweigh the benefit of total resection, and a conservative surgical approach with resection of as much of the tumor as possible without attempted removal of the portion involving the hypothalamus and adjuvant radiation is warranted (Muller et al., 2011; Elowe-Gruau et al., 2013). Thus, to date there is no evidence to support limited resection in tumors that do not invade the hypothalamus (grades 0 and 1) and radical excision should be attempted for the majority of these lesions. Overall, the approach to craniopharyngioma should be tailored to both the individual patient's clinical condition and the location of the tumor to determine a treatment paradigm that is both safe and durable.

References

Bartlett, J.R., 1971. Craniopharyngiomas – a summary of 85 cases. J. Neurol. Neurosurg. Psychiatr. 34, 37–41.

Caldarelli, M., Massimi, L., Tamburrini, G., Cappa, M., Rocco, C., 2005. Long-term results of the surgical treatment of craniopharyngioma: the experience at the Policlinico Gemelli, Catholic University, Rome. Childs. Nerv. Syst. 21, 747–757.

Chakrabarti, I., Amar, A.P., Couldwell, W., Weiss, M.H., 2005. Long-term neurological, visual, and endocrine outcomes following transnasal resection of craniopharyngioma. J. Neurosurg. 102, 650–657.

Clark, A.J., Cage, T.A., Aranda, D., Parsa, A.T., Auguste, K.I., Gupta, N., 2012. Treatment-related morbidity and the management of pediatric craniopharyngioma. J. Neurosurg. Pediatr. 10, 293–301.

Cushing, H., 1932. Intracranial Tumors. Charles C Thomas, Baltimore.

Dandy, Walter E., 1945. Surgery of the Brain. W. F. Prior Company, Inc, Hagerstown. Print, p 562.

Defoort-Dhellemmes, S., Moritz, F., Bouacha, I., Vinchon, M., 2006. Craniopharyngioma: ophthalmological aspects at diagnosis. J. Pediatr. Endocrinol. Metab. 19 (Suppl. 1), 321–324.

Duff, J., Meyer, F.B., Ilstrup, D.M., Laws, E.R., Schleck, C.D., Scheithauer, B.W., 2000. Long-term outcomes for surgically resected craniopharyngiomas. Neurosurgery 46, 291–302; discussion 302–305.

Elliott, R.E., Hsieh, K., Hochm, T., Belitskaya-Levy, I., Wisoff, J., Wisoff, J.H., 2010. Efficacy and safety of radical resection of primary and recurrent craniopharyngiomas in 86 children. J. Neurosurg. Pediatr. 5, 30–48.

Elliott, R.E., Jane Jr, J.A., Wisoff, J.H., 2011. surgical management of craniopharyngiomas in children: meta-analysis and comparison of transcranial and transsphenoidal approaches. Neurosurgery 69, 630–643.

Elowe-Gruau, E., Beltrand, J., Brauner, R., Pinto, G., Samara-Boustani, D., Thalassinos, C., Busiah, K., Laborde, K., Boddaert, N., Zerah, M., Alapetite, C., Grill, J., Touraine, P., Sainte-Rose, C., Polak, M., Puget, S., 2013. Childhood craniopharyngioma: hypothalamus-sparing surgery decreases the risk of obesity. J. Clin. Endocrinol. Metab. 98, 2376–2382.

Fahlbusch, R., Honegger, J., Paulus, W., Huk, W., Buchfelder, M., 1999. Surgical treatment of craniopharyngiomas: experience with 168 patients. J. Neurosurg. 90, 237–250.

Fischer, E.G., Welch, K., Belli, J.A., Wallman, J., Shillito, J.J., Winston, K.R., Cassady, R., 1985. Treatment of craniopharyngiomas in children: 1972–1981. J. Neurosurg. 62, 496–501.

Gautier, A., Godbout, A., Grosheny, C., Tejedor, I., Coudert, M., Courtillot, C., Jublanc, C., De Kerdanet, M., Poirier, J.Y., Riffaud, L., Sainte-Rose, C., Van Effenterre, R., Brassier, G., Bonnet, F., Touraine, P., 2012. on behalf of the Craniopharyngioma Study Group Prs and Drs Anne Bachelot, Anne-Laure Boch Raja Brauner Jean-Claude Carel Anne Colobert Helene Crosnier Vonny Derennes Pierre Doyard Francoise Getin Isabelle Guilhem Muriel Hoang Claire Josseaume. J. Clin. Endocrinol. Metab. 97, 1258–1267. Markers of recurrence and long-term morbidity in craniopharyngioma: a systematic analysis of 171 patients.

Gordy, P.D., Peet, M.M., Kahn, E.A., 1949. The surgery of the craniopharyngiomas. J. Neurosurg. 6, 503–517.

Grant, F.C., 1948. Surgical experience with tumors of the pituitary gland. J. Am. Med. Assoc. 136, 668–672.

Hardy, J., 1971. Transsphenoidal hypophysectomy. J. Neurosurg. 34, 582–594.

Hoff, J.T., Patterson, R.H., 1972. Craniopharyngiomas in children and adults. J. Neurosurg. 36, 299–302.

Hoffman, H.J., Silva, M.D., Humphreys, R.P., Drake, J.M., Smith, M.L., Blaser, S.I., 1992. Aggressive surgical management of craniopharyngiomas in children. J. Neurosurg. 76, 47–52.

Hofmann, B.M., Höllig, A., Strauss, C., Buslei, R., Buchfelder, M., Fahlbusch, R., 2012. Results after treatment of craniopharyngiomas: further experiences with 73 patients since 1997. J. Neurosurg. 116, 373–384.

Honegger, J., Barocka, A., Sadri, B., Fahlbusch, R., 1998. Neuropsychological results of craniopharyngioma surgery in adults: a prospective study. Surg. Neurol. 50, 19–28; discussion 28–29.

Honegger, J., Buchfelder, M., Fahlbusch, R., 1999. Surgical treatment of craniopharyngiomas: endocrinological results. J. Neurosurg. 90, 251–257.

Ingraham, F.D., Matson, D.D., McLaurin, R.L., 1952. Cortisone and ACTH as an Adjunct to the Surgery of Craniopharyngiomas. N. Engl. J. Med. 246, 568–571.

Ingraham, F.D., Scott, H.W., 1946. Craniopharyngiomas in children. J. Pediatr. 29, 95–116.

Jane Jr, J.A., Kiehna, E., Payne, S.C., Early, S.V., Laws Jr, E.R., 2010a. Early outcomes of endoscopic transsphenoidal surgery for adult craniopharyngiomas. Neurosurg. Focus 28, E9.

Jane Jr, J.A., Laws, E.R., 2006. Craniopharyngioma. Pituitary 9, 323–326.

Jane, J.A., Prevedello, D.M., Alden, T.D., Laws, E.R., 2010b. The transsphenoidal resection of pediatric craniopharyngiomas: a case series. J. Neurosurg. Pediatr. 5, 49–60.

Kouri, J.G., Chen, M.Y., Watson, J.C., Oldfield, E.H., 2000. Resection of suprasellar tumors by using a modified transsphenoidal approach. J. Neurosurg. 92, 1028–1035.

Kramer, S., McKissock, W., Concannon, J.P., 1961. Craniopharyngiomas. Treatment by combined surgery and radiation therapy. J. Neurosurg. 18, 217–226.

Laws, E.R., 1980. Transsphenoidal microsurgery in the management of craniopharyngioma. J. Neurosurg. 52, 661–666.

Leng, L.Z., Greenfield, J.P., Souweidane, M.M., Anand, V.K., Schwartz, T.H., 2012. Endoscopic, endonasal resection of craniopharyngiomas. Neurosurgery 70, 110–124.

Lichter, A.S., Wara, W.M., Sheline, G.E., Townsend, J.J., Wilson, C.B., 1977. The treatment of craniopharyngiomas. Int. J. Radiat. Oncol. Biol. Phys. 2, 675–683.

Louis, D.N., Ohgaki, H., 2007. WHO classification of tumours of the central nervous system. World Health Organization.

Mallucci, C., Pizer, B., Blair, J., Didi, M., Doss, A., Upadrasta, S., Newman, W., Avula, S., Pettorini, B., 2012. Management of craniopharyngioma: the Liverpool experience following the introduction of the CCLG guidelines. Introducing a new risk assessment grading system. Childs. Nerv. Syst. 28, 1181–1192.

Matson, D.D., Crigler, J.F., 1960. Radical treatment of craniopharyngioma. Ann. Surg. 152, 699–704.

Matson, D.D., Crigler Jr, J.F., 1969. Management of craniopharyngioma in childhood. J. Neurosurg. 30, 377–390.

Merchant, T.E., Kiehna, E.N., Sanford, R.A., Mulhern, R.K., Thompson, S.J., Wilson, M.W., Lustig, R.H., Kun, L.E., 2002. Craniopharyngioma: the St. Jude Children's Research Hospital experience 1984–2001. Int. J. Radiat. Oncol. Biol. Phys. 53, 533–542.

Mortini, P., Losa, M., Pozzobon, G., Barzaghi, R., Riva, M., Acerno, S., Angius, D., Weber, G., Chiumello, G., Giovanelli, M., 2011. Neurosurgical treatment of craniopharyngioma in adults and children: early and long-term results in a large case series. J. Neurosurg., 1–10.

Muller, H.L., 2011. Consequences of craniopharyngioma surgery in children. J. Clin. Endocrinol. Metab. 96, 1981–1991.

the study committee of KRANIOPHARYNGEOM Muller, H.L., Gebhardt, U., Teske, C., Faldum, A., Zwiener, I., Warmuth-Metz, M., Pietsch, T., Pohl, F., Sorensen, N., Calaminus, G., 2000. 2011. Post-operative hypothalamic lesions and obesity in childhood craniopharyngioma: results of the multinational prospective trial KRANIOPHARYNGEOM 2000 after three year follow-up. Eur. J. Endocrinol. 165, 17–24.

Müller, H.L., Gebhardt, U., Schröder, S., Pohl, F., Kortmann, R.-D., Faldum, A., Zwiener, I., Warmuth-Metz, M., Pietsch, T., Calaminus, G., Kolb, R., Wiegand, C., Sörensen, N., 2010. Analyses of treatment variables for patients with childhood craniopharyngioma – results of the multicenter prospective trial KRANIOPHARYNGEOM 2000 after three years of follow-up. Horm. Res. Paediatr. 73, 175–180.

Puget, S., Garnett, M., Wray, A., Grill, J., Habrand, J.-L., Bodaert, N., Zerah, M., Bezerra, M., Renier, D., Pierre-Kahn, A., Sainte-Rose, C., 2007. Pediatric craniopharyngiomas: classification and treatment according to the degree of hypothalamic involvement. J. Neurosurg. Pediatr. 106, 3–12.

Regine, W.F., Kramer, S., 1992. Pediatric craniopharyngiomas: long term results of combined treatment with surgery and radiation. Int. J. Radiat. Oncol. Biol. Phys. 24, 611–617.

Richmond, I.L., Wara, W.M., Wilson, C.B., 1980. Role of radiation therapy in the management of craniopharyngiomas in children. Neurosurgery 6, 513–517.

Russell, R., Pennybacker, J., 1961. Craniopharyngioma in the elderly. J. Neurol. Neurosurg. Psychiatr. 24, 1–13.

Sands, S.A., Milner, J.S., Goldberg, J., Mukhi, V., Moliterno, J.A., Maxfield, C., Wisoff, J.H., 2005. Quality of life and behavioral follow-up study of pediatric survivors of craniopharyngioma. J. Neurosurg. Pediatr. 103, 302–311.

Schoenfeld, A., Pekmezci, M., Barnes, M.J., Tihan, T., Gupta, N., Lamborn, K.R., Banerjee, A., Mueller, S., Chang, S., Berger, M.S., Haas-Kogan, D., 2012. The superiority of conservative resection and adjuvant radiation for craniopharyngiomas. J. Neurooncol. 108, 133–139.

Symon, L., Pell, M.F., Habib, A.H., 1991. Radical excision of craniopharyngioma by the temporal route: a review of 50 patients. Br. J. Neurosurg. 5, 539–549.

Tomita, T., Bowman, R.M., 2005. Craniopharyngiomas in children: surgical experience at Children's Memorial Hospital. Childs. Nerv. Syst. 21, 729–746.

Tytus, J.S., Seltzer, H.S., Kahn, E.A., 1955. Cortisone as an aid in the surgical treatment of craniopharyngiomas. J. Neurosurg. 12, 555–564.

Van Effenterre, R., Boch, A.-L., 2002. Craniopharyngioma in adults and children: a study of 122 surgical cases. J. Neurosurg. 97, 3–11.

Yasargil, M.G., Antic, J., Laciga, R., de Preux, J., Fideler, R.W., Boone, S.C., 1976. The microsurgical removal of intramedullary spinal hemangioblastomas. Report of twelve cases and a review of the literature. Surg. Neurol., 141–148.

Yasargil, M.G., Curcic, M., Kis, M., Siegenthaler, G., Teddy, P.J., Roth, P., 1990. Total removal of craniopharyngiomas. J. Neurosurg. 73, 3–11.

Zhang, Y.Q., Ma, Z.Y., Wu, Z.B., Luo, S.Q., Wang, Z.C., 2008. Radical resection of 202 pediatric craniopharyngiomas with special reference to the surgical approaches and hypothalamic protection. Pediatr. Neurosurg. 44, 435–443.

Zuccaro, G., 2005. Radical resection of craniopharyngioma. Childs. Nerv. Syst. 21, 679–690.

CHAPTER

35

Controversies: Extended Endoscopic vs. Open Transcranial Approaches

Khaled Krisht, Walavan Sivakumar, William Couldwell

Department of Neurosurgery, Clinical Neurosciences Center, University of Utah, Salt Lake City, UT, USA

"Neurosurgeons are more at home in the cranial cavity than in the nose and, besides, we feel that we can deal more radically with a tumor in this way; we no longer content ourselves with merely relieving pressure on the optic nerves to prevent blindness." ***Ernest Sachs, 1949***

INTRODUCTION

Craniopharyngiomas pose a challenge for complete resection via transcranial and transsphenoidal means because of their difficult anatomical location and proximity to vital neurovascular structures. Despite the advancements made in microscopic transsphenoidal microsurgery for the resection of craniopharyngiomas, its use usually remains limited to intrasellar tumors or those lesions with a subdiaphragmatic origin (Laws Jr, 1994; Maira et al., 1995; Fahlbusch et al., 1999; Chakrabarti et al., 2005; Jane et al., 2010). After the introduction of the extended transsphenoidal transplanum approach by Weiss in the 1980s, many surgeons began to approach select cases of suprasellar craniopharyngiomas via a transsphenoidal route as well. The introduction of the transnasal endoscope-assisted or purely endoscopic approach to the sellar region in the early 1990s helped to redefine the surgical management of craniopharyngiomas, adding yet another important stand-alone or adjunct tool to the neurosurgeon's armamentarium (Jho and Carrau, 1997; Cappabianca et al., 1998; Doglietto et al., 2005; Prevedello et al., 2007). Locatelli et al. (2004) first reported the endoscopic endonasal approach for the resection of craniopharyngiomas in 2004. In their study, five pediatric patients with recurrent cystic craniopharyngiomas were successfully treated, without any recurrences reported at 48 months' follow-up. Incorporating the endoscope into Weiss's transplanum extended approach resulted in the extended endoscopic endonasal approach to these tumors (Couldwell et al., 2004). With the endoscope, a sharper panoramic view of the anterior cranial fossa was obtained, with clear visualization of small structures in difficult anatomical corridors and at challenging angles. The introduction of

Craniopharyngiomas
http://dx.doi.org/10.1016/B978-0-12-416706-3.00035-0

endoscopy and its advancements, however, has not entirely supplanted microscopy. The operating microscope for both transsphenoidal and transcranial approaches remains an important tool for accessing difficult craniopharyngioma cases and, in certain instances, is the preferred method. The introduction of the extended approach and endoscopy to transsphenoidal surgery has changed modern-day surgical treatment of craniopharyngiomas. While there is no defined standard of surgical care for these difficult lesions, there are many case series that support either extended transsphenoidal microscopy, endoscopy, or a combination of both modalities. The standard transcranial approaches, however, remain essential for addressing select cases of craniopharyngiomas, which creates much discourse on when to use an endoscope versus a microscope, when to use both modalities, and when to resort to a transcranial route. The aim of this chapter is to highlight the advantages and disadvantages of each modality for the resection of craniopharyngiomas, and to clarify the future course of craniopharyngioma surgery.

THE INTRODUCTION OF ENDOSCOPY: A GAME CHANGER

There is no doubt that the resection of a craniopharyngioma remains one of the most challenging tumor cases for a neurosurgeon. Subtotal resection with adjuvant radiotherapy has a lower likelihood of causing acute post-operative pituitary dysfunction at the cost of higher rate of recurrence, whereas gross total resection (GTR) carries the risk of panhypopituitarism and hypothalamic syndrome. Although the desired degree of resection for various age groups is still the subject of much controversy, there is a general theoretical consensus that the more tumor is resected, the lower is the chance of future recurrence and the better the overall outcome and survival benefit (Fahlbusch et al., 1999; Cappabianca et al., 2000; Hadad et al., 2006; de Divitiis et al., 2007; Gardner et al., 2008; Cavallo et al., 2009).

The microscopic transsphenoidal approach has been the workhorse approach for small midline intrasellar lesions with midline suprasellar extension for many years. This is facilitated by intrasellar expansion and cystic tumors. More extensive lesions extending into the suprasellar space were previously addressed from above via a transcranial frontotemporal or subfrontal approach, or a combination of both transcranial and transsphenoidal approaches. With the advent of endoscopy, however, many surgeons today would argue that a ventral extended endoscopic approach with the magnified and precise visual delineation of small hidden neurovascular structures allows more aggressive resection with careful scanning of structures (Figure 35.1). It also offers the advantage of better visualization of the involved anatomical structures, especially in lesions extending behind the pituitary stalk, and with extension up into the third ventricle (Cappabianca et al., 2000; Cavallo et al., 2008; Gardner et al., 2008; Kassam et al., 2008b,c; Komotar et al., 2013). The extended endoscopic endonasal transsphenoidal approach to the planum sphenoidale has changed the historical indications of the transsphenoidal approach, making it a potential surgical route for the removal of different types of suprasellar lesions (Couldwell et al., 2004; Dusick et al., 2005; Cappabianca et al., 2008; Kaptain et al., 2008; Kassam et al., 2008b,c). This approach allows the surgeon to immediately face the tumor after the dural opening without brain retraction, and permits the direct visualization of the anterior skull base anatomy via a straight route. This is even more attractive in cases of recurrent craniopharyngiomas previously operated

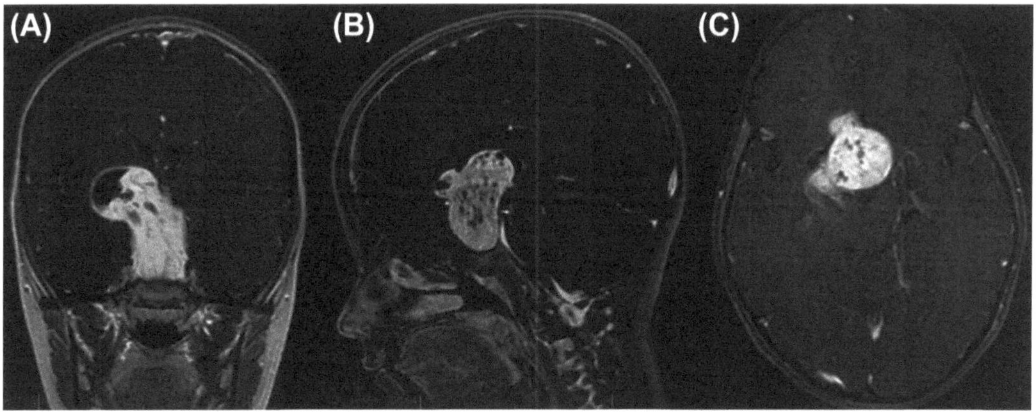

FIGURE 35.1 **Advantage endoscope.** This 9-year-old girl with a large enhancing sellar and suprasellar cystic lesion extending into the third ventricle presented with worsening coordination, especially on her left side, and tilting of her head. Coronal **A,** sagittal **B,** and axial **C** T1-weighted MRI with gadolinium contrast demonstrates the extent of the tumor. An extended transsphenoidal approach via a sublabial incision was performed to remove the tumor. An angled endoscope was used for visualization of residual tumor within the right superior quadrant of the resection cavity that was not visible to the operating microscope.

on via a transcranial route, bypassing scar tissue and potential adherences that may hinder the progress of surgery (Coppens and Couldwell, 2010).

The advantage of the purely endoscopic transsphenoidal approach is the wider multi-angled close-up view that it affords showing more accurate anatomy, which enhances the surgeon's understanding of the neurovascular anatomy including the optic apparatus (Halves and Bushe, 1979; Cappabianca et al., 2000; Dusick et al., 2005; Frank et al., 2006; Kassam et al., 2008b; Cavallo et al., 2009). It also allows for the more direct access to the retro-sellar and intraventricular spaces, which are difficult to access transcranially. In fact, it is a superb approach for tumors extending into the third ventricle as it offers a complete view of the lower and upper third ventricle. Surgeons using a predominantly microscopic trans-sphenoidal approach with endoscopic assistance have, in fact, noted the angled endoscope's importance in allowing the visualization of tight hidden spaces that could not be seen with a microscope and in resolving uncertainties during the dissection phase of surgery.

In select cases of craniopharyngiomas that are midline with sellar and suprasellar involvement, the transsphenoidal approach may prove to be safer with better visual outcomes than the transcranial interhemispheric transcallosal approach. In a meta-analysis study by Komotar et al. (2013) endonasal approaches, whether microscopic or endoscopic, had a higher rate of GTR compared with transcranial approaches (66.9% vs. 48.3%, $P < 0.003$), less visual disturbance (56.2% vs. 33.1%, $P < 0.003$), and a trend towards a lower recurrence rate. In one of the largest case series on outcomes after extended endoscopic endonasal surgery for craniopharyngiomas by Gardner et al. (2008), 11 of 16 patients underwent planned GTR. This was achieved in 8/11 patients with no recurrence after a mean follow-up time of 34 months. Fourteen of 16 patients presented with vision loss, of which 93% had improvement or complete recovery and one remained stable. Eighteen percent of patients developed

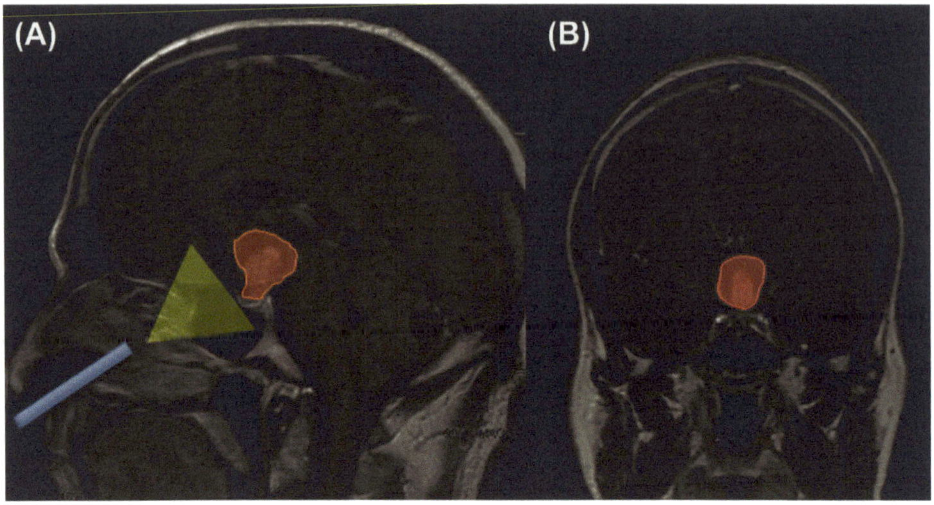

FIGURE 35.2 Sagittal **A,** and coronal **B** views of a midline suprasellar lesion, which can be easily accessed via an extended endoscopic approach. The blue line represents the trajectory of the endoscope toward the suprasellar region; the yellow triangle represents the angle of view in the sagittal plane that is available via the extended endoscopic approach; red shading indicates the suprasellar region that includes the lesion.

new panhypopituitarism, and 8% developed permanent diabetes insipidus. In a retrospective case series, Jane et al. (2010) evaluated 12 patients who underwent endoscopic transsphenoidal surgery for craniopharyngioma. They noted a 75% GTR rate when assessed on the first post-operative magnetic resonance imaging studies. Eighty-three percent of patients, however, achieved a near-total resection (95% of original tumor). Permanent diabetes insipidus occurred in 44% of patients and 67% of patients developed panhypopituitarism after surgery. Visual improvement was noted in 78% of patients with pre-operative visual deficits.

The general consensus regarding the use of an extended endoscopic approach favors its application for small midline tumors especially with endonasal involvement (Figure 35.2). Larger, midline tumors with significant suprasellar extension may still be addressed through a purely endoscopic approach, but at the cost of a higher rate of cerebrospinal fluid (CSF) leak.

THE SHORTCOMINGS OF ENDOSCOPY

While the extended endoscopic endonasal approach has proven to be just as effective as its microscopic counterpart in exposing the anterior skull base and perhaps somewhat more effective in visualizing difficult-to-see angles, it is not without shortcomings. First, endoscopic approaches can be difficult to complete in children with non-pneumatized sphenoid sinuses and with a small sella (Komotar et al., 2013). These make the passage of an endoscope through the sphenoid sinus very difficult and limit the space for passing instruments.

Intracavitary bleeding is another drawback, which can blind the operator in a cavity where the maneuverability of surgical instruments is not as seamless as with the microscope (Cappabianca et al., 2000, 2008; Cavallo et al., 2008; Komotar et al., 2013). Maneuverability with endoscopic surgery becomes quite problematic when bipolar forceps are required at different angles for the dissection of perforating vessels (Kouri et al., 2000; de Divitiis et al., 2007; Kim et al., 2011). Also, the lack of a speculum, which is used with microscopic surgery, precludes the surgical corridor through which instruments can be introduced and removed without injury to the mucosa.

Another disadvantage is that the approach requires a learning curve with two surgeons adept at endoscopic and skull base techniques (Cappabianca et al., 1998, 2008; Frank et al., 2006; de Divitiis et al., 2007; Cote et al., 2013; Komotar et al., 2013). While the endoscope offers superior wide-angle vision, the perimeter of the image is distorted, and in most instances, endoscopic approaches are performed with two-dimensional vision. These shortcomings may be overcome with experience (Cote et al., 2013), but the time to execute tasks under endoscopic vision is longer than that with three-dimensional microscopic vision. These may be overcome in the future with the routine employment of three-dimensional endoscopes. At present, some fully trained neurosurgeons are reluctant to learn endoscopy because of the learning curve and the time and effort required to become proficient. Even with sufficient training, endoscopic closure after a CSF leak is fraught with difficult reconstruction techniques that continue to challenge many surgeons, as the defect created in the skull base needs adequate closure. CSF leak remains one of the major limitations of the extended endoscopic approach for craniopharyngioma resection; its incidence in many studies has been noted to be significantly greater than in transcranial approaches (Hirsch, 1952; Frank et al., 2006; de Divitiis et al., 2007; Gardner et al., 2008; Stamm et al., 2008; Jane et al., 2010). In these extensive approaches, the subarachnoid space is intentionally exposed and approached through a wide dural opening, making CSF leak in extended approaches much more likely than in conventional transsphenoidal approaches. Early retrospective reviews report rates of CSF leaks of 20% to 30%, and some have reported rates as high as 58% (Gardner et al., 2008).

Complex skull base reconstruction techniques have evolved over time to help address the common problem of CSF leak. Simple fascia and bone overlays have been replaced by more sophisticated closures involving inlay and overlay fascial grafts, bone reconstruction and pedicled rotation flaps, which have resulted in fewer incidents of CSF leak in newer studies (Hadad et al., 2006; Fortes et al., 2007; Gardner et al., 2008; Kassam et al., 2008a; Oliver et al., 2008; Prevedello et al., 2009; Shah et al., 2009; Kim et al., 2011). In recent reports of endonasal craniopharyngioma resection, CSF leak rates as low as 0% to 4% have been reported (Kassam et al., 2008c). The narrow working corridor and lack of three-dimensional perception make techniques for suturing fascia lata and other dural substitutes difficult. In addition to the crowded working space and lack of appropriate instrumentation, a higher rate of CSF leak is attributed to several other factors, including the high CSF flow and protein content of craniopharyngiomas, prior radiation, history of previous endoscopic surgery, large dural defects, large resection volumes, opening of the cisterns and ventricles, and obesity (Zimmer and Theodosopoulos, 2009). The use of specialized instruments, curved needles, and self-tying sutures has lowered the technical difficulty of endoscopic closure of skull base defects (Cukurova et al., 2008; Kassam et al., 2008c). Further experience and technological advancements within the field of endoscopic skull base surgery will allow a higher rate of watertight closures in the future.

ENDOSCOPY-ASSISTED MICROSCOPIC EXTENDED TRANSSPHENOIDAL RESECTION

Endoscopy-assisted microscopic extended transsphenoidal resection has been advocated by many as the surest and safest way to achieve maximal safe resection. Proponents argue that it avoids unnecessary brain retraction, manipulation of many neurovascular structures, blind dissection around the inferior and posterior surfaces of the optic nerves (a common point of adherence for many craniopharyngiomas especially in a prefixed chiasm) and that it combines the advantages of both microscopic and endoscopic surgery to ensure adequate instrument maneuverability as well as detailed visualization of blind spots around neurovascular structures (Liu et al., 2003; Laws et al., 2005; Kim et al., 2011; Paluzzi et al., 2012). In a study by Kim et al. (2011), 18 patients with suprasellar craniopharyngiomas underwent microscopic extended transsphenoidal surgery with endoscopic assistance for visualization of portions of the tumors that could not be properly visualized with the microscope. Total resection was achieved in all patients, and all visual symptoms improved. Pre-operative hypopituitarism improved in two patients, whereas it remained stable in 15 patients who had it pre-operatively. Permanent diabetes insipidus was present in 16% post-operatively. No CSF leak was observed in the dural suture technique of fascia lata groups but it occurred in three patients in the conventional closure method without using suture. According to the authors, the former technique could be more precisely applied when using the microscope.

OPEN TRANSCRANIAL APPROACHES

While the indications for extended endoscopic approaches for the resection of craniopharyngioma have expanded over the years, the role of transcranial surgery for tackling craniopharyngiomas remains an important mainstay in certain instances. The pterional (frontotemporal) approach may be used for large retrochiasmatic craniopharyngiomas with significant anterior and posterior extension. It is the best route to craniopharyngiomas involving primarily large suprasellar lesions because it provides the shortest distance to the suprasellar region. This is also the preferred method in patients with a prefixed chiasm, because the tumor can be resected beneath the chiasm by coming in from a more lateral trajectory. A combined pterional and subfrontal approach allows access to both anterior and posterior portions of the tumor (Mori et al., 2007; Zimmer and Theodosopoulos, 2009). In cases of a post-fixed chiasm, a subfrontal approach may be used; it can be supplemented with a trans-lamina terminalis route to access the third ventricle. Alternatively, a frontal interhemispheric approach may be used as well. The transcallosal approach is advocated primarily for craniopharyngiomas arising from within the third ventricle or with marked superior extension within the third ventricle. The transcallosal route may also be applied for the planned staged resection of the superior component of a large tumor extending superiorly into the third or lateral ventricles in conjunction with a pterional or subfrontal approach. In the aforementioned scenario, it is advisable to start with the pterional approach to help achieve brain relaxation by opening the basal cisterns and rendering the inferior portion of the tumor mobile after dissecting it from the optic apparatus and anterior cerebral artery complex and then resorting to the transcallosal approach to complete the resection (Wilson, 1979; Kobayashi et al., 1987; Barrow et al., 1992; Patterson, 1996; Couldwell and Weiss, 1998).

Purely intraventricular craniopharyngiomas with hydrocephalus may be approached via a transcortical transventricular route through the foramen of Monro (Chamoun and Couldwell, 2013) (Figure 35.3); this avoids the pituitary infundibulum and hypothalamus while providing optimal visualization of the lesion. In the senior author's experience, the key to determining whether the tumor lies wholly within the third ventricle is careful review of the pre-operative imaging and location of the pituitary stalk. If the stalk remains in its native position, there is a higher likelihood that the tumor lies within the ventricle in contrast to deforming the floor of the ventricle. In our experience, the endoscope can be a very helpful adjunct to microscopy in exploring blind angles within the ventricle.

Transcranial approaches are also very useful in patients with recurrent craniopharyngiomas whose tumors were initially resected via a transsphenoidal approach to avoid ventral arachnoid scar (Laws Jr, 1994; Fahlbusch et al., 1999; Dusick et al., 2005; Jane et al., 2010). Another important advantage of the transcranial approach is the lower rate of post-operative CSF leak, which results because the surgeon has the ability to more easily reconstruct the anterior skull base floor with a pericranial flap or synthetic dural

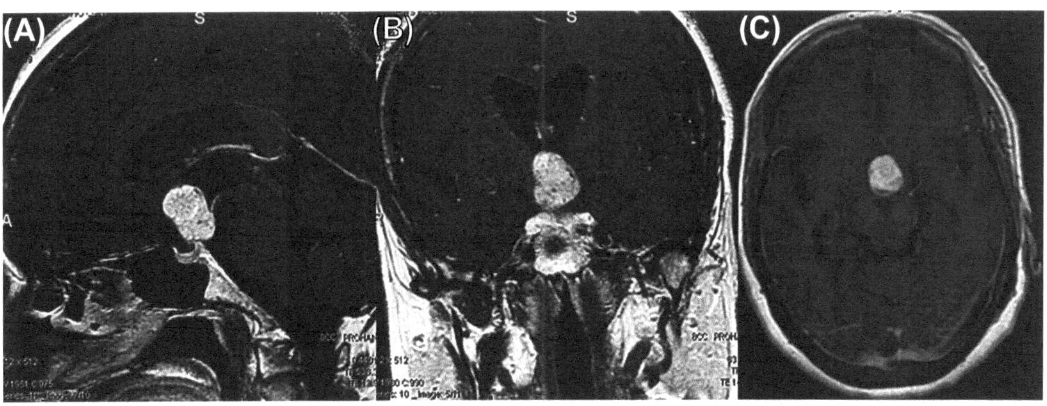

FIGURE 35.3 **Advantage open microsurgical transventricular approach.** This is a 66-year-old woman with progressive headache and confusion. MRI of the brain with gadolinium contrast demonstrated a solid enhancing suprasellar lesion with extension into the third ventricle. Sagittal **A,** coronal **B,** and axial **C** T1-weighted, gadolinium-enhanced MRI demonstrates the extent of the tumor. An open microscopic microsurgical approach via a transventricular approach was chosen using a right frontal craniotomy. Complete resection of the lesion was achieved. *Figures reproduced with permission from Chamoun R, Couldwell WT. Transcortical–transforaminal microscopic approach for purely intraventricular craniopharyngioma. Neurosurg Focus (Suppl) 34(1): Video 4, 2013.* (*Chamoun and Couldwell, 2013*).

substitutes. The space for maneuvering suturing instruments is larger and offers the depth perception of an operating microscope. Similarly with the open transsphenoidal approach, vascular pedicle flaps are easier to develop, and suturing techniques are less cumbersome (Bushe and Halves, 1978; Fortes et al., 2007; Kassam et al., 2008c; Prevedello et al., 2009).

In cases in which there is significant optic nerve compression from above with visual compromise, a transcranial pterional approach to directly decompress the optic nerve is a quicker and more effective way to safeguard a patient's deteriorating vision. For lesions with significant lateral extension into the mesiotemporal region and posterior extension into the posterior fossa, the transcranial pterional approach and its modifications (orbitozygomatic and transzygomatic) allow a more visible and controlled access (Figure 35.4) (Maira et al., 1995; Zimmer and Theodosopoulos, 2009).

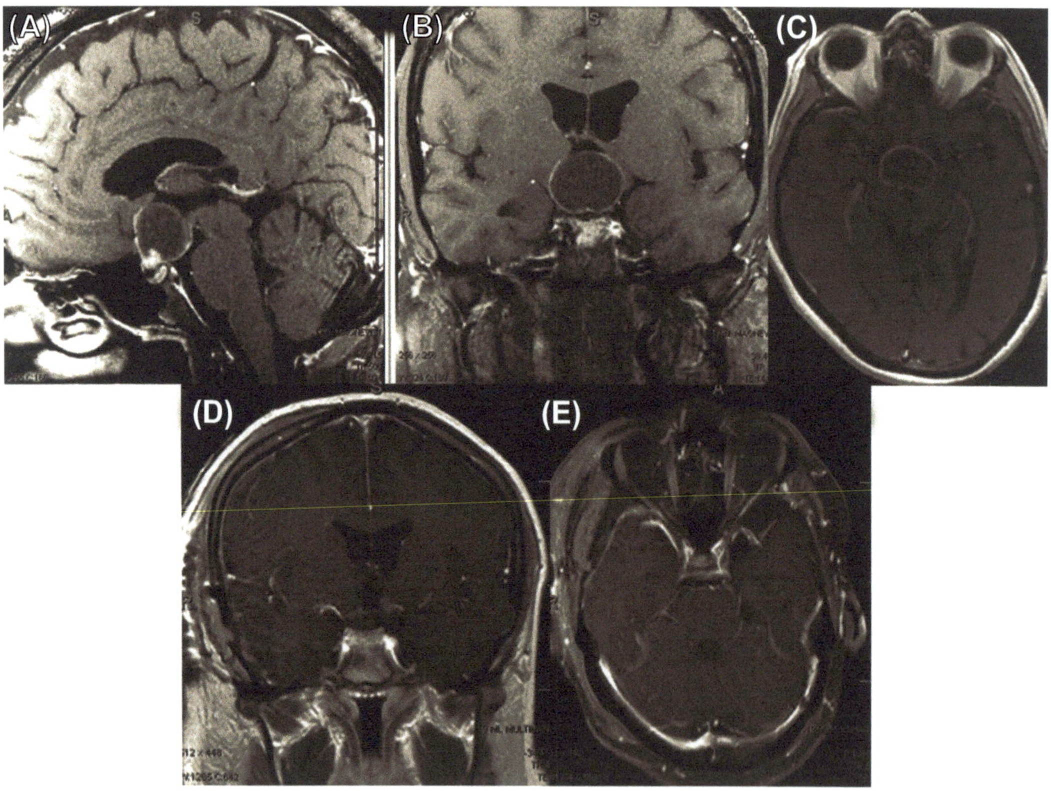

FIGURE 35.4 **Advantage microscope.** This 41-year-old man presented with severe bitemporal hemianopsia and vision loss in both eyes. An MRI of the brain with gadolinium contrast demonstrated an enhancing, cystic, partially solid suprasellar lesion with compression of the optic apparatus. Sagittal **A**, coronal **B**, and axial **C** T1-weighted, gadolinium-enhanced MRI demonstrates the extent of the rumor. This tumor was completely removed through an open right frontotemporal approach. The post-operative coronal **D**, and axial **E** T1-weighted MRI with gadolinium enhancement shows complete resection of the lesion.

MINIMALLY INVASIVE TRANSCRANIAL APPROACHES

A common argument in favor of pursuing transsphenoidal endoscopic and/or microscopic approaches to midline craniopharyngiomas is that these approaches are less invasive and have a shorter recovery time. During recent decades, however, minimally invasive approaches have been described for select lesions in the anterior cranial fossa and parasellar region. The supraorbital craniotomy, through an eyebrow incision, involves a small craniotomy flap cut flush to the orbital roof (Mori et al., 2007; Brydon et al., 2008; Zimmer and Theodosopoulos, 2009). Keeping the head in a slightly extended position with early release of CSF affords the same exposure of the subfrontal area with minimal brain retraction. A variation of the latter approach is a transorbitotomy through an eyelid incision, with a similar exposure but slightly improved superior exposure and a shortened distance to the parasellar area (Andaluz et al., 2008). Careful pre-operative planning is of the essence to avoid inadvertent entry into the frontal sinus, especially in cases where there is CSF egress. Neuronavigation is very helpful in planning the craniotomy and avoiding the sinus. The degrees of operative freedom are more limited with these approaches, which must be kept in mind with particular attention to the extension of tumor.

DISADVANTAGES OF TRANSCRANIAL APPROACHES

An open transcranial approach with poor visualization of the sella may be inadequate with tumors that extend into the sella turcica. In such cases an adjunct ventral approach, either open or endoscopic transsphenoidal may be helpful, since 50% of recurrences of craniopharyngioma occur in the pituitary fossa, which is not adequately exposed via a pterional approach (Patterson, 1996; Couldwell and Weiss, 1998; Mori et al., 2007; Zimmer and Theodosopoulos, 2009). The surgeon approaching a craniopharyngioma from above is blinded by the inferior part of the optic nerve as well as the chiasm and internal carotid artery. Neurovascular structures as well as the pituitary stalk and their anatomical relationships may not be fully appreciated without the endoscope, which may make patients undergoing open transcranial surgery more prone to neurovascular injury and pituitary dysfunction. In addition, with the transcranial approach, the risk of wound infection and seizures is higher.

CONCLUSION

In conclusion, the applications of endoscopic endonasal skull base surgery approaches have expanded to include pathological conditions that would not have been contemplated through a transsphenoidal route a few years ago. Early results from many case series seem to confirm the safety and efficacy of endoscopic surgery and extended endoscopic surgery. Further refinements in reconstructive techniques and improvement in instrumentation are the key to curtailing the rate of CSF leak and improving overall patient outcomes. Meanwhile, the continued use of the microscopic transsphenoidal technique with the assistance of the endoscope remains a viable method for addressing ventral midline craniopharyngiomas while upholding the advantages of both methods. Endoscopy may one day become the gold standard for addressing midline craniopharyngiomas, but this will require improvements in technique and instrumentation as well as dedication on the part of skull base trainees to become acquainted with the endoscope and develop their skills early in their careers. Although the transcranial approach is becoming less popular for the resection of craniopharyngiomas, it will always have a role to play in tackling larger lesions with lateral extensions, and recurrent lesions previously resected via the transsphenoidal route.

References

Andaluz, N., Romano, A., Reddy, L.V., Zuccarello, M., 2008. Eyelid approach to the anterior cranial base. J. Neurosurg. 109 (2), 341–346.

Barrow, D., Tindall, G., Tindall, S., 1992. Combined simultaneous transsphenoidal transcranial operative approach to selected sellar tumors. Perspect. Neurol. Surg. 3, 49–57.

Brydon, H.L., Akil, H., Ushewokunze, S., Dhir, J.S., Taha, A., Ahmed, A., 2008. Supraorbital microcraniotomy for acute aneurysmal subarachnoid haemorrhage: results of first 50 cases. Br. J. Neurosurg. 22 (1), 40–45.

Bushe, K.A., Halves, E., 1978. [Modified technique in transsphenoidal operations of pituitary adenomas. Technical note (author's transl)]. Acta Neurochir. (Wien) 41 (1–3), 163–175.

Cappabianca, P., Alfieri, A., de Divitiis, E., 1998. Endoscopic endonasal transsphenoidal approach to the sella: towards functional endoscopic pituitary surgery (FEPS). Minim. Invasive Neurosurg. 41 (2), 66–73.

Cappabianca, P., Alfieri, A., Colao, A., Cavallo, L.M., Fusco, M., Peca, C., Lombardi, G., de Divitiis, E., 2000. Endoscopic endonasal transsphenoidal surgery in recurrent and residual pituitary adenomas: technical note. Minim. Invasive Neurosurg. 43 (1), 38–43.

Cappabianca, P., Cavallo, L.M., Esposito, F., De Divitiis, O., Messina, A., De Divitiis, E., 2008. Extended endoscopic endonasal approach to the midline skull base: the evolving role of transsphenoidal surgery. Adv. Tech. Stand. Neurosurg. 33, 151–199.

Cavallo, L.M., Prevedello, D., Esposito, F., Laws Jr., E.R., Dusick, J.R., Messina, A., Jane Jr., J.A., Kelly, D.F., Cappabianca, P., 2008. The role of the endoscope in the transsphenoidal management of cystic lesions of the sellar region. Neurosurg. Rev. 31 (1), 55–64; discussion 64.

Cavallo, L.M., Prevedello, D.M., Solari, D., Gardner, P.A., Esposito, F., Snyderman, C.H., Carrau, R.L., Kassam, A.B., Cappabianca, P., 2009. Extended endoscopic endonasal transsphenoidal approach for residual or recurrent craniopharyngiomas. J. Neurosurg. 111 (3), 578–589.

Chakrabarti, I., Amar, A.P., Couldwell, W., Weiss, M.H., 2005. Long-term neurological, visual, and endocrine outcomes following transnasal resection of craniopharyngioma. J. Neurosurg. 102 (4), 650–657.

Chamoun, R., Couldwell, W.T., 2013. Transcortical-transforaminal microscopic approach for purely intraventricular craniopharyngioma. Neurosurg. Focus (1 Suppl.), 34. Video 4.

Coppens, J.R., Couldwell, W.T., 2010. Staged use of the transsphenoidal approach to resect superior third ventricular craniopharyngiomas. Minim. Invasive Neurosurg. 53 (1), 40–43.

Cote, M., Kalra, R., Wilson, T., Orlandi, R.R., Couldwell, W.T., 2013. Surgical fidelity: comparing the microscope and the endoscope. Acta Neurochir. (Wien) 155 (12), 2299–2303.

Couldwell, W., Weiss, M.H., 1998. The transnasal transsphenoidal approach. In: Apuzzo, M. (Ed.), Surgery of the Third Ventricle, Second ed. Williams & Wilkins, Philadelphia, pp. 553–574.

Couldwell, W.T., Weiss, M.H., Rabb, C., Liu, J.K., Apfelbaum, R.I., Fukushima, T., 2004. Variations on the standard transsphenoidal approach to the sellar region, with emphasis on the extended approaches and parasellar approaches: surgical experience in 105 cases. Neurosurgery 55 (3), 539–547; discussion 547–550.

Cukurova, I., Cetinkaya, E.A., Aslan, I.B., Ozkul, D., 2008. Endonasal endoscopic repair of ethmoid roof cerebrospinal fluid fistula by suturing the dura. Acta Neurochir. (Wien) 150 (9), 897–900; discussion 900.

de Divitiis, E., Cappabianca, P., Cavallo, L.M., Esposito, F., de Divitiis, O., Messina, A., 2007. Extended endoscopic transsphenoidal approach for extrasellar craniopharyngiomas. Neurosurgery 61 (5 Suppl. 2), 219–227 discussion 228.

Doglietto, F., Prevedello, D.M., Jane Jr., J.A., Han, J., Laws Jr, E.R., 2005. Brief history of endoscopic transsphenoidal surgery – from Philipp Bozzini to the First World Congress of Endoscopic Skull Base Surgery. Neurosurg. Focus 19 (6), E3.

Dusick, J.R., Esposito, F., Kelly, D.F., Cohan, P., DeSalles, A., Becker, D.P., Martin, N.A., 2005. The extended direct endonasal transsphenoidal approach for nonadenomatous suprasellar tumors. J. Neurosurg. 102 (5), 832–841.
Fahlbusch, R., Honegger, J., Paulus, W., Huk, W., Buchfelder, M., 1999. Surgical treatment of craniopharyngiomas: experience with 168 patients. J. Neurosurg. 90 (2), 237–250.
Fortes, F.S., Carrau, R.L., Snyderman, C.H., Prevedello, D., Vescan, A., Mintz, A., Gardner, P., Kassam, A.B., 2007. The posterior pedicle inferior turbinate flap: a new vascularized flap for skull base reconstruction. Laryngoscope 117 (8), 1329–1332.
Frank, G., Pasquini, E., Doglietto, F., Mazzatenta, D., Sciarretta, V., Farneti, G., Calbucci, F., 2006. The endoscopic extended transsphenoidal approach for craniopharyngiomas. Neurosurgery 59 (1 Suppl 1), ONS75–83.
Gardner, P., Kassam, A., Snyderman, C., Mintz, A., Carrau, R., Moossy, J.J., 2008. Endoscopic endonasal suturing of dural reconstruction grafts: a novel application of the U-Clip technology. Technical note. J. Neurosurg. 108 (2), 395–400.
Gardner, P.A., Kassam, A.B., Snyderman, C.H., Carrau, R.L., Mintz, A.H., Grahovac, S., Stefko, S., 2008. Outcomes following endoscopic, expanded endonasal resection of suprasellar craniopharyngiomas: a case series. J. Neurosurg. 109 (1), 6–16.
Hadad, G., Bassagasteguy, L., Carrau, R.L., Mataza, J.C., Kassam, A., Snyderman, C.H., Mintz., A., 2006. A novel reconstructive technique after endoscopic expanded endonasal approaches: vascular pedicle nasoseptal flap. Laryngoscope 116 (10), 1882–1886.
Halves, E., Bushe, K.A., 1979. Transsphenoidal operation on craniopharyngiomas with extrasellar extensions. The advantage of the operating endoscope [proceedings]. Acta Neurochir. Suppl. (Wien) 28 (2), 362.
Hirsch, O., 1952. Successful closure of cerebrospinal fluid rhinorrhea by endonasal surgery. AMA Arch. Otolaryngol. 56 (1), 1–12.
Jane Jr., J.A., Kiehna, E., Payne, S.C., Early, S.V., Laws Jr., E.R., 2010. Early outcomes of endoscopic transsphenoidal surgery for adult craniopharyngiomas. Neurosurg. Focus 28 (4), E9.
Jho, H.D., Carrau, R.L., 1997. Endoscopic endonasal transsphenoidal surgery: experience with 50 patients. J. Neurosurg. 87 (1), 44–51.
Kaptain, G.J., Vincent, D.A., Sheehan, J.P., Laws Jr., E.R., 2008. Transsphenoidal approaches for the extracapsular resection of midline suprasellar and anterior cranial base lesions. Neurosurgery 62 (6 Suppl. 3), 1264–1271.
Kassam, A.B., Gardner, P.A., Snyderman, C.H., Carrau, R.L., Mintz, A.H., Prevedello, D.M., 2008a. Expanded endonasal approach, a fully endoscopic transnasal approach for the resection of midline suprasellar craniopharyngiomas: a new classification based on the infundibulum. J. Neurosurg. 108 (4), 715–728.
Kassam, A.B., Prevedello, D.M., Thomas, A., Gardner, P., Mintz, A., Snyderman, C., Carrau, R., 2008b. Endoscopic endonasal pituitary transposition for a transdorsum sellae approach to the interpeduncular cistern. Neurosurgery 62 (3 Suppl 1), 57–72; discussion 72–74.
Kassam, A.B., Thomas, A., Carrau, R.L., Snyderman, C., Vescan, A., Prevedello, D., Mintz, A., Gardner, P., 2008c. Endoscopic reconstruction of the cranial base using a pedicled nasoseptal flap. Neurosurgery 63 (1 Suppl. 1), ONS44–52; discussion ONS52–53.
Kim, E.H., Ahn, J.Y., Kim, S.H., 2011. Technique and outcome of endoscopy-assisted microscopic extended transsphenoidal surgery for suprasellar craniopharyngiomas. J. Neurosurg. 114 (5), 1338–1349.
Kobayashi, T., Nakane, T., Kageyama, N., 1987. Combined trans-sphenoidal and intracranial surgery for craniopharyngioma. Prog. Exp. Tumor Res. 30, 341–349.
Komotar, R.J., Starke, R.M., Raper, D.M., Anand, V.K., Schwartz, T.H., 2013. Endoscopic endonasal compared with anterior craniofacial and combined cranionasal resection of esthesioneuroblastomas. World Neurosurg. 80 (1–2), 148–159.
Kouri, J.G., Chen, M.Y., Watson, J.C., Oldfield, E.H., 2000. Resection of suprasellar tumors by using a modified transsphenoidal approach. Report of four cases. J. Neurosurg. 92 (6), 1028–1035.
Laws Jr., E.R., 1994. Transsphenoidal removal of craniopharyngioma. Pediatr. Neurosurg. 21 (Suppl. 1), 57–63.
Laws, E.R., Kanter, A.S., Jane Jr., J.A., Dumont, A.S., 2005. Extended transsphenoidal approach. J. Neurosurg. 102 (5), 825–827; discussion 827–828.
Liu, J.K., Weiss, M.H., Couldwell, W.T., 2003. Surgical approaches to pituitary tumors. Neurosurg. Clin. N. Am. 14 (1), 93–107.
Locatelli, D., Levi, D., Rampa, F., Pezzotta, S., Castelnuovo, P., 2004. Endoscopic approach for the treatment of relapses in cystic craniopharyngiomas. Childs Nerv. Syst. 20 (11–12), 863–867.

Maira, G., Anile, C., Rossi, G.F., Colosimo, C., 1995. Surgical treatment of craniopharyngiomas: an evaluation of the transsphenoidal and pterional approaches. Neurosurgery 36 (4), 715–724.

Mori, K., Osada, H., Yamamoto, T., Nakao, Y., Maeda, M., 2007. Pterional keyhole approach to middle cerebral artery aneurysms through an outer canthal skin incision. Minim. Invasive Neurosurg. 50 (4), 195–201.

Oliver, C.L., Hackman, T.G., Carrau, R.L., Snyderman, C.H., Kassam, A.B., Prevedello, D.M., Gardner, P., 2008. Palatal flap modifications allow pedicled reconstruction of the skull base. Laryngoscope 118 (12), 2102–2106.

Paluzzi, A., Gardner, P., Fernandez-Miranda, J.C., Snyderman, C., 2012. The expanding role of endoscopic skull base surgery. Br. J. Neurosurg. 26 (5), 649–661.

Patterson, R.H., 1996. The role of transcranial surgery in the management of pituitary adenoma. Acta Neurochir. Suppl. 65, 16–17.

Prevedello, D.M., Doglietto, F., Jane Jr., J.A., Jagannathan, J., Han, J., Laws Jr., E.R., 2007. History of endoscopic skull base surgery: its evolution and current reality. J. Neurosurg. 107 (1), 206–213.

Prevedello, D.M., Barges-Coll, J., Fernandez-Miranda, J.C., Morera, V., Jacobson, D., Madhok, R., dos Santos, M.C., Zanation, A., Snyderman, C.H., Gardner, P., Kassam, A.B., Carrau, R., 2009. Middle turbinate flap for skull base reconstruction: cadaveric feasibility study. Laryngoscope 119 (11), 2094–2098.

Sachs, E., 1949. Diagnosis and treatment of brain tumors and care of the neurosurgical patient. St. Louis: C.V. Mosby Company, p. 292.

Shah, R.N., Surowitz, J.B., Patel, M.R., Huange, B.Y., Snyderman, C.H., Carrau, R.L., Kassam, A.B., Germanwala, A.V., Zanation, A.M., 2009. Endoscopic pedicled nasoseptal flap reconstruction for pediatric skull base defects. Laryngoscope 119 (6), 1067–1075.

Stamm, A.C., Vellutini, E., Harvey, R.J., Nogeira Jr., J.F., Herman, D.R., 2008. Endoscopic transnasal craniotomy and the resection of craniopharyngioma. Laryngoscope 118 (7), 1142–1148.

Wilson, C., 1979. Neurosurgical management of large invasive pituitary tumors. In: Tindall, G., Collins, W. (Eds.), Clinical Management of Pituitary Disorders. Raven Press, New York, pp. 335–342.

Zimmer, L.A., Theodosopoulos, P.V., 2009. Anterior skull base surgery: open versus endoscopic. Curr. Opin. Otolaryngol. Head Neck Surg. 17 (2), 75–78.

CHAPTER

36

Controversies: Endoscopic Resection

Heather J. McCrea, Tong Yang*, Theodore H. Schwartz*,†*

*Departments of Neurosurgery; †Otolaryngology, Head and Neck Surgery, Weill Cornell Medical College, New York Presbyterian Hospital, New York, NY, USA

"There is perhaps no other primary brain tumor that evokes passion, emotion, and as a result, controversy than does the craniopharyngioma." **James Rutka, 2002**

INTRODUCTION

Craniopharyngiomas have engendered much controversy over the years. These tumors are difficult to classify, being both benign in histology but malignant in invasiveness, require different treatment algorithms in adults versus children, respond well to radiation in some circumstances and not well to radiation in others, and are located in the center of the brain and skull base, making surgery difficult and leading to multiple surgical approaches over the years. In this chapter we will focus on the controversies surrounding surgical approach, particularly those that have arisen in recent years with the advent of the endonasal, endoscopic, extended approaches (Table 36.1). These minimal access approaches provide unparalleled and unprecedented views above the sella into the suprasellar cistern and roof of the third ventricle, precisely the most difficult areas from which to remove craniopharyngiomas and thus have changed the landscape and playing field with regards to choosing the best surgical approach. Not only are there controversies in the choice of approach, these also exist in the choice of closure technique and adjuvant maneuvers associated with endonasal surgery, and these will be addressed in this chapter as well.

TABLE 36.1 Advantages of Endoscopic vs. Open Approach

Endoscopic advantages	Open advantages
Reduced brain retraction	Reduced risk of CSF leak
Improved visual outcomes	Better lateral visualization
Reduced risk of seizures	
Better superior visualization	
Minimally invasive	

Craniopharyngiomas
http://dx.doi.org/10.1016/B978-0-12-416706-3.00036-2

SURGICAL APPROACH

Surgical approaches for craniopharyngioma depend on the location and extension of the tumor. Most craniopharyngiomas are found in the sellar and parasellar regions. Although craniopharyngiomas are benign tumors, their deep location and locally aggressive nature have made them challenging to treat. Additionally, they often occur adjacent to or infiltrate critical structures, including the optic chiasm, hypothalamus, pituitary stalk, anterior cerebral artery complex, and local perforating vessels. The two main approaches typically employed to access this region are a transcranial approach or a transsphenoidal approach. The transsphenoidal approach uses a microscope or endoscope to maximize visualization. The relationship of the tumor to the sella, chiasm, and floor of the third ventricle, as well as the amount of lateral extension, help guide the choice of surgical approach.

Yasargil et al. outlined six typical craniopharyngioma configurations and recommended surgical approaches specific to each of these (Yasargil et al., 1990). Other systems of categorizing craniopharyngiomas have determined the degree of aggressiveness for planned surgery based on a grading system of hypothalamic involvement on MRI (Puget et al., 2007). This decision-making surgical approach is based on the high morbidity of hypothalamic damage, particularly in the pediatric population. Transcranial approaches may be subdivided into pterional (frontotemporal with or without orbitozygomatic osteotomy), interhemispheric transcallosal, subfrontal (with or without translaminal), transcortical-transventricular, or combination approaches (Liu et al., 2005; Komotar et al., 2009). Each approach has strengths and weaknesses, and specific tumors may be more amenable to specific approaches.

Originally, the transsphenoidal approach was reserved for tumors with an intrasellar or infradiaphragmatic location (Yasargil et al., 1990). Approximately 94–95% of tumors have a suprasellar component, with 20–41% being purely suprasellar and 53–75% being both supra- and intrasellar (Karavitaki et al., 2006). This suprasellar component limited the utility of the transsphenoidal approach until recent advances in technique took place. Extended transsphenoidal approaches, first utilizing the operating microscope and more recently incorporating the endoscope, have significantly increased the variety and size of craniopharyngiomas that can be successfully removed via this approach (Cappabianca et al., 2002; Frank et al., 2006; Gardner et al., 2008; Schwartz et al., 2008; Jane Jr et al., 2010). With the transsphenoidal approach, after bone and dural opening, the tumor is typically the first structure encountered, thus removing potential complications resulting from brain retraction. Additionally, the endoscope has significantly improved the surgical corridor through which surgeons operate in this approach by improving illumination and field of view. The limitation imposed by lack of pneumatization in the pediatric sphenoid sinus appears to be of minimal concern, with most patients undergoing pneumatization sufficient for use of the transsphenoidal route by age 4 years (Banu et al., 2013). Even if complete pneumatization is not encountered, there is often soft cancellous bone that can be easily drilled to widen the sinus. Additionally, the rate of CSF leak in these procedures, a significant concern during development of this technique, is now low (0% in a recent series from our institution) (Patel et al., 2013).

TRANSCRANIAL VS. TRANSSPHENOIDAL APPROACH

Comparing outcomes of the transcranial or transsphenoidal approaches is difficult. This is a relatively rare disease, and although there are a significant number of papers discussing the operative approach to craniopharyngioma, they are restricted primarily to single-institution case series without any randomization. Some series include large numbers from high-volume centers, but these series typically lack controls or have groups that are not comparable between treatment strategies. The surgical approach employed is typically based on a combination of surgeon preference, anatomy and size of the tumor, and the view of the surgeon as to the limitations of each approach with respect to the patient's tumor. Additionally, for the transsphenoidal approach, the choice of microscope versus endoscope for visualization during surgery is currently entirely based on surgeon preference and experience with each technique. Two reviews compare open craniotomy to the transsphenoidal approach. A meta-analysis of published series from 1990–2010 by Elliott et al. included significant numbers of children treated via a transsphenoidal or transcranial approach (Elliott et al., 2011). They identified 2955 patients in 48 studies treated with a transcranial (TC) approach and 373 patients in 13 studies treated with either a microscopic or endoscopic transsphenoidal approach. The groups treated with both approaches were not equivalent, with the transcranial group having "less visual loss, more frequent hydrocephalus and increased intracranial pressure, larger tumors, and more suprasellar disease" pre-operatively. Not surprisingly given the difference in presentation, they found that post-operatively the transcranial group had "lower rates of gross total resection, more frequent recurrence after gross total resection, higher neurological morbidity, more frequent diabetes insipidus, less improvement, and greater deterioration in vision" (Elliott et al., 2011). In contrast, overall survival percentages, operative mortality, and obesity/hyperphagia were found not to differ between groups. The authors of this meta-analysis concluded that it was not valid to compare the two approaches directly and that the approach should be determined based on tumor characteristics (Elliott et al., 2011).

Komotar et al. performed a review of published reports and compared the endoscope-assisted transsphenoidal approach to transsphenoidal microscope-based and transcranial microscope-based approaches (Komotar et al., 2012). They identified 88 studies with 3470 patients from 1995–2010 and found that patients treated via the transsphenoidal endoscopic approach "had a significantly greater rate of gross total resection (66.9% vs. 48.3%; $P < 0.003$) and improved visual outcome (56.2% vs. 33.1%; $P < 0.003$)" compared to those treated with an open approach. The transsphenoidal microscope group was similar in outcome to the transsphenoidal endoscope group. Complications varied depending on the approach, with transcranial routes having a 10.1% risk of hydrocephalus, 8.5% risk of seizure, 2.9% risk of hemiparesis/stroke, 2.6% risk of CSF leak, and 2.3% risk of meningitis. The transsphenoidal microscopic approach had a CSF leak risk of 9.0% and risk of meningitis of 1.8% (Komotar et al., 2012). Although the rate of CSF leak was higher with transsphenoidal approaches (18.4% in the endoscopic group and 9.0% in the microscope group) than the open transcranial group (2.6%; $P < 0.003$), the rate of seizure was higher in the transcranial group (8.5%) and did not occur in the endoscopic or microscopic transsphenoidal groups ($P < 0.003$). Additionally, transsphenoidal approaches had a greater rate of improved visual outcome than open approaches. It is worth noting that the average tumor size was smaller in the transsphenoidal microscope and endoscope groups than in the transcranial group, but this difference was not statistically significant. The main bias of these meta-analyses is that cases are not randomized. Hence, smaller cases may be selected for transsphenoidal surgery and larger or more eccentric tumors selected for transcranial surgery. Thus the results may be poorer for the transcranial cases since they are applied to a different group of tumors. These data suggest, however, that for small midline tumors, the endonasal approach may be superior with respect to visual function, assuming the CSF leak rate can be kept < 5%. The literature is calling for a study of transcranial results for tumors that would be considered for endonasal endoscopic surgery in order to compare both approaches more fairly.

While most series analyzed in these meta-analyses include only open transcranial or only transsphenoidal cases, there are a few series that include both approaches. One series by Chakrabarti et al. with 86 patients treated from 1984–1994 included 68 patients undergoing a transnasal approach and 18 patients treated with a transcranial approach (Chakrabarti et al., 2005). The authors concluded that a transnasal approach led to good outcomes in intrasellar cases, or even in cases with suprasellar extension when the tumors included a cystic component. Another report with 57 patients used a transsphenoidal approach for intrasellar tumors or those that were partially intrasellar and a pterional approach for completely suprasellar tumors (Maira et al., 1995). This series had 61% transsphenoidal cases and 39% pterional and showed gross total resection in 66% of transsphenoidal patients and 94% of pterional patients. "Good clinical outcome" was observed in 100% and 91% of cases, respectively. Given the different types of tumors in the two approach cohorts, it is difficult to directly compare the success of these two techniques. In these papers, where a single surgeon selects cases for a given approach, the selection bias issues are even more profound. Similarly, a series with 148 patients (including 39.2% pterional and 23.6% transsphenoidal) had tumor size < 2 cm in 60% of transsphenoidal cases and 22.3% of open transcranial cases (Fahlbusch et al., 1999). Thus, a larger number of transsphenoidal cases had small tumors, making the gross total resection rate of 85.7% for transsphenoidal and 45.7% for open transcranial difficult to compare. More recently, the same group published their experience with 73 patients treated since 1997, which used the transsphenoidal approach on 35.6% of patients (26 patients total) (Hofmann et al., 2012). Transsphenoidal patients had an 88.5% gross total resection rate while transcranial patients had a rate of 79.5%. The transsphenoidal approach was used for subdiaphragmatic tumors, but tumors with significant suprasellar calcification were excluded from this approach. In a further series of 121 patients, the transsphenoidal approach was utilized in 26 of these patients for intrasellar lesions, and a rate of gross total resection of 31% and 15% was demonstrated for transsphenoidal and transcranial approaches, respectively (Fischer et al., 1990).

Overall, both transsphenoidal and open craniotomy approaches may be of utility in craniopharyngioma. Craniotomy has risk of brain retraction, seizures, optic nerve manipulation, and visual deterioration. In contrast, transsphenoidal endonasal approaches have a risk of CSF leak and sinusitis, though this complication is decreasing with surgeon experience and the improved closure techniques described below. For midline tumors that extend to the roof of the third ventricle, the endonasal approach may provide a superior view of the top of the tumor, while tumors that extend lateral to the carotid artery may require a craniotomy for complete excision.

ENDOSCOPIC VS. MICROSCOPIC TRANSSPHENOIDAL APPROACHES

For those patients undergoing a transsphenoidal approach, the surgeon may choose to utilize either a microscope or an endoscope for visualization. The microscope has a limited field of view but, given its binocular vision, it allows a 3-D view. In contrast, the endoscope allows a wider field of view, and angled scopes allow for visualization of areas that would be impossible to see with the microscope. Angled scopes become particularly useful in the case of larger cavities, as they can provide a wider and more panoramic view. One limitation of the endoscope is that it does not allow 3-D vision. However, 3-D scopes are under development, and this will likely remove one concern that users may have about endoscopes (Fraser et al., 2009; Roth et al., 2011).

There are no series directly comparing the endoscopic transsphenoidal approach to the microscopic transsphenoidal approach for craniopharyngioma, as cases series utilizing the endoscopic approach tend to only include patients with this approach. The meta-analysis done by Komotar et al. does include a comparison of these two approaches (Komotar et al., 2012). While both endoscopic and microscopic transsphenoidal approaches showed a greater rate of visual improvement than open transcranial approaches, the endoscopic approach did show a trend toward an even higher rate of improvement than the microscopic approach (56.2% improved vs. 44% improved). In contrast, the rate of CSF leak and rate of hypopituitarism were significantly higher with the endoscopic approach than the microscopic transsphenoidal approach (18.4% vs. 9.0%, $P = 0.024$ and 47.1% vs. 12.8%, $P < 0.003$, respectively). It is worth noting that many of the endoscopic studies included in this analysis were conducted at the time that the endoscopic technique was developing, and there is a steep learning curve to this technique. Recent studies suggest a lower CSF rate than this analysis with CSF leak rates ranging from 0–3.8% (Jane Jr. et al., 2010; Leng et al., 2012; Patel et al., 2013). Likewise, endoscopic surgeons tend to tackle larger and more complex tumors than microscopic surgeons, who may tackle such tumors through a craniotomy, not being familiar with endoscopic techniques.

Gross total resection rates were similar for both groups; 69.1% for transsphenoidal microscopic and 66.9% for transsphenoidal endoscopic (Komotar et al., 2012). This difference was not significant. It should be noted that there were some differences in presenting characteristics between the two groups. The endoscopic group had a higher incidence of visual disturbance, diabetes insipidus, and hypopituitarism pre-operatively and a lower rate of mixed solid and cystic tumors. The endoscopic group also had a higher rate of planned post-operative radiation therapy. Post-operatively, follow-up times were shorter for the endoscope group, likely a further indication that many cases included were from the early years of this technique (Komotar et al., 2012). Nevertheless, the authors concluded that the endoscopic technique was effective and safe. They advocate the use of this technique for most craniopharyngiomas that do not have significant extension lateral to the carotid arteries.

We find that the endoscopic approach is useful even for larger tumors in the case of a surgeon who is experienced with this technique. Increased visualization, especially through the use of angled endoscopes allows for better visualization within the sellar and suprasellar regions, and the development of the 3-D endoscope will provide a significant advance by allowing for depth perception with the endoscope. Although the field would benefit from direct comparisons of microscopic versus endoscopic transsphenoidal approaches, given the strong surgeon preference for one technique or the other, it is unlikely that studies such as these will ever be performed.

GROSS TOTAL RESECTION VS. SUBTOTAL RESECTION AND RADIATION

While differences in cohort characteristics make the rate of gross total resection between approaches challenging to compare directly, the question of whether to aim for a gross total resection also remains controversial. Most would agree that gross total resection should be employed if morbidity and mortality are low, but the morbidity of gross total resection and whether this morbidity should be accepted for the sake of total excision remains controversial, especially in the pediatric population. The two main treatment strategies include aggressive gross total resection or a more limited surgical resection/decompression with adjuvant radiation treatment. Gross total resection (determined radiographically) has a significantly lower rate of recurrence; 10-year recurrence is 0–62%, versus 25–100% for subtotal resection (Karavitaki et al., 2006). Adjuvant radiotherapy after partial resection has recurrence rates of 10–63% (Karavitaki et al., 2006). Surgery for recurrence is considered more challenging due to adhesions and scarring, and morbidity is higher and resection rates lower in repeat resection. In Yasargil's series, surgical mortality was 11.8% for children and 8.2% for adults in primary cases, and 31.6% for children and 38.5% in adults undergoing secondary surgery. Good clinical outcome was seen in 72.5% of children and 80.3% of adults with primary surgery and 31.6% of children and 38.5% of adults with secondary surgery (Yasargil et al., 1990). In a more recent endoscopic series, 22 patients with recurrent or residual craniopharyngioma were treated between 2004 and 2008 (Cavallo et al., 2009). The cohort included both patients with prior transcranial and transsphenoidal approaches. Nine patients (40.9%) had total removal, eight patients (36.4%) had near-total removal (> 95%), four patients (18.2%) had subtotal removal (> 70%), and one patient (4.5%) had partial removal (< 50%). This series had no mortality or major complication "including behavior changes," and CSF leak was seen in 13.6% of cases.

In the modern era, 10-year survival rates for craniopharyngioma are high (83–92.7%) (Karavitaki et al., 2006), making quality of life post treatment a significant concern. As a result, some authors have advocated using radiation as an adjuvant treatment in order to limit quality of life morbidities associated with aggressive resection (Cavazzuti et al., 1983; Merchant et al., 2006). However, the cognitive side effects of radiation, especially in children, are also of concern (Merchant et al., 2006). Common morbidities to consider include pituitary dysfunction, hypothalamic injury, and visual injury. Hypopituitarism is easily treated with hormone replacement, but this morbidity can still be challenging without careful adherence to hormone therapy. Hypothalamic injury can be particularly devastating, especially in children, and has been a major concern resulting in a recommendation for a more limited resection (Puget et al., 2007).

Several large case series discuss the outcomes of craniopharyngiomas resected at a particular institution or by a particular surgeon. Yasargil's series included 144 patients, including 70 children, treated between 1967–1989 and achieving gross total resection in 90% of cases (Yasargil et al., 1990). Of note, computed tomography (CT) was only used after 1976, so one potential bias in this study is that gross total resection was based on the surgeon's estimate. In this study, 7% had recurrence and 67.4% had "good" outcomes. Another pediatric series included 50 patients from 1975–1989 with surgeon's estimate of 90% gross total resection and a 34% recurrence rate (Hoffman et al., 1992). Another large series from France included 122 patients (29 children) from 1975–2000 (Van Effenterre and Boch, 2002). In this series, a 59% gross total resection rate was achieved (based on surgeon's estimate), with a mortality of 2.5%, recurrence rate of 23.8%, and excellent result in 85%. Duff's group included 121 patients (32 children) from 1974–1991, based their gross total resection rate on imaging, and achieved a rate of 57% (Duff et al., 2000). The recurrence rate was 24%, and 60.3% resulted in "good outcome." Another series during this era considered 168 patients from 1983–1997 and included 148 undergoing primary surgery and 30 children (Fahlbusch et al., 1999). Of those undergoing primary surgery, 49.3% had a gross total resection. Similar to Yasargil's series, mortality depended on whether the patient had prior surgery, with 1.1% mortality for primary transcranial cases and 10.5% for recurrent ones. Ten-year overall survival after primary surgery was 92.7%, and 79% were independent without impairment. This group published a follow-up series of 73 patients (1997–2005) which had a gross total resection rate of 83.1% and 0% mortality (Hofmann et al., 2012). Comparison of these studies is significantly limited by variation in tumor anatomy and invasion, pre-operative symptoms, surgeon experience, and assessment of extent of resection.

One recent series includes only pediatric patients and focuses on morbidity associated with hypothalamic injury. It included 66 patients treated from 1984–2001, and had a 50% rate of gross total resection and a 53% recurrence rate (Puget et al., 2007). Of the 66 patients, 45 were available for interview, and in this group 76% reported normal development. Morbidity in this series was related to hypothalamic injury, underscoring the importance of the hypothalamus in development for pediatric patients. Surgeon experience also significantly affected post-operative outcome ($P = 0.035$). In the same publication, this group discussed a cohort of 22 children followed prospectively from 2002–2004. In this cohort, a pre-operative grading system taking into account hypothalamic invasion was used to determine whether the child would undergo gross total resection, complete resection avoiding the hypothalamus, or subtotal resection. Patients with remaining tumor were treated with radiation. This cohort had no cases of behavioral dysfunction, hyperphagia, or morbid obesity with a mean follow-up of 1.2 years. The authors suggest that hypothalamic injury is the greatest morbidity for pediatric patients and that this can be minimized by determining the planned extent of resection based on the degree of hypothalamic involvement.

A recent systematic review of the literature on pediatric craniopharyngioma identified 109 studies, with data on extent of resection for 531 patients (Clark et al., 2012). The author found that increased rates of new endocrine dysfunction, panhypopituitarism, and new neurological deficits were associated with gross total resection when compared with biopsy. New neurological deficits were not associated with subtotal resection. Diabetes insipidus was increased with gross total resection compared to subtotal resection, but adding radiation to subtotal resection did increase the rate of panhypopituitarism over subtotal resection alone.

The author of this study was unable to assess differences in hypothalamic dysfunction or quality of life in those treated with different modalities (Clark et al., 2012).

Overall, while gross total resection is often achievable with acceptable mortality, the surgeon must consider the extent of morbidity associated with each approach. Tumor recurrence rates are significantly higher with subtotal resection than gross total resection if adjuvant radiation is not used. One recent prospective pediatric study demonstrated that gross total resection had an 80% risk reduction of recurrence when compared to incomplete resection. In the modern era, however, most patients with a subtotal resection can be treated with adjuvant radiation with acceptable recurrence rates. Although aggressive surgical resection and sectioning of the pituitary stalk to achieve gross total resection leads to panhypopituitarism, radiation may also lead to panhypopituitarism in a delayed fashion. Additionally, in patients with stable home situations/follow-up, hormone replacement therapy is a viable option to treat panhypopituitarism or diabetes insipidus. Radiation also carries a risk of secondary malignancy and cognitive damage, particularly in the pediatric population, while aggressive surgical resection increases the risk of hypothalamic morbidity, a cause for significant concern especially in the pediatric population. Though there is no clear consensus that applies to all patients, the emerging view is that craniopharyngiomas should be treated by experienced surgeons with the overall goal of gross total resection while minimizing hypothalamic injury but accepting panhypopituitarism and that radiation should be employed in cases with subtotal resection (Rutka, 2002; Boop, 2007, 2012).

ENDOSCOPIC CLOSURES: WHICH TECHNIQUE IS BEST?

Concern for CSF leak has traditionally been one of the limiting factors preventing more extensive resections via a transsphenoidal route, and early rates of CSF leak in endoscopic cases were very high. Improvements in closure techniques have provided significant advances and reduced the rate of CSF leak; however, differences exist between closures done by different groups. The Pittsburgh group favors a multilayer closure with a nasoseptal flap held in place with a Foley catheter balloon and no use of lumbar drainage, and they report a CSF leak rate of 6.2% with this approach (Hadad et al., 2006; Patel et al., 2010). Another group recommends a tiered approach to closure with utilization of gelfoam, abdominal fat, mucoperiosteum from the middle turbinate, or a multilayer closure including fat, fascia lata, bone, and mucoperiosteum from the middle turbinate (Sciarretta et al., 2010). The approach chosen depends on the degree of CSF leak encountered, with the spectrum ranging from gelfoam used in the absence of a CSF leak to the multilayer closure used for larger sellar or supradiaphragmatic defects. Utilizing this strategy, this group reports an 8% rate of post-operative CSF leak in the cohort of patients with either an overt intra-operative CSF leak or thin diaphragma sellae (i.e., patients at high risk of post-operative rupture and CSF leak) (Sciarretta et al., 2010). The Jefferson group advocates the use of a "bilayer button" closure for high-flow cranial base defects (Luginbuhl et al., 2010). In this approach, two pieces of fascia lata, an inlay portion and an onlay graft, are sutured together and placed with the inlay portion intradural and the onlay portion extradural. The inlay portion is 25–30% larger than the defect while the onlay portion is 5–10% larger than the opening and sutured in the center of the inlay portion (Luginbuhl et al., 2010). In some cases a nasoseptal flap was then employed over this closure, and fibrin or biologic glue is applied either over the nasoseptal flap or directly onto the button closure if no graft is employed. Use of the button closure reduced CSF leak rates in this high-risk population from 45% to 10% (Luginbuhl et al., 2010). Currently, this group advocates routine use of a vascularized nasoseptal flap to cover the "button graft," which further decreases their CSF leak rate. The Toronto group employs a multilayer closure technique which incorporates the use of DuraGen (Integra LifeSciences), followed by one or two layers of autologous fascia lata placed as an intradural inlay and an extradural outlay, fibrin glue or BioGlue (CryoLife Inc.), and fat (Dehdashti et al., 2009). This group holds the entire closure in place through the use of a 14-French Foley catheter, and more recently has included a nasoseptal flap as part of the closure as well. They noted a CSF fistulae rate of 18% but did comment that no CSF leaks were seen in the seven patients in which the nasoseptal flap was incorporated with the multilayer closure (Dehdashti et al., 2009). Additionally, a small series attempting to treat post-operative CSF leak while avoiding re-operation suggested that repeated endoscopic endonasal injections of fibrin glue in awake patients in an outpatient operating room were successful in controlling post-operative leak (Cavallo et al., 2013). In some cases this approach was combined with lumbar drainage.

At Cornell, the choice of closure approach depends on the size and extent of the tumor as well as the extent of suprasellar extension. However, for suprasellar craniopharyngiomas we start with a "gasket seal" closure, which consists of a fascia lata graft which is buttressed in place with a piece of MEDPOR (Garcia-Navarro et al., 2011; Leng et al., 2012). This is covered with a nasoseptal flap and held in place with DuraSeal (Covidien). A lumbar drain is left open after surgery for 24 hours at 5 cc/h. This technique has lowered our CSF leak rate dramatically compared with the multilayer closure to essentially 0% (Mascarenhas et al., 2013).

In a retrospective analysis of 209 consecutive patients treated with the Cornell algorithm, including 11 craniopharyngiomas, 84 patients (40%) had no intra-operative CSF leak and no post-operative CSF leak while 125 patients (60%) that had an intra-operative CSF leak achieved a 0% rate of post-operative CSF leak (Patel et al., 2013). During the development of these techniques, the rate of CSF leak in transplanum transtuberculum approaches for suprasellar and sellar-suprasellar lesions of all pathologies with each closure technique and combination of techniques was assessed. Mascarenhas et al. report that leak rates varied from 11% with fat graft only to 4.2% with gasket seal only. CSF leaks were improved to 1.8% by combining fat graft and nasoseptal flap, and to 0% with gasket seal plus nasoseptal flap. Additionally, CSF leak rates improved from 6.3% in the first half of the series to 0% in the second half, suggesting the significant learning curve associated with the endoscopic approach and appropriate closure of this approach (Mascarenhas et al., 2013).

It is impossible to compare CSF leak rates associated with the varying closure techniques described above, as there is variability in terms of both types of tumors resected and the way in which CSF leak rates are reported. For instance, some groups report the rate for all cases while others report the rates only in high-risk cases such as those with an identified intra-operative leak. There are no studies directly comparing the variety of techniques developed. However, multiple groups appear to attain good results through utilization of a nasoseptal flap combined with an additional closure strategy of their choice. It is also clear that the rate of CSF leak in endoscopic procedures has significantly decreased since the development of the endoscopic approach, and the reduction in leak rates appears to be a result of both increased surgical experience and advances in closure technique.

THE USE OF LUMBAR DRAINS

At our institution, we have found that the risk of CSF leak can be reduced by the placement of a pre-operative lumbar drain in the case of larger tumors, and the routine injection of fluorescein (Akorn, Inc.) into the cerebrospinal fluid pre-operatively allows for better identification and treatment of CSF leaks at the time of initial surgery (Placantonakis et al., 2007; Jakimovski et al., 2013). Patients should be pre-treated with dexamethasone and diphenhydramine prior to intrathecal injection of fluorescein in order to minimize risk of seizure or radiculopathy. Our protocol involves the withdrawal of 10 ml of CSF, mixing it with 0.25 ml of 10% fluorescein, and intrathecal injection of this mixture. At our institution, the determination of lumbar drain placement depends on the size of the tumor and the extent of suprasellar extension. Patients with a tumor ≥ 2.5 cm with ≥ 1 cm suprasellar extension have a lumbar drain placed pre-operatively, while those with tumors < 2.5 cm or with < 1 cm suprasellar extension will have fluorescein injected via a lumbar puncture only (Patel et al., 2013). Lumbar drainage is continued for 24 hours post-operatively at a rate of 5 ml/h, and the lumbar drain is removed in the evening of the first post-operative day. Mehta and Oldfield, though focusing on pituitary macroadenomas rather than craniopharyngiomas, similarly found that the risk of CSF leak was reduced by placement of a pre-operative lumbar drain (Mehta and Oldfield, 2012). In their series, they compared 114 cases of pituitary macroadenomas without CSF drainage to 44 cases with pre-operative placement of a lumbar drain in order to drain CSF during tumor removal, and found that the rate of intra-operative CSF leak was reduced from 41% to 5% ($P < 0.001$). However, the rate of post-operative CSF leakage was similar in both groups (5%), since operative repair, closure techniques, and post-operative lumbar drainage were utilized for those with a CSF leak.

Not all authors, however, support the use of lumbar drains, with Laws et al. responding to the above study with a comment that "in the past five years, in 356 transsphenoidal operations for pituitary macroadenoma" they have used lumbar drains only seven times, to slowly deliver suprasellar portions, and have a CSF leak rate of 3.4%, lower than that reported by Mehta and Oldfield (Laws et al., 2013). They additionally argue that lumbar drains are not without morbidity, and describe their "personal experience with symptomatic intractable post-lumbar puncture headache, radiculopathies (usually transient), and retained fragments of catheter" and describe a particularly bad case of retained catheter followed by laminectomy to remove catheter which was complicated by wound infection, sepsis, and death (Laws et al., 2013). Cases such as these are obviously extremely rare, but it is worth noting that lumbar drains are not completely benign procedures. In addition to the complications described above, prolonged use of lumbar drains may put patients at risk of infection (especially with any leakage around the drain site or disconnection) and pneumocephalus, and immobility from prolonged usage could increase the risk of deep venous thrombosis and pulmonary embolism. Thus, the surgeon should carefully consider the tumor at hand when determining whether a lumbar drain is warranted and how long to maintain such a drain post-operatively. For correctly selected tumors, lumbar drains can be a very useful tool, and at our institution, we balance the risk/benefit ratio by utilization of the algorithm outlined above and attempt to minimize post-operative lumbar drain complications by early post-operative removal.

CONCLUSIONS

There are no randomized controlled studies comparing different operative approaches for craniopharyngiomas of comparable size and location. Transcranial microscopic, transsphenoidal microscopic, and transsphenoidal endoscopic (endoscopic endonasal) approaches may all be considered as reasonable operative approaches to craniopharyngioma depending on the particular tumor and the goals of surgery. Many microscopic studies include patients collected over a long period of time and some pre-date the use of modern imaging which allows better pre-operative planning and assessment of post-operative residual tumor. Endoscopic series are more recent and have more limited follow-up time, precluding a good assessment of long-term recurrence rates. Despite the limitations in the studies, some conclusions can be made. All three strategies seem to be effective, suggesting that the decision as to which type of procedure should be determined on the basis of the anatomy of the tumor and the surgeon's experience and comfort level with each technique. Additionally, the transcranial route has a higher rate of seizures and injury through brain retraction, while the transsphenoidal route, particularly the endoscopic transsphenoidal route, has a higher rate of CSF leak, at least in less experienced hands. This rate of leakage has significantly improved with advances in closure technique and surgeon experience. Visual deterioration after surgery may also be more frequent following a transcranial approach.

When performed by a surgeon with experience in this technique, the endoscopic transsphenoidal approach is a safe and effective approach in correctly selected tumors. Although suprasellar extension was previously thought to favor a transcranial approach, advancement in CSF closure techniques and the increased view provided by the endoscope have allowed many of these tumors to safely be treated via a transsphenoidal endoscopic approach. The main restriction for the endoscopic transsphenoidal approach at this time is significant lateral extension beyond the carotid arteries. In addition, there is a steep learning curve for the endoscopic transsphenoidal approach, suggesting that surgeons should choose the approach with which they are most comfortable. Those beginning to use the endoscopic approach may wish to restrict resection to smaller tumors with a midline intrasellar location until comfort level is increased as larger tumors with suprasellar extension are more technically challenging.

References

Banu, M.A., Guerrero-Maldonado, A., McCrea, H.J., Garcia-Navarro, V., Souweidane, M.M., Anand, V.K., Heier, L., Schwartz, T.H., Greenfield, J.P., 2013. Impact of skull base development upon endonasal endoscopic surgical corridors. J. Neurosurg. Pediatr. 13 (2), 155–169.

Boop, F.A., 2007. Craniopharyngioma. J. Neurosurg. 106 (suppl. 1), 1–2.

Boop, F.A., 2012. Craniopharyngioma. J. Neurosurg. Pediatr. 10 (4), 291–292.

Cappabianca, P., Cavallo, L.M., Colao, A., Del Basso De Caro, M., Esposito, F., Cirillo, S., Lombardi, G., de Divitiis, E., 2002. Endoscopic endonasal transsphenoidal approach: outcome analysis of 100 consecutive procedures. Minim. Invas. Neurosurg. 45 (4), 193–200.

Cavallo, L.M., Prevedello, D.M., Solari, D., Gardner, P.A., Esposito, F., Snyderman, C.H., Carrau, R.L., Kassam, A.B., Cappabianca, P., 2009. Extended endoscopic endonasal transsphenoidal approach for residual or recurrent craniopharyngiomas. J. Neurosurg. 111 (3), 578–589.

Cavallo, L.M., Solari, D., Somma, T., Savic, D., Cappabianca, P., 2013. The awake endoscope-guided sealant technique with fibrin glue in the treatment of post-operative cerebrospinal fluid leak after extended transsphenoidal surgery: technical note. World Neurosurg., S1878–8750, 00066–1.

Cavazzuti, V., Fischer, E.G., Welch, K., Belli, J.A., Winston, K.R., 1983. Neurological and psychophysiological sequelae following different treatments of craniopharyngioma in children. J. Neurosurg. 59 (3), 409–417.

Chakrabarti, I., Amar, A.P., Couldwell, W., Weiss, M.H., 2005. Long-term neurological, visual, and endocrine outcomes following transnasal resection of craniopharyngioma. J. Neurosurg. 102 (4), 650–657.

Clark, A.J., Cage, T.A., Aranda, D., Parsa, A.T., Sun, P.P., Auguste, K.I., Gupta, N., 2012. Treatment-related morbidity and the management of pediatric craniopharyngioma: a systematic review. J. Neurosurg. Pediatrics. 10 (4), 293–301.

Dehdashti, A.R., Ganna, A., Witterick, I., Gentili, F., 2009. Expanded endoscopic endonasal approach for anterior cranial base and suprasellar lesions: indications and limitations. Neurosurgery 64 (4), 677–687.

Duff, J.M., Meyer, F.B., Ilstrup, D.M., Laws Jr, E.R., Schleck, C.D., Scheithauer, B.W., 2000. Long-term outcomes for surgically resected craniopharyngiomas. Neurosurgery 46 (2), 291–304.

Elliott, R.E., Jane Jr, J.A., Wisoff, J.H., 2011. Surgical management of craniopharyngiomas in children: meta-analysis and comparison of transcranial and transsphenoidal approaches. Neurosurgery 69 (3), 630–643.

Fahlbusch, R., Honegger, J., Paulus, W., Huk, W., Buchfelder, M., 1999. Surgical treatment of craniopharyngiomas: experience with 168 patients. J. Neurosurg. 90 (2), 237–250.

Fischer, E.G., Welch, K., Shillito Jr., J., Winston, K.R., Tarbell, N.J., 1990. Craniopharyngiomas in children: long-term effects of conservative surgical procedures combined with radiation therapy. J. Neurosurg. 73 (4), 534–540.

Frank, G., Pasquini, E., Doglietto, F., Mazzatenta, D., Sciarretta, V., Farneti, G., Calbucci, F., 2006. The endoscopic extended transsphenoidal approach for craniopharyngiomas. Neurosurgery 59 (1 Suppl 1), 75–83.

Fraser, J.F., Allen, B., Anand, V.K., Schwartz, T.H., 2009. Three-dimensional neurostereoendoscopy: subjective and objective comparison to 2-D. Minim. Invasive. Neurosurg. 52 (1), 25–31.

Garcia-Navarro, V., Anand, V.K., Schwartz, T.H., 2011. Gasket seal closure for extended endonasal endoscopic skull base surgery: efficacy in a large case series. World Neurosurg 80 (5), 563–568.

Gardner, P.A., Prevedello, D.M., Kassam, A.B., Snyderman, C.H., Carrau, R.L., Mintz, A.H., 2008. The evolution of the endonasal approach for craniopharyngiomas. J. Neurosurg. 108 (5), 1043–1047.

Hadad, G., Bassagasteguy, L., Carrau, R.L., Mataza, J.C., Kassam, A., Snyderman, C.H., Mintz, A., 2006. A novel reconstructive technique after endoscopic expanded endonasal approaches: vascular pedicle nasoseptal flap. Laryngoscope 116 (10), 1882–1886.

Hoffman, H.J., De Silva, M., Humphreys, R.P., Drake, J.M., Smith, M.L., Blaser, S.I., 1992. Aggressive surgical management of craniopharyngiomas in children. J. Neurosurg. 76 (1), 47–52.

Hofmann, B.M., Hollig, A., Strauss, C., Buslei, R., Buchfelder, M., Fahlbusch, R., 2012. Results after treatment of craniopharyngiomas: further experiences with 73 patients since 1997. J. Neurosurg. 116 (2), 373–384.

Jakimovski, D., Bonci, G., Attia, M., Shao, H., Hofstetter, C., Tsiouris, A.J., Anand, V.K., Schwartz, T.H., 2013. Incidence and significance of intra-operative cerebrospinal fluid leak in endoscopic pituitary surgery using intrathecal fluorescein. World Neurosurg., S1878–8750 (13), 00297–0.

Jane Jr, J.A., Kiehna, E., Payne, S.C., Early, S.V., Laws Jr, E.R., 2010. Early outcomes of endoscopic transsphenoidal surgery for adult craniopharyngiomas. Neurosurg. Focus 28 (4), E9.

Karavitaki, N., Cudlip, S., Adams, C.B., Wass, J.A., 2006. Craniopharyngiomas. Endocr. Rev. 27 (4), 371–397.

Komotar, R.J., Roguski, M., Bruce, J.N., 2009. Surgical management of craniopharyngiomas. J. Neurooncol. 92 (3), 283–296.

Komotar, R.J., Starke, R.M., Raper, D.M., Anand, V.K., Schwartz, T.H., 2012. Endoscopic endonasal compared with microscopic transsphenoidal and open transcranial resection of craniopharyngiomas. World Neurosurg. 77 (2), 329–341.

Laws, E.R., De Los Reyes, K., Rincon-Torroella, J., 2013. Lumbar drains in transsphenoidal surgery. J. Neurosurg. 118 (2), 481.

Leng, L.Z., Greenfield, J.P., Souweidane, M.M., Anand, V.K., Schwartz, T.H., 2012. Endoscopic, endonasal resection of craniopharyngiomas: analysis of outcome including extent of resection, cerebrospinal fluid leak, return to pre-operative productivity, and body mass index. Neurosurgery 70 (1), 110–124.

Liu, J.K., Cole, C., Kestle, J.R., Brockmeyer, D.L., Walker, M.L., 2005. Cranial base strategies for resection of craniopharyngioma in children. Neurosurg. Focus 18 (6A), E9.

Luginbuhl, A.J., Campbell, P.G., Evans, J., Rosen, M., 2010. Endoscopic repair of high-flow cranial base defects using a bilayer button. Laryngoscope 120 (5), 876–880.

Maira, G., Anile, C., Rossi, G.F., Colosimo, C., 1995. Surgical treatment of craniopharyngiomas: an evaluation of the transsphenoidal and pterional approaches. Neurosurgery 36 (4), 715–724.

Mascarenhas, L., Moshel, Y.A., Bayad, F., Szentirmai, O., Salek, A.A., Leng, L.Z., Hofstetter, C.P., Placantonakis, D.G., Tsiouris, A.J., Anand, V.K., Schwartz, T.H., 2013. The transplanum transtuberculum approaches for suprasellar and sellar-suprasellar lesions: avoidance of cerebrospinal fluid leak and lessons learned. World Neurosurg. (13), S1878–8750, 00297–0.

Mehta, G.U., Oldfield, E.H., 2012. Prevention of intra-operative cerebrospinal fluid leaks by lumbar cerebrospinal fluid drainage during surgery for pituitary macroadenomas. J. Neurosurg. 116 (6), 1299–1303.

Merchant, T.E., Kiehna, E.N., Kun, L.E., Mulhern, R.K., Li, C., Xiong, X., Boop, F.A., Sanford, R.A., 2006. Phase II trial of conformal radiation therapy for pediatric patients with craniopharyngioma and correlation of surgical factors and radiation dosimetry with change in cognitive function. J. Neurosurg. 104 (Suppl. 2), 94–102.

Patel, K.S., Komotar, R.J., Szentirmai, O., Moussazadeh, N., Raper, D.M., Starke, R.M., Anand, V.K., Schwartz, T.H., 2013. Case-specific protocol to reduce cerebrospinal fluid leakage after endonasal endoscopic surgery. J. Neurosurg. 119 (3), 661–668.

Patel, M.R., Stadler, M.E., Snyderman, C.H., Carrau, R.L., Kassam, A.B., Germanwala, A.V., Gardner, P., Zanation, A.M., 2010. How to choose? Endoscopic skull base reconstructive options and limitations. Skull Base 20 (6), 397–404.

Placantonakis, D.G., Tabaee, A., Anand, V.K., Hiltzik, D., Schwartz, T.H., 2007. Safety of low-dose intrathecal fluorescein in endoscopic cranial base surgery. Neurosurgery 61 (Suppl. 3), 161–165.

Puget, S., Garnett, M., Wray, A., Grill, J., Habrand, J.L., Bodaert, N., Zerah, M., Bezerra, M., Renier, D., Pierre-Kahn, A., Sainte-Rose, C., 2007. Pediatric craniopharyngiomas: classification and treatment according to the degree of hypothalamic involvement. J. Neurosurg. 106 (Suppl. 1), 3–12.

Roth, J., Fraser, J.F., Singh, A., Bernardo, A., Anand, V.K., Schwartz, T.H., 2011. Surgical approaches to the orbital apex: comparison of endoscopic endonasal and transcranial approaches using a novel 3D endoscope. Orbit 30 (1), 43–48.

Rutka, J.T., 2002. Craniopharyngioma. J. Neurosurg. 97 (1), 1–2.

Schwartz, T.H., Fraser, J.F., Brown, S., Tabaee, A., Kacker, A., Anand, V.K., 2008. Endoscopic cranial base surgery: classification of operative approaches. Neurosurgery 62 (5), 991–1005.

Sciarretta, V., Mazzatenta, D., Ciarpaglini, R., Pasquini, E., Farneti, G., Frank, G., 2010. Surgical repair of persisting CSF leaks following standard or extended endoscopic transsphenoidal surgery for pituitary tumor. Minim. Invasive. Neurosurg. 53 (2), 5–59.

Van Effenterre, R., Boch, A.L., 2002. Craniopharyngioma in adults and children: a study of 122 surgical cases. J. Neurosurg. 97 (1), 3–11.

Yasargil, M.G., Curcic, M., Kis, M., Siegenthaler, G., Teddy, P.J., Roth, P., 1990. Total removal of craniopharyngiomas. J. Neurosurg. 73 (1), 3–11.

Index

Note: Page numbers followed by "b", "f" and "t" indicate boxes, figures and tables respectively.

D

T

Kolibri 360 GmbH
Ferdinand-Jühlke-Straße 7
99095 Erfurt, Deutschland
produktsicherheit@kolibri360.de